Handbook of Epilepsy Treatment

Handbook of Epilepsy Treatment

Simon Shorvon, MA, MB BChir, MD, FRCP

Professor of Neurology and Clinical Subdean, UCL Institute of Neurology, University College London
Consultant Neurologist, National Hospital for Neurology and Neurosurgery, Queen Square London

THIRD EDITION

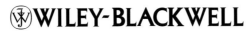

WILEY-BLACKWELL

A John Wiley & Sons, Ltd., Publication

This edition first published 2010 © 2000, 2005, 2010 by Simon Shorvon

Blackwell Publishing was acquired by John Wiley & Sons in February 2007. Blackwell's publishing program has been merged with Wiley's global Scientific, Technical and Medical business to form Wiley-Blackwell.

Registered office: John Wiley & Sons Ltd, The Atrium, Southern Gate, Chichester, West Sussex, PO19 8SQ, UK

Editorial offices: 9600 Garsington Road, Oxford, OX4 2DQ, UK

The Atrium, Southern Gate, Chichester, West Sussex, PO19 8SQ, UK

111 River Street, Hoboken, NJ 07030-5774, USA

For details of our global editorial offices, for customer services and for information about how to apply for permission to reuse the copyright material in this book please see our website at www.wiley.com/wiley-blackwell

The right of the author to be identified as the author of this work has been asserted in accordance with the Copyright, Designs and Patents Act 1988.

Wiley also publishes its books in a variety of electronic formats. Some content that appears in print may not be available in electronic books.

Designations used by companies to distinguish their products are often claimed as trademarks. All brand names and product names used in this book are trade names, service marks, trademarks or registered trademarks of their respective owners. The publisher is not associated with any product or vendor mentioned in this book. This publication is designed to provide accurate and authoritative information in regard to the subject matter covered. It is sold on the understanding that the publisher is not engaged in rendering professional services. If professional advice or other expert assistance is required, the services of a competent professional should be sought.

The contents of this work are intended to further general scientific research, understanding, and discussion only and are not intended and should not be relied upon as recommending or promoting a specific method, diagnosis, or treatment by physicians for any particular patient. The publisher and the author make no representations or warranties with respect to the accuracy or completeness of the contents of this work and specifically disclaim all warranties, including without limitation any implied warranties of fitness for a particular purpose. In view of ongoing research, equipment modifications, changes in governmental regulations, and the constant flow of information relating to the use of medicines, equipment, and devices, the reader is urged to review and evaluate the information provided in the package insert or instructions for each medicine, equipment, or device for, among other things, any changes in the instructions or indication of usage and for added warnings and precautions. Readers should consult with a specialist where appropriate. The fact that an organization or Website is referred to in this work as a citation and/or a potential source of further information does not mean that the author or the publisher endorses the information the organization or Website may provide or recommendations it may make. Further, readers should be aware that Internet Websites listed in this work may have changed or disappeared between when this work was written and when it is read. No warranty may be created or extended by any promotional statements for this work. Neither the publisher nor the author shall be liable for any damages arising herefrom.

Library of Congress Cataloging-in-Publication Data

Shorvon, S. D. (Simon D.)

Handbook of epilepsy treatment / Simon Shorvon. – 3nd ed.

p. ; cm.

Includes bibliographical references and index.

ISBN 978-1-4051-9818-9

1. Epilepsy–Handbooks, manuals, etc.   2. Anticonvulsants–Handbooks, manuals, etc.   I. Title.

[DNLM: 1. Epilepsy–therapy.   WL 385 S559h 2010]

RC372.S528 2010

616.8′5306–dc22

2010015320

A catalogue record for this book is available from the British Library.

Set in 9.25 on 11.5pt Minion by Toppan Best-set Premedia Limited
Printed and bound in Singapore by Markono Print Media Pte Ltd.

01   2010

Contents

Preface to the Third Edition

This monograph is part of the series of handbooks that are produced to accompany the large multi-authored reference books published by Wiley-Blackwell. The third edition of the reference text *Treatment of Epilepsy* was published in 2009 (edited by myself, Emilio Perucca and Jerome Engel), and this handbook is now also in its third edition.

As we now enter the second decade of the age of the internet, the first question to address when contemplating a writing project is a fundamental one – are books of this nature still required? In an age where information is now readily available at a click of a Google button, does a book have a function frozen as it is in form and in content, not unlike, some would argue, the fossilized remains of past life forms? This is a question that is already central to medical publishing. My own opinion on this matter is, however, clear – books that concentrate and filter information are both necessary and desirable, in the field of epilepsy treatment, as much as anywhere else, for at least three reasons:

1 Accuracy of information: comprehensive as the internet is, accurate it is not. There exists on the web much information that is phoney, wild and irresponsible, many data that are inaccurate or uncorroborated, and much opinion that has more to do with kite-flying than medical science. A book can avoid these snake-pits.

2 Condensation of information into a short and concise form, in one easily accessible place: this I have tried to do here, avoiding repetition, redundancy or excessive verbiage. Whether this is successfully achieved is a judgement for the reader, but the condensation of data in the book is surely an overwhelming advantage over the diffuse nature of the information highway (now less of a discrete path than a horizonless moor).

3 Consistency of perspective and approach: this book is written from a single perspective – that of the practising neurologist who specializes in epilepsy. This is not a scientific, theoretical or populist, but a medical, text. Its audience is the practising doctor who sees patients with epilepsy in the clinic. The internet, by its all inclusive nature, cannot take such a singular approach.

This is the justification for embarking on a third edition. The first two editions of the handbook were published 10 and 4 years ago, were both generously received and, I hope, fulfilled at least in part their purpose of informing and improving epilepsy therapy. However, in epilepsy, as in all of medicine, treatment moves on, knowledge has increased and fashions have changed and, in the short span of these handbooks, much new information has arrived on the desks of physicians. The writing of a third edition is an opportunity to reflect these changes, and also, sad to say, to correct the all too obvious deficiencies of the previous editions.

As I noted in the previous edition, this book contains pretty much everything I know about epilepsy therapy. It is a worrying thought that all one's professional knowledge can be compressed into a couple of megabytes (the draft manuscript of the whole book amounted to less than five megabytes, and could be saved onto a memory stick smaller than my fingernail, but this is the rather humbling reality). Another concern is that this is a single author text, with the danger of bias and prejudice. My defence is that the disadvantages of single-authorship need to be weighed against the advantages of coherence and lack of omission, repetition or inconsistency. Avoiding these in the writing of this book has been a constant preoccupation.

The aim of this edition is exactly the same the aim of the previous editions, and so is cited verbatim from the second edition:

> The aim is to summarize the many and various treatments of epilepsy in a clear yet comprehensive, and concise yet balanced and practical manner. Surgical as well as medical therapy is included, as is the treatment of epilepsy in adults and children. Rare as well as common clinical problems are covered, and rarely – as well as commonly -used therapies. It is intended to be a hands-on text which will guide clinical

practice and rational therapy, and to be a source of ready reference; a catalogue of epilepsy therapy. There is an emphasis on factual information, which I have tried to give in a parsimonious and easily-digested form, but one that still gives the reader a clear idea of the scientific basis of current practice. This scientific perspective is important and, where possible, the text has endeavoured to be science- and evidence-based. In some areas of therapy an evidence base, however, is lacking (perhaps especially in the area of epilepsy surgery), and data informing longer-term outcome, risk and benefit in particular are missing. In these areas the book inevitably reflects the author's own prejudices and anecdotal experience.

The book is embedded in the experience gained from my own clinical practice, now over 30 years of specialization in epilepsy at the National Hospital for Neurology and Neurosurgery, Queen Square, London, and is heavily influenced by this. The book also reflects the work of the International League Against Epilepsy, on whose executive committee I have served now for more than 17 years. These influences provide the context and a distinctive perspective, which I hope adds coherence and interest.

I mentioned, in the previous edition, three developments in epilepsy therapy that had occurred in the years leading up to 2005, and that I considered to deserve special mention. The first was molecular genetics – but now 5 years later one has to admit that in the therapeutic arena the impact has been less than hoped for. The goal of therapy tailored to an individual's genomic make-up, which 5 years ago was trumpeted by colleagues and seemed within reach, now seems entirely unrealizable in the foreseeable future. The second was the plethora of guidelines – this torrent continues to flow, and now, in my personal opinion, the downsides of this outweigh the advantages. This fashion for guidelines risks bland uniformity and guideline fatigue. Does the wearying audience really need the further imposition of more of these? The third thread of contemporary therapy identified in the last edition was the importance of patient involvement in medical decisions. This remains an important prerogative and in this edition too the importance of two-way communication and of patient choice is emphasized.

There are a series of significant changes to this edition, which it is hoped will improve the book. First, the structure has changed, which reflects the greater attention to the causes of and the syndromes of epilepsy (now separate chapters), as well as more detail on principles of therapy, and a greater emphasis on tables to summarize and extract data. Second, since the last edition there have been licensed at least five new antiepileptic drugs and a large range of novel drugs is also in the process of development. The widely predicted famine in the field of epilepsy therapy that so many foresaw in the past decade has resolutely failed to materialize. Indeed, it is probably true to say that there have been more novel and exciting therapies in current development since the publication of the last edition than at any time in the history of epilepsy therapy. It is not, I hope, too panglossian to think that these have incrementally improved treatment of many patients. Finally, the scientific information about drug therapy has again improved, due to advances in clinical and molecular chemistry, and this is also incorporated where possible in this book. Developments in the surgical therapy of epilepsy have been less impressive, but there are some areas of incremental change that I hope also to have recorded.

As in the last edition, a number of editorial decisions have been made that should be noted here. The summary of factual information in table form (for easy reference) is a deliberate policy, but it should be recognized that, especially in relation to pharmacological and pharmacokinetic data, conflicting information commonly exists. This can lead to contention, and the tables include what I consider to be the most reliable data. It is important also to recognize that data do vary, and in some places the data in the tables are not universally applicable. Second, the contentious decision has been made, in the interests of readability and clarity, to omit citations to the literature from the text. In the age of PubMed and Medline, literature is now easily tracked, and citations can also be found in the relevant chapters of the associated textbook. In place of this, a 'further reading' section, listing key articles, books and review articles, with an emphasis on recent publications, has been included; this seemed to me to be of more general utility. Finally, the reader should know that this book, like its predecessor, is conceptually, and in many places actually, a condensation of the multi-authored textbook (*Treatment of Epilepsy*, edited by Shorvon SD, Perucca E, Engel J, Blackwell Publishing Ltd, Oxford, 2009). Much of the information in this handbook has its basis in the textbook (that indeed is a rationale of this handbook) and the borrowing has often been heavy, sometimes word for word, and the influence great. I would like to acknowledge here my debt of gratitude to my co-editors of this textbook, Professor Emilio Perucca and Professor Pete Engel, and also to all the contributors to the multi-authored textbook (listed in the acknowledgement section), for without their work this book would not exist. The textbook remains a landmark in the bibliography of epilepsy therapy.

Finally, thanks too are due to the production crew at Wiley-Blackwell, Rebecca Huxley and Martin Sugden for their expert guidance and assistance, and Lynne and Matthew, for whom the writing of this book has meant lost time and the smoke of much midnight oil.

Finally, I repeat the *health warning* of the second edition: although every effort has been made in the preparation of this book to ensure that the details given are correct, it is possible that errors have been overlooked (e.g. in pharmaceutical or pharmacokinetic data). The reader is advised to refer to published information from the pharmaceutical companies and other reference works to check accuracy.

Simon Shorvon
London 2010

Acknowledgements

In the preparation of the text of this book, I am heavily indebted to the contributors to the textbook *The Treatment of Epilepsy*. The *Handbook of Epilepsy Treatment* is modelled on this sister book, and the text and tables are in places borrowed and transposed from this book. I thank Blackwell Publishing Ltd for permission for this, and also offer my thanks and acknowledgement to the following individuals who were the contributors to the *Treatment of Epilepsy* and whose work has therefore influenced and contributed to the writing of this Handbook:

Luis Almeida; Meriem Amarouche; Hiba Arif; Fiona Arnold; Giuliano Avanzini; Fabrizio Alestrieri; Nicholas Barbaro; Michel Baulac; Gregory Bergey; Meir Bialer; Gretchen Birbeck; Victor Biton; Blaise Bourgeois; Christine Bower Baca; Martin Brodie; Eylert Brodtkorb; Christine Bulteau; Richard Byrne; Carol Camfield; Peter Camfield; Gregory Cascino; Edward Chang; Joshua Chern; Catherine Chiron; Maria Roberta Cilio; Hannah Cock; Aaron Cohen-Gadol; Youseff Comair; Mark Cook; Helen Cross; Olivier Delalande; Marc Dichter; Jelena Djordjevic; W. Edwin Dodson; Georg Dorfmüller; Jennifer Dorward; Robert Duckrow; Mervyn Eadie; Christian Elger; Brent Elliott; Jerome Engel Jr; Kai Eriksson; Edward Faught; Colin Ferrie; Andrew Fisher; Lars Forsgren; Silvana Franceschetti; Jacqueline French; Itzhak Fried; Tracy Glauser; Karolien Goffin; Christina Gurnett; Leena Haataja; Yvonne Hart; Jason Hauptman; Dale Hesdorffer; Lawrence Hirsch; Martin Holtkamp; Rüdiger Hopfengärtner; Svein I. Johannessen; Marilyn Jones-Gotman; Julien Jung; Mithri Junna; Reetta Kälviäinen; Andres Kanner; Christian Kaufman; Tapani Keränen; Neil Kitchen; Eric Kossoff; Günter Krämer; Patrick Kwan; James Leiphart; Ilo Leppik; Howan Leung; Nita Limdi; Anthony Linklater; John Livingston; Wolfgang Löscher; Andrew McEvoy; Harry Mansbach; Gary W. Mathern; Fumisuke Matsuo; François Mauguière; Hartmut Meierkord; Anil Mendiratta; Isabelle Merlet; Andrew Michell; Roberto Michelucci;

Miri Neufeld; Dang Nguyen; Karen Nilsen; Gerald Novak; Andre Palmini; Elena Pasini; Philip Patsalos; Doreen Patsika; Emilio Perucca Webster Pilcher; Charles Polkey; Kurupath Radhakrishnan; Aldo Ragazzoni; Stefan Rampp; Sylvain Rheims; Awais Riaz; Catherine Riney; David Roberts; Philipp von Rosenstiel; Philippe Ryvlin; Rajesh Sachdeo; Josemir Sander; Steven Schachter; Dieter Schmidt; Matti Sillanpää; Gagandeep Singh; Michael Smith; Patricio Soares-da-Silva; Ernest Somerville; Susan Spencer; Edoardo Spina; Hermann Stefan; John Stern; Rainer Surges; Carlo Alberto Tassinari; Nancy Temkin; Torbjörn Tomson; Françoise Tonner; Eugen Trinka; Christopher Uff; Susan Usiskin; Barbara Van de Wiele; Koen Van Laere; Wim Van Paesschen; Federico Vigevano; Matthew Walker; Jörg Wellmer; Nicholas Wetjen; James White; Steve White; Tom Whitmarsh; Gabriele Wohlrab; Stephen Wroe; Isaac Yang; Gaetano Zaccara; Federico Zara.

I also am grateful for permission to reproduce the illustrations, text and tables from the following sources.

Figures

Fig 1.1 and fig 1.2 The figures are redrawn from Forsgren L 2004. Epidemiology and prognosis of epilepsy and its treatment. In: Shorvon SD *et al.* (eds) *The Treatment of Epilepsy* (2nd edn). Blackwell Publishing, Oxford: 21–42. The figures are based on data from: Jensen P 1986. *Acta Neurol Scand*, **74**: 150–155; Olafsson E *et al.* 1996. *Epilepsia* 37: 951–955; Fosgren L *et al.* 1996. *Epilepsia*, **37**: 224–229; Hauser WA *et al.* 1993. *Epilepsia*, **34**: 453–468; Sidenvall R *et al.* 1993. *Acta Paediatr*, **82**: 62–65.

Fig 4.1 Redrawn from Lennox WG 1960. *Epilepsy and related disorders*. Boston: Little Brown.

Fig 4.2 Derived from Scaravilli F 1980. Structure, Function and Connection. In: Scaravilli F (ed) *Neuropathology in Epilepsy*. London: Scientific Publishing Company plc, p. 20.

Fig 4.4 Derived from Dean G and Shorvon S 2010. Porphyria. In: *The Causes of Epilepsy* Eds: Shorvon S,

Guerrini R, Andermann F. Cambridge: Cambridge University Press (in press).

Fig 5.1 From Shorvon SD 2004. The choice of drugs and approach to drug treatments in partial epilepsy. In: Shorvon SD *et al.* (eds) *The Treatment of Epilepsy* (2nd edn). Oxford: Blackwell Science Ltd, p. 322.

Fig 5.2 Adapted from Shorvon SD 2004. The choice of drugs and approach to drug treatments in partial epilepsy. In: Shorvon SD *et al.* (eds). *The Treatment of Epilepsy* (2nd edn). Oxford: Blackwell Science Ltd, p. 323.

Fig 5.3 From Hart Y *et al.* Recurrence after the first seizure. *Lancet* 1990: **336**: 1271–1274.

Fig 5.4 From Hart Y *et al.* Recurrence after the first seizure. *Lancet* 1990: **336**: 1271–1274.

Fig 5.5 From MRC Antiepileptic Drug Withdrawal Study Group. 1991. *Lancet* 191; **37**: 1175–1180.

Fig 5.2 Adapted from Shorvon SD 2004. The choice of drugs and approach to drug treatments in partial epilepsy. In: Shorvon SD *et al.* (eds). *The Treatment of Epilepsy* (2nd edn). Oxford: Blackwell Science Ltd, p. 323.

Fig 5.3 From Hart Y *et al.* Recurrence after the first seizure. *Lancet* 1990: **336**: 1271–1274.

Fig 5.4 From Hart Y *et al.* Recurrence after the first seizure. *Lancet* 1990: **336**: 1271–1274.

Fig 5.5 From MRC Antiepileptic Drug Withdrawal Study Group. 1991. *Lancet* 191; **37**: 1175–1180.

Fig 6.1 From: Wallace H *et al.* Age-specific incidence and prevalence rates of treated epilepsy in an unselected population of 2,052,922 and age-specific fertility rates of women with epilepsy. *Lancet.* 1998; 6; **352**: 1970–1973.

Fig 7.1 From: Richens A *et al.* 1985. In: Williams DC and Marks V (eds) *Biochemistry in Clinical Practice*. Amsterdam: Elsevier.

Fig 8.1 From: Kutt H 1995. In: Levy R *et al.* (eds) *Antiepileptic Drugs* (4th edn) Raven Press, New York.

Fig 8.2 Adapted from: Mattson RH 1998. In: Engel J and Pedley TA (eds) *Epilepsy: A Comprehensive Textbook*, Vol 2. New York: Lippencott-Raven, 1497.

Fig 8.3 From: Rupp R *et al.* 1979. *Br J Clin Pharmacol*, **7** (Suppl. 1): 219–234.

Fig 8.4 From: Almeida *et al.* 2009. Eslicarbazepine. In: Shorvon S, Perucca E and Engel J (eds). *The Treatment of Epilepsy* (3rd edn). Oxford: Blackwell Publishing Ltd, p. 486.

Fig 8.5 From: Wilenski AJ *et al.* 1982. *Eur J Clin Pharmacol*, **23**: 87–92.

Fig 8.6 from Michelucci R and Tassinari CA 2004. Phenobarbital, primidone and other barbituates. In: Shorvon SD *et al.* (eds) *The Treatment of Epilepsy* (2nd edn). Oxford: Blackwell Science Ltd, 461–474.

Fig 8.7 Derived from; Imai J *et al.* 2000. *Pharmacogenetics*. **10**: 85–89.

Fig 8.8 From: Richens A and Dunlop A 1975. *N Engl J Med*, **2**: 347–348.

Fig 8.9 From: Michelucci R, Pasini E, Tassinari CA 2009. Phenobarbital, primidone and other barbiturates. In Shorvon S, Perucca E and Engel J (eds). *The Treatment of Epilepsy* (3rd edn). Oxford: Blackwell Publishing Ltd, p. 587.

Fig 8.10 With grateful thanks to Mr James Acheson.

Fig 8.11 From: Camfield P, Camfield C 2009. Benzodiazepines used primarily for chonic treatment (clobazam, clonazepam, clorazepate and nitrazepam). In: Shorvon S, Perucca E and Engel J (eds). *The Treatment of Epilepsy* (3rd edn). Oxford: Blackwell Publishing Ltd, p. 423.

Fig 8.12 From: Shorvon S, Piracetam 2009. In: *The Treatment of Epilepsy* (3rd edn). Edited by Shorvon S, Perucca E and Engel J. Oxford: Blackwell Publishing Ltd, p. 620.

Fig 8.13 From: Noyer M, Gillard M, Matagne A, Henichart J-P, Wulfert E. *Eur J Pharm* 1995; **286**: 137–146.

Fig 9.1 From Kapur J and MacDonald RL 1997. *J Neuroscience*, **17**: 7532–7540.

Fig 9.2 From Lothman EW 1990. *Neurology*, **40** (Suppl. 2): 13–23.

Fig 10.1 From: Wellmer J, Elger E. 2009. MRI in presurgical evaluation of epilepsy. In: Shorvon S, Perucca E and Engel J (eds). *The Treatment of Epilepsy* (3rd edn). Oxford: Blackwell Publishing Ltd, p. 811.

Fig 10.2, 10.3 From: Cook MJ, Fish DR, Shorvon SD, Straughan K, Stevens JM. Hippocampal volumetric and morphometric studies in frontal and temporal lobe epilepsy. *Brain*. 1992 115 Pt 4:1001–1015.

Fig 10.4, 10.5, 10.14, 10.15, 10.16, 10.17, 10.18, 10.19, 10.20, 10.21 From: Fish D 1996. The role of scalp electoencephalography evaluation for epilepsy surgery. In: Shorvon SD *et al.* *The Treatment of Epilepsy* (1st edn) Oxford: Blackwell Science Ltd, 542–561.

Fig 10.6 From: Spencer SS and Lamoureux D 1996. Invasive electoencephalography evaluation for epilepsy surgery. In: Shorvon SD *et al.* *The Treatment of Epilepsy* (1st edn) Oxford: Blackwell Science Ltd.

Fig 10.7 From: Spencer S *et al.* 2009. In: Shorvon S, Perucca E and Engel J (eds). *The Treatment of Epilepsy* (3rd ed). Oxford: Blackwell Publishing Ltd, pp. 767–804.

Fig 10.8 From: Raymond AA *et al.* 1994. *Neurology*, 44: 1841–1845.

Fig 10.9 From: Olivier A. 1996. Surgery of mesial temporal epilepsy. In: Shorvon SD *et al. The Treatment of Epilepsy* (1st edn). Oxford: Blackwell Science Ltd, 689–698.

Fig 10.10 From: Kitchen ND and Thomas DGT 1996. Stereotactic neurosurgery for epilepsy. In: Shorvon SD *et al. The Treatment of Epilepsy* (1st edn). Oxford: Blackwell Science Ltd, 759–771.

Fig 10.11, 10.12 From: Kitchen ND *et al.* 2004. Resective surgery of vascular and infective lesions for epilepsy. In: Shorvon SD *et al.* (eds). *The Treatment of Epilepsy* (2nd edn). Oxford: Blackwell Science Ltd, 742–762.

Fig 10.13 From: Schweitzer JS and Spencer DD 1996. Surgery of congenital, traumatic and infectious lesions and those of uncertain aetiology. In: Shorvon SD *et al. The Treatment of Epilepsy* (1st edn). Oxford: Blackwell Science Ltd, 669–688.

Fig 10.22 From: Gates JR and De Paola L 2004. Corpus callosum section for epilepsy. In: Shorvon SD *et al. The Treatment of Epilepsy* (2nd edn). Oxford: Blackwell Science Ltd, 798–811.

Fig 10.23 From: Selway R and Dardis R 2004. Multiple subpial transection for epilepsy. In: Shorvon SD *et al. The Treatment of Epilepsy* (2nd edn). Oxford: Blackwell Science Ltd, 812–823.

Fig 10.24 From: Schachter S 2004. Vagal nerve stimulation. In: Shorvon SD *et al. The Treatment of Epilepsy* (2nd edn). Oxford: Blackwell Science Ltd, 873–883.

Table

Tables 2.2, 2.3, 2.7 These tables (and also borrowings of text) are derived from Duncan JS, Fish DR and Shorvon SD 1995. *Clinical Epilepsy*. Edinburgh: Churchill Livingstone.

Table 2.9 From: Commission for the Classification and Terminology of the International Leagues Against Epilepsy. 1981. Proposal for revised clinical and electroencephalographic classification of epileptic seizures. *Epilepsia* 1981: 22: 489–501.

Table 3.1 From: Commission for the Classification and Terminology of the International Leagues Against Epilepsy. Proposal for revised classification of epilepsies and epileptic syndromes. *Epilepsia*, 1989: 30: 389–399.

Table 3.2 Derived from Loiseau P *et al.* Survey of seizure disorders in the French southwest. I. Incidence of epileptic syndromes. *Epilepsia* 1990: 31: 391–396.

Table 3.5 This table (and also borrowings of text) are derived from Duncan JS, Fish DR and Shorvon SD 1995. *Clinical Epilepsy*. Edinburgh: Churchill Livingstone.

Table 4.6 Derived from Zara F. Genetic counselling in epilepsy. In: Shorvon SD, Perucca E, Engel J (eds), *The Treatment of Epilepsy*, 3rd edn. Oxford: Blackwell Publishing, 2009. p. 355.

Table 4.7 Derived from Roach E *et al.* Tuberous sclerosis complex consensus conference: revised clinical diagnostic criteria. *J Child Neurol* 1998: 13: 624–628.

Table 4.9 Derived from Gutmann DH *et al.* The diagnostic evaluation and multidisciplinary management of neurofibromatosis 1 and neurofibromatosis 2. *JAMA* 1997 278:51–57.

Table 4.11 Derived from Kennedy PG. Viral encephalitis: causes, differential diagnosis, and management. *J Neurol Neurosurg Psychiat* 2004 75 (suppl. 1): 110–155.

Table 4.13 From Nelligan A. 2010. Drug-induced seizures. In: Shorvon SD, Guerrini R, Andermann F (eds), *The Causes of Epilepsy*. Cambridge: Cambridge University Press: in press.

Table 5.7 Derived from Perucca E *et al.* Assessing risk to benefit ratio in antiepileptic drug therapy. *Epilepsy Res.* 2000 41: 107–139.

Table 5.8 Derived from McCorry D *et al.* Current drug treatment of epilepsy in adults. *Lancet Neurology* 2004; 3: 729–735.

Table 5.13 Derived from Moran D *et al.* Epilepsy in the United Kingdom: seizure frequency and severity, antiepileptic drug utilization and impact on life in 1652 people with epilepsy. *Seizure* 2004 13: 425–433.

Table 5.17 Derived from Chadwick D 2004. Management of epilepsy in remission. In: Shorvon SD *et al.* (eds) *The Treatment of Epilepsy* (2nd edn) Oxford: Blackwell Science Ltd.

Table 5.18 From Elliott B, Amarouche M, Shorvon S. 2009. Psychiatric features of epilepsy and their management. In: Shorvon SD, Perucca E, Engel J (eds), *The Treatment of Epilepsy* (3rd edn). Oxford: Blackwell Publishing, 2009. p. 278.

Table 5.19 Derived from Zaccara G, Balestrieri F, Ragazzoni A. 2009. Management of side effects of antiepileptic drugs. In: Shorvon SD, Perucca E, Engel J (eds), *The Treatment of Epilepsy* (3rd edn). Oxford: Blackwell Publishing, 289–299.

Table 5.20 Derived from Zara F. 2009. Genetic counselling in epilepsy. In: Shorvon SD, Perucca E, Engel J (eds), *The Treatment of Epilepsy* (3rd edn). Oxford: Blackwell Publishing Ltd, p. 357.

Table 6.1 From Livingston JH. 2009. Management of epilepsies associated with specific diseases in children. In: Shorvon SD, Perucca E, Engel J Jr, eds. *The Treatment of Epilepsy* (3rd edn). Oxford: Blackwell Publishing Ltd, pp. 195–202.

Table 6.2 From Kossoff EH, Jennifer L. Dorward JL. 2009. Ketogenic diets. In: Shorvon SD, Perucca E, Engel J Jr, eds (2009). *The Treatment of Epilepsy*. (3rd edn). Oxford: Blackwell Publishing Ltd, pp. 301–310.

Table 6.3 From Kossoff EH, Jennifer L. Dorward JL. Ketogenic diets. In: Shorvon SD, Perucca E, Engel J Jr, eds. *The Treatment of Epilepsy* (3rd edn). Oxford: Blackwell Publishing Ltd, pp. 301–310.

Table 6.5 Derived from Arif J, Mendiratta A, Hirsch L. 2009. Management of epilepsy in the elderly. In: Shorvon SD, Perucca E, and Engel J Jr (edn). *The Treatment of Epilepsy*. (3rd edn). Oxford: Blackwell Publishing Ltd, pp. 203–218.

Table 7.2 From: Spina E. 2009. Drug interactions. In: Shorvon SD, Perucca E, Engel J Jr, eds. *The Treatment of Epilepsy* (3rd edn). Oxford: Blackwell Publishing Ltd, p. 364.

Table 8.1 Modified from: Patsalos PN, Perucca E. *Lancet Neurol* 2003; **2**: 347–356; Perucca E. *Br J Clin Pharmacol* 2006; **61**: 246–255.

Table 8.2 Modified from: Patsalos PN, Perucca E. *Lancet Neurol* 2003; **2**: 347–356; Perucca E. *Br J Clin Pharmacol* 2006; **61**: 246–255.

Table 8.3 Modified from: Patsalos PN, Perucca E. *Lancet Neurol* 2003; **2**: 473–481; Perucca E. *Br J Clin Pharmacol* 2006; **61**: 246–255.

Table 8.4 Modified from: Patsalos PN, Perucca E. *Lancet Neurol* 2003; **2**: 473–481; Perucca E. *Br J Clin Pharmacol* 2006; **61**: 246–255.

Table 8.5 Data from Mattson RH *et al.* 1992. *N Engl J Med*, **327**: 765–771.

Table 8.6 From Dalby MA, Clobazam 2004. In: Shorvon SD, Perucca E, Fish D, Dodson E. *The Treatment of Epilepsy* (2nd edn). Oxford: Blackwell Science Ltd, 358–364.

Table 8.7 Derived from Browne T 1983. Ethosuximide (zarontin) and other succinimides. In: Browne T and Feldman R (eds) Epilepsy, Diagnosis and Management. Boston: Little, Brown: 215–224.

Table 8.8 Derived from Chadwick D 1994. *Lancet*, **343**: 89–91.

Table 8.9 From: Biton V, Fountain N, Rosenow F, *et al.* *Epilepsia* 2009 **50** (Suppl. 4): 109.

Table 8.10 Derived from Brodie MJ, Richens A and Yuen AWC 1995. *Lancet*, **345**: 476–479; Reunanen OM, Dam M and Yuen AWC 1996. *Epilepsy Res*, **23**: 149–155; Steiner TJ, Dellaportas CI, Findley LJ *et al.* 1999. *Epilepsia*, **40**: 601–607.

Table 8.11 Derived from Schachter S 1995 *J Epilepsy*, **8**: 201–210.

Table 8.12 Derived from Messenheimer JA, Giorgi L and Risner ME 2000. The tolerability of lamotrigine in children. *Drug Saf*, **22**: 303–312.

Table 8.16 Derived from Sadek A and French JA 2001 *Epilepsia* **42** (Suppl. 4): 40–43.

Table 8.18 Derived from Barcs G, Walker EB and Elger CE *et al.* 2000. *Epilepsia*, **41**: 1597–1607; Glauser TA, Nigro M, Sachdeo R *et al.* 2000. *Neurology*, **54**: 2237–2244.

Table 8.20 Data from: Loiseau P, Brachet Liermain A, Legroux M, Jogeix M. *Nouv Presse Med* 1977; **16**: 813–817; Patsalos PN, Berry DJ, Bourgeois BF, *et al.* *Epilepsia* 2008; **49**: 1239–1276; Schmidt D, Einicke I, Haenel F. *Arch Neurol* 1986; **43**: 263–265.

Table 8.22 From: Brodie M 2004. *Epilepsia*, **45** (Suppl. 6): 19–27.

Table 8.23 Derived from Leppik *et al.* 1999. *Epilepsy Res*, **33**: 235–246.

Table 8.24 From Shorvon SD 1996. *Epilepsia*, **37**: S18–22.

Table 8.25 From Shorvon SD 1996. *Epilepsia*, **37**: S18–22.

Table 8.26 From Ben-Menarchem E 1997. *Exp Clin Invest Drugs*, **6**: 1088–1089.

Table 8.27 From Ben-Menarchem E 1997. *Exp Clin Invest Drugs*, **6**: 1088–1089.

Table 8.28 From Ben-Menachem E and French J 1998. In: Engel J and Pedley TA (eds) *Epilepsy: A Comprehensive Textbook, Vol 2*. New York: Lippencott-Raven, 1613.

Table 8.29 From Seino M and Fujitani B Zonisamide. 2004. In: Shorvon SD *et al.* (eds) *The Treatment of Epilepsy* (2nd edn) Oxford: Blackwell Science Ltd, 548–559.

Table 8.30 From Seino M and Fujitani B Zonisamide. 2004. In: Shorvon SD *et al.* (eds) *The Treatment of Epilepsy* (2nd edn) Oxford: Blackwell Science Ltd, 548–559.

Tables 9.1, 9.2, 9.4, 9.5 Derived from: Shorvon S 1994. *Status Epilepticus: Its Clinical Features and Treatment in Children and Adults.* Cambridge: Cambridge University Press.

Table 9.3 Derived from: Tan R, Neligan A, Shorvon SD. 2010 *Epilepsy Res* In press.

Tables 9.6, 9.7, 9.8 Derived from: Walker MC, Shorvon SD. 2009. In: Shorvon S, Perucca E and Engel J (eds). *The Treatment of Epilepsy* (3rd edn). Oxford: Blackwell Publishing Ltd, pp. 231–247.

Table 10.10 From Schachter SC. 2009. Vagal nerve stimulation. In: Shorvon SD, Perucca E, and Engel J (eds), *The Treatment of Epilepsy* (3rd edn). Oxford: Blackwell Publishing Ltd, 1017–1024.

Tables 10.11, 10.12 From: Schachter SC 2004. Vagus nerve stimulation. In: Shorvon SD *et al.* (eds) *The Treatment of Epilepsy* (2nd edn) Oxford: Blackwell Science Ltd, 873–883.

1 Definitions and Epidemiology

Epilepsy is – rather like headache – a *symptom* of neurological dysfunction. It has many forms and underlying causes, and also biological and non-biological facets that extend well beyond the simple occurrence of seizures. Treatment approaches vary considerably in the different types of epilepsy and, in this section of the book, the various clinical forms and causes of epilepsy are described.

The forms of epilepsy can be described and classified in four main ways: (1) by seizure type; (2) in the case of partial (focal) seizures, by the anatomical site of seizure onset; (3) by syndrome; and (4) by aetiology. Each system has its value. In Chapter 2 the seizure type and anatomical substrate are described, in Chapter 3 the epilepsy syndromes and in Chapter 4 the causes of epilepsy.

What is not available, given our current state of knowledge, is a description, or classification, of the types of epilepsy according to molecular mechanisms. Such a 'pathophysiological' classification would be highly desirable and is the challenge for the future.

Definitions

Epileptic seizure (epileptic fit)

Epileptic seizures are defined as 'the transient clinical manifestations that result from an episode of epileptic neuronal activity'. The epileptic neuronal activity is a specific dysfunction, characterized by abnormal synchronization, excessive excitation and/or inadequate inhibition, and can affect small or large neuronal populations (aggregates). The clinical manifestations are sudden, transient and usually brief. They include motor, psychic, autonomic and sensory phenomena, with or without alteration in consciousness or awareness. The symptoms depend on the part of the brain involved in the epileptic neuronal discharge, and the intensity of the

Handbook of Epilepsy Treatment, 3rd Edition. By Simon Shorvon. Published 2010 by Blackwell Publishing Ltd.

discharge. The signs of a seizure vary from the only too evident wild manifestations of a generalized convulsion, to the subtle changes, apparent only to the patient, of some simple partial seizures. Some neuronal epileptic discharges, detectable by electroencephalography, are not accompanied by any evident symptoms or signs and this complicates definition. For most purposes these 'subclinical' or 'interictal' changes are not considered to be epileptic seizures, although the physiological changes can be identical to overt attacks, and the difference is largely one of degree. Furthermore, subtle impairment of psychomotor performance can be demonstrated due, for example, to interictal spiking, of which the patient may be unaware.

Epilepsy

Epilepsy is 'a disorder of brain characterized by an ongoing liability to recurrent epileptic seizures'. This definition is unsatisfactory for various reasons. First, it is difficult clearly to define, in many cases, to what extent recurrent attacks are likely – a definition based on crystal-ball gazing is inherently unsatisfactory. In the clinical setting, for pragmatic reasons, a 'liability to further attacks' is often said to be present when two or more spontaneous attacks have occurred, on the basis that this means that more are likely. However, this arbitrary definition is inadequate, for example, in patients after a single attack who have a clear liability to further seizures, for patients who have had more than one provoked attack (see below), or for those whose epilepsy has remitted and whose liability for further attacks has lapsed. Furthermore, in physiological terms, the distinction between single and recurrent attacks is often meaningless. A second problem is that 'epilepsy' occurs with a wide variety of cerebral pathologies; similar to 'anaemia' or 'headache' it is a symptom masquerading as a disease.

The standard definition is also inadequate in epileptic states in which physiological changes occur without obvious seizures. In these so-called epileptic encephalopathies, alterations in cognition and other cortical functions are major features unrelated to overt seizures (examples include the Landau–Kleffner syndrome and the childhood epileptic encephalopathies). Patients with subclinical discharges sometimes exhibit cognitive, psychological or behavioural change. There are also certain non-epileptic conditions where differentiation from epilepsy is problematic. These are sometimes called borderline conditions, and include certain psychiatric conditions, some cases of migraine and some forms of movement disorder. Finally, the fact of 'having epilepsy' involves far more than the risk of recurrent seizures, but incorporates prejudice and stigmatization, and psychosocial and developmental issues that may, indeed, be more problematic than the seizures themselves. A comprehensive definition should ideally incorporate these broader psychosocial, developmental and cognitive aspects

There are furthermore types of overt epileptic seizure that do not warrant a diagnosis of epilepsy. These include isolated first seizures in which no liability to recurrence can be demonstrated, some provoked seizures, febrile seizures, and the 'early seizures' after acute brain injury.

Epilepsy syndrome

An epileptic syndrome is defined as 'an epileptic disorder characterized by a cluster of signs and symptoms customarily occurring together' (see chapter 3). Different syndromes have different prognoses and require different treatment approaches. They are commonly diagnosed in children (and indeed up to 70% of childhood epilepsy may be categorized into epilepsy syndromes) but more rarely so in adult epilepsy.

Status epilepticus

This is defined as a condition in which epileptic seizures continue, or are repeated without recovery, for a period of 30 minutes or more. This is the maximal expression of epilepsy, and often requires emergency therapy (see chapter 9). There are physiological and neurochemical changes that distinguish status epilepticus from ordinary epileptic seizures. Recent debate has revolved around the minimum duration of seizures necessary to define this condition, with suggestions ranging from 10 min to 60 min; the usual 30 min is to some extent a compromise. As with the definitions of epilepsy and of epileptic seizures, there is a range of boundary conditions associated with status epilepticus that do not fall easily into the simple clinical definitions.

Febrile seizures

A febrile seizure is an epileptic attack occurring in children age under 5 years (usually between 2 and 5 years) in the setting of a rise in body temperature. For most purposes, such seizures are not included within the rubric of 'epilepsy', because they are very common (2–5% of children in the west have at least one febrile seizure, and 9% in Japan), presumably have a specific physiological basis that is distinct from epilepsy, and have clinical implications that are very different from those of epilepsy. Febrile seizures are discussed further on pp. 28–30.

Epileptic encephalopathy

An 'epileptic encephalopathy' is a term used to describe a clinical state in which epilepsy is a prominent feature, and in which changes in cognition or other cerebral functions are, at least in part, likely to be due to ongoing epileptic processes in the brain. The epileptic encephalopathies are more common in children than in adults.

Idiopathic, symptomatic, provoked and cryptogenic epilepsy

Epilepsy can have many causes. These are terms used to describe the causes of epilepsy and are dealt with in more detail later (see chapter 3).

Active epilepsy and epilepsy in remission

A person is said to have active epilepsy when at least one epileptic seizure has occurred in the preceding period (usually 2–5 years). Conversely, epilepsy is said to be in remission when no seizures have occurred in this preceding period. The period of time used in these definitions varies in different studies, and furthermore some definitions of remission require the patient not only to be seizure free but also off medication. An interesting question, and one of great importance to those with epilepsy, is after what period of remission can the person claim no longer to have the condition? Logically, the condition has remitted as soon as the last seizure has occurred, but this cannot be known except retrospectively. In practice, it is reasonable to consider epilepsy to have ceased in someone off therapy if 2–5 years have passed since the last attack.

Acute symptomatic, remote symptomatic and congenital epilepsy

A categorization of epilepsy has been used for epidemiological studies that divided epilepsy into three types: acute symptomatic epilepsy, where there is an acute cause; remote symptomatic, where there is a cause that

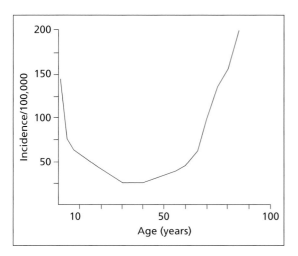

Figure 1.1 Age-specific incidence rates based on combined results from studies in the USA, Iceland and Sweden.

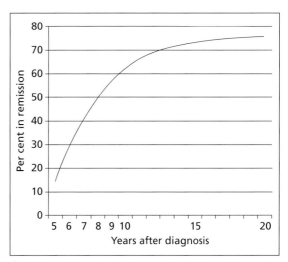

Figure 1.2 Proportion of patients in 5-year remission by years after diagnosis of epilepsy (figures based on four population-based studies).

has been present for at least 3 months; and idiopathic, where the cause is not known. This classification has been severely criticized and is, in the view of the author, of little value and should not now be used.

Frequency and population features of epilepsy

Epilepsy is a common condition. Its incidence is in the region of 80 cases per 100 000 persons per year, with different studies showing rates varying between 50 and 120 per 100 000 per year. Its point prevalence is about 4–10 cases per 1000 persons. The prevalence is higher in developing countries, perhaps due to poorer perinatal care and standards of nutrition and public hygiene, and the greater risk of brain injury, cerebral infection and congenital/developmental disorders The frequency of epilepsy is also slightly higher in lower socioeconomic classes. However, more striking than any differences in frequency is the fact that epilepsy occurs in all parts of the world and can affect all strata in a population. Males may be slightly more likely to develop epilepsy than females, and there are no differences in rate in large ethnic populations. The incidence of seizures is age dependent, with the highest rates in the first year of life and a second peak in late life (Figure 1.1). About 40% of patients develop epilepsy below the age of 16 years and about 20% over the age of 65 years. In recent times, the rate in children has been falling, possibly owing to better

Table 1.1 The characteristics of epilepsy in a population of 1 000 000 people (approximate estimates).

Incident cases (new cases each year)	
Febrile seizures (annual incidence rate 50/100 000)	500
Single seizures (annual incidence rate 20/100 000)	200
Epilepsy (annual incidence rate 50/100 000)	500
Prevalent cases (cases with established epilepsy)	
Active epilepsy (prevalence rate 5/1000)	5000
Epilepsy in remission	15 000
Severity of cases (in patients taking antepileptic drugs; seizures in previous year) (%)	
More than one seizure per week	10
Between one seizure per week and one per year	40
No seizures	50
Type of seizure (%)	
Partial seizures alone	15
Partial and secondarily generalized	60
Generalized tonic–clonic	20
Other generalized seizures	5
Medical care required (in prevalent cases) (%)	
Occasional medical attention	65
Regular medical attention	30
Residential or institutional care	5

Table 1.2 The main aetiological categories of epilepsy and an estimate of their approximate relative frequency.

Main category	Subcategory	Subcategory	Frequency (%)[a]
Idiopathic epilepsy		Pure epilepsies due to single gene disorders	<1
		Pure epilepsies with complex inheritance[b]	10–20
Symptomatic epilepsy	Predominately genetic or developmental causation	Severe childhood epilepsy syndromes	<1
		Progressive myoclonic epilepsies	<1
		Neurocutaneous syndromes	<1
		Other neurological single gene disorders	<1
		Disorders of chromosome function	<1
		Developmental anomalies of cerebral structure[c]	<5
	Predominately acquired causation	Hippocampal sclerosis	10–30
		Perinatal and infantile causes	5
		Cerebral trauma	5–10
		Cerebral tumour	5–10
		Cerebral infection	<5
		Cerebrovascular disorders[d]	10–30
		Cerebral immunological disorders	<5
		Degenerative and other neurological conditions	<5
Provoked epilepsy		Provoking factors[e]	<10
		Reflex epilepsies	<5
Cryptogenic epilepsies			20–40

[a]Figures adjusted to account for the increased identification of hippocampal sclerosis/genetic disorders/congenital malformations possible with modern neuroimaging and genetics, which were not available to most of the population-based studies.
[b]Idiopathic generalized epilepsies and benign partial epilepsies.
[c]Including cortical dysplasias and other congenital cerebral malformations.
[d]Ischaemic (approximately 80%) and haemorrhagic (approximately 20%).
[e]Provoking factors play a role in many epilepsies, but the figure here is an estimate of the proportion of cases in which provoking factors are the predominant cause.

public health and living standards and better perinatal care. Conversely, the rate in elderly people is rising largely due to cerebrovascular disease.

An isolated (first and only) seizure occurs in about 20 people per 100 000 each year. The cumulative incidence of epilepsy – the risk of an individual developing epilepsy in his or her lifetime – is between 3 and 5%. The fact that prevalence is much lower than cumulative incidence demonstrates that in many cases epilepsy remits. In fact the prognosis is generally good and, within 5 years of the onset of seizures, 50–60% of patients will have entered long remission (Figure 1.2). However, in about 20% of cases, epilepsy, once developed, never remits. Fertility rates are reduced by about 30% in women with epilepsy (see pp. 136–137).

Mortality of epilepsy

Standardized mortality rates are also two to three times higher in patients with epilepsy than in others in the population. The excess mortality is due largely to the underlying cause of the epilepsy. However, some deaths are directly related to seizures and there are higher rates of accidents, sudden unexpected deaths and suicides among patients with epilepsy when compared with the general population. The rates of death are highest in the first few years after diagnosis, reflecting the underlying cerebral disease (tumour, stroke, etc.). In chronic epilepsy, the more severe the epilepsy, the higher the mortality rate, an excess due largely to sudden unexpected death in epilepsy (SUDEP), and rates of SUDEP range from about one death per 2500 person-years in mild epilepsy to one death per 100 person-years among those with severe and intractable epilepsy. Life expectancy estimates at a population level have recently been calculated, showing a reduction of expectancy in idiopathic/cryptogenic epilepsy of up to 2 years and in symptomatic epilepsy of up to 10 years.

Features of epilepsy in a population

Table 1.1 shows an approximate breakdown of epilepsy in a typical western population of 1 000 000 people. This gives some indication of the burden of epilepsy. In populations of patients on therapy for epilepsy, about two-thirds had 'mild epilepsy' (i.e. seizures less than once a month) that required only minor medical input, and 50% had no seizures in the prior 12 months. However, about 5–10% had seizures at a greater than weekly frequency, required frequent medical attention for their epilepsy and incurred significant medical costs.

As mentioned above, almost every brain disorder can cause epileptic seizures and aetiology differs greatly in different populations, geographical locations and different age groups. The aetiologies of epilepsy are described in Chapter 4. The main aetiological categories of epilepsy and their approximate frequency in a typical western population are given in Table 1.2.

About a third to half of children and about a fifth of adults with epilepsy have additional learning disabilities.

Epilepsy occurs in about 20% of those with learning disability (7–18% of those with intelligence quotients [IQs] rated between 50 and 70, and 35–44% in those with IQ ratings <50), equating to a prevalence rate of 1.2 per 1000. Of adults with newly diagnosed epilepsy, 18% show additional dementia, 6% motor disabilities (usually hemiplegia due to stroke) and 6% severe psychiatric disorders. About 1 in 15 with epilepsy is dependent on others for daily living because of epilepsy and the associated handicaps. In terms of direct medical care costs, epilepsy accounts for about 0.25% of general practitioner costs, 0.63% of hospital costs and 0.95% of pharmaceutical costs in the UK National Health Service. Epilepsy results in social exclusion and isolation, and causes problems in education, employment, personal development, personal relationships and family life, and dependency. These secondary handicaps are to a large extent culturally determined. Taking a broad brush, the World Health Organization (WHO) has estimated that epilepsy causes 6.4 million disability-adjusted life-years (DALYs) and 1.32 million years of life lost (YLL) worldwide, second among neurological diseases only to stroke and dementia in its impact. Stigmatization of patients with epilepsy is common, and social attitude change would alleviate many of the problems encountered by patients with epilepsy; this is as important as any medical therapy.

2 Seizure Type and Anatomical Location of Seizures

Seizure type

Epilepsy is a variable condition, and one way of describing and categorizing the multifarious forms is to consider the seizure type – the clinical and electroencephalographic (EEG) forms of the seizures themselves.

The International League Against Epilepsy (ILAE) has systematized the process of description by formulating a seizure type classification. The first ILAE classification of seizure type was proposed in 1964 and accepted in 1969, and since then there have been several revisions (the most influential in 1981). This is the most widely accepted classification of epilepsy and has been the bedrock of epilepsy description over the last 50 years. The ILAE classification uses only two criteria – the clinical form of the seizure and the EEG abnormality – and is this an entirely descriptive classification, with few pretensions.

The 1981 ILAE classification divides seizures into generalized and partial categories (Table 2.1). Generalized seizures are those that arise from large areas of the cortex in both hemispheres, and in which consciousness is always lost. Generalized seizures are subdivided into seven categories. Partial seizures are those that arise in specific, often small, loci of cortex in one hemisphere. They are divided into simple partial seizures, which occur without alteration of consciousness, and complex partial seizures, in which consciousness is impaired or lost.

A secondarily generalized seizure is a seizure with a partial onset (the aura) that spreads to become a generalized attack. Simple partial seizures may spread to become complex partial seizures and either can spread to become secondarily generalized. Although this is a classification based entirely on clinical and EEG phenomenology, it should be realized that some of the generalized seizure types occur only in specific types of epilepsy, and this is discussed further below. Partial seizures invariably imply focal brain pathology, although this may not necessarily be demonstrated by conventional clinical investigation.

About two-thirds of newly diagnosed epilepsies are partial and/or secondarily generalized.

The limitations of a classification based only on clinical and EEG appearance should not be underestimated, and the current classification is inadequate for many clinical and research purposes. The more recent ILAE Classification of the Epilepsies and Epileptic Syndromes was devised to be more comprehensive, but is in fact hardly used in routine practice (see pp. 19–21). There have been other criticisms of the ILAE Classification of Seizure Type. The subdivision of partial seizures on the basis of consciousness is criticized because of the difficulty of deciding in many cases whether or not consciousness is altered. Many seizures do not fit well into any of the categories. Treatment can greatly modify the clinical form. With advances in imaging and neurophysiology, it has become clear that some generalized seizures do in fact have underlying focal brain disorders. Conversely some partial seizures are underpinned by a large neuronal network akin to that of some generalized epilepsies and hardly justify the term 'focal'. In this book, devoted to therapy, a damning criticism of the classification is that, as a general rule, the seizure type classification does not help in choosing treatment or defining prognosis. There are obvious exceptions (e.g. the use of valproate or ethosuximide in generalized absence attacks) but the lack of treatment specificity for individual categories is striking.

The ILAE classifications of seizure type and of the epilepsies and epileptic syndromes are currently undergoing revision and are increasingly challenged by alternative systems. However, the main value of the ILAE Classification of Seizure Type lies in its widespread clinical acceptance and, in spite of all its problems, this classification has become adopted universally in clinical practice.

Handbook of Epilepsy Treatment, 3rd Edition. By Simon Shorvon.
Published 2010 by Blackwell Publishing Ltd.

Table 2.1 The 1981 International League Against Epilepsy (ILAE) Classification of Seizure Type.

I Partial (focal, local) seizures
  A Simple partial seizures
    1 With motor signs
    2 With somatosensory or special sensory symptoms
    3 With autonomic symptoms or signs
    4 With psychic symptoms
  B Complex partial seizures
    1 Simple partial onset followed by impairment of consciousness
    2 With impairment of consciousness at onset
  C Partial seizures evolving to secondarily generalized seizures (tonic–clonic, tonic or clonic)
    1 Simple partial seizures evolving to generalized seizures
    2 Complex partial seizures evolving to generalized seizures
    3 Simple partial seizures evolving to complex partial seizures evolving to generalized seizures
II Generalized seizures (convulsive and non-convulsive)
  A Absence seizures
    1 Absence seizures
    2 Atypical absence seizures
  B Myoclonic seizures
  C Clonic seizures
  D Tonic seizures
  E Tonic–clonic seizures
  F Atonic seizures (astatic seizures)
III Unclassified epileptic seizures

Partial seizures

Simple partial seizures

Simple partial seizures are defined as partial seizures in which consciousness is not impaired. They are due to focal cerebral disease. Any cortical region may be affected, the most common sites being the frontal and temporal lobes. The symptomatology is useful in predicting the anatomical localization of the seizures. The form of the seizures usually has no pathological specificity. Partial seizures occur at any age. Most simple partial seizures last only a few seconds.

Motor manifestations

The most common manifestations are jerking (clonus), spasm or posturing. These occur in epilepsies arising in frontal or central regions, although they can also occur with spread of the epileptic discharges from other regions.

The clonic jerks can spread from one part of the body to another (the so-called jacksonian march) as the focal discharges spread along the motor cortex of the brain. Speech arrest occurs if the simple partial seizure involves the speech areas, and anarthria, dysarthria or choking sensations can occur in seizures involving areas of the brain involved with muscles of articulation.

Turning (known usually as 'version') of the head or eyes, or less commonly rotation of the whole body, can occur in epilepsy arising in many cortical areas. It is of little localizing value unless it is the first symptom in a seizure and in full consciousness, in which case the epilepsy arises usually from the contralateral anterior frontal lobe.

Todd's paralysis (or paresis) is a term used to refer to a reversible unilateral weakness that occurs after a partial seizure involving the motor cortex. It can last minutes or hours, but is never prolonged beyond 24 hours (prolonged paralysis indicates that cortical damage has occurred, unrelated to epilepsy itself). The occurrence of Todd's paralysis has reliable localizing value, indicating that the epilepsy arises in the contralateral motor cortex.

Somatosensory or special sensory manifestations (simple hallucinations)

These take the form of tingling or numbness, or less commonly as an electrical shock-like feeling, burning, pain or a feeling of heat. The epileptic focus is usually in the central or parietal region, although similar symptoms occur with spread from epileptic foci in other locations. Simple visual phenomena such as flashing lights and colours occur if the calcarine cortex is affected. A rising epigastric sensation is the most common manifestation of a simple partial seizure arising in the mesial temporal lobe.

Autonomic manifestations

Autonomic symptoms such as changes in skin colour, blood pressure, heart rate, pupil size and piloerection can be isolated phenomena in simple partial seizures, but more commonly are a component of generalized or complex partial seizures of frontal or temporal origin.

Psychic manifestations

Psychic simple partial seizures can take various forms, and are more common in complex partial than in simple partial seizures. They can occur in epilepsy arising from a temporal, frontal or parietal focus. There are six principal categories:

1 *Dysphasic symptoms* occur if cortical speech areas (frontal or temporoparietal) are affected. Speech usually ceases or is severely reduced, and postictal dysphasia is a very reliable sign localizing the seizure discharge to the dominant hemisphere. Repetitive vocalization with formed words may occur during a complex partial seizure of origin in the non-dominant temporal lobe. Palilalia can occur in epilepsy arising in the dominant hemisphere. Dysphasia should be distinguished where possible from anarthria (speech arrest), which suggests a fronto-central origin.

2 *Dysmnestic symptoms* (disturbance of memory) may take the form of flashbacks, déjà vu, jamais vu or panoramic experiences (recollections of previous experiences, former life or childhood), and are most common in mesial temporal lobe seizures. However, similar symptoms also occur in inferior frontal or lateral temporal lobe seizures. The epileptic déjà vu is distinguished from the non-epileptic form by its intensity and its association with a sense of dreaminess and detachment.

3 *Cognitive symptoms* include dreamy states and sensations of unreality or depersonalization, and occur primarily in temporal lobe seizures.

4 *Affective symptoms* include fear (the most common symptom), depression, anger and irritability. Elation, erotic thoughts, serenity or exhilaration may occur. Affective symptomatology is most commonly seen with mesial temporal lobe foci. Laughter (without mirth) is a feature of the automatism of seizures (known as gelastic seizures) which arise in frontal areas, and are a consistent feature of the epilepsy associated with hypothalamic hamartomas.

5 *Illusions* of size (macropsia, micropsia), shape, weight, distance or sound are usually features of temporal or parieto-occipital epileptic foci.

6 *Structured hallucinations* of visual, auditory, gustatory or olfactory forms, which can be crude or elaborate, are usually due to epileptic discharges in the temporal or parieto-occipital association areas. Hallucinations of taste, usually an unpleasant taste, are usually a symptom of temporal lobe epilepsy. Visual hallucinations can vary greatly in sophistication from simple colours or flashing lights in epilepsy arising in the calcarine cortex to complex visual perceptual hallucinations in posterior temporal association areas. Auditory hallucinations also vary in complexity, and most commonly occur in seizures arising in Herschel gyrus. Vertigo is a common perceptual change in temporal lobe epilepsy and, unlike vertigo of vestibular origin, epileptic vertigo is rarely associated with nausea and is usually not severe or incapacitating.

The scalp EEG, both interictally and also during a simple partial seizure, is often normal, because the epileptic disturbance is too small or too deep to be detected by the scalp electrodes. If an interictal abnormality is present, it will take the form of spikes, sharp waves, focal slow activity or suppression of normal rhythms. Before the seizure, the interictal EEG may show a sudden reduction in the frequency of interictal spike or sharp waves. Ictal abnormalities can take the form of rhythmic theta activity, focal spike–wave activity or runs of fast activity (13–30 Hz).

Complex partial seizures

Complex partial seizures arise from the temporal lobe in about 60% of cases, the frontal lobe in about 30% and other cortical areas in about 10% of cases. The clinical features reflect the anatomical site of onset of the seizures, and the clinical features characteristic of specific sites of onset are described on pp. 12–18. Complex partial seizures vary considerably in duration. In one series of temporal lobe epilepsy, the ictal phase lasted 3–343 seconds (mean 54 s), the postictal phase 3–767 s and the total seizure duration 5–998 s (mean 128 s), although longer seizures (occasionally lasting hours) are sometimes encountered.

Complex partial seizures of temporal or frontal lobe origin can have three components.

Auras

These are equivalent to simple partial seizures, and can take any of the forms described above. The aura is usually short-lived, lasting a few seconds or so, although in rare cases a prolonged aura persists for minutes, hours or even days. Many patients experience isolated auras as well as full-blown complex partial seizures.

Altered consciousness

This follows the aura or evolves simultaneously. The altered consciousness takes the form of an absence and motor arrest, during which the patient is motionless and inaccessible, and appears vacant or glazed (the so-called 'motionless stare'). Sometimes there are no outward signs at all, and at other times there may be associated spasms, posturing or mild tonic jerking.

Automatisms

Automatisms are defined as involuntary motor actions that occur during or in the aftermath of epileptic seizures, in a state of impaired awareness. The patient is totally amnesic for the events of the automatism. Sometimes the actions have purposeful elements, are affected by the environment and can involve quite complex activity. Automatisms should be distinguished from postictal confusion. Automatisms are most common in temporal and frontal lobe seizures. They are usually divided into:

• *Oroalimentary:* orofacial movements such as chewing, lip smacking, swallowing or drooling. These are most common in partial seizures of mesial temporal origin.

• *Mimicry:* including displays of laughter or fear, anger or excitement.

• *Gestural:* fiddling movements with the hands, tapping, patting or rubbing, ordering and tidying movements. Complex actions such as undressing are quite common, as are genitally directed actions. These too are most common in temporal lobe epilepsy.

• *Ambulatory automatisms:* walking, circling, running.

• *Verbal automatisms:* meaningless sounds, humming, whistling, grunting, words that may be repeated, formed sentences. If these occur in temporal lobe epilepsy, it indicates that the epilepsy is arising in the non-dominant lobe.

• *Responsive automatisms:* quasi-purposeful behaviour, seemingly responsive to environmental stimuli.

• *Violent behaviour* can occur in an automatism, and is best considered as a response in an acutely confused person. It is especially likely if the patient is restrained. The violent actions of the epileptic automatism are never premeditated, never remembered, never highly coordinated or skilful, and seldom goal directed; these are useful diagnostic features in a forensic context.

In about 10–30% of seizures, the scalp EEG is unchanged and, in the rest, runs of fast activity, localized spike–wave complexes, spikes or sharp waves or slow activity may occur, or the EEG may simply show flattening (desynchronization). The patterns can be focal (indicating the site or origin of the seizure), lateralized, bilateral or diffuse.

Partial seizures evolving to secondarily generalized seizures

Partial seizures (simple, complex or simple evolving to complex) may spread to become generalized. The partial seizure is often experienced as an aura in the seconds before the generalized seizure. The generalized seizure usually takes a tonic–clonic form.

Generalized seizures

Consciousness is almost invariably impaired from the onset of the attack (owing to the extensive cortical and subcortical involvement), motor changes are bilateral and more or less symmetrical, and the EEG patterns are bilateral and grossly synchronous and symmetrical over both hemispheres.

Typical absence seizures (petit mal seizures)

The seizure comprises an abrupt loss of consciousness (the absence) and cessation of all motor activity. Tone is usually preserved, and there is no fall. The patient is not in contact with the environment, is inaccessible and often appears glazed or vacant. The attack ends as abruptly as it starts, and previous activity is resumed as if nothing had happened. There is no confusion, but the patient is often unaware that an attack has occurred. Most absence seizures (>80%) last less than 10 s. Other clinical phenomena including blinking, slight clonic movements of the trunk or limbs, alterations in tone and brief automatisms can occur, particularly in longer attacks. The attacks can be repeated, sometimes hundreds of times a day, often cluster and are often worse when the patient is awakening or drifting off to sleep.

Absences may be precipitated by fatigue, drowsiness, relaxation, photic stimulation or hyperventilation. Typical absence seizures develop in childhood or adolescence and are encountered almost exclusively in the syndrome of idiopathic generalized epilepsy (see pp. 22–24). Variations from this typical form include the myoclonic absence, and absence with perioral myoclonia or eyelid myoclonia. Whether or not these are distinct entities is controversial (see pp. 22–23).

The EEG during a typical absence has a very striking pattern. A regular, symmetrical and synchronous 3 Hz spike–wave paroxysm is the classic form, although in longer attacks and in older patients the paroxysms may not be entirely regular and frequencies vary between 2 and 4 Hz. The interictal EEG has normal background activity and there may be intermittent short-lived bursts of spike–wave. These spike–wave paroxysms can frequently be induced by hyperventilation and less commonly by photic stimulation.

The features useful in differentiating a complex partial seizure and a typical absence are shown in Table 2.2.

Atypical absence seizures

Atypical absence seizures, similar to typical absence seizures, take the form of loss of awareness (absence) and hypomotor behaviour. They differ from typical absences in clinical form, EEG, aetiology and clinical context (Table 2.3). Their duration is longer, loss of awareness is often incomplete and much less marked, and associated tone changes are more severe than in typical absence

Table 2.2 Clinical features that help differentiate typical absence seizures from complex partial seizures.

	Typical absence seizure	Complex partial seizure
Age of onset	Childhood or early adult	Any age
Aetiology/syndrome	Idiopathic generalized epilepsy	Any focal aetiology (or cryptogenic epilepsy)
Underlying focal anatomical lesion	None	Limbic structures, neocortex
Duration of attack	Short (usually <10 s)	Longer, usually several minutes
Other clinical features	Slight (blinking, nodding or mild loss of tone)	Can be prominent, including aura, automatism
Patient aware that an attack has occurred	Often not	Almost always
Postictal	None	Confusion, headache, emotional disturbance are common
Frequency	May be very numerous (hundreds a day) and cluster	Usually less frequent
Ictal and interictal EEG	3 Hz spike–wave	Variable focal disturbance
Photosensitivity	10–30%	None
Effect of hyperventilation on EEG	Often marked increase	None, modest increase

Table 2.3 Clinical features that help differentiate typical and atypical absence seizures.

	Typical absence seizure	Atypical absence seizure
Context	No other neurological signs or symptoms	Usually in context of learning difficulty, and other neurological abnormalities
Aetiology	Idiopathic generalized epilepsy	Lennox–Gastaut syndrome and other secondarily generalized and cryptogenic generalized epilepsies
Consciousness	Totally lost	Often only partially impaired
Focal signs in seizures	Nil	May be present
Onset/offset of seizures	Abrupt	Often gradual
Coexisting seizure types	Sometimes tonic–clonic and myoclonic	Mixed seizure disorder common, all seizure types

seizures. The onset and cessation of the attacks are not so abrupt. Amnesia may not be complete and the patient may be partially responsive. The patient appears relatively inaccessible, may be ambulant although often stumbling or clumsy and needing guidance or support, and there can be atonic, clonic or tonic phenomena, autonomic disturbance and automatism. The attacks can wax and wane and can be of long duration.

The ictal EEG shows usually diffuse but often asymmetrical and irregular spike–wave bursts at 2–2.5 Hz, and sometimes fast activity or bursts of spikes and sharp waves. The background interictal EEG is usually abnormal, with continuous slowing, spikes or irregular spike–wave activity, and the ictal and interictal EEGs may be similar. The seizures are often not induced by hyperventilation or photic stimulation.

Atypical absences occur in the symptomatic epilepsies, and are usually associated with learning disability, other neurological abnormalities or multiple seizure types. They form part of the Lennox–Gastaut syndrome and may occur at any age.

Myoclonic seizures

A myoclonic seizure is a brief contraction of a muscle, muscle group or several muscle groups due to a cortical discharge. It can be single or repetitive, varying in severity from an almost imperceptible twitch to a severe jerking resulting, for example, in a sudden fall or the propulsion of hand-held objects (the 'flying saucer' syndrome). Recovery is immediate, and the patient often maintains that consciousness was not lost. During a myoclonic jerk, the electromyogram shows biphasic or polyphasic potentials of 20–120 ms in duration followed by tonic contraction or hypotonia. Myoclonus can be induced by action, noise, startle, photic stimulation or percussion.

Myoclonic seizures occur in very different types of epilepsy. They are one of the three seizure types in the syndrome of Idiopathic Generalized Epilepsy (the other two being absence and tonic–clonic seizures) and in this syndrome the myoclonus usually has a strong diurnal pattern, occurring mainly in the first few hours after waking or when dropping off to sleep. Myoclonic seizures also occur in the epileptic encephalopathies (e.g. the Lennox–Gastaut syndrome) and in epilepsy associated with other forms of childhood myoclonic encephalopathy. Focal myoclonus is a feature of focal occipital lobe epilepsy and epilepsy arising in the central areas (and if continuous is named epilepsia partialis continua). Generalized myoclonus can also occur in symptomatic epilepsies due to cerebral anoxia, cerebral infections, hereditary or acquired metabolic disease, drugs, toxins or poisoning. Myoclonus is also the major seizure type in the progressive myoclonic epilepsies. Epileptic myoclonus needs to be differentiated from non-epileptic myoclonus of spinal and subcortical origin.

The ictal EEG usually shows a generalized spike, spike–wave or polyspike–wave discharge, which is often asymmetrical or irregular, and frequently has a frontal predominance. The cortical origin of some myoclonic jerks can, however, be detected only on back averaging of the EEG. The interictal EEG varies with the cause, being usually normal in idiopathic generalized epilepsy, and abnormal in other types of myoclonic epilepsy showing generalized changes.

Clonic seizures

Clonic seizures consist of clonic jerking that is often asymmetrical and irregular. Clonic seizures are most frequent in neonates, infants or young children, and are always symptomatic. In older children and adults, tonic-clonic seizures can be modified by therapy to take the form of a clonic seizure. The EEG may show fast activity (10 Hz), fast activity mixed with larger-amplitude slow waves, or more rarely polyspike–wave or spike–wave discharges. These should not be confused with bilateral clonic jerking (with or without loss of consciousness, even if involving all four limbs), which is a form of partial seizure arising in the frontal lobe.

Tonic seizures

Tonic seizures take the form of a tonic muscle contraction with altered consciousness without a clonic phase. The tonic contraction causes the following: extension of the neck; contraction of the facial muscles, with the eyes opening widely; upturning of the eyeballs; contraction of the muscles of respiration; and spasm of the proximal upper limb muscles, causing the abduction and elevation of the semiflexed arms and the shoulders. If the tonic contractions spread distally, the arms rise up and are held as if defending the head against a blow, and the lower limbs become forcibly extended or contracted in triple flexion. There may be a cry followed by apnoea. The spasm may fluctuate during the seizure, causing head nodding or slight alterations in the posture of the extended limbs, and autonomic changes can be marked. Tonic seizures last less than 60 s.

The ictal EEG may show flattening (desynchronization), fast activity (15–25 Hz) with increasing amplitude (to about 100 mV) as the attack progresses, or a rhythmic 10 Hz discharge similar to that seen in the tonic phase of the tonic–clonic seizure. On a scalp recording, however, the ictal EEG changes are often obscured by artefact from muscle activity and movement. The interictal EEG is seldom normal, usually showing generalized changes.

Tonic seizures occur at all ages in the setting of diffuse cerebral damage and learning disability, and are invariably associated with other seizure types. Tonic seizures are the characteristic and defining seizure type in the Lennox–Gastaut syndrome, and this is their usual clinical setting. They should be differentiated from partial motor seizures, which can also show predominantly tonic features, and from partially treated tonic–clonic seizures.

Tonic–clonic seizures (grand mal seizures)

This is the classic form of epileptic attack, the 'convulsion' or 'fit' that typifies epilepsy in the public imagination. It has a number of well-defined stages. It is sometimes preceded by a prodromal period during which an attack is anticipated, often by an ill-defined vague feeling or sometimes more specifically, e.g. by the occurrence of increasing myoclonic jerking. If an aura then occurs (in fact a simple or complex partial seizure) in the seconds before the full-blown attack, this indicates that the tonic–clonic seizure is secondarily generalized. The seizure is initiated by loss of consciousness, and sometimes the epileptic cry. The patient will fall if standing, there is a brief period of tonic flexion, and then a longer phase of rigidity and axial extension, with the eyes rolled up, the jaw clamped shut, the limbs stiff, adducted and extended, and the fists either clenched or held in the main d'accoucher position. Respiration ceases and cyanosis is common. This tonic stage lasts on average 10–30 s and is followed by the clonic phase, during which convulsive movements, usually of all four limbs, jaw and facial muscles, occur; breathing can be stertorous and saliva (sometimes blood stained owing to tongue biting) may froth from the mouth. The convulsive movements decrease in frequency (eventually to about four clonic jerks per second), and increase in amplitude as the attack progresses.

Autonomic features such as flushing, changes in blood pressure, changes in pulse rate and increased salivation are common. The clonic phase lasts between 30 and 60 s and is followed by a further brief tonic contraction of all muscles, sometimes with incontinence. The final phase lasts between 2 and 30 min and is characterized by flaccidity of the muscles. Consciousness is slowly regained. The plantar responses are usually extensor at this time and the tendon jerks are diminished. Confusion is invariable in the postictal phase. The patient often has a severe headache, feels dazed and extremely unwell, and often lapses into deep sleep. On awakening minutes or hours later, there may be no residual symptoms or, more commonly, persisting headache, dysthymia, lethargy, muscle aching and soreness (including stiffness of the jaw).

Tonic–clonic seizures can occur at any age and are encountered in many different types of epilepsy, including idiopathic generalized epilepsy, symptomatic generalized epilepsies, epileptic encephalopathies, and in various epilepsy syndromes, febrile convulsions and acute symptomatic seizures. They have no pathological specificity.

The interictal EEG has a variable appearance, depending on the cause of the tonic–clonic seizures. During the tonic phase, the ictal EEG may show generalized flattening (desynchronization). This is followed by low-voltage fast activity and then 10 Hz rhythms appear and increase in amplitude (recruiting rhythms). These are followed some seconds later by slow waves increasing in amplitude and decreasing in frequency from 3 Hz to 1 Hz. During the clonic phase, the slow waves are interrupted by bursts of faster activity (at about 10 Hz) corresponding to the clonic jerks and, as the phase progresses, the slow waves widen and these bursts become less frequent. With scalp recordings, however, these EEG patterns will often be obscured by artefact from muscle and movement. As the jerks cease, the EEG becomes silent and then slow delta activity develops. This persists for a variable period and the EEG background rhythms then slowly increase in frequency. Minutes or hours usually elapse before the EEG activity returns to normal. In patients with Idiopathic Generalized Epilepsy, the EEG in the preictal period may show increasing abnormalities with spike–wave or spike paroxysms.

Atonic seizures

The most severe form is the classic drop attack (astatic seizure) in which all postural tone is suddenly lost, causing collapse to the ground like a rag doll. The tone change can be more restricted, resulting, for example, in nodding of the head, a bowing movement or sagging at the knees. The seizures are short and followed by immediate recovery. Longer (inhibitory) atonic attacks can develop in a stepwise fashion with progressively increasing nodding, sagging or folding.

The seizures occur at any age, and are always associated with diffuse cerebral damage and learning disability, and are common in severe symptomatic epilepsies (especially in the Lennox–Gastaut syndrome and in myoclonic astatic epilepsy).

The ictal EEG shows irregular spike–wave, polyspike–wave, slow wave or low-amplitude fast activity, or a mixture of these, and may be obscured by movement artefact. The interictal EEG usually shows diffuse abnormalities.

Unclassifiable seizures

Up to a third of seizures in many clinical series are considered unclassifiable using the current ILAE classification scheme, taking forms that do not conform to the typical clinical and EEG patterns described above.

The clinical context of the different seizure types

The clinical context of the different seizure types is summarized in Table 2.4. It is also important to recognize that treatment can markedly modify the form of an epileptic attack, and this can cause confusion. The seizures can be shortened, and the aura and the phasic nature of a prolonged seizure can be lost. Tonic–clonic seizures can, for example, be modified and appear more like clonic or atonic attacks.

Classification of partial seizures by anatomical site of seizure onset

From the point of view of epilepsy surgery, it is clearly imperative to have a classification of partial seizures based on anatomical localization. Thus, various subclassifications of partial seizures have been devised based on the anatomical site of seizure onset. About 60% of complex partial seizures have their origin in the temporal lobe and about 40% are extratemporal and, although less well studied, a similar pattern probably also applies in the

Table 2.4 The usual clinical contexts in which different seizure types occur.

Seizure type	Clinical context
Partial seizures	
Simple, complex, secondarily generalized	Epilepsies due to any focal or multifocal cerebral pathology and in cryptogenic partial epilepsy
Generalized seizures	
Typical absence seizures	Idiopathic generalized epilepsy
Atypical absence seizures	Lennox–Gastaut syndrome
	Other severe cryptogenic or secondarily generalized epilepsies
Myoclonic seizures	Idiopathic generalized epilepsy Progressive myoclonus epilepsies Myoclonic epilepsy syndromes of childhood Occasionally in focal occipital or frontal lobe epilepsies
Clonic, tonic, atonic	Lennox–Gastaut syndrome Other epileptic encephalopathies Occasionally in focal frontal or parietal lobe epilepsy
Tonic–clonic seizures	Epilepsy due to generalized or diffuse cerebral pathologies or in cryptogenic generalized epilepsy

case of simple partial seizures. Although the epilepsy arising in each region can have characteristic clinical features, in practice the distinction is often blurred, owing to the non-specific nature of many epileptic symptoms and the tendency for seizures arising in one cortical area to spread rapidly to another. Of even more importance is the fact, often ignored in too facile a view of the anatomical basis of seizures, that some seizures have a very extended anatomical basis and arise simultaneously in different but connected structures. This is particularly true of limbic seizures (including some mesial temporal and frontal lobe seizures). To talk about strict anatomical localization in these seizures is fanciful and oversimplistic – and this is a mistake often made.

Over-interpretation of the anatomical basis of symptoms should be avoided – and is responsible for many cases of expensive presurgical investigation and failed surgery.

Partial seizures arising in the temporal lobe

Sixty per cent of partial seizures are said to arise in the temporal lobes, and these are an important target for surgical therapy. Having said this, the temporal lobe seizure is often based on an extended neural network, extending beyond the mesial temporal structures. As a result of this, subclassification, e.g. into opercular, temporal polar, basal or limbic types, seems seldom to be valid or useful. The distinction into two categories – mesial temporal and lateral temporal – is more widely accepted, even though symptomatology overlaps owing to rapid spread from lateral to mesial cortex (and vice versa) and because of the widely distributed nature of temporal lobe seizures. This categorization has some utility in clinical practice.

Epilepsy arising in the mesial temporal lobe (limbic epilepsy)

The seizures take the form of simple or complex partial seizures. The simple partial seizures usually last for a matter of seconds only. The complex partial seizures typically evolve relatively gradually (compared with extratemporal seizures) over 1–2 min, have an indistinct onset with initially at least some retention of awareness, and last longer than most extratemporal complex partial seizures (2–10 min). The typical complex partial seizure of temporal lobe origin has three components (Table 2.5).

Aura

An aura can occur in isolation (in which case, the seizure is categorized as a 'simple partial seizure') or it can be the initial manifestation of a complex partial seizure. Typically, auras of mesial temporal origin are made up of visceral, autonomic, cephalic, gustatory, dysmnestic or affective symptoms. The most common symptoms are a rising epigastric sensation (the most common), an abnormal sense of taste (almost invariably unpleasant) or smell, déjà vu and a dreamy sensation. Fear is the most common affective symptom, although other complex emotional feelings occur. Common autonomic features in mesial temporal seizures include changes in skin colour (pallor or flushing), blood pressure, heart rate, pupil size and piloerection.

Table 2.5 Complex partial seizures of mesial temporal lobe origin.

Tripartite seizure pattern (aura, absence, automatism; although only one feature may be present in any individual)

Partial awareness commonly preserved, especially in early stages, and slow evolution of seizure

Auras common and include visceral, cephalic, gustatory, dysmnestic, affective, perceptual or autonomic phenomena

Dystonic posturing of the contralateral upper limb and ipsilateral automatisms common

In seizures arising in the dominant temporal lobe, speech arrest during the seizures and dysphasia postictally. In seizures involving non-dominant temporal lobe, speech or vocalizations during the seizure

Seizures typically last >2 min, with a slow evolution and gradual onset/offset

Autonomic changes (e.g. pallor, redness and tachycardia) common

Automatisms usually take an oroalimentary (lip smacking, chewing, swallowing) or gestural form (e.g. fumbling, fidgeting, repetitive, motor actions, undressing, walking, sexually directed actions, walking, running), and are sometimes prolonged

Postictal confusion common

Seizures tend to cluster

Secondary generalization (to tonic–clonic seizure) infrequent

In patients with hippocampal sclerosis:
– Past history of febrile convulsions
– Onset in mid-childhood or adolescence
– Initial response to therapy, lost after several years

Absence

Motor arrest or absence is prominent especially in the early stages of seizures arising in mesial temporal structures, and more so than in extratemporal lobe epilepsy. The patient stops ongoing activity, looks blank and stares (the 'motionless stare'). A 'dreamy' state is highly characteristic. Speech usually ceases or is severely reduced if the seizure is in the dominant temporal lobe. In the non-dominant lobe, speech may be retained throughout the seizure or meaningless repetitive vocalizations can occur.

Automatisms

The automatisms of mesiobasal temporal lobe epilepsy are typically less violent than in frontal lobe seizures, and are usually oroalimentary (e.g. lip smacking, chewing, swallowing) or gestural (e.g. fumbling, fidgeting, repetitive motor actions, undressing, circling, walking, sexually directed actions, running), and sometimes prolonged. The automatisms are often unilateral, occurring ipsilaterally to the side of the seizure. Ipsilateral upper limb automatisms combined with contralateral upper limb tonic/dystonic spasm are a reliable and very useful lateralizing sign.

Postictal confusion and headache are common after a temporal lobe complex partial seizure, and if dysphasia occurs this is a useful lateralizing sign indicating seizure originating in the dominant temporal lobe. Amnesia is the rule for the absence and the automatism – and, if the patient can recall the automatism, the seizure must be arising outside the mesial structures, usually in the fontal cortex. Secondary generalization is much less common than in extratemporal lobe epilepsy.

The most common pathology underlying this type of epilepsy is hippocampal sclerosis (Ammon horn sclerosis, mesial temporal sclerosis). This is strongly associated (in about 50% of cases) with a history of febrile convulsions and the development of complex partial seizures in late childhood or adolescence. Other aetiologies include dysembryoplastic neuroepithelial tumours (DNETs), other benign tumours, arteriovenous malformations, cavernomas, gliomas, cortical dysplasias or gliotic damage as a result of encephalitis or head injury. Severe seizures, and especially status epilepticus, can also result in hippocampal sclerosis.

The EEG in mesial temporal lobe epilepsy often shows anterior or mid-temporal spikes. Superficial or deep sphenoidal electrodes can assist in their detection in some cases. Other changes include intermittent or persisting slow activity over the temporal lobes. The EEG signs can be unilateral or bilateral. Modern magnetic resonance imaging (MRI) will frequently reveal the abnormality underlying the epilepsy.

Epilepsy arising in the lateral temporal neocortex

There is considerable overlap between the clinical and EEG features of mesial and lateral temporal lobe epilepsy, due presumably to rapid spread and dissemination of discharges between these two anatomical areas. However, differences in degree exist (Table 2.6). Simple auditory phenomena such as humming, buzzing, hissing and roaring may occur if the discharges occur in the superior

Table 2.6 Complex partial seizures of lateral temporal lobe origin.

Features overlap with those of complex partial seizures of mesial temporal origin (see Table 2.5) with the following differences in emphasis:
• Motor arrest and absence less prominent
• Aura more likely to take the form of complex perceptual changes, visual or auditory hallucinations
• Tonic posturing or jerking more common
• More frequent secondary generalization

Table 2.7 Clinical features of complex partial seizures of frontal lobe origin that help differentiation from seizures of temporal lobe origin.

Frequent attacks with clustering

Brief stereotyped seizures (<30 s)

Nocturnal attacks common

Sudden onset and cessation, with rapid evolution and awareness lost at onset

Absence of complex aura

Version of head or eyes common

Prominent motor activity (posturing, jerking and tonic spasm)

Prominent complex bilateral motor automatisms involving lower limbs (can be bizarre and misdiagnosed as pseudoseizures)

Absence of postictal confusion

Frequent secondary generalization

History of status epilepticus

temporal gyrus (Herschel gyrus), and olfactory sensations, which are usually unpleasant and difficult to define, with seizures in the sylvian region. More complex hallucinatory or illusionary states are produced with seizure discharges in association areas, e.g. structured visual hallucinations, complex visual patterns, musical sounds and speech. Illusions of size (macropsia, micropsia), shape, weight, distance or sound can occur. A cephalic aura can also occur in focal temporal lobe seizures, although this is more typical of a frontal lobe focus. Affective, visceral or psychic auras are less common than in mesial temporal lobe epilepsy.

Lateral temporal lobe seizures typically have more motor activity, less prominent motor arrest and may more frequently secondarily generalize because of spread outside the temporal lobe. It is sometimes claimed that consciousness may be preserved for longer than in a typical mesial temporal seizure, but this distinction is seldom useful clinically. The automatisms can be unilateral and have more prominent motor manifestations than in mesial temporal lobe epilepsy. Postictal phenomena, amnesia for the attack and the psychiatric accompaniments are indistinguishable from those of the mesial temporal form.

There is usually a detectable underlying structural pathology, the most common being a glioma, angioma, cavernoma, hamartoma, DNET, other benign tumour, cortical dysplasia and post-traumatic change. There is no association with a history of febrile convulsions. The age of onset of the epilepsy will depend on the aetiology.

The interictal EEG often shows spikes over the temporal region, maximal over the posterior or lateral temporal rather than inferomesial electrodes. MRI will reliably demonstrate the other structural lesions responsible for the epilepsy.

Partial epilepsy arising in non-temporal lobe structures

Epilepsy arising in the frontal lobe

Seizures of frontal lobe origin can take the form of complex partial seizures, simple partial seizures and secondarily generalized attacks. About 30% of complex partial seizures arise in the frontal lobe.

The clinical and EEG features of the complex partial seizures overlap with those of temporal lobe origin, not least because of the rapid spread from seizure foci in the frontal lobe (especially the orbitofrontal cortex) to the mesial temporal lobe, and the widely distributed anatomical location of some seizures. There are, however, several core features that are strongly suggestive of a frontal lobe origin (Table 2.7).

Typically, complex partial seizures of frontal lobe origin are frequent with a marked tendency to cluster. The attacks are brief, with a sudden onset and offset, without the gradual evolution of the temporal lobe seizure. Some types of frontal lobe seizure occur largely or exclusively during sleep, and in some patients the epilepsy comprises frequent short nocturnal attacks (sometimes mistaken for parasomnias). The tripartite pattern of aura/absence/automatism is seldom as well defined in frontal lobe as in mesial temporal lobe complex partial seizures. A brief non-specific 'cephalic aura' can occur, but not the rich range of auras of temporal lobe epilepsy. The absence (motor arrest) is usually short, and may be obscured by the prominent motor signs of the automatism. There are marked qualitative differences between frontal and temporal lobe automatisms, although these are not always specific enough to be reliably of diagnostic value. Frontal lobe automatisms, typically gestural, involve the lower limbs, especially comprising bilateral leg movements (e.g. cycling, stepping, kicking) rather than oroalimentary and upper limb automatisms. The behaviour in the automatism is sometimes highly excited, violent or bizarre, and not infrequently leads to a misdiagnosis of non-epileptic attacks (pseudoseizures). In some frontal seizures, posturing of the limbs or muscle spasm predominates. Urinary incontinence is frequent in frontal lobe complex partial seizures, as is vocalization. The automatisms are usually short, with minimal postictal confusion, and recovery is usually rapid. Frontal lobe partial seizures have a more marked tendency to evolve into secondarily generalized seizures than do those of temporal lobe origin, and the evolution is also more rapid. There is also commonly a history of status epilepticus, of both the tonic–clonic and the non-convulsive types.

The manifestations of complex partial seizures from different frontal lobe regions may differ, but, because of rapid spread of discharges, there is considerable overlap between types, and attempts to classify according to site of origin have been uniformly unsatisfactory. Various patterns of frontal lobe partial seizures occur, many with marked motor manifestations (clonic jerking or posturing) either bilateral or contralateral. Note that consciousness is sometimes retained in the presence of bilateral limb jerking, and these attacks are commonly misdiagnosed as non-epileptic attacks. Apparently generalized tonic–clonic seizures, without lateralizing features, are particularly characteristic of seizures arising in the cingulate or dorsolateral cortex, but can occur from other frontal lobe locations. Version of the head and eyes is common in many types of frontal lobe (and less frequently in temporal lobe epilepsy), and is sometimes the only seizure manifestation ('versive seizures'). When version occurs in full consciousness at the onset of a seizure, this is useful evidence of a focus in the contralateral frontal dorsolateral anterior convexity, but in other situations the direction of version is of little lateralizing value. Occasionally, version is so marked

that the patient actually circles round. Drop attacks or freezing attacks are not uncommon in partial seizures arising especially mesially or anteriorly. Autonomic features are common in frontal lobe epilepsy, and may occasionally be an isolated manifestation of an epileptic focus. Dysphasia in frontal seizures is often accompanied by versive or clonic movements. In epileptic discharges from the perisylvian areas, the aphasia is often preceded by numbness in the mouth and throat, or salivation, swallowing or laryngeal symptoms. Mesial frontal foci can result in absence seizures which can be almost indistinguishable from generalized absences. Seizures arising in the dorsolateral convexity sometimes take the form of a sudden assumption of an abnormal posture (usually bilateral and asymmetrical) with or without loss of consciousness, lasting a second or two only and which cluster, with numerous attacks over a few minutes.

The scalp EEG in frontal lobe epilepsy is often rather disappointing. This is partly because the large area of frontal cortex is covered by relatively few scalp electrodes and also because much of the frontal cortex is hidden in sulci or on the medial or inferior surfaces of the frontal lobe which are distant from the dorsolaterally placed electrodes. Many frontal lobe seizures either fail to show a focus, or demonstrate only widespread and poorly localized foci. Apparently generalized irregular or bilateral and synchronous spike–wave or polyspike discharges with anterior predominance can occur. Sometimes, the interictal and ictal EEGs show non-specific generalized slow activity only.

Epilepsy arising in the central (peri-rolandic) region

The primary manifestations are motor or sensory (Table 2.8). The motor features can take the form of jerking, dystonic spasm, posturing or occasionally paralysis, often with clear consciousness (i.e. simple partial seizures). The jerking can affect any muscle group, usually unilaterally, the exact site depending on the part of the precentral gyrus involved in the seizure, and the jerks may 'march' (the Jacksonian march) from one part of the body to another as the discharge spreads over the motor cortex. The seizure discharge may remain limited to one small segment for long periods of time, and when it does spread it is typically very slow (in contrast to the very fast spread in more anterior frontal lobe seizures). The clonic jerks consist of brief tetanic contractions of all the muscles that cooperate in a single movement. The seizures spread through the cortex, producing clonic movements according to the sequence of cortical

Table 2.8 Partial seizures of central origin.

Often no loss of consciousness (simple partial seizure)

Contralateral clonic jerking (which may or may not march)

Contralateral tonic spasm

Posturing, which is often bilateral, and version of head and eyes

Speech arrest and involvement of bulbar musculature (producing anarthria or choking, gurgling sounds)

Contralateral sensory symptoms

Short, frequently recurring attacks which cluster

Prolonged seizures with slow progression, and episodes of epilepsia partialis continua

Postictal Todd's paresis

Table 2.9 Parietal and occipital lobe epilepsy.

Somatosensory symptoms (e.g. tingling, numbness or more complex sensations – may or may not march)

Sensation of inability to move

Illusions of change in body size/shape

Vertigo

Gustatory seizures

Elementary visual hallucinations (e.g. flashes, colours, shapes, patterns)

Complex visual hallucinations (e.g. objects, scenes, autoscopia, often moving)

Head turning (usually adversive, with sensation of following or looking at the visual hallucinations)

Visual–spatial distortions (e.g. of size [micropsia, macropsia], shape, position)

Loss or dulling of vision (amaurosis)

Eyelid fluttering, blinking, nystagmus

representation. A seizure that begins in the hand usually passes up the arm and down the leg and, if it begins in the foot, it passes up the leg and down the arm. A seizure beginning in the face is most likely to originate in the mouth because of the correspondingly large area of cortical representation. In seizures arising anywhere in the central region, head and eye version is common. Arrest of speech (anarthria) may occur if the motor area of the muscles of articulation is affected (phonatory seizure) and is usually associated with spasm or clonic movements of the jaw. After focal seizure activity, there may be localized paralysis in the affected limbs (Todd's paralysis), which is usually short-lived.

If the seizure is initiated in or evolves to affect supplementary motor areas, posturing of the arms may develop, classically with adversive head and eye deviation, abduction and external rotation of the contralateral arm, and flexion at the elbows. There may also be posturing of the legs, and speech arrest or stereotyped vocalizations. Consciousness is usually maintained unless secondary generalization occurs. The classic posture is named by Penfield the 'fencing posture' (resembling as it does the *en garde* position), but other postures also occur. The posturing is often bilateral and asymmetrical. The fencing posture or fragments of it can also occur in seizures originating in various other frontal and temporal brain regions, presumably due to spread of the seizure discharge to the supplementary motor cortex. In contrast

to Jacksonian seizures, supplementary motor area seizures are often very brief, occur frequently and in clusters, sometimes hundreds each day, and are sometimes also precipitated by startle.

Somatosensory or special sensory manifestations (simple hallucinations) occur if the seizure discharge originates in, or spreads to, the post-central region. Typically, these take the form of tingling, numbness, an electric shock-like feeling, a tickling or crawling feeling, burning, pain or a feeling of heat. These symptoms are usually accompanied by jerking, posturing or spasms because the epileptic discharges usually spread anteriorly. The sensory symptoms may remain localized or march in a Jacksonian manner. Ictal pain is occasionally a prominent symptom and can be severe and poorly localized.

Interictal and ictal scalp EEGs in focal epilepsy in central regions are often normal because the focus may be small and buried within the central gyri.

Epilepsy arising in the parietal and occipital lobes
Focal seizures arise from foci in these locations less commonly than from frontal, central or temporal lobe regions. The typical manifestations of the seizures are subjective sensory and visual disturbances (Table 2.9).

Additional features are common owing to spread to adjacent cortical regions.

Parietal lobe seizures typically comprise sensory manifestations. These may be tingling or a feeling of electricity, which can be confined or march in a jacksonian manner. Sensations of sinking, choking or nausea can occur. There may be accompanying loss of tone or a sensation of paralysis. Illusions of bodily distortion are characteristic, such as a feeling of swelling or shrinking, or lengthening or shortening, particularly affecting the tongue, mouth or extremities. Ictal pain typically, but not exclusively, occurs in parietal seizures. Ictal apraxia, alexia and agnosia have been reported. Sexual feelings can occur sometimes with erection or ejaculation. Gustatory seizures have their origin in the suprasylvian region (adjacent to the mouth and throat primary sensory region). Ictal vertigo also originates in the suprasylvian region. Transient postictal sensory deficits or spatial disorientation occurs.

Seizures from the occipital, parieto-occipital and temporo-occipital cortex are usually characterized by visual symptoms. Elementary visual hallucinations (sensations of colours, shapes, flashes and patterns) are most common, which can be intermittent, stationary, or appear to move across the visual field and to grow. More complex stereotyped hallucinations/illusions can take the form of scenes, animals, people (including self-images), or topographical or spatial distortion, alterations of size and shape, perseveration or repetition of visual objects, or the break-up of visual objects or movement. Vision commonly blacks out in occipital lobe seizures, one of the few examples of negative epileptic symptomatology. The blindness is typically accompanied by the development of illusions of lights or colours. Forced head and eye turning are common, with the patient believing that the visual hallucination is being tracked voluntarily. Rapid blinking or eyelid flutter is frequent in some types of occipital seizures. Headache and nausea are common, and the attacks are not infrequently misdiagnosed as migraine. In the benign occipital epilepsies (especially of Panayiotopoulos syndrome, p. 26), the seizures can be very prolonged, but most focal seizures in adults last seconds or minutes only. Studies have shown that there are no clinical or EEG features that help differentiate epilepsy arising in the medial or lateral occipital cortex. Occasionally, occipital seizures denote mitochondrial disease (including Alpers disease), Lafora body disease, coeliac disease or metabolic disorders.

The EEG in occipital or parietal epilepsy can be normal or show appropriate focal discharges, although often the epileptic disturbance is poorly localized without correlation to the ictal symptoms. Occipital spike–wave is characteristic of some types of focal occipital seizures, which can be confused with idiopathic generalized epilepsy.

3 Epilepsy Syndromes

ILAE Classification of the Epilepsies and Epilepsy Syndromes

In an attempt to encompass a broader range of clinical features than is possible in a classification of seizure type, the ILAE published, in 1985, and revised in 1989, a *Classification of the Epilepsies and Epileptic Syndromes* (Table 3.1). An epileptic syndrome is defined as 'an epileptic disorder characterized by a cluster of signs and symptoms customarily occurring together'. The relationship between the epilepsy syndrome and the underlying disease is complex. Although some syndromes represent a single disease, others can be the result of many diseases. A good example of the latter is the Lennox–Gastaut syndrome. Furthermore, the same underlying disease can manifest as different epileptic syndromes, an example being tuberous sclerosis. The syndromes are often age specific, and over time in individual patients one epileptic syndrome can evolve into another. Similarly, the same seizure type can occur in very different syndromes (e.g. myoclonic seizures in the benign syndrome of juvenile myoclonic epilepsy and the refractory syndromes of the progressive myoclonic epilepsies). The advantages of the classification are its flexibility, the potential for change and expansion, and the acknowledgement of the complex interplay of factors underlying epilepsy.

There are, however, also disadvantages. First, the classification is a complex system with very clumsy terminology, and for this reason alone has not gained widespread clinical usage, especially in non-specialist settings. A second problem is the maintenance of the distinction between focal and generalized epilepsies, which in many types of epilepsy is difficult to justify and presumes an unrealistic level of knowledge of the underlying physiological processes. It is perhaps in recognition of this problem that the third category has been introduced, although it might have been better to avoid this distinction altogether. A third problem is that, in the attempt to

be all inclusive, this classification becomes unwieldy. Common syndromes are mixed in with those that are extremely rare and syndromes with an identity that is contentious are also included. In normal clinical practice, the majority of epilepsy cases seen (66% in one series) will fall into categories 1.2, 2.3 and 4.1, each of which is a poorly defined 'non-specific' category – which undermines the purpose and value of the scheme. Another problem is the arbitrary nature of some categories (notably 3 and 4). This results in the grouping of epilepsies that have little else in common. Finally, it is difficult to justify the full epithet 'syndrome' for some of the idiopathic conditions listed. Some prefer to see the idiopathic generalized epilepsies, for example, as a 'neurobiological continuum' whereas others have split the conditions into at least 10 subdivisions. The incidence of different syndromes presenting in one study is shown in Table 3.2.

The categorization is also of limited value from the perspective of therapy. Most of the categories can be treated by most of the available drug therapies (there are exceptions discussed under the relevant sections of this book) and this lack of specificity is disappointing.

Localization-related epilepsies and syndromes
These epilepsies and syndromes are sometimes referred to as the partial or focal epilepsies.

Idiopathic localization-related epilepsies and syndromes
Three conditions are included here, one of them being benign childhood epilepsy with centrotemporal spikes (see pp. 24–25), which is said to account for up to 15% of childhood epilepsies, and two much less common syndromes, childhood epilepsy with occipital paroxysms (see p. 26) and primary reading epilepsy. Other genetic and idiopathic syndromes will no doubt be added as knowledge advances, such as the recently described syndrome of dominantly inherited, nocturnal, frontal lobe epilepsy.

Symptomatic localization-related epilepsies and syndromes
This category includes the large number of epilepsies due to specific focal cerebral lesions (e.g. tumour, stroke) in

Handbook of Epilepsy Treatment, 3rd Edition. By Simon Shorvon. Published 2010 by Blackwell Publishing Ltd.

Table 3.1 International classification of epilepsies and epileptic syndromes.

1 Localization-related (focal, local, partial epilepsies and syndromes)
  1.1 Idiopathic (with age-related onset)
   • Benign childhood epilepsy with centrotemporal spike
   • Childhood epilepsy with occipital paroxysms
   • Primary reading epilepsy
  1.2 Symptomatic epilepsy
   • Chronic epilepsia partialis continua of childhood (Kojewnikow syndrome)
   • Syndromes characterized by seizures with specific modes of precipitation
  1.3 Cryptogenic

2 Generalized epilepsies and syndromes
  2.1 Idiopathic (with age-related onset – listed in order of age)
   • Benign neonatal familial convulsions
   • Benign neonatal convulsions
   • Benign myoclonic epilepsy in infancy
   • Childhood absence epilepsy (pyknolepsy)
   • Juvenile myoclonic epilepsy (impulsive petit mal)
   • Epilepsy with grand-mal seizures (GTCSs) on awakening
   • Other generalized idiopathic epilepsies not defined above
   • Epilepsies with seizures precipitated by specific modes of activation
  2.2 Cryptogenic or symptomatic (in order of age)
   • West syndrome (infantile spasms, Blitz–Nick–Salaam–Krämpfe syndrome)
   • Lennox–Gastaut syndrome
   • Epilepsy with myoclonic–astatic seizures
   • Epilepsy with myoclonic absences
  2.3 Symptomatic
    2.3.1 Non-specific aetiology
     • Early myoclonic encephalopathy
     • Early infantile epileptic encephalopathy with suppression burst
     • Other symptomatic generalized epilepsies not defined above
    2.3.2 Specific syndromes
     • Epileptic seizure may complicate many disease states
     Under this heading are diseases in which seizures are a presenting or predominant feature

3 Epilepsies and syndromes undetermined whether focal or generalized
  3.1 With both generalized and focal seizures
   • Neonatal seizures
   • Severe myoclonic epilepsy in infancy
   • Epilepsy with continuous spike–waves during slow-wave sleep
   • Acquired epileptic aphasia (Landau–Kleffner syndrome)
   • Other undetermined epilepsies not defined above
  3.2 Without unequivocal generalized or focal features. All cases with generalized tonic–clonic seizures in which clinical and EEG findings do not permit classification as clearly generalized or localization related such as in many cases of sleep GTCSs are considered not to have unequivocal generalized or focal features

4 Special syndromes
  4.1 Situation-related seizures (*Gelegenheitsanfälle*)
   • Febrile convulsions
   • Isolated seizures or isolated status epilepticus
   • Seizures occurring only when there is an acute metabolic or toxic event due to factors such as alcohol, drugs, eclampsia, non-ketotic hyperglycaemia

GTCS, generalized tonic–clonic seizure.

Table 3.2 Annual incidence of different categories of epilepsy (from a prospective study in south-west France).

International classification of epilepsies and epilepsy syndromes: category	Annual incidence per 100 000 population
1.1 Idiopathic localization-related epilepsy	1.68
1.2 Symptomatic localization-related epilepsy	17.11
2.1 Idiopathic generalized epilepsies	6.65
2.2 Symptomatic generalized epilepsies	1.15
3 Epilepsies and syndromes undetermined whether focal or generalized	2.92
4 Situation-related seizures	37.33[a]

[a]Acute symptomatic epilepsy, 25.37; isolated unprovoked seizure, 11.70; television epilepsy, 0.26.

which epilepsy is a variable feature. The epilepsies are divided into anatomical site and are described below. Chronic epilepsia partialis continua is also included, rather strangely, in this category.

Cryptogenic localization-related epilepsies and syndromes

This category has been created to include symptomatic focal epilepsies in which the aetiology is unknown. With increasingly sophisticated neuroimaging techniques, the number of cases falling into this category has become much smaller than when the classification was first proposed.

Generalized epilepsies and syndromes

These conditions, similar to the localization-related epilepsies, are divided into subcategories on the basis of presumed aetiology.

Idiopathic generalized epilepsies and syndromes

The idiopathic generalized epilepsies (also called the primary generalized epilepsies) are genetic conditions in which epilepsy is the major clinical feature. Encompassed within this rubric are a variety of age-related syndromes, although to what extent the subdivisions are specific entities or simply a biological continuum is a matter of

controversy. These common conditions are considered in more detail on pp. 24–26.

Cryptogenic or symptomatic generalized epilepsies

This category includes the epileptic encephalopathies in which epilepsy is a major clinical feature of a diffuse encephalopathic condition. Included in this category are conditions described elsewhere in this book: West syndrome (see pp. 28–29), the Lennox–Gastaut syndrome (see pp. 29–30), epilepsy with myoclonic astatic seizures (see p. 24) and epilepsy with myoclonic absences. Also included are the rare myoclonic syndromes and epileptic encephalopathies of infancy. The relative nosological position of many of these conditions is often unclear, and there is considerable overlap between the core conditions. Also included here are the epilepsies due to malformations, inborn errors of metabolism, and hereditary or congenital disorders.

Epilepsies and syndromes undetermined as to whether they are focal or generalized

The existence of this category is an acknowledgement that the differentiation between focal epilepsy and generalized epilepsy is not always easy to make. The category is divided into those syndromes with both focal and generalized seizures, and those without unequivocal generalized or focal features. Included in the first subdivision is a miscellany of 'syndromes', including neonatal seizures (which have a variety of forms that overlap with other categories), infantile myoclonic epilepsy, electrical status epilepticus during slow-wave sleep (ESES) and the Landau–Kleffner syndrome, which are epileptic encephalopathies of unknown pathophysiology. In the second subdivision are those epilepsies with tonic–clonic seizures in which clinical and EEG features do not allow categorization into focal or generalized groups.

Special syndromes

This category includes the 'situational-related syndromes' (reflex epilepsy), febrile seizures (see pp. 26–28), isolated seizures (including single seizures and isolated status epilepticus) and the acute symptomatic seizures precipitated by acute toxic or metabolic events.

The epilepsy syndromes

There are a number of syndromes identified in the ILAE *Classification of the Epilepsies and Epilepsy Syndromes* that are common or important and these are briefly reviewed here.

Some have no specific identifiable cause, some a single cause and others can result from various identifiable conditions. It must be recognized that there is overlap between some of these syndromes and there is considerable disagreement about the exact nosology. It is assumed that the cryptogenic or idiopathic cases have a complex polygenic genetic basis, although environmental influences also play a part. Most of these syndromes are highly age specific and assume characteristic clinical forms regardless of cause. These may be best conceptualized as generic age-related responses of disordered brain function or development.

Neonatal seizures

The clinical and EEG features, the cause and the pathophysiology of seizures in the neonatal period differ from those in later life. Clinical signs are necessarily confined to motor features and are usually focal or multifocal, reflecting the immature synaptic connections in the neonatal brain. The EEG changes are variable and nonspecific. Seizures can take the form of tonic attacks, clonic seizures, unilateral focal seizures, electrographic seizures without overt clinical changes and so-called subtle seizures. The seizures can have mild or atypical features such as grimacing, staring, eye movements, posturing or pedalling movements.

Neonatal seizures occur in about 1% of all infants, with a higher frequency (up to 23%) in premature babies. Although there is no doubt that most neonatal seizures are 'epileptic', some subtle and some tonic seizures are not associated with any EEG changes and may be subcortical in origin and the result of abnormal brain-stem release mechanisms. There are a large variety of potential causes, the most common being hypoxic–ischaemic encephalopathy, intracranial haemorrhage, neonatal infection and metabolic disorders (especially hypocalcaemia, hypomagnesaemia and hypoglycaemia). The development of neonatal seizures is an ominous sign, not only because they often indicate cerebral disease but also because the seizures themselves possibly damage the developing brain.

The prognosis depends largely on the underlying cause. Overall, the immediate mortality rate is about 15%, 37% develop neurological deficits and only 48% of infants develop normally. Prognosis is worse in premature infants, especially those with a gestational age <31 weeks.

If the seizures are considered non-epileptic, antiepileptic drug treatment is not indicated. Indeed, medication may worsen the phenomenon by decreasing the level of cortical inhibition over subcortical structures. Whether genuine (cortical) but slight (subtle) epileptic seizures

Table 3.3 Some subdivisions of idiopathic generalized epilepsy.

Epilepsy with myoclonic absences
Childhood absence epilepsy (pyknolepsy)
Juvenile absence epilepsy
Juvenile myoclonic epilepsy
Epilepsy with grand-mal seizures on awakening
Absence epilepsy with perioral myoclonia

require treatment is uncertain. Not uncommonly, such seizure manifestations remit spontaneously after days or weeks and the usefulness of treatment in this situation is difficult to assess. Opinions vary about the need to treat infants with EEG evidence of seizure activity without overt clinical signs. There is also disagreement about the duration of therapy, although most would aim for as short a period as possible. Many neonatal seizures are self-limiting and over-long treatment carries its own risks. Specific treatment is outlined on pp. 89–90.

Idiopathic generalized epilepsy

The term 'idiopathic generalized epilepsy' (IGE; also known as primary generalized epilepsy) is used to denote a very common and important group of conditions, with a probable genetic basis, and in which there is a characteristic clinical and electrographic pattern. It has been estimated that patients with IGE account for about 10–20% of all those with epilepsy. The identification of the genetic basis of IGE has proved elusive. This was the first 'pure' epilepsy in which an intensive genetic search was undertaken, on the basis that there may be a single underlying gene (albeit with markedly variable penetrance). None was found, and it is now believed that the syndromes of IGE have a polygenic basis, but disappointingly still no common susceptibility gene has been found. There is current interest in the possibility that deletions or duplications (copy number variations) might be the cause of some of these cases. A contentious and unresolved issue, which itself may have confounded the search for genes, is the extent to which the 'syndrome' can or should be subcategorized. Nowhere in the study of epilepsy is there more divergence of opinion than between those who view this epilepsy type as a 'biological continuum' (possibly with a unitary genetic mechanism) and those who subdivide according to clinical pattern. It is not currently possible to know where nosological reality exists. Table 3.3 shows commonly proposed subdivisions, but, even in this matter, different authorities

Table 3.4 Clinical features of idiopathic generalized epilepsy.

Onset in childhood or early adult life

Positive family history

Generalized seizure types – myoclonus, generalized absence (petit mal) and generalized tonic–clonic seizures

Normal EEG background

Paroxysms of generalized EEG discharges, either 3 Hz spike-and-wave or polyspike bursts, often exacerbated by over-breathing and photosensitivity

A diurnal pattern of seizure recurrence, with seizures especially on waking and during sleep

Normal intellect and low co-morbidity

Absence of identifiable underlying structural aetiology

Excellent response to therapy with sodium valproate

subdivide to different extents. It is a dearly held expectation that, when the genetic basis is clarified, a more definitive subclassification will become apparent based on genotypic–phenotypic correlation, but such a belief may be over-optimistic.

Core clinical features shared to a greater or lesser extent by these syndromes (at least those with onset in later childhood or early adult life) are shown in Table 3.4. The treatment of the idiopathic generalized epilepsies is described on pp. 90–91.

Childhood absence epilepsy

Childhood absence epilepsy (pyknolepsy) appears in the early and middle years of childhood (peak age 6–7 years), more commonly in girls than in boys and usually in children without learning disability or other neurological problems. It accounts for between 1 and 3% of newly diagnosed epilepsies and up to 10% of childhood epilepsies. The absence seizures usually last 10–15 s, and are so brief that in many cases they pass unrecognized for long periods. Many can occur in a day, and the seizures tend to cluster. The loss of consciousness is usually complete, and the patient is unaware that a seizure has occurred. Eyes, if closed at onset, open after 2–3 s. The seizures can be induced by hyperventilation. The classic EEG pattern is monotonous, generalized 3 Hz spike–wave. In a series of 194 patients with typical clinical features and EEG, approximately a third also had generalized tonic–clonic seizures (GTCSs) at some point and absence status occurred in 15%. The prognosis is good,

and rapid remission on therapy is expected in 80% or more of patients. When followed up after 18 years of age, only about 20% of previously diagnosed patients are still having seizures. Prognosis is better in those with onset of seizures before the age of 12 years; they have a more rapid response to therapy, a low chance of GTCSs and a high remission rate. GTCSs can develop, usually after years of exclusively absence seizures and usually in those whose response to therapy is incomplete. The nosological boundaries between this and the other syndromes of IGE are indistinct, and how often tonic–clonic seizures occur depends on the inclusiveness of the diagnostic criteria; the frequency is reported to be between 3 and 35%. The genetic basis is unknown in spite of serious attempts to identify susceptibility genes.

'Phantom absence' is a term used to describe the phenomenon of short-lived EEG bursts of spike and wave without any obvious clinical signs. These may be quite common in some IGE syndromes and also seem to be associated with a relatively high incidence of absence status. There may be very subtle clinical signs, but sometimes even quite prolonged EEG bursts seem to occur without any noticeable clinical change. It is considered by some that phantom absences are particularly common in patients with the syndrome of epilepsy with grand-mal seizures (GTCSs) on awakening (see p. 24) and in others the occurrence of phantom absence and tonic–clonic seizures is itself a separate syndrome (IGE with phantom absences).

Juvenile myoclonic epilepsy

Juvenile myoclonic epilepsy (JME; also known as impulsive petit mal, Janz syndrome) is the most common subtype of idiopathic generalized epilepsy, and accounts for up to 10% of all epilepsies. The characteristic seizures are brief myoclonic jerks, occurring in the first hour or so after waking, and usually in bursts. These are sudden, shock-like jerks, affecting mainly the shoulders and arms, usually but not always symmetrically. It may not be clear whether consciousness is retained or lost. In 80% of cases, the myoclonus develops between the ages of 12 and 18 years (and always between 6 and 25 years), but may be unrecognized initially and taken to be early morning clumsiness. In about 80% of cases, GTCSs also occur, usually months or years after the onset of myoclonus, and it is these that often lead to the diagnosis.

It is worth enquiring specifically about myoclonus in anyone presenting with generalized epilepsy. The tonic–clonic seizures are usually infrequent (average two per year). About a third of patients also develop typical absence seizures (usually very brief, lasting 2–5 s) and again usually on waking. Almost invariably, the absence seizures occur in patients with both myoclonus and tonic–clonic seizures. About 5% of patients exhibit strong photosensitivity, and the myoclonus (and other seizures) can be precipitated by photic stimuli. The seizures (myoclonus and GTCSs) often have other clear precipitants such as lack of sleep, alcohol, hypoglycaemia or poor compliance with medication. Myoclonic jerks may evolve into myoclonic status, and the tonic–clonic seizures are also often preceded by increasing myoclonus. About 50% of cases show interictal abnormalities – 3 Hz spike–wave or faster polyspike–wave at 4–6 Hz – which can be symmetrical or asymmetrical. The background EEG is normal. In about a third of untreated cases, EEG shows a photoparoxysmal response. Intelligence is normal and there is usually no other neurological morbidity or co-morbidity. It has been claimed that patients show typical personality traits, but whether this is really the case is unclear. Complete response to treatment can be expected in 80–90% of cases, but lifelong therapy may be needed. Appropriate drug therapy is important (see pp. 90–91) because carbamazepine, vigabatrin, tiagabine and phenytoin can exacerbate myoclonus. Imaging is normal, although there is an isolated unconfirmed report of quantitative MRI cortical volume change. The genetics of JME have been controversial; a non-single gene has been found to account for cases (except in rare atypical family clusters) and JME is now generally assumed to have polygenic inheritance. A family history of epilepsy is found in about 25% of cases, and in about 5% of close relatives (of whom a third have JME and most of the others have other IGE subtypes). The risk of epilepsy in offspring is about 5%.

Other IGE variants with myoclonus

Other types of myoclonic IGE subtypes are less well defined, and their nosological position less clear cut. Myoclonic absences occur at a younger age, have a male predominance, an EEG initially at least indistinguishable from that of typical absence epilepsy, are associated with intellectual disturbance and are much more resistant to drug therapy; other seizure types evolve in two-thirds of cases. Eyelid myoclonia with or without absence is a photosensitive IGE variant, characterized by very short attacks comprising jerking of the eyelids and upward deviation of the eyes. There may or may not be associated absence seizures. The peak age of onset is 6 years; there is usually a strong family history and a marked female preponderance. Many attacks per day can occur, and the children may induce attacks, which are associated with a pleasurable sensation, by photic stimulation. Tonic–clonic seizures develop in adolescence or adult life. The EEG shows 4–6 Hz polyspike–wave, which can be triggered by eye opening, and also marked photosensitivity. Benign myoclonic epilepsy is a rare condition, occurring in infancy or early childhood, with spontaneous remission in most cases and without long-term sequelae.

Epilepsy with grand-mal seizures on waking

This condition overlaps considerably with other generalized epilepsies, especially with JME, in which most affected people also have GTCSs on awakening. The EEG pattern is a generalized spike–wave. Whether this syndrome represents a discrete entity or simply part of the spectrum of other forms of IGE has been the subject of discussion for several decades, without clear resolution.

Myoclonic–astatic epilepsy (myoclonic astatic petit mal)

This is an ill-defined syndrome with myoclonic and astatic (atonic) seizures, and an EEG signature of fast (>3 Hz) spike–wave. Repeated episodes of non-convulsive status epilepticus are reported in severe cases, and usually associated with intellectual regression, qualifying the condition as an epileptic encephalopathy. Young children often have seizures with falls, which can have serious consequences. The EEG changes reported in different series are also variable. The delineation of this symptom complex as a 'syndrome' is rather muddled, and cases that overlap with benign myoclonic epilepsy, on the one hand, and the Lennox–Gastaut syndrome, on the other, are reported. Idiopathic and symptomatic forms are proposed, and severity and outcome with respect both to epilepsy and to cognitive function are very variable. However, severe epilepsy with falls and episodes of non-convulsive status requires expert attention, and a 'syndrome' tag assists communication. Recently, missense mutations on the *SCN1A* and *GABRG2* genes have been described in children with a phenotype consistent with myoclonic–astatic epilepsy, and advances in an understanding of the genetic bases of the early childhood epilepsies may help clarify the basis of this syndrome.

Benign partial epilepsy with centrotemporal spikes

Benign partial epilepsy with centrotemporal spikes (BECTS; also known as rolandic epilepsy or benign epilepsy with rolandic spikes) is the most common 'idiopathic' epilepsy syndrome, accounting for perhaps

Table 3.5 Benign epilepsy with centrotemporal spikes.

15% of all childhood epilepsy
Age of onset 5–10 years
Simple partial seizures with frequent secondary
    generalization
Partial seizures involve the face, oropharynx and upper limb
Seizures typically during sleep and infrequent
No other neurological features; normal intelligence
Family history
EEG shows typical centrotemporal spikes
Excellent response to antiepileptic drugs
Excellent prognosis with remission by mid-teenage years

15% of all epilepsies (Table 3.5). The peak age of onset is 5–8 years and over 80% of cases have onset between 4 and 10 years. The condition is the result of age-related, genetically determined, neuronal hyperexcitability in the rolandic area, causing characteristic giant EEG spikes and seizures, although it is estimated that less than 10% of children with the EEG disturbance actually have seizures. The seizures are infrequent – about 10% of cases have only a single attack and 50% only a few attacks. Less than 20% of cases have 20 or more seizures, and the total duration of seizure activity is 3 years or more in only 10%. About 50% of children have seizures only while asleep (typically in non-rapid eye movement [REM] sleep at the onset of sleep or just before awakening), about 40% both during the day and at night, and in 10% seizures occur exclusively during the day. The daytime seizures usually occur when the child is tired or bored (e.g. on a long car journey).

The seizures are highly characteristic, usually beginning with spasm and clonic jerking of one side of the face and/or throat muscles. In many cases, the seizures sometimes evolve to secondarily generalized tonic–clonic attacks. The motor features include speech arrest and a gurgling or guttural sound, and profuse salivation is also characteristic. There are also often sensory symptoms involving one side of the mouth and the throat. The arm or rarely the legs can be involved. In most cases consciousness is preserved until the seizures generalize.

The EEG shows focal spikes that originate most often in the centrotemporal regions, although, on repeated EEG recordings, the spikes often wander. The waveform and distribution are characteristic. In a small number of patients (probably less than 10%, although figures vary), a generalized spike–wave is seen. There are no associated neurological disturbances and intellect is normal. The epilepsy remits in almost all cases, usually by the age of 12 years, with no long-term sequelae. It is assumed that there is a genetic basis to the condition, although no genetic abnormality has been consistently described, and polygenic inheritance is likely. One family has been described with autosomal dominant inheritance and linkage to chromosome 15q14. The family history is positive for seizures of various types in 40% of cases. The treatment of BECTS is described on p. 91.

The prognosis of the typical condition is good, neurological development and cognitive function are generally normal, and the seizures remit in more than 95% of cases. There are, however, children in whom the condition appears to evolve into other seizure syndromes and who develop intractable seizures and neuropsychological deficit.

The overlap, even of BECTS, which seems a relatively specific symptom complex, and other syndromes, is an illustration of the boundary problems that exist in all epilepsy syndromes. Transitional cases have been labelled atypical benign partial epilepsy (ABPE) or pseudo-Lennox–Gastaut syndrome, and some authorities consider BECTS, ESES and the Landau–Kleffner syndrome to be part of a spectrum. Others consider febrile seizures, Panayiotopoulos syndrome and BECTS all to be manifestations of a continuum (the benign childhood seizure susceptibility syndrome). Atypical features include bouts of status epilepticus, atypical absence seizures, atonic seizures, and cognitive and behavioural impairment combined with an EEG pattern of slow spike–wave. Similarly, although patients with BECTS are lesion free, patients who manifest the same phenotype have been shown to have hippocampal atrophy, cortical dysplasia, lesions of corpus callosum, porencephalic cysts and toxoplasmosis.

Childhood epilepsy with occipital paroxysms (benign occipital epilepsy; Gastaut-type idiopathic childhood occipital epilepsy)

This is a well-defined syndrome, with mean age of onset of 8 years (3–15 years), in which seizures occur with prominent visual symptomatology, including hemianopia and amaurosis, abstract simple and complex visual hallucinations, forced eyelid closure, blinking, eye deviation and prominent postictal headaches, sometimes with nausea and vomiting. The visual symptomatology typically comprise coloured visual spots of light or coloured patterns, growing and moving from the periphery to the centre of the visual field as the seizure progresses. Consciousness is usually preserved but there may be secondary generalization. The EEG shows prominent occipital epileptiform spike–wave activity which appears after eye closure and is suppressed by eye opening. There are often frequent seizures (several a day) before treatment but the condition has an excellent prognosis with full remission in 60% of cases after several years of therapy. The condition needs to be differentiated from migraine and also from symptomatic occipital epilepsies, which include those due to mito-chondrial disease (Alpers disease, and mitochondrial encephalomyopathy, lactic acidosis and stroke-like episodes [MELAS]), coeliac disease or cortical dysplasia. Seizures show a complete response to carbamazepine in over 90% of cases, and some patients require long-term treatment.

Early onset benign occipital epilepsy (synonym: Panayiotopoulos syndrome)

This is another syndrome with age of onset between 1 and 14 years (mean 4–5 years). Prevalence is estimated to be 2–3 cases/1000 children, and in one study it accounted for 28% of all benign focal epilepsies of childhood. Panayiotopoulos considers the condition to be due to diffuse maturation-related epileptogenicity activating emetic centres and the hypothalamus. The clinical presentation is distinctive. In the core syndrome, seizures take the form of eye deviation, nausea, retching and vomiting, with subsequent evolution into impaired consciousness and then clonic hemiconvulsions in 25% and convulsions in 20%. The convulsions are often nocturnal and awareness may or may not be altered. Other autonomic features occur including incontinence of urine, pallor, hyperventilation and headache. Typically, the seizures are prolonged, often lasting several hours, and are therefore classified as episodes of status epilepti-cus (taking the form of absence or autonomic status epilepticus). Despite this high incidence of status, the prognosis for the syndrome is excellent and at least 75% of patients have fewer than five attacks in total (25% have only a single attack). The interictal EEG shows occipital spikes, which can be continuous. The EEG discharges are abolished by eye opening (the fixation-off phenomenon) and continue to be seen for years after the cessation of seizures. The boundaries of the syndrome are less well defined than in other syndromes, and the condition can evolve into other seizure types. It is considered by some authorities to be part of the spectrum of BECTS or the

benign childhood seizure susceptibility syndrome. Some cases are included in which the prolonged seizures consist only of vomiting, or of syncopal or prominent autonomic symptoms. This syndrome is often misdiagnosed as migraine, and also needs to be differentiated from other occipital epilepsies. The epilepsy usually remits over time without adverse sequelae, although a minority of cases evolve to other forms of epilepsy.

Usually, continuous antiepileptic drug treatment is not needed but a small night-time dose of carbamazepine, valproate or benzodiazepines will usually suppress all seizures. In the acute phase when seizures are prolonged, rectal diazepam should be given. Parents should be counselled about the condition and the acute manage-ment of the seizures.

Other benign partial epilepsy syndromes

There are a number of other predominantly childhood syndromes with partial epilepsy that are best divided according to anatomical origin of the seizures. Epilepsy with occipital calcifications is an occipital epilepsy syndrome in which there is more severe epilepsy and a poorer outcome. Many cases are associated with coeliac disease, which may be demonstrable only on jejunal biopsy. Other rarer but interesting childhood benign focal syndromes have been described, sometimes in a handful of families only, and include: benign partial epilepsy in infancy, idiopathic photosensitive occipital lobe epilepsy, idiopathic frontal lobe epilepsy, familial temporal lobe epilepsy, autosomal dominant rolandic epilepsy with speech dyspraxia and benign focal seizures in adolescents.

Febrile seizures

Febrile seizures are defined as epileptic events that occur in the context of an acute rise in body temperature, usually in children aged between 6 months and 5 years, in whom there is no evidence of intracranial infection or other defined intracranial cause (Table 3.6). They are common. About 2–5% of children (7% in Japan and up to 14% in the Mariana Islands) will have at least one attack, and it has been estimated that between 19/1000 and 41/1000 infants with fever will convulse. The first febrile seizure happens in the second year of life in 50% and in the first 3 years in 90%; 4% occur before 6 months and 6% after 6 years of age. Boys are slightly more likely to have febrile seizures than girls. In over 85%, the seizures are generalized and usually brief. Febrile seizures are usually subdivided into simple and complex forms. Complex febrile seizures are those that last more than

Table 3.6 Febrile seizures.

2–5% of all children

Peak age of onset 2–4 years

10–20% of children have existing neurodevelopmental problems

Probably genetic basis to some cases

Tonic–clonic seizures

Usually at onset of fever

35% of children have a second febrile seizure and 15% a third (recurrence more likely with early age of onset, positive family history)

Prognosis worse in complex seizures (prolonged or focal; 30% of all febrile seizures)

May induce hippocampal sclerosis and subsequent temporal lobe epilepsy

Risk of subsequent epilepsy small (2–10%; more likely if onset <13 months, complex convulsion or existing neurodevelopmental problems)

15 min and have strongly unilateral features or those that recur within a single illness. Up to a third of all febrile convulsions are classifiable as complex. The important risk factors seem to be an acute temperature rise, and viral infection is the underlying cause of the fever in 80%. The seizure usually occurs early, almost always within the first 24 hours of the viral illness, and in about a quarter of cases is the first recognizable sign of the illness. Seventy-five per cent of children affected have a temperature >39°C. There is a family history of febrile convulsions in at least 25% of cases, and some families have an autosomal dominant pattern of inheritance. One population study has shown an association between febrile convulsions and polymorphisms in the *SCN1A* gene, and similar abnormalities have been found in families with generalized epilepsy with febrile seizures (GEFS+). The empirical risk for further seizures is 10–15% if there is one affected sibling, rising to 50% if a parent and a sibling have a history of febrile seizures.

These essentially benign seizures need to be differentiated from the 5–10% of first seizures with fever in which the seizure is in fact due to viral or bacterial meningitis, and other cases where the fever lights up an existing latent predisposition to epilepsy. In neither of these situations

should the term 'febrile convulsion' be used, because both carry significantly different clinical implications.

Obviously, in all cases, the aetiology of the fever should be established. Febrile seizures occurring before 6 months of age in particular raise the possibility of bacterial meningitis, and urgent lumbar puncture is indicated. In older children, investigation depends on the clinical circumstances, but may include lumbar puncture or brain scanning.

The outcome of febrile seizures has been the subject of intensive study, which has concentrated on three aspects: the risk of recurrent febrile convulsions, the risk of neurological or developmental deficit, and the risk of subsequent non-febrile epilepsy. Although parents, on witnessing the first febrile convulsion, almost invariably feel that the child is about to die, the mortality risk from febrile convulsions is negligible.

About 35% of susceptible children will have a second febrile seizure and 15% three or more. Recurrence is more common if the initial convulsion was at a young age, in those in whom the convulsion occurred at a relatively low temperature (<39°C), and in those with prolonged initial convulsions. However, even in recurrent attacks, the outcome in relation to longer-term neurological function is usually excellent. In fact, the mental and neurological development of children after a febrile convulsion is usually entirely normal, provided that there were no pre-existing developmental problems. In about 10–20% of children, subsequent neurodevelopment problems are noted, but these usually reflect pre-existing problems and are not due to the convulsions. Occasionally, prolonged convulsions cause acute cerebral damage (the HHE – hemiplegia, hemiatrophy, epilepsy – syndrome typically develops after febrile status) and, the longer the duration of the attack, the more likely is cerebral damage. It is for this reason that seizures continuing for 15 min or more require emergency therapy.

The occurrence of febrile seizures is also associated with the later development of subsequent epilepsy. The risk of epilepsy is small – about 2–10% in children with a history of febrile seizures, compared with 0.5% in those who have not had a febrile seizure. The risk is higher in those with pre-existing neurodevelopmental dysfunction, and in some of these cases the febrile seizure is simply the first manifestation of an existing predisposition to epilepsy. The risk of subsequent epilepsy is somewhat higher after complex febrile seizures (10–20%), compared with single febrile seizures (2–7.5%).

It has been proposed that febrile convulsions cause hippocampal sclerosis and, by this mechanism, subsequent temporal lobe epilepsy. Certainly, at least 50% of those with temporal lobe epilepsy and MRI evidence of hippocampal sclerosis have a history of febrile convulsions, although distinguishing cause from consequence is difficult. However, there are indisputable animal experimental data showing that focal status epilepticus can result in subsequent hippocampal damage, and human studies of serial MRI after a febrile convulsion have also demonstrated the development of hippocampal atrophy. The risk of seizure-induced hippocampal sclerosis has been estimated to be about 3% after complex febrile seizure and less than 1% after all febrile seizures. As a result of this risk, febrile seizures should be treated as a medical emergency, and specific treatment measures are outlined on pp. 92–93.

West syndrome

West syndrome (Table 3.7) is a severe epileptic encephalopathy, with an incidence of 1–2/4000 live births, and a family history in 7–17%. The condition is defined by the occurrence of a typical form of epileptic seizure (infantile spasm) and EEG (hypsarrhythmia). The infantile spasms take the form of sudden, generally bilateral and symmetrical contractions of the muscles of the neck, trunk or limbs. The spasms grow in frequency as the condition evolves and, at its peak, seizures occur hundreds of times a day. The spasms show a strong tendency to cluster, with intensity waxing and waning during the cluster. In the most common type, the flexor muscles are predominantly affected, and the attack takes the form of sudden flexion with arms and legs held in adduction (the so-called salaam attacks). Extensor spasms are less common, and are rarely the sole type of seizure. Mixed flexor–extensor spasms commonly occur. Severity is variable, and slight spasms consisting of head nodding and upward eye deviation or 'shrugging' of the shoulders are often overlooked; it is a common experience to find that, when recorded on video-EEG, the actual number of attacks is usually far in excess of that reported by parents or carers. The stereotyped and repetitive nature is important diagnostically, and even mild but repetitive movements in an infant should raise diagnostic suspicion. About 5–10% of spasms are unilateral, and these are invariably associated with focal cerebral pathology.

The peak age of onset is 4–6 months, and the spasms rarely develop before the age of 3 months; 90% develop in the first year of life. The EEG shows the characteristic pattern of hypsarrhythmia in its fully developed form. Modified EEG forms frequently occur.

In the past up to a third of patients who developed West syndrome were thought to have normal neurodevelopment before the onset of infantile spasms (idiopathic or cryptogenic cases). However, with advances in MRI, underlying dysplasia and congenital anomalies are found in increasing proportions of cases previously categorized as cryptogenic. Positron emission tomography (PET) studies furthermore show unifocal or multifocal abnormalities in over 95% of cases, which in the presence of normal MRI are claimed to be due to subtle dysplastic lesions. A wide variety of conditions has been reported to cause this encephalopathy (Table 3.8), the most common of which are: tuberous sclerosis (7–25% of all cases), neonatal ischaemia and infections (about 15% of all cases), lissencephaly and pachygyria, and hemimegalencephaly (about 10% of cases), Down syndrome and acquired brain insults.

Table 3.7 West syndrome.

1–2 cases/4000 live births
Age-specific epileptic encephalopathy
Variety of causes
Age of onset 4–8 months
Seizures take the form of infantile spasms (salaam attacks)
EEG shows hypsarrhythmia pattern
Response to corticosteroids or vigabatrin
Spasms remit on therapy or spontaneously
Prognosis poor; 5% die in acute phase; learning difficulty and continuing epilepsy are common sequelae
20% cryptogenic, 80% symptomatic

Table 3.8 Some causes of West syndrome.

Neurocutaneous syndromes (especially tuberous sclerosis, Sturge–Weber syndrome)
Cortical dysplasia (many types)
Congenital chromosomal disorders (many types)
Inherited metabolic disorders (many types)
Mitochondrial disease
Neonatal and infantile infections
Hypoxic–ischaemic encephalopathy
Tumours and vascular disorders
Trauma
Degenerative disorders

The term 'idiopathic West syndrome' has been used to describe the condition in some patients who recover spontaneously after a brief course of infantile spasms. Probably less than 5% of patients with West syndrome have the truly idiopathic form. Other features include: normal psychomotor development at the onset of the infantile spasm; symmetrical hypsarrhythmia with absence of focal EEG abnormalities (spike-and-slow-wave focus) after intravenous diazepam; and reappearance of hypsarrhythmia between successive spasms in a cluster in an ictal record. Patients with truly idiopathic West syndrome can show normal subsequent neurological and cognitive development, and it has been proposed that this subgroup represents a form of benign epilepsy of childhood. There is no relationship between the severity of the spasms and the prognosis.

Intellectual impairment is the second cardinal clinical feature of symptomatic West syndrome. There is often some evidence of developmental retardation before the onset of the spasms, and occasionally prior epilepsy, but, as the spasms develop, the child's behaviour and responsiveness are rapidly impaired. Previously gained visual and social skills disappear, and severe regression and autistic withdrawal are common.

West syndrome takes a terrible place among the childhood epilepsies because of its severe prognosis in terms of seizure recurrence and mental development, rapid deterioration of psychomotor status and resistance to conventional antiepileptic drug treatment. About 5% of children die in the acute phase of spasms, and the death rate was much higher before the introduction of adrenocorticotrophic hormone (ACTH) therapy. On treatment, the spasms remit in almost all cases, with few cases having attacks after the age of 3 years. However, both the development of the child and the ultimate neurological status are usually impaired. Of the survivors 70–96% have learning difficulty (which in over 50% is severe) and chronic epilepsy develops in 35–60%. The epilepsy can be severe, and evolve into the Lennox–Gastaut syndrome. The treatment of West syndrome is described on p. 93.

Lennox–Gastaut syndrome

This term denotes an ill-defined, age-specific, epileptic encephalopathy with a wide range of causes (Table 3.9). It was first proposed in 1966 to describe the severe epilepsies of childhood in which multiple types of seizure are associated with slow spike–wave EEG discharges (2–3 Hz). Although some take the view that this is a specific syndrome, others disagree and view the

Table 3.9 Lennox–Gastaut syndrome.

Epileptic encephalopathy – 1–5% of all childhood epilepsies

Age of onset 1–7 years

40% cryptogenic, 60% symptomatic (identifiable underlying cause)

Learning disability, sometimes severe

Multiple seizure types – atypical absence, tonic, atonic, tonic–clonic, myoclonic

Episodes of non-convulsive status epilepticus common (75% of patients)

Seizures precipitated by sedation and lack of stimulation

Characteristic EEG pattern – slow spike–wave (≤ 2.5 Hz), abnormal background, bursts of fast (≥ 10 Hz) activity in non-REM sleep

Evolution over time

<5% seizure remission

Poor response to antiepileptic therapy

REM, rapid eye movement.

clinical and EEG patterns as simply a reflection of severe epilepsy in childhood associated with learning disability. In favour of the latter view is the fact that there are many underlying causes, there is no specific histopathological change or specific treatment, and it can evolve from other epilepsy syndromes (e.g. West syndrome, neonatal convulsions). This is a nosological jungle and the fine distinctions proposed by epileptologists are of largely academic interest only. There are few areas of more nosological confusion, even in epileptology (a subject blighted by esoteric and largely pointless argument about classification). Whatever else, the term has acquired wide currency and is used to denote a profoundly handicapping clinical symptom complex.

The Lennox–Gastaut syndrome accounts for between 1 and 5% of all childhood epilepsies, and occurs in up to 15% of institutionalized patients with learning disability. The age of onset is usually between 1 and 7 years, although apparent adult-onset cases are recorded. It can develop from West syndrome, myoclonic astatic epilepsy or neonatal seizures. Many identifiable cerebral lesions can underlie the encephalopathy (Table 3.10), although in at

Table 3.10 Underlying aetiology in symptomatic Lennox–Gastaut syndrome.

Cortical dysplasia (many types)
Neurocutaneous syndromes (tuberous sclerosis, Sturge–Weber syndrome, hypothalamic hamartoma, other forms)
Inherited metabolic disorders
Evolution from neonatal seizures or West syndrome
Ischaemic–hypoxic injury
Trauma

least a third no cause is identifiable (these cases are termed 'cryptogenic Lennox–Gastaut syndrome'). About a third of cases are due to malformations of brain development. About 20–30% of cases evolve from West syndrome and, when associated with frequent tonic seizures, these patients carry a particularly poor prognosis.

The epilepsy is very severe, with seizures usually occurring many times a day. These take the form of atypical absence, tonic, myoclonic, tonic and tonic–clonic seizures, and later complex partial and other seizure types develop. The most characteristic are tonic attacks, which occur most often in non-REM (but not REM) sleep and in wakefulness. They result in falls and the patients are prone to repeated head, facial and orthopaedic injuries. Tonic seizures are said to occur in between 17 and 95% of cases, depending on the nosological inclusivity of the report. Atypical absence and tonic–clonic seizures are also universal, as are episodes of convulsive and more typically non-convulsive status. Indeed, non-convulsive status (atypical absence status) may last hours or days and be repeated on an almost daily basis. Consciousness may be little affected in these periods (which can be referred to by carers as 'off days'), although the patients are usually obtunded to some extent, and there may be additional signs such as alteration of muscle tone, myoclonic jerks or increased sialorrhoea.

The EEG shows a characteristic pattern. The signature of the condition is the presence interictally of long bursts of diffuse slow (1–2.5 Hz) spike–wave activity, widespread in both hemispheres, roughly bilaterally synchronous but often asymmetrical. The spike–wave is not induced by hyperventilation and there is no photosensitivity. The background activity is abnormal with an excess of slow activity and diminished arousal or sleep potentials. Bursts of fast (>10 Hz) activity, especially during non-REM sleep, sometimes without clinical manifestations and sometimes with tonic attacks, are also highly characteristic and are indeed a diagnostic requirement by some authorities. The ictal EEG reflects the seizure type, although the ictal EEG during atypical absence attacks is often very similar to the apparently interictal EEG, and the distinction between ictal and interictal states, as alluded to above, can be difficult, with periods of non-convulsive status merging into the baseline state.

Learning disability is the other major feature of the condition. The intellectual impairment may be profound. At least 50% of cases have an IQ <50. There may be a slow deterioration in skills, although progression is not particularly marked, and sometimes better control of the epilepsy results in intellectual improvement.

Subcategories of the syndrome have been proposed although these do not influence treatment strategies. Differentiation from the severe myoclonic epilepsies of childhood, and atypical or severe cases of 'benign partial epilepsy', can be problematic but, as the syndromic definition is vague, so inevitably is the syndromic differentiation. The prognosis for control of seizures and for the development of intellectual impairment is grave.

According to some authors, long remissions from seizures or intellectual improvement occur in up to 15% of cases, although case definitions have not been uniform, and this seems optimistic. However, seizures do improve in adult life, and rarely is the epilepsy as ferocious as in early childhood. Persisting motor slowness and intellectual disability are, however, almost invariable. Many patients require institutional care in childhood and in adult life, and are dependent on carers for daily activities. Life expectancy has not been studied, but the encephalopathy is essentially static, and many patients live a stable adult life. Poor prognosis is associated with symptomatic aetiology, early age of onset, frequent tonic seizures and episodes of non-convulsive status, and a persistently slow EEG background. Conversely, a better outcome is found in those with onset after the age of 4 years, normal neuroimaging, EEG responsiveness to hyperventilation and faster spike–wave components (>3 Hz). The treatment of the Lennox–Gastaut syndrome is described on p. 94–95.

Syndrome of electrical status epilepticus during slow wave sleep

ESES (continuous spike–wave of slow sleep [CWES]; Table 3.11) refers to an epileptic encephalopathy characterized by the presence of generalized 1–3 Hz spike–wave discharges occupying 85% or more of the EEG of non-

Table 3.11 Electrical status epilepticus during slow-wave sleep.

Childhood epileptic encephalopathy
Age of onset 1–14 years
0.5% of children with epilepsy
EEG shows continuous epileptic activity during non-REM sleep (≥85% of time)
Overt seizures occur during wakefulness and sleep
Learning disability present in most cases
30% of children have an identifiable cause
Overlap with Landau–Kleffner syndrome and BECTS
Epilepsy often remits by age of 16 years

BECTS, benign epilepsy with centrotemporal spikes.

Table 3.12 Landau–Kleffner syndrome.

Uncommon form of epileptic encephalopathy
Pathogenesis uncertain
Onset between age 1 and 14 years (usually 4–7 years)
Dysphasia, fluctuating – often severe
Associated behavioural disorder and learning disability in some cases
EEG shows focal epileptiform patterns often amounting to electrographic status epilepticus; also ESES
75% have overt seizures, often not frequent or severe, various types
Overlap with ESES and BECTS
Prognosis is variable
Treatment with antiepileptic drugs, ACTH/corticosteroids and/or multiple subpial transection

ACTH, adrenocorticotrophic hormone; BECTS, benign epilepsy with centrotemporal spikes; ESES, electrical status epilepticus during slow-wave sleep.

REM sleep. Of children with epilepsy, 0.5% show this EEG pattern. The condition is diagnosed during childhood (1–14 years) with a peak age of onset between 3 and 5 years. About 30% of children showing this pattern have identifiable brain pathology such as previous meningitis or brain anoxia, hydrocephalus and developmental lesions, and one pair of affected monozygous twins has also been reported. There are no specific clinical signs during sleep. Overt seizures occur in daytime and at night, and can take various forms, both focal and generalized. Episodes of status are common. The EEG pattern usually occurs in children with severe epilepsy and learning difficulty. Furthermore, many children exhibit the symptoms of the Landau–Kleffner syndrome, and some authorities consider the two conditions to be synonymous. However, ESES is also seen in cases of the Lennox–Gastaut syndrome and in some cases of BECTS. Indeed, whether this is a specific epileptic syndrome or simply a reflection of severe epilepsy is uncertain. ESES is largely a childhood phenomenon, and the EEG pattern usually disappears by the age of 16 years.

The EEG pattern is usually resistant to conventional antiepileptic therapy, and often long-term corticosteroids or ACTH is recommended, albeit without any clear evidence of efficacy. Intravenous immunoglobulin therapy has also been used. Oral antiepileptic drugs are given to control seizures. Any first-line antiepileptic can be used and therapy follows conventional lines, although carbamazepine can exacerbate the nocturnal EEG disturbance. The EEG disturbance and seizures remit by the mid-teens. Cognition improves but most children do not gain normal functioning, especially in relation to speech and attention.

Landau–Kleffner syndrome

The Landau–Kleffner syndrome is a childhood epileptic encephalopathy in which persisting aphasia develops in association with severe EEG abnormalities and epilepsy (Table 3.12). It is an uncommon condition with a male predominance and usually with no family history. Onset occurs at between 18 months and 13 years, in most cases between 4 and 7 years. The aetiology and pathogenesis of the syndrome, if indeed these are unitary, are unknown. The condition develops in children who were previously developmentally normal, and presents with a progressive aphasia, developing gradually over months or subacutely over weeks, although acute presentations are also encountered. Verbal comprehension and expressive speech both become severely affected. The children can become almost mute.

Rather fruitless and inconclusive discussion has revolved around whether or not this is a true aphasia or an auditory agnosia, but the language disturbance seems particularly to involve the decoding of spoken words. The aphasia fluctuates, and indeed during the course of the condition speech can become quite normal, only to relapse again. Other inconsistent features include behavioural disorder, personality disturbance and intellectual decline. Overt epileptic seizures occur in about 75% of cases, and are usually mild, but 15% of cases have episodes of overt status epilepticus. The epilepsy, but not the EEG disturbance, is usually controlled by simple antiepileptic therapy. The EEG shows repetitive high-voltage spikes or spike–wave discharges in a generalized, focal/ multifocal (temporal/bitemporal) distribution, particularly affecting the speech areas of the brain. EEG studies have shown the origin of spikes to be over the dorsal surface of the superior temporal gyrus. The EEG abnormality is usually severe, and furthermore is activated by slow-wave sleep, and may become continuous, evolving into the ESES pattern. The pathophysiology of the speech disturbance is unclear. It is tempting to see this as a manifestation of continuous focal epileptic activity disrupting language (i.e. a functional disturbance, a form of nonconvulsive status epilepticus), and there is a general correlation between the course of the speech disturbance and the EEG changes, although this is not always very close.

Imaging is usually normal, although cases with neurocysticercosis, polymicrogyria and cerebral tumour have been described. The long-term prognosis is variable. Some children make a complete recovery after years of aphasia, and others are left with permanent, sometimes severe, speech disturbance and mental impairment. The EEG changes usually recover, although ESES may persist.

It is suggested that this syndrome is a form of BECTS, on the basis of EEG similarities, although its manifestations are much more severe, severe and its prognosis is generally far worse than that of the classic BECTS syndrome.

The treatment of the Landau–Kleffner syndrome is described on p. 95.

4 The Causes of Epilepsy

It is possible to divide the causes of epilepsy into four main categories (Table 4.1):

1 Idiopathic epilepsy: defined as 'an epilepsy of predominately genetic origin and in which there is no gross neuroanatomical or neuropathological abnormality'. A small number of new mendelian idiopathic epilepsy syndromes have been delineated in the past 10 years, but these have been in single families, and the genetic basis for the vast majority of idiopathic cases is currently unknown. It seems likely that these are the result of more complex non-Mendelian genomic or developmental mechanisms.

2 Symptomatic epilepsy: defined as 'an epilepsy of an acquired or genetic cause, associated with neuroanatomical or neuropathological abnormalities indicative of underlying disease or condition'. Included in this category are the developmental and congenital disorders with cerebral pathological changes, whether genetic or acquired (or indeed cryptogenic) in origin.

3 Provoked epilepsy: defined here as 'an epilepsy in which a specific systemic or environmental factor is the predominant cause of the seizures and in which there are no gross causative neuroanatomical or neuropathological changes'. Some 'provoked epilepsies' will have a genetic basis and some an acquired basis. The reflex epilepsies are included in this category as well as the epilepsies with a marked seizure precipitant.

4 Cryptogenic epilepsy: defined here as 'an epilepsy of presumed symptomatic nature in which the cause has not been identified'. The number of such cases is diminishing, but currently this is still an important category, accounting for at least 40% of adult – onset cases of epilepsy.

Obviously, such a categorization has difficulties, not least being the fact that epilepsy is often multifactorial

(graphically illustrated by Lennox in 1960 as multiple tributaries feeding into the stream that is the patient phenotype – Figure 4.1). Even in the presence of a major aetiology, other factors (genetic and environmental) can play a part in its clinical manifestations. The range of aetiology varies in different age groups, patient groups and geographical locations. Broadly speaking, congenital and perinatal conditions are the most common causes of early childhood-onset epilepsy, whereas in adult life epilepsy is more likely to be due to external non-genetic causes, but this distinction is by no means absolute. In late adult life vascular disease is increasingly common. In certain parts of the world, endemic infections – including tuberculosis (TB), cysticercosis, human immunodeficiency virus (HIV) and viral diseases – are common causes. The specific 'epilepsy syndromes' are also highly age dependent.

Idiopathic epilepsy

Heredity plays a very important part in the production of epilepsy – a fact noted by Hippocrates 2000 years ago and only recently fully appreciated again. The idiopathic epilepsies are likely to have a strong genetic basis, usually polygenic or oligogenic in nature (although it has to be said that absolute proof of this is somewhat lacking). Gene expression can be variable and influenced by developmental and to a lesser extent environmental factors, and the epilepsies are often also age dependent. Single-gene disorders probably underlie only 1–2% of all epilepsies, and usually in these conditions there are additional neurological or systemic features. It is useful to categorize the 'pure' epilepsies separately from the epilepsies associated with other neurological defects, although this distinction, like most in medicine, is somewhat artificial and transitional cases occur in a grey area between categories. Epilepsies due to some developmental anomalies have genetic and acquired forms but are included here for the sake of convenience.

Handbook of Epilepsy Treatment, 3rd Edition. By Simon Shorvon. Published 2010 by Blackwell Publishing Ltd.

Table 4.1 An aetiological classification of epilepsy.

Main category	Subcategory	Subcategory
Idiopathic epilepsy		Pure epilepsies due to single-gene disorders Pure epilepsies with complex non-Mendelian genomic mechanisms
Symptomatic epilepsy	Predominately genetic or developmental causation	Some of the severe childhood epilepsy syndromes Progressive myoclonic epilepsies Neurocutaneous syndromes Other neurological single-gene disorders Disorders of chromosome function Developmental anomalies of cerebral structure
	Predominately acquired causation	Hippocampal sclerosis Perinatal and infantile causes Cerebral trauma Cerebral tumour Cerebral infection Cerebrovascular disorders Cerebral immunological disorders Degenerative and other neurological conditions
Provoked epilepsy		Provoking factors Reflex epilepsies
Cryptogenic epilepsies		

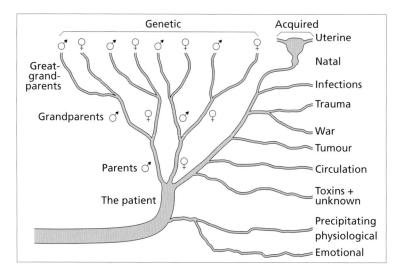

Figure 4.1 The multifactorial nature of epilepsy was illustrated by Lennox as the analogy of a river in which many different streams (causes) contribute to the occurrence of a seizure.

Pure epilepsies as a result of single-gene disorders

Pure epilepsies resulting from single-gene disorders are generally rare conditions, described in families (sometimes single families), but are potentially important for the mechanistic light that they may throw on the more common polygenic epilepsies. Interestingly, almost all of the genes identified that contribute to susceptibility to epilepsy are genes that code for ion channels (Table 4.2). In this sense, epilepsy has been recognized in recent years to be one of a burgeoning group of neurological disorders with intermittent symptoms that have underlying ion channel genetic defects.

Table 4.2 The single-gene 'pure epilepsies'.

Syndrome	Genes implicated[a]
Benign familial neonatal convulsions	*KCNQ2, KCNQ3*
Generalized epilepsy with febrile seizures +	*SCN1A, SCN1B, GABRG2*
ADNFLE	*CHRNA2, CHRNA4, CHRNB2*
Severe myoclonic epilepsy of infancy	*SCN1A, GABRG2*
Autosomal dominant partial epilepsy with auditory features	*LGI1*
Idiopathic generalized epilepsy, especially the juvenile myoclonic epilepsy and childhood absence epilepsy subtypes	*GABRA1, GABRG2, CLCN2, CACNB4. CACNA1H, SCN1A, EFHC1*
Benign familial neonatal–infantile seizures	*SCN2A*

[a]Mutations in these genes have been clearly associated with the disease in family linkage studies.

Benign familial neonatal convulsions:

The syndrome of benign familial neonatal convulsions is a condition that is inherited in an autosomal dominant fashion and is due to mutations of the voltage-gated potassium channel genes *KCNQ2* and *KCNQ3*. The abnormalities of these genes result in reduced potassium conductance and hence enhanced neuronal excitability. Why the effects are restricted to the first few weeks of life is unclear. One plausible hypothesis is that the mutated channels are replaced by other potassium channels that are upregulated early in life. The seizures are usually controlled by phenobarbital, phenytoin or valproate.

Autosomal dominant nocturnal frontal lobe epilepsy:

Autosomal dominant nocturnal frontal lobe epilepsy (ADNFLE) was the first 'pure epilepsy' in which the causal gene was found. Various mutations in the α_4-, α_2- and β_2-subunits of the nicotinic acetylcholine receptor have been identified in families with this interesting condition. Their condition is inherited in an autosomal dominant pattern with about 75% penetrance (in most

families). There is often a strong family history and apparently unaffected members in a family can have subtle nocturnal events, mistaken as simply restlessness or normal sleep phenomena. The patients have purely nocturnal frontal lobe seizures – sometimes many each night – without daytime seizures and without other symptoms. The seizures are brief, lasting less than 1 min, and are clustered around the onset and end of sleep. The seizures take the form of spasms with various motor and hyperkinetic features, and consciousness may be preserved. The onset is in childhood and the seizures persist, albeit with varying severity. Magnetic resonance imaging (MRI) is negative and the interictal EEG can show frontal abnormalities but is often normal. As a result of their bizarre form, the seizures can be misdiagnosed as parasomnias or even pseudoseizures (in spite of the fact that pseudoseizures never arise from sleep), and are not uncommonly resistant to therapy. Carbamazepine is the usual first-choice drug therapy, but, in cases not responsive to carbamazepine, any of the conventional antiepileptic drugs can be used.

Generalized epilepsy with febrile seizures plus

Generalized epilepsy with febrile seizures plus (GEFS+) is a heterogeneous form of epilepsy inherited in an autosomal dominant fashion, with age-specific manifestations and variable penetrance (penetrance of about 60% was found in the original families). Many different mutations have been described in either the α- or the β-subunits of the voltage-gated sodium channel genes *SCNIA* and *SCNIB*, and more recently the γ_2-subunit of the γ-aminobutyric acid A (GABA$_A$) receptor *GABRG2* gene in families from many places in the world. Functional studies have confirmed that these mutations confer abnormal membrane excitability. Febrile seizures are the most common feature, and seizures precipitated by fever tend to occur throughout childhood. Afebrile seizures of varying types, generalized tonic–clonic, myoclonic, atypical absence and less commonly focal seizures, develop later in childhood. Status epilepticus can occur. The severity during the active phase is very variable, but the condition often remits by late childhood or early adult life. The phenotype is so broad that it is arguable whether this condition really deserves the epithet 'syndrome'.

A really interesting question is how often sporadic mutations of the sodium channel γ-aminoglutamic acid (GABA)-receptor genes underlie sporadic febrile convulsions or even cryptogenic epilepsy, and this is a subject of active research. Another intriguing aspect of GEFS+ is its marked phenotypic variability, both within and across families. Digenic or oligogenic inheritance has been postulated to explain some of this variability. The seizures are treated along conventional lines for secondarily generalized epilepsy, and the prognosis is variable, with spontaneous remission of seizures in some cases and intractable epilepsy in others.

Dravet syndrome

Dravet syndrome (severe myoclonic epilepsy of infancy [SMEI]) is a severe form of epilepsy in which many (but not all) patients have mutations in the *SCNIA* gene, the same gene that causes the more benign GEFS+, and indeed there are families in which both phenotypes coexist. Furthermore, despite the frequency of a family history, curiously, the mutations are in the vast majority of cases new. Seizures develop between the ages of 2 and 9 months. These are often prolonged attacks, at least initially, taking the form of unilateral clonic or tonic–clonic seizures, and are precipitated by fever or even hot baths. Myoclonic seizures develop later (usually in the second year of life) but may not be a prominent feature. They take the form of massive myoclonia or erratic (segmental) myoclonia, and can be precipitated by photic stimuli. Focal seizures, atypical absence and episodes of convulsive and non-convulsive status epilepticus are common. Prolonged episodes of non-convulsive status can be mistaken for non-epileptic deterioration. Other motor signs and intellectual difficulties occur and the epilepsy is entirely intractable to treatment. The diagnosis, with seizures precipitated by fever, is highly characteristic. However, diagnostic confusion can occur with: febrile seizures (initially at least); immunization encephalopathy as whooping cough immunization is given at a similar age; degenerative diseases; the Lennox–Gastaut syndrome; and myoclonic–astatic epilepsy. There are also transitional cases sharing features of Dravet syndrome and other childhood epileptic encephalopathies. The prognosis is very poor with intractable epilepsy, early death, severe retardation or institutionalization in all cases. Therapy follows conventional lines.

Other single-gene 'pure epilepsy' syndromes

A ragbag of other single-gene epilepsy syndromes has been described, in either single or a few families, and include: familial adult myoclonic epilepsy (in a few families from Japan); familial autosomal recessive idiopathic myoclonic epilepsy of infancy (in an Italian family); X-linked infantile spasms; benign familial infantile convulsions; familial partial epilepsy with variable foci (linked to 22q); autosomal dominant epilepsy with auditory features (linked to 10q); familial temporal lobe epilepsies; and autosomal recessive rolandic epilepsy with paroxysmal exercise-induced dystonia and writer's cramp. Autosomal dominant rolandic epilepsy with speech dyspraxia (ADRESD) is a rare condition with an unknown genetic basis but which exhibits anticipation, suggesting that it may be a triplet repeat syndrome.

Pure epilepsies with complex (presumed polygenic) inheritance

Pure epilepsies with complex inheritance are far more common than the single-gene epilepsies. These conditions are divided into the idiopathic generalized epilepsies (IGEs) and the benign partial epilepsies of childhood, and have been the subject of intensive genetic study, but to date no common susceptibility genes have been identified. These conditions are probably best conceptualized as polygenic disorders in which the phenotype is the result of interactions between susceptibility genes and developmental and probably to a lesser extent environmental effects. There has also been recent interest in the possibility that some cases are due to copy number variations rather than mutations or single nucleotide polymorphism. There is often no strong family history, and genetic studies have to be conducted using case–control methodology in large populations. The phenotypes are wide, and the concept of epilepsy syndromes as discrete entities that are clinically homogeneous and biologically distinct frequently cannot be sensibly sustained. More attractive is the concept of the neurobiological continuum, in which there are widely varying phenotypes with complex and probably multiple genetic mechanisms and also overlapping phenotypes caused by different gene abnormalities. To confuse the picture further, many of these phenotypes can result from a range of identifiable acquired and congenital brain disorders (symptomatic cases). In this sense, the epilepsy syndrome can be thought of as a genetically determined endpoint response of dysfunctional brain tissue to an acquired insult. The extent to which other cryptogenic epilepsies have a genetic basis is less clear, but some authorities have proposed that the contribution of 'genetic influences' to epilepsy in broad terms is about 60%.

Symptomatic epilepsy of genetic or congenital origin

Over 250 single-gene and chromosomal disorders result in neurological disorders in which epilepsy is part of the phenotype (listed on the OMIN database). Most are rare or very rare, manifest initially in childhood, and present for diagnosis to paediatric neurological services rather than to an epilepsy specialist. In only a few of these conditions does epilepsy have distinctive features or it is a predominant or consistent feature: exceptions are the progressive myoclonus epilepsies and some neurocutaneous syndromes. Some of the conditions associated with epilepsy are shown in Table 4.3.

The inborn errors of metabolism are conditions in which biochemical defects are inherited, usually in an autosomal recessive fashion, and in which the epilepsy is one symptom within a much broader spectrum of learning disability, and neurological and systemic features. These include conditions with intermittent or persistent metabolic changes, including hypoglycaemia, hyperammonaemia, hypocalcaemia, hyperglycinaemia, metabolic acidosis, ketoacidosis, abnormal amino acid or oligosaccharide profile, mucopolysaccharidoses and lipid storage diseases. Epilepsy is particularly found in Angelman syndrome, Tay–Sachs disease, Niemann–Pick disease type C, Krabbe disease, amino acid disorders and glycogen storage disorders. In a substantial number of cases presenting with epilepsy and learning disability, on a congenital basis, no cause can be identified. Porphyria is another important cause with geographical variation.

Angelman syndrome

This condition, with a frequency of about 1 in every 10 000–20 000 births, accounts for about 6% of all those with learning disability and epilepsy. The condition usually presents with developmental delay apparent between 6 and 12 months of age. It is characterized by dysmorphic features, grave learning disability and motor handicap, severe epilepsy, a characteristic motor disturbance with 'puppet-like' movements due to truncal ataxia and titubation, a happy demeanour with a rather specific behavioural phenotype and severe speech disturbance. There is a characteristic morphology with protruding jaw, wide mouth and widely spaced teeth, occipital depression and blue eyes. Epilepsy is present in 85–90% of cases, and typically can include episodes of absence or myoclonic status, myoclonus, absence and tonic–clonic seizures. Partial seizures with occipital symptomatology also seem common. Jerky movements, additional to ataxia, can occur and can be due to unrecognized myoclonus or myoclonic status. Angelman syndrome is one cause of the Lennox–Gastaut syndrome. In about 80% of cases defects are present in the chromosome 15q11–q13 region, and involve a deletion, maternal disomy, imprinting defect or

Table 4.3 Some single-gene disorders causing epilepsy.

Agenesis of the corpus callosum
Alpers disease
Aminoacidurias
Angelman disease
Argininosuccinicaciduria
Disorders of biotin and folate metabolism
Carnitine palmitoyltransferase 11 deficiency
Choreoacanthocytosis (neuroacanthocytosis)
Dentato-rubro-pallido-luysian atrophy
D-Glycine acidaemia
Familial cavernoma
Fructose-1,6-diphosphatase deficiency
Fumarase deficiency
Glucocerebrosidase deficiency (Gaucher disease)
Hexosaminidase A deficiency
Huntington disease
Isovaleric acidaemia
Krabbe disease (galactosylceramidase deficiency)
Lafora body disease
Maple syrup urine disease
Menkes disease
Methylmalonic aciduria
Mitochondrial diseases (MERFF, MELAS, Leigh syndrome)
Mucopolysaccharidoses
Neuronal ceroid lipofuscinoses
Niemann–Pick disease
Non-ketotic hyperglycinaemia
Ornithine transcarbamylase deficiency
Periventricular heterotopia
Peroxisomal enzyme deficiencies
Phenylalanine hydroxylase deficiency (phenylketonuria)
Porphyria
Proprionic acidaemia
Pyridoxine deficiency
Pyruvate dehydrogenase deficiency
Respiratory chain disorders
Rett syndrome
Sialidoses
Tuberous sclerosis
Unverricht–Lundborg disease
Urea cycle disorders
Wolf–Hirschhorn syndrome

MERFF, myoclonic epilepsy with ragged red fibres; MELAS, myoclonic epilepsy, lactic acidosis and stroke-like episodes.
List excludes the single-gene disorders causing 'pure epilepsy'– see Table 4.2.

rarely translocation. This region contains a cluster of GABA-receptor subunit genes. Iatrogenic mutations in the *UBE3A* gene are found in about 10% of cases. Diagnostic genetic testing is available. About 80% of cases can be identified via the methylation test, and mutation testing of the *UBE3A* gene can be used in cases where the methylation test is negative. MRI is normal and EEG usually shows large–amplitude slow spike–wave. The lifespan is probably normal. Treatment of the epilepsy follows conventional lines, and has no specific features.

Gaucher disease

Gaucher disease (glucocerebrosidase deficiency, glucosylceramidase deficiency) is caused by deficient activity of the lysosomal enzyme glucosylceramidase and the resultant accumulation of its undegraded substrate, glucosylceramide, and other glycolipids. In the central nervous system (CNS) glucosylceramide originates from the turnover of membrane gangliosides. There is a wide phenotypic range, and the condition is usually divided into five subtypes. The frequency is about 1 case per 50 000–100 000 live births. There is a marked founder effect in some populations and the condition is particularly common in Ashkenazi Jewish populations, Swedish populations and the Jenin Arabs. Only types 2 and 3 are primarily neurological disorders. Type 2 has onset of disease before the age of 2 years, and presents as regression, profound psychomotor delay and a rapidly progressive course, with death in the first 4 years of life. Type 3 has a more slowly progressive course, and death occurs in the second to fourth decades. Seizures occur and may take the form of progressive myoclonic epilepsy. The diagnosis of Gaucher disease relies on demonstration of deficient glucosylceramidase enzyme activity in peripheral blood leucocytes or other nucleated cells. Mutation analysis for the common mutations is available. Family studies can be carried out.

Lysosomal disorders (lipidoses)

The most important lipidosis resulting in epilepsy is due to mutation of the hexosaminidase A (*HEXA*) gene. At least 90 different disease-causing mutations have been identified, of which 6 account for 98% of all cases in the Ashkenazi Jewish population but less than 50% in the non-Jewish cases. Defects in the enzyme result in a spectrum of disorders caused by the intralysosomal storage of the glycosphingolipid GM2 ganglioside. The diagnosis depends on the demonstration of deficient hexosamini-

dase A enzyme activity in the serum or white blood cells (with normal hexosaminidase B activity). The acute infantile condition Tay–Sachs disease presents in the first year of life with severe regression, visual deterioration, severe seizures and progressive enlargement of the head. An exaggerated startle response and startle-induced seizures occur. Death is inevitable by the age of 4 years. The condition is relatively common in Ashkenazi Jewish populations (91 in 3000 live births and carrier rates of 1 in 30), and 100 times less common in non-Jewish or Sephardic Jewish populations. The juvenile form begins with ataxia and then progressive intellectual decline with seizures and death by the age of 20 years. The adult forms do not commonly cause epilepsy.

Menkes syndrome

This X-linked recessive disorder is the result of mutations in the ATPase copper transport gene *ATP7A*. A range of mutations has been found, which result in an abnormal ATPase transport protein and low copper concentrations in tissue. Classic Menkes disease presents around the age of 2 months with severe neurological regression and epilepsy, and other features including characteristic changes in the hair (kinky hair), autonomic and gastrointestinal dysfunction, and other abnormalities. Death occurs between 7 months and 3 years. A few patients have been described with a mild condition, with ataxia, tremor, weakness, mild intellectual impairment and seizures developing in mid to late childhood. Diagnosis is by measurement of copper and ceruloplasmin. Genetic testing is also available, including prenatal testing. Treatment of the underlying condition consists of subcutaneous injections of copper histidine or copper chloride (250–500 mg/day). If given within 10 days of birth, developmental outcome can be normalized.

Neuroacanthocytosis

Neuroacanthocytosis (choreoacanthocytosis) is a progressive neurological disorder with prominent epilepsy, motor dysfunction, myopathy, cognitive and behavioural changes, and acanthocytosis of the red blood cells. The condition is inherited in an autosomal recessive manner. Seizures are observed in almost half of affected individuals, are often the initial manifestation and can be very severe. Chorea and dystonia are common, particularly affecting the facial and buccal muscles, causing dysarthria and dysphagia, with resulting weight loss. Habitual tongue and lip biting are characteristic. Progressive cognitive and behavioural changes have strong frontal lobe features. The mean age of onset is about 35 years of age, but the disease can present at any time between 10 and 70 years of age. The diagnosis of choreoacanthocytosis depends upon the presence of characteristic MRI atrophy of the caudate nuclei and T2-signal increase in the caudate and putamen. Acanthocytes are present in 5–50% of the red cells, and it is usually advised that acanthocytes are searched for on fresh smears on six separate occasions before the condition is excluded. Increased serum concentration of muscle creatine phosphokinase is observed in most cases. Acanthocytes also occur in McCleod syndrome and abetalipoproteinaemia with vitamin E deficiency. Muscle biopsy reveals central nuclei and atrophic fibres. Missense, frameshift, nonsense, splice-site and deletion mutations in the *VPS13A* gene are associated with some cases. Molecular genetic testing is currently available only on a research basis. Acanthocytosis needs to be differentiated clinically from Huntington disease, Lesch–Nyhan disease and pantothenate kinase-associated neurodegeneration (PKAN; Hallervorden–Spatz syndrome). There is no effective curative therapy and treatment is symptomatic and palliative. The disease runs a chronic progressive course, leading to major disability within a few years and death after 10 years or more. Treatment of the epilepsy follows conventional lines and has no specific features.

Niemann–Pick disease type C

Niemann–Pick disease type C (NPC) is a lipid storage disease presenting in infants, children or adults. NPC is inherited in an autosomal recessive manner and has a frequency of about 1 in 150 000. The classic presentation occurs in middle to late childhood with the insidious onset of ataxia, vertical supranuclear gaze palsy, dementia, dystonia and seizures. The seizures are partial or generalized, or both. The epilepsy is often refractory to medical therapy, but improves if survival is prolonged, presumably reflecting neuronal loss. About 20% of affected children have cataplexy induced by laughing. Dysarthria and dysphagia eventually become disabling, making oral feeding impossible. Adults are more likely to present with dementia or psychiatric symptoms. The diagnosis of NPC is confirmed by bone marrow biopsy, which shows lipid-laden histiocytes, the biochemical demonstration of impaired cholesterol esterification and positive filipin staining in cultured fibroblasts. The diagnosis is often delayed substantially because 'routine' screening tests for metabolic disease, such as urine screens

and lysosomal enzyme panels, are negative. In about 90% of cases NPC is caused by an identifiable mutation in the *NPC1* gene (and a handful of cases have been described with *NPC2* gene mutations). Molecular genetic testing is available.

Organic acidurias and aminoacidurias

These are autosomal recessive conditions. The most common is phenylketonuria caused by defects in phenylalanine hydrolase, and over 400 disease-causing mutations in the gene have been described. The prevalence shows marked geographical and racial differences, ranging between 1 in 2600 and 1 in 200 000 live births, and carrier rates between 1 in 26 and 1 in 225 (in Turkey and Finland, respectively). It can and should be detected by neonatal screening, and early dietary treatment will prevent any abnormalities. If the condition is missed, learning disability, epilepsy, microcephaly, and motor and behavioural disturbances occur. A less common cause of phenylalaninaemia is tetrahydrobiopterin deficiency. Other acidurias in which epilepsy occurs include argininosuccinicaciduria, tyrosinaemia and histidinaemia. They commonly result in epilepsy associated with learning disability and other neurological and systemic features. Diagnosis is made by screening blood and urine for abnormal amino acids.

Lactic acidosis is present in blood and urine in Leigh syndrome. This is usually due to X-linked or autosomal recessive nuclear gene mutations of one of the mitochondrial respiratory chain complex I or IV enzymes or pyruvate dehydrogenase (X-linked *PDHA1* gene). About 30% are due to mutations in mitochondrial DNA, which have been identified in at least 11 mitochondrial genes. The diagnostic features are a subacute encephalopathy, seizures (myoclonic or tonic–clonic), and progressive dementia with cerebellar and brain-stem signs. Motor abnormalities include hypotonia, spasticity, ataxia, involuntary movements and bulbar problems. Vomiting, hyperventilation and abnormalities of thermoregulation are common. Optic atrophy, pigmentary retinopathy, deafness and cardiomyopathy are sometimes present. On imaging, basal ganglia lucencies are highly characteristic, and proton magnetic resonance spectroscopy (MRS) can detect high cerebral lactic acid levels. High alanine levels are found in plasma. The condition typically presents in infancy after a viral disease, but less commonly can occur at any age. Leigh syndrome-like conditions also occur without the full complement of features, and the complex 'neurogenic weakness, ataxia and retinitis pigmentosa'

(NARP) is considered to be part of the spectrum of this condition. Genetic testing is available.

Peroxisomal disorders

At least 17 autosomal recessive disorders are described due to abnormalities of 11 genes coding for peroxisomal enzymes. These enzymes act as metabolic pathways in the oxidation of long-chain fatty acids, necessary for myelin production. Zellweger syndrome and neonatal adrenoleucodystrophy are examples, presenting as severe seizure disorders that often start in the neonatal period and include all seizure types, one of which is infantile spasm. Other features include poor feeding, severe intellectual regression, bony stippling (chondrodysplasia punctata), retinal dystrophy, hearing loss, hypotonia and dysmorphic features (including high palate, high forehead and shallow orbital ridges). The EEG is severely abnormal. In some cases polymicrogyria is present. The diagnosis is made by measuring serum long-chain fatty acids in plasma, and then fibroblast culture. Mutations in 11 different *PEX* genes – those that encode peroxins – have been identified. Mutations of *PEX1* is the most common cause, and sequencing of exons 13 and 15 will reveal at least one mutation in about 50% of patients. Such testing is clinically available. Later in life, X-linked adrenoleucodystrophy is the most common peroxisomal disorder, but seizures are the presenting symptom in only a minority, and are sometimes secondary to hypoglycaemia associated with adrenal failure.

Porphyria

The porphyrias are a group of conditions in which there are deficiencies in one of the eight enzymes of the haem biosynthetic pathway (the porphyrin pathway; four of the enzymes are located in the mitochondria and the other four in the cytosol). The enzyme deficiency leads to underproduction of haem and the accumulation of porphyrins which are haem precursors. It is this accumulation, rather than the deficiency of haem, that causes the symptoms in most cases. The disorders are sometimes inherited and sometimes secondary to severe liver disease (porphyria cutaneous tarda). The inherited conditions are classified into the acute porphyrias (hepatic porphyrias) and cutaneous (erythropoietic) porphyrias, depending on the site of accumulation of porphyrins or precursors.

Neurological disturbance, including epilepsy, is a feature of the inherited acute porphyrias (hepatic porphyrias), and the major symptoms including pain are due to acute neurological dysfunction. There are three acute porphyrias that cause epilepsy and other neurological symptoms: acute intermittent porphyria (AIP), variegate porphyria and hereditary co-proporphyria (HCP). In AIP, seizures occur in about 5% of cases.

AIP is the most common hepatic porphyria and the most commonly associated with epilepsy. This condition is inherited in an autosomal dominant fashion and is caused by a deficiency of porphobilinogen deaminase (synonym – hydroxymethylbilane synthase [HMB synthase] and uroporphyrinogen I synthase).

Most people with this deficiency are asymptomatic (i.e. are carriers). Furthermore, in symptomatic individuals, the deficiency often becomes evident only when the susceptible individual is exposed to provoking factors, including: intercurrent infection, hormonal changes (especially oestrogen or progesterone changes), low calorific diet or other dietary changes, or medicinal drugs. The drugs that can induce or worsen an attack are those that induce aminolaevulinic acid (ALA) synthetase or porphobilinogen (PBG) deaminase in the liver, and these include most enzyme-inducing antiepileptic drugs, which should therefore be avoided. Oral contraceptives, some analgesics, some cardiovascular and antihypertensive drugs, ergotamine derivatives, chloramphenicol, erythromycin, rifampicin, trimethoprim, ketoconazole, nitrofurantoin and sulphonamide antibiotics are among the other drugs that frequently precipitate attacks. The clinical and biochemical features of the acute attacks of variegate porphyria are identical to AIP, except for cutaneous photosensitivity which occurs in a third of cases. Seizures are relatively common in the acute attacks, although chronic epilepsy is seldom a problem.

The diagnosis of acute porphyria depends on demonstrating increased levels of urinary δ-ALA and PBG in urine which establishes one of the acute porphyrias. The diagnosis of AIP is confirmed if there is a deficiency of PBG deaminase in red blood cells, a test that is not, however, always positive in all patients. In some patients, only hepatic PBG deaminase is deficient, requiring liver biopsy to confirm the diagnosis. Estimations of PBG deaminase in red blood cells are a sensitive way of detecting latent porphyria in asymptomatic family members.

In an acute attack, the measurement of PBG in a random urine sample is a useful screening test, and, if positive, followed by a 24-hour collection of δ-ALA, PBG and/or porphyrin. Estimation of faecal porphyrins distinguishes between variegate porphyria and HCP (Tables 4.4 and 4.5). Interpretation of the tests can be complex.

Table 4.4 The diagnostic tests in the acute porphyrias associated with epilepsy.

	Urine ALA and PBG levels	Urine porphyrin levels	Faecal prophyrin levels	Red cell porphyrin levels
Acute intermittent porphyria	Normal	Increased URO (may be normal if not in an acute attack)	Normal	Normal
Variegate porphyria	Increased (may be normal if not in an acute attack)	Increased COPRO	Increased COPRO and PROTO	Normal
Hereditary coproporphyria	Increased (may be normal if not in an acute attack)	Increased COPRO	Increased COPRO	Normal

ALA, aminolaevulinic acid; COPRO , coproporphyrins; PBG, porphobilinogen; PROTO, protoporphyrins; URO, uroporphyrins.

Table 4.5 Antiepileptic drug use in acute intermittent porphyria.

Drugs that are unsafe and should be avoided
Carbamazepine and oxcarbazepine
Lamotrigine
Ethosuximide/methsuximide
Felbamate
Phenytoin
Phenobarbital and other barbiturates
Valproic acid

Drugs that can be used (with care)
Clonazepam and other benzodiazepines
Gabapentin
Levetiracetam
Pregabalin
Vigabatrin

Genetic testing can confirm the disease, but as there are many different mutations in the PBG deaminase gene it is not used widely for screening purposes. Detection is easier if the familial mutation has been identified. Members of a family can be tested to identify asymptomatic cases in order to counsel about avoiding precipitants.

Treatment is with high oral or intravenous glucose intake, intravenous haematin (Panhematin) or haem arginate (NormoSang) and control of electrolyte disturbance. Provoking drugs should be immediately discontinued.

Prevention is possible with simple measures. Patients at risk of attacks should eat a normal or high-carbohydrate diet. Dieting or weight loss should be avoided or carried out only under medical supervision and a diet with 90% of the normal haem intake is recommended. Non-enzyme-inducing drugs such as gabapentin, pregabalin, topiramate and levetiracetam are safer than conventional therapy for chronic epilepsy. For acute therapy, diazepam and clonazepam are relatively safe. Magnesium sulphate has also traditionally been used.

Pyridoxine deficiency

Pyridoxine deficiency is due to a recessively inherited defect in the enzyme glutamic acid decarboxylase. It presents in infancy with neonatal convulsions and EEG disturbance. It responds rapidly to pyridoxine, and is, rarely among the inborn errors of metabolism, entirely curable if the diagnosis is made in time. Indeed, pyridoxine should be given to any neonate with seizures if no other cause is clearly present.

Rett syndrome

This is an X-linked dominant disorder, almost always presenting in girls. The defect is in the *MECP2* gene, which controls RNA production. Birth and development in the first 6 months are normal. In the classic phenotype, the children then decline with severe mental regression with autistic features, motor disturbances with highly characteristic manual stereotopies, and eventually total quadraparesis, apnoeic attacks, and a complex disturbance of breathing and a tendency for gastric regurgitation. Short stature, growth failure, wasting and microcephaly are typical. Language is severely affected and speech may cease altogether. Epilepsy occurs in over 50% of identified cases, and tends to develop when the disease has stabilized. The seizures take many forms and include episodes of convulsive status epilepticus. The latter can be precipitated by inhalation due to gastric regurgitation. Often, however, the epilepsy is not severe, and can be controlled by relatively small doses of conventional antiepileptic therapy. MRI does not show specific features, but EEG is often severely abnormal with predominant slow activity, spikes and spike–wave, and frequent electrographic seizures. It has recently become clear that the phenotype is much wider than in the classic descriptions, and it is recognized that some adult women with only mild intellectual disability have the same genetic defect. Most cases are due to mutations in one of several mutation hotspots in the *MECP2* gene. Atypical cases exist with mutations in the *CDKL5* gene. Occasional male cases survive who have either a 47,XXY karyotype with a normal *MECP2* gene on one X chromosome, or somatic mosaicism. Males with 47,XY and *MECP2* mutations die in the first years of life. Diagnostic genetic testing is available.

Urea cycle disorders

Various autosomal recessive disorders of urea cycle enzymes occur, with a prevalence of about 1 in 30 000 live births, resulting in abnormalities of protein breakdown and consequential hyperammonaemia. There are five urea cycle enzymes and one co-factor, and defects in each are described. The severity of the conditions vary, with some rapidly fatal. Ornithine transcarbamylase (OTC) deficiency is the most common deficiency, with a frequency of about 1 in 80 000 live births. It is an X-linked trait, with marked phenotypical variation. Male homozygotes usually present in infancy with severe neonatal hyperammonaemic encephalopathy, whereas female heterozygotes may be virtually asymptomatic. In mild or moderately affected cases, epilepsy is common, associated sometimes with ataxia, tremor and other motor abnormalities. A significant number of carrier females exist, presumably due to X-chromosome inactivation. These patients can also have epilepsy, and are at risk of hyperammonaemic crises precipitated, for example, by pregnancy, drugs such as corticosteroids or valproate, or intercurrent infection. The hyperammonaemic episodes are characterized by encephalopathy, vomiting, lethargy, behavioural and psychiatric disturbances, and sleep disorder. The encephalopathy is sometimes misdiagnosed as non-convulsive status epilepticus, and this can be a disastrous if further valproate is given. The diagnosis can be made by the demonstration of a high serum ammonia, and valproate withdrawal and/or treatment of the intercurrent illness will reverse the clinical picture. Genetic testing is possible, by linkage analysis (with linkage established in the family before individual testing), and the disease can be confirmed by enzymatic testing on hepatic tissue.

Progressive myoclonic epilepsies

This is a rather specific phenotype, which can be caused by a variety of genetically determined neurological disorders (Table 4.6). In most parts of the world there are six common underlying conditions: mitochondrial disorders, Unverricht–Lundborg disease, dentato-rubro-pallido-luysian atrophy (DRPLA), Lafora body disease, neuronal ceroid lipofuscinosis and sialidosis. The term 'progressive myoclonic epilepsy' (PME) should be confined to those cases where the predominant clinical symptom is myoclonus. This needs to be differentiated from other progressive encephalopathies with myoclonus and from the so-called progressive myoclonic ataxias.

There are marked geographical variations in the frequency, but in most countries the condition is uncommon, accounting for less than 1% of all referrals to tertiary epilepsy services.

Baltic myoclonus (Unverricht–Lundborg disease)

This is the most benign form of PME. It is an autosomal recessive disorder due to mutations in the *EPM1* gene coding for the cystatin B protein, a protease inhibitor. The most common mutation is an unstable expansion of a dodecamer repeat. There is marked geographical variation, with the condition being especially common in Finland (where the incidence is in excess of 1 in 20 000 people), Scandinavia and the Baltic regions, due to founder effects in these isolated populations. Myoclonic movements first develop, usually between the ages of 6 and 15 years, and the condition slowly progresses. Initially the myoclonus is easy to control, but eventually it becomes intractable and disabling. Other seizures are infrequent, although tonic–clonic seizures may be the presenting symptom, and are usually easily controlled. Ataxia and tremor also develop and become major clinical features. There is a very slow intellectual decline, but this can be mild. Death used to occur between the ages of 30 and 40 years, but with improved treatment survival now is often into the seventh decade. The EEG has an interesting pattern, sometimes showing spike–wave on waking at 3–5 Hz and with photosensitivity. Diagnosis can be made by genetic testing.

Table 4.6 Causes of progressive myoclonic epilepsy.

Disease	Age at onset		Suggestive clinical features	Suggestive laboratory features	Genetics	Gene(s)
Unverricht–Lundborg disease	8–13 years		Severe myoclonus, mild dementia and ataxia	None identified	AR	*CSTB*
Lafora disease	10–18 years		Severe myoclonus, occipital seizures, inexorable dementia, Lafora bodies	Lafora bodies in skin biopsies	AR	*EPM2A* *EPM2B*
Myoclonus epilepsy and ragged red fibres (MERRF)	Variable		Deafness, optic atrophy, myopathy, myoclonus	Ragged red fibres, increased level of pyruvate and lactate (blood)	Mitochondrial	*tRNA^{lys}*
Sialidoses	Type I	8–20 years	Severe myoclonus, tonic–clonic seizures, ataxia, cherry-red spot, visual failure	Elevated urinary sialyloligosaccharides, deficiency of neuroaminidase in leucocytes and cultured skin fibroblasts	AR	*NEU*
	Type II	10–30 years	Severe myoclonus, ataxia, cherry-red spot, visual failure, dysmorphic features, hearing loss	Elevated urinary sialyloligosaccharides, deficiency of neuroaminidase and β-galactosidase in leucocytes and cultured skin fibroblasts	AR	*PPGB*
Neuronal ceroid lipofuscinoses	CLN2	2.4–4 years	Myoclonic, tonic–clonic, atonic or atypical absence seizures, psychomotor delay and ataxia, visual failure	Curvilinear, rectilinear or fingerprint lipidic inclusions in skin biopsy at electron microscopy	AR	*TPP1*
	CNL3	5–10 years	Myoclonus and tonic–clonic seizures, macular degeneration, optic atrophy, dementia		AR	*CLN3*
	CNL4	15–50 years	Generalized seizures, myoclonic jerks, extrapyramidal symptoms		AR/AD	–
Dentato-rubro-pallido-luysian dysptrophy (DRPLA)*	Variable		Seizures, myoclonus, ataxia, chorea, dementia	None identified	AD	*ATN1*

These are the more common causes. The condition can also be due to: biotin-responsive progressive myoclonus, coeliac disease, Gaucher disease, GM2 gangliosidosis (juvenile type), hexosaminidase deficiency, Huntington disease, juvenile neuroaxonal dystrophy, Menkes disease, phenylketonuria, tetrahydrobiopterin deficiencies.
AD, autosomal dominant; AR, autosomal recessive.
*DRPLA is caused by an expanded trinucleotide repeat in the *ATN1* gene

Dentato-rubro-pallido-luysian atrophy

DRPLA is inherited in an autosomal dominant fashion. It occurs with markedly varying frequency around the world, being particularly common in Japan (a frequency of 0.2–0.7 per 100 000 people) and in northern Europe. It is a triplet-repeat disorder involving the *ATN1* gene, which is of uncertain function. The normal repeat number is between 6 and 35 and the condition is present with full penetrance when the repeat number is >48. DRPLA is a slowly progressive disorder in which ataxia, choreoathetosis, dementia and behavioural changes, myoclonus and epilepsy occur. In common with other triplet-repeat disorders, significant 'anticipation' is exhibited, and there is marked phenotypic variation even within a family. Fifty per cent of cases present tonic–clonic seizures and myoclonus, some present with ataxia–athetosis–chorea and others with dementia in a 'pseudo-Huntington' form.

The condition can present at any time from infancy to late adult life, the mean age of onset being 30 years. The mode of presentation of the condition is age dependent, and there is also an inverse relationship between the age of onset of symptoms and the number of repeats. Individuals with onset before age 20 years invariably have epilepsy and frequently present with PME, although other forms of generalized seizures (tonic, clonic or tonic–clonic seizures) occur. Seizures are rare in individuals with onset after age 40. The diagnosis of DRPLA rests on a positive family history, the characteristic clinical findings, and the detection of an expanded trinucleotide repeat in the *ATN1* gene. The CAG repeat length in individuals with DRPLA ranges from 48 to 93. Molecular genetic testing is widely available. Diffuse high-intensity areas deep in the white matter are often observed on T2-weighted MRI in individuals with adult-onset DRPLA of long duration.

Lafora body disease

Lafora body disease, an autosomal recessive condition mostly reported from southern Europe, is characterized by the presence of Lafora bodies, which are periodic acid–Schiff (PAS)-positive intracellular polyglucosan inclusions found in neurons, sweat glands and a variety of other sites. The age of onset is between 6 and 19 years (usually 12–17 years), although many patients have a history of isolated febrile or non-febrile seizures earlier in childhood, and the disease presents with progressive myoclonic and associated tonic–clonic and partial seizures. The partial seizures often have occipital or visual symptomatology, typically with ictal blindness and visual hallucinations. The seizure disorder becomes progressively more severe, and status epilepticus is common. There is also a rapidly progressive and severe dementia. Ataxia and dysarthria also occur.

The condition is progressive, although often in a stepwise form, and death occurs within 2–10 years of the onset of the disease, by which time the myoclonus is severe and disabling. The EEG may show spike–wave initially at 3 Hz, with faster frequencies developing over time, and focal occipital spike discharges, although these are not a reliable diagnostic finding. The myoclonus is not associated with EEG change and this helps differentiate early cases from myoclonus in IGE. Later EEG signs include slowing of background activity and the loss of normal sleep patterns. Up to 80% of patients have a mutation in the *EPM2A* gene, which codes for laforin, a tyrosine phosphatase protein. Fourteen different mutations in 24 families are now known. A second gene, *EPM2B*, has been identified, which codes for malin, a ubiquitin ligase protein. A third locus has recently been described in one family. The diagnosis can be confirmed by histological examination of the skin (which should include ecrine glands) and liver or muscle biopsy, but genetic testing has now rendered this largely unnecessary.

Mitochondrial cytopathy (myoclonic epilepsy with ragged red fibres)

Mitochondrial cytopathy (myoclonic epilepsy with ragged red fibres [MERRF]) is caused by a range of point mutations or deletions of mitochondrial DNA, or nuclear genes linked to mitochondrial function, which result in dysfunction of the mitochondrial respiratory chain. On the inner mitochondrial membrane there are over 70 different polypeptides that form the respiratory chain and 13 of these polypeptides are encoded by mitochondrial DNA; defects have been described in all of these. Two classic phenotypes (MERFF and mitochondrial encephalopathy with lactic acidaemia and stroke [MELAS]) occur, in which seizures are a common and important symptom, although intermediate and transitional cases are not uncommon. In a third mitochondrial disorder, Leigh syndrome and neuropathy, ataxia and retinitis pigmentosa (NARP) continuum, seizures are also common but not a predominant feature.

The full range of the phenotypes of mitochondrially inherited defects is probably not known, and it certainly seems possible that some cryptogenic epilepsies will have mitochondrial defects as yet undetected. The inheritance is, of course, usually maternal. Mitochondrial disease can result in forms of epilepsy other than PME. Other forms of myoclonus are characteristic and can be either focal or multifocal, but partial seizures and tonic–clonic seizures are also not infrequently encountered.

The mitochondrial cytopathy that typically causes PME is the syndrome of MERRF. This is a multisystem disorder with a very variable phenotype, in which myoclonic seizures are often the first symptom, followed by generalized epilepsy, myopathy, ataxia and dementia. Other features are short stature, deafness, optic atrophy, retinopathy, ophthalmoparesis and cardiomyopathy with Wolff–Parkinson–White syndrome. The clinical features are variable, even within families. The EEG shows spike–wave at 2–5 Hz with a slow background. Ragged red fibres are found on muscle biopsy in 80% of cases, and biochemical analysis will show decreased activity in respiratory chain enzymes. MRI may show atrophy, T2 signal change and basal ganglia calcification. In 90% of cases the genetic defect is an A-to-G transition at nucleotide 8344 in the tRNA^{lys} gene of mitochondrial (mt)DNA, and some other cases are caused by *T8356C* or *G8363A* mutations. Genetic testing is available. Heteroplasmy is responsible for some of the phenotypical variation and can complicate genetic diagnosis.

Alpers disease (progressive neuronal degeneration of childhood with liver disease and poliodystrophy)

This condition has now been found to be due to a mitochondrial defect, inherited by nuclear DNA mutations. Most cases are due to mutations in the *POLG1* gene (and less often in the *COX II* gene), causing a deficiency in mitochondrial DNA polymerase γ (POLG) catalytic activity – similar to that in another mitochondrial syndrome MNGIE. It is a rare condition (<1/200 000 births) inherited in an autosomal recessive fashion, presenting usually in infancy or early childhood with intractable seizures and developmental arrest. Late-onset cases occasionally occur, in childhood or early adult life, presenting typically with status epilepticus. Other signs include dementia, spasticity, peripheral neuropathy, optic atrophy and gastrointestinal disturbance. Liver dysfunction is usually evident and severe hepatic failure is common. The seizures in Alpers disease characteristically take the form of tonic–clonic status epilepticus or epilepsia partialis continua (EPC). As with other mitochondrial disorders, the seizures can have visual features and the EEG and imaging abnormalities are often posterior in location. Antiepileptic therapy follows conventional lines, but the seizures are invariably severe and intractable. The prognosis is poor with death usually within a short time of diagnosis.

Neuronal ceroid lipofuscinosis

The neuronal ceroid lipofusinoses (NCLs) are a group of inherited lysosomal storage disorders that may present with progressive myoclonic epilepsy, and mental and motor deterioration. These are the most common of the hereditary progressive neurodegenerative diseases, occurring generally in about 1/25 000 live births, but with marked geographical variation and a particularly high frequency in Finland. The phenotypes are categorized by age of onset: infantile neuronal ceroid lipofuscinosis (INCL), late-infantile (LINCL), juvenile (JNCL), adult (ANCL) and northern epilepsy (NE). Myoclonic epilepsy is a feature of all types. Almost all cases are inherited in an autosomal recessive manner although an autosomal dominant form of adult-onset NCL has been described. Carriers show no symptoms. In Santavuori disease (INCL), infants are normal at birth and then develop retinal blindness and seizures by 2 years of age, followed by progressive mental deterioration, and usually death in the first decade (although longer survival is possible with some mutations). Jansky–Bielschowsky disease (LINCL) appears typically between 2 and 4 years of age, usually starting with myoclonic epilepsy, followed by developmental regression, dementia, ataxia, blindness, and extrapyramidal and pyramidal signs. Death is usually between 6 and 30 years of age.

Batten disease (JNCL) develops between 4 and 10 years of age with rapidly progressing visual loss. Epilepsy, taking the form of tonic–clonic seizures, complex partial seizures or myoclonic seizures, typically appears between age 5 and 18 years. Other features include dementia and extrapyramidal features, and behavioural disturbance and psychosis. Death occurs between the late teens and the fourth decade.

Kufs disease (ANCL) usually develops around 30 years of age, with death occurring about 10 years later. There are two major phenotypes. In type A, patients present with PME with dementia, ataxia, and late-occurring pyramidal or extrapyramidal signs. Seizures are often uncontrollable. In type B, behavioural abnormalities and dementia are the presenting signs, sometimes associated with motor dysfunction, ataxia, extrapyramidal signs and suprabulbar signs. Visual failure does not occur. Northern epilepsy is characterized by tonic–clonic or complex partial seizures, learning disability and motor dysfunction. Onset occurs between 5 and 10 years of age.

The diagnosis of an NCL is based on clinical findings, electron microscopy of biopsied tissues and, in some instances, assay of enzyme activity or enzyme levels, and molecular genetic testing. Causative mutations in a variety of genes (*NCL* and *MFSD8* genes) have been identified, which vary geographically. MRI shows atrophy and sometimes T2 hyperintensity, and visually evoked responses (VEPs) and electroretinogram (ERG) responses are abnormal. White cells are vacuolated. Electron microscopy of white blood cells, skin, conjunctiva or other tissues typically reveals lysosomal storage material, manifest as fingerprint, curvilinear profiles or granular osmophilic deposits. The levels of enzyme products of each of the six genes can also be assayed. There are six causative genes – *PPT1*, *CLN2*, *CLN3*, *CLN5*, *CLN6* and *CLN8* – and over 140 mutations described. There is a marked geographical variation in the genetic abnormalities, with *CLN8* abnormalities found only in Finland, for example. Genetic testing, and also prenatal testing, for each are available.

Sialidosis

Sialidosis is less common than the other causes of PME. There are at least two variants. All cases are inherited in an autosomal recessive manner. Type 1 sialidosis (cherry-red spot myoclonus syndrome) is due to *N*-acetylneuraminidase deficiency: a gene has been mapped to chromosome 6p21.3, which results in defective cleavage, and thus accumulation, of oligosaccharides, typically with inclusion bodies with vacuolation. It has a juvenile or adult onset and is characterized by action myoclonus and an intention tremor, gradual visual failure and later tonic–clonic seizures. There is little in the way of mental deterioration. In type 2 sialidosis (also known as galactosidase), there are defects in β-galactosidase activity in addition to those in *N*-acetylneuraminidase. Timing of the onset varies from infancy to the second decade, and clinical features include severe myoclonus, tonic–clonic seizures, dysmorphic features, coarse facies, corneal clouding, skeletal dysostosis, cardiac involvement, organomegaly and dementia. One gene has been mapped to chromosome 20. The genetic basis of this disorder is complex and not completely elucidated, and involves both the gene for Neu-1 and the gene for cathepsin A, which forms a complex with Neu-1. Diagnosis is confirmed by finding elevated urinary sialyloligosaccharides and by assaying enzyme activity in leucocytes and cultured skin fibroblasts.

Neurocutaneous syndromes

The so-called neurocutaneous conditions often result in epilepsy. Tuberous sclerosis complex, Sturge–Weber syndrome and neurofibromatosis (type 1) are the most important, and are not uncommonly encountered in epilepsy clinics. Other rare conditions causing epilepsy include hypomelanosis of Ito, epidermal naevus syndrome, hereditary haemorrhagic telangiectasia, Parry–Romberg syndrome, midline linear naevus syndrome, incontinentia pigmenti and Klippel–Trénaunay–Weber syndrome.

Tuberous sclerosis

Tuberous sclerosis or tuberous sclerosis complex (TSC) is a common and important cause of epilepsy. The incidence may be as high as 1 in 5800 live births and there is a high spontaneous mutation rate (1 in 25 000). It is inherited in an autosomal dominant fashion, and is usually caused by mutations of the *TSC1* or *TSC2* genes, both tumour-suppressor genes. Mutations of *TSC1* tend to result in a milder disease with fewer tubers, and less severe epilepsy, renal and retinal disease, although there is a large overlap in the phenotypical manifestations of mutations in either gene. To date, about 300 unique *TSC1* or *TSC2* mutations have been identified in almost 400 separate patients/families. The *TSC1* mutations are primarily small deletions, insertions or nonsense mutations; in contrast, *TSC2* mutations also include significant numbers of missense mutations, large deletions and rearrangements. Between 60 and 80% of patients with TSC have an identifiable *TSC1* or *TSC2* mutation. The condition is a form of cortical dysplasia, and the histological appearance of the tumours shows similar features to other forms of focal cortical dysplasia. There is considerable clinical variability in the manifestations of tuberous sclerosis, and the extent to which some other forms of cortical dysplasia represent forme fruste cases will no doubt be established by modern genetic studies.

Epilepsy is the presenting symptom in 80% or more of patients. It can take the form of neonatal seizures, West syndrome, Lennox–Gastaut syndrome, or adult-onset partial or generalized seizures. About two-thirds of patients present with seizures before the age of 2 years, with motor seizures, drop attacks or infantile spasms. About 25% of all cases of West syndrome are due to tuberous sclerosis. The skin is abnormal in almost all patients, and skin lesions include: hypomelanotic macules (87–100% of patients), facial angiofibromas (47–90%), shagreen patches (20–80%), fibrous facial plaques and subungual fibromas (17–87%). The facial angiofibromas cause disfigurement, but none of the skin lesions results in more serious medical problems. CNS tumours are the leading cause of morbidity and mortality. The brain lesions can be distinguished on the basis of MRI studies and comprise subependymal glial nodules (90% of cases), cortical tubers (70% of cases) and subependymal giant cell astrocytomas (6–14% of cases). Linear streaks seen on MRI represent disordered neuronal migration.

Subependymal giant cell astrocytomas progressively enlarge, causing pressure and obstruction, and result in significant morbidity and mortality. Psychiatric disorders are common and include autism, hyperactivity or attention deficit hyperactivity disorder, and aggression. At least 50% of patients have developmental delay or learning disability. An estimated 80% of children with TSC have an identifiable renal lesion by the age of 10 years. Five different renal lesions occur in TSC: benign angiomyolipoma (70% of affected individuals), epithelial cysts (20%), oncocytoma (benign adenomatous hamartoma) (<1%), malignant angiomyolipoma (<1%) and renal cell carcinoma (<1%). Cardiac rhabdomyomas are present in 47–67% of patients with TSC. Lymphangiomyomatosis of the lung is estimated to occur in 1–6% of cases and primarily affects women between the ages of 20 and 40 years. The retinal lesions are hamartomas (elevated mulberry lesions or plaque-like lesions) and achromic patches (similar to the hypopigmented skin lesions). One or more of these lesions may be present in up to 75% of patients and are usually asymptomatic. Status epilepticus, renal disease and bronchopneumonia are the leading causes of premature death.

Diagnostic criteria are shown in Table 4.7. Molecular genetic testing for diagnostic confirmation and prenatal testing of the *TSC1* and *TSC2* genes are available but complicated by the large size of the two genes, the large number of disease-causing mutations and the high rate of somatic mosaicism (10–25%).

The epilepsy is treated with conventional antiepileptic drugs, but in at least a third of cases is highly resistant to treatment. It is claimed, on the basis of uncontrolled studies, that vigabatrin is especially helpful in infantile spasm due to tuberous sclerosis, and this is a niche indication for this drug. Occasionally, surgical resection of individual lesions is curative. Presurgical work-up follows the normal principles of epilepsy surgery, and outcome is best when data from different modalities of investigation are convergent, when there is a single seizure type and a single large tuber, and when one cortical tuber is larger or calcified. Anterior callosotomy is sometimes useful to alleviate drop attacks or severe generalized epilepsy.

Table 4.7 Diagnostic criteria of tuberous sclerosis.

Major features
Facial angiofibromas or forehead plaque
Non-traumatic ungual or periungual fibromas
Hypomelanotic macules (three or more)
Shagreen patch (connective tissue naevus)
Multiple retinal nodular hamartomas
Cortical tuber
Subependymal nodule
Subependymal giant cell astrocytoma
Cardiac rhabdomyoma, single or multiple
Lymphangiomyomatosis
Renal angiomyolipoma

Minor features
Multiple randomly distributed pits in dental enamel
Hamartomatous rectal polyps
Bone cysts
Cerebral white matter radial migration lines
Gingival fibromas
Non-renal hamartoma
Retinal achromic patch
'Confetti' skin lesions
Multiple renal cysts

Definite tuberous sclerosis complex (TSC): two major features or one major feature plus two minor features.

Probable TSC: one major feature plus one minor feature.

Possible TSC: one major feature or two or more minor features.

There is no curative therapy for tuberous sclerosis. However, control of seizures and treatment of individual lesions can greatly improve quality of life. It is important to monitor patients regularly for the development of lesions – a screening protocol is shown in Table 4.8. Patients with retinal lesions seldom develop progressive visual loss, so regular ophthalmological evaluations are unnecessary. The skin lesions (with the exception of the facial angiolipomas) also seldom require therapy. Early identification of an enlarging giant cell astrocytoma permits its removal before symptoms develop and before it becomes locally invasive, and is the rationale for regular neuroimaging of children and adolescents with documented subependymal nodules.

Neurofibromatosis type 1

Neurofibromatosis type 1 (NF1) is a common, dominantly inherited genetic disorder, occurring in about 1 in 3000 live births. Almost half of all cases are new

Table 4.8 Screening protocol for patients with tuberous sclerosis.

- Renal ultrasonography (1–3 yearly – and then renal CT/MRI, if large or numerous renal tumours are detected)
- Cranial CT/MRI (1–3 yearly)
- Regular neurodevelopmental/behavioural evaluations
- Periodic ocular, cardiological, dermatological, ophthalmological evaluations
- Echocardiography, electroencephalography, chest CT (if symptomatic)

mutations. The mutation rate for the NF1 gene is about 1 in 10 000, among the highest known for any human gene. It is a large gene, and many different mutations have resulted in the clinical manifestations. Although the penetrance is essentially complete, the clinical manifestations are extremely variable. In NF1, the incidence of epilepsy is about 5–10%. The epilepsy can take various forms and present at any age. Infantile spasms due to NF1 are said to have a more favourable outcome than other symptomatic types. MRI can show heterotopia, other dysplastic lesions and congenital changes, but epilepsy can occur even if there are no overt MRI abnormalities.

Diagnostic criteria are listed in Table 4.9. Multiple café-au-lait spots occur in almost all patients with intertriginous freckling. Numerous benign cutaneous or subcutaneous neurofibromas are usually present in adults. Plexiform neurofibromas are less common but can cause disfigurement and may compromise function or even jeopardize life. Ocular manifestations include optic gliomas, which may lead to blindness, and Lisch nodules (innocuous iris hamartomas). Scoliosis, vertebral dysplasia, pseudarthrosis and overgrowth are the most serious bony complications of NF1. Other medical concerns include vasculopathy, hypertension, intracranial tumours and malignant peripheral nerve sheath tumours.

About half of those with NF1 have a learning disability. Many of the manifestations are age related, e.g. optic gliomas develop in the first 4 years of life. The rapidly progressive (dysplastic) form of scoliosis almost always develops between 6 and 10 years of age, although milder forms of scoliosis without vertebral anomalies typically occur during adolescence. Malignant peripheral nerve sheath tumours (neurofibrosarcomas) usually occur in adolescents and adults. Neurofibromas can occur in almost any organ in the body. The total number of

Table 4.9 Diagnostic criteria for neurofibromatosis type 1 (NF1).

Two or more of the following features (National Institutes of Health criteria):

Six or more café-au-lait macules >5 mm in greatest diameter in prepubertal individuals and >15 mm in greatest diameter in postpubertal individuals

Two or more neurofibromas of any type or one plexiform neurofibroma

Freckling in the axillary or inguinal regions

Optic glioma

Two or more Lisch nodules (iris hamartomas)

Bone lesion such as sphenoid dysplasia or thinning of the long bone cortex, pseudarthrosis

First-degree relative (parent, sib, or offspring) with NF1

Only about half the patients with NF1 with a known family history of NF meet these criteria for diagnosis by age 1 year, but almost all do by age 8 years because many features of NF1 increase in frequency with age. Children who have inherited NF1 from an affected parent can usually be identified within the first year of life because diagnosis requires just one feature in addition to a positive family history.

neurofibromas seen in adults with NF1 varies from a few to hundreds or even thousands. Additional cutaneous and subcutaneous neurofibromas continue to develop throughout life, although the rate of appearance may vary greatly from year to year. Many patients with NF1 develop only cutaneous manifestations of the disease and Lisch nodules, but the frequency of more serious complications increases with age. Cerebrovascular abnormalities in NF1 typically present as stenoses or occlusions of the internal carotid, middle cerebral or anterior cerebral artery. Small telangiectatic vessels form around the stenotic area and appear as a 'puff of smoke' ('moya-moya') on cerebral angiography. There is no curative treatment, but annual follow-up by a physician familiar with the condition is important. This should include annual ophthalmological examination in childhood, less frequent examination in adults, regular developmental assessment by screening questionnaire (in childhood), regular blood pressure monitoring and other studies, as indicated by clinically apparent signs or symptoms. Genetic counselling and testing are available, but are complex and need to be carried out by units experienced in the condition.

The treatment of epilepsy follows conventional medical lines, and in most cases the epilepsy is easily controlled. Surgical therapy usually has no role in the management of the epilepsy.

Sturge–Weber syndrome

This is an uncommon sporadic developmental disorder, of uncertain causation. The principal clinical features are a unilateral or bilateral port wine naevus, epilepsy, hemiparesis, mental impairment and ocular signs. The port wine naevus is usually, but not exclusively, in the distribution of the trigeminal nerve. It can cross the midline and spread into the dermatomal distribution of the upper cervical nerve. If it affects the lip or the gum the naevus can be enlarged. In 15% of cases the naevus is bilateral.

The epilepsy can be focal or generalized. It is often the earliest symptom, and most patients with Sturge–Weber syndrome develop seizures within the first year of life (at least 70%) and almost all have developed epilepsy before the age of 4 years. Adult-onset epilepsy can, however, occur occasionally. The early seizures are often triggered by fever. The seizures take the form of partial or multifocal attacks, often with frequent and severe secondary generalization. Convulsive status occurs in over half the cases. Seizures developing in the neonatal period can be very difficult to control and carry a poor prognosis. The hemiplegia and mental impairment deteriorate in a step-like fashion following a severe bout of seizures, and in Sturge–Weber syndrome there is little doubt that brain damage can result directly from epileptic attacks, presumably by ischaemic or excitotoxic mechanisms. Severe learning disability is now less common due to better control of the epilepsy. Similarly, outcome is better in the few patients in whom epilepsy is absent. In addition to the seizures and motor disturbance, there can be other neurological features. Ophthalmological complications (80%) include increased intraocular pressure with glaucoma or buphthalmos. Homonymous field defects are common, particularly when the cerebral lesion is in the occipital region (as is frequently the case), and episcleral haemangiomas, choroidal naevi and colobomas of the iris can occur. The underlying brain pathology is a cerebral angiomatosis (often occipital) sometimes with gyral calcification. The affected cerebral hemisphere is often atrophic and gliotic. The lesion is probably the result of abnormal persistence of embryonic primordial vascular plexus.

The epilepsy should be treated aggressively to prevent neurological deterioration. There are no specific features to the choice of drug or drug regimen, but control of seizures is important to prevent neurological deterioration. High doses of antiepileptic drugs may be required. Status epilepticus should be vigorously treated, because failure to rapidly control the status often results in a permanent and significant worsening of the neurological deficit. Resective surgery (lesionectomy, hemispherectomy or lobectomy) can greatly improve quality of life and seizures, and should be given early consideration in any patient in whom control of seizures is poor. Surgical resection of abnormal tissue is worthwhile, particularly if carried out early in life and early in the course of the condition.

Epilepsies in disorders of chromosome structure

Epilepsy is also a feature of two common chromosomal abnormalities: Down syndrome and fragile X syndrome. It also takes a highly characteristic form in the rare ring chromosome 20. Other uncommon chromosomal abnormalities in which epilepsy is found include: trisomy 12p, 8, 13; ring chromosome 14; partial monosomy 4p (Wolf–Hirschhorn syndrome); inverted duplication of pericentromeric chromosome 15; and Klinefelter syndrome (where epilepsy occurs in about 10% of cases). In all these conditions, there are additional behavioural and intellectual disabilities, and characteristic dysmorphic features. The seizures often take multiple forms, including myoclonus, and are of variable severity. Genetic testing is available for most conditions. In addition to these large-scale chromosomal abnormalities, it is becoming clear that smaller changes (deletions, duplications, translocations etc – copy number variations) are also the cause of epilepsy in cases hitherto considered 'cryptogenic'.

Down syndrome

The Down syndrome phenotype occurs in about 1 in every 650 live births. It is usually caused by trisomy of chromosome 21, and triplication of 21q22.3 results in the typical phenotype. In 95% of cases the cause is a nondysjunction, and in about 4% an unbalanced translocation. About 1% of cases are due to mosaicism. The risk of trisomy increases with maternal age. Epilepsy is present in up to 12% of cases and EEG abnormalities in more than 20%. Epilepsy typically develops either in the first year of life, due to perinatal or congenital complications, or in the third decade, possibly due to the development of Alzheimer disease-like neuropathological changes. The epilepsy is very variable and can take multiple forms, reflecting the complex pathogenesis. West syndrome is common, and Down syndrome can also cause febrile seizures and the Lennox–Gastaut syndrome. Usually the epilepsy is rather non-specific, although frequent, small, brief, partial seizures seem particularly common in adults. Startle-induced seizures are, however, a characteristic feature. Treatment follows conventional medical lines, and the prognosis and response to treatment vary with type and cause. Surgical therapy for epilepsy has no role in this syndrome. Genetic testing and prenatal screening are available.

Fragile X syndrome

Fragile X syndrome is a condition resulting from an increased number of CGG repeats (typically >200) in the *FMR1* gene (at Xq27.3) accompanied by aberrant methylation of the gene. It is an X-linked condition in which the presenting symptom is usually learning disability, which is moderate in affected males and mild in affected females. Fragile X syndrome occurs in about 1 in 4000 male births and is the most common identified cause of learning disability. Carrier rates in females (CAG repeats of approximately 50–200) may be as high as 1 in 250, with some geographical and racial variation. Developmental delay is noticed from infancy, and manifests with abnormalities of speech, abnormal behaviour, typically with tantrums, hyperactivity and autism. Dysmorphic features include abnormal craniofacies, with typically a long face, prominent forehead, large ears and prominent jaw. After puberty macro-orchidism, strabismus and rather abnormal behaviour are evident. Heterozygotic females show a milder but similar phenotype. Seizures are present in a quarter of cases and EEG abnormalities in a half. The seizures usually develop before the age of 15 years, sometimes remitting in the second decade of life and can take various forms (both generalized and partial) with equally variable non-specific EEG findings. Repeat numbers vary, and mosaicism is common, and these may account for the variable clinical features. Genetic testing and prenatal testing are widely available. The methylation status of the gene can also be identified using Southern blot. Identification of the abnormal protein is not usually required. The epilepsy is treated by conventional medical means and is often easily controlled.

Ring chromosome 20

This is a rare condition, but one in which epilepsy is the predominant feature, and it has a highly characteristic phenotype. The locus of fusion between the deleted short and long arms of the chromosome is at p13q13, p13q13.3.3 or p13q13.33. Seizures begin between infancy and 14 years of age, typically with episodes of non-convulsive status epilepticus. These episodes are characterized by confusion, staring, and perioral and eyelid myoclonus. The seizures can be very severe, occurring daily, and are drug resistant. The prolonged seizures may be misdiagnosed as non-epileptic behavioural disturbance. The EEG during episodes shows high-voltage, rhythmic, notched, slow-activity waves. Mental regression and learning disability are present in addition to epilepsy. This is a sporadic condition that can be identified by genetic testing. Mosaicism is common and at least 100 mitoses may need to be examined before excluding the condition. The seizures can be highly resistant to therapy, which follows conventional lines. The treatment of non-convulsive status epilepticus is outlined on pp. 303–307.

Epilepsies as a result of developmental anomalies of cerebral structure (the 'cortical dysplasias')

Cortical dysplasia (synonyms: cortical dysgenesis, malformations of cortical development) is a term that is applied to developmental disorders of the cortex producing structural change (Table 4.10). Some of these conditions are caused by identifiable genetic abnormalities. Others are caused by environmental influences such as infection, trauma, hypoxia, or exposure to drugs or toxins. In most cases the cause is unclear. The form of dysplasia consequent on environmental insults depends not only on the nature of the insult, but also on the stage of development at which it occurred. Cortical malformations can be due to abnormal neuronal and glial proliferation, abnormal neuronal migration or abnormal synaptogenesis, cortical organization or programmed cell death.

The true prevalence of these conditions, previously thought to be rare, has only become apparent with the widespread use of MRI, which can detect cortical dysplasia in cases previously classified as cryptogenic epilepsy. Epilepsy is a leading feature of these conditions, usually, but not always, in association with learning disability and other neurological findings.

Drug therapy follows conventional lines (as for any focal epilepsy), but, in many cases, the epilepsy can be refractory to treatment. Cortical dysplasia is the underlying cause of the epilepsy in up to 30% of children and 10% of adults referred to epilepsy centres for intractable

Table 4.10 Types of cortical dysplasia.

Abnormalities of gyration
Agyria (lissencephaly), macrogyria, pachygyria spectrum (focal or diffuse) (*LIS1*, *RELN*, *ARX* and *DCX* genes)
Polymicrogyria
Cobblestone complex (*FCMD* gene)
Schizencephaly (*EMX2* gene)
Minor gyral abnormalities

Heterotopias
Periventricular nodular heterotopia (*FLNA* gene)
Subcortical nodular heterotopia
Subcortical band heterotopia (*DCX* and *LIS1* gene)

Other gross malformations
Megalencephaly and hemimegalencephaly
Agenesis of corpus callosum
Anencephaly and holoprosencephaly
Microcephaly

Cortical dysgenesis associated with neoplasia
Dysembryoneuroepithelial tumour
Ganglioglioma
Gangliocytoma

Other cortical dysplasias
Hypothalamic hamartoma
Focal cortical dysplasia
Tuberous sclerosis (*TSC1* and *TSC2* genes)
Microdysgenesis

This is an arbitrary classification, based largely on neuroimaging appearances; the categories overlap.

epilepsy. At the other extreme, easily controlled epilepsy is not uncommon with mild forms of dysplasia. The surgical therapy of cortical dysplasia is described on pp. 349–351.

Hemimegalencephaly

Hemimegalencephaly describes a gross structural abnormality that can be the end-result of various cerebral processes and insults. One cerebral hemisphere is enlarged and structurally abnormal with thickened cortex, reduced sulcation, and poor or absent laminar organization. Giant neurons are found throughout the brain and in 50% of cases balloon cells are found. The condition can occur in isolation, associated with other cortical dysplasias, or as part of other syndromes (notably tuberous sclerosis or other rarer neurocutaneous syndromes, such as epidermal naevus syndrome, Klippel–Trenaunay–Weber syndrome, NF1 or hypomelanosis of Ito). The restriction of the abnormality to one hemisphere may be

a result of somatic mosaicism, and it has been suggested that the condition is due to defects in the process of programmed cell death (apoptosis) in early fetal life.

Hemimegalencephaly always results in severe epilepsy presenting in early life, accompanied by learning disability, hemiplegia and hemianopia. The epilepsy can take the form of neonatal seizures, West syndrome, the Lennox–Gastaut syndrome or other less specific focal forms. Status epilepticus is common and a frequent cause of death in the early years. Medical treatment follows conventional lines, but is often unsuccessful. Surgical therapy (hemispherectomy or hemispherotomy) can be curative, and this is an important condition to identify early, because early surgery will prevent seizures, mitigate cognitive decline, and improve social behaviour and adjustment

Focal cortical dysplasia

Focal cortical dysplasia is a common form of dysplasia, important to identify because of its potential for surgical therapy. The term encompasses a variety of subtypes with different histological appearances, possibly as a result of formation at different stages of embryogenesis. In some, the cortical lamination is normal, but in others there may be associated macrogyria and polymicrogyria. Focal dysplasia can occur in any part of the cortex, and varies greatly in size. There are often widespread minor dysplastic abnormalities, associated with some forms of focal cortical dysplasia, although in the Taylor form, diagnosed by the histological presence of 'balloon cells', the dysplastic changes are more limited.

Dysplastic tissue generates epileptic discharges directly and seizures have been recorded by depth electrodes within dysplastic areas, possibly due to deranged GABA-ergic inhibition. Epilepsy is the leading symptom, and other features depend on the extent of the lesion and include learning disability and focal deficits. Focal cortical dysplasia underlies neonatal seizures, West syndrome or the Lennox–Gastaut syndrome, but more typically does not take a syndromic form and presents in childhood or adult life as less specific focal or secondarily generalized epilepsy. Episodes of EPC or tonic–clonic or partial status epilepticus are common. Interictal EEG can show rather typical, continuous, focal, slow-wave activity. The MRI signs are increased signal on T2 imaging and FLAIR (fluid attenuation inversion recovery), blurring of the grey–white junction and simplified sulcation in the Taylor type, and similar but often more widespread changes in other types. Some cases of focal cortical dysplasia respond well to conventional antiepileptic drug therapy but others are highly resistant. Therapy should conform to the usual principles and there is nothing particularly specific about drug choice or usage. Surgical resection is possible in restricted and particularly small lesions, and surgical work-up follows conventional principles. The Taylor form responds particularly well to surgery.

Schizencephaly

Schizencephaly refers to the presence of clefts in the cortex, stretching from the surface to the ventricle. The clefts are subdivided into open-lip schizencephaly (in which the walls of the cleft are separated) and closed-lip schizencephaly (in which the walls of the cleft are not separated). The clefts can be unilateral or bilateral and they are usually perisylvian in location. Schizencephaly is often associated with polymicrogyria and less often with other focal cortical dysplastic anomalies, corpus callosum agenesis or septo-optic dysplasias. The cortex may or may not have normal lamination. The pathogenesis in some cases is a failure of migration and in others an environmental insult causing focal necrosis of developing cortex. The causes are heterogeneous, and include germline mutations of the homeobox gene *EMX2* and environmental insults during development, including radiation, infection and ischaemia.

The clinical presentation can be very variable. Epilepsy is the most common symptom (>90% of cases), associated usually but by no means always with learning disability or cognitive changes. Focal neurological deficit is common in extensive or bilateral cases. Medical therapy follows conventional lines and, generally speaking, surgical resection is not possible.

Agyria–pachygyria band spectrum

Lissencephaly, pachygyria, agyria and subcortical band heterotopia are descriptive terms denoting abnormalities of cortical gyration, and are grouped together because they show an interconnected genetic basis: in all of these, the gyration is simplified and the cortex is thickened. Lissencephaly (literally meaning smooth brain) is the most severe form, in which gyration is grossly diminished or even absent. Subcortical band heterotopia (synonym: subcortical laminar heterotopia, band heterotopia, double cortex syndrome) denotes the presence of a band of grey matter sandwiched by white matter below the cortical grey matter. The band may be thin or thick and can merge with overlying cortex, in which case the cortex takes a macrogyric form. When the bands are thin and clearly separated from the cortical ribbon, the ribbon itself may appear normal. Thicker bands are usually

associated with macrogyria. Macrogyria refers to thickened cortex and can occur as an isolated phenomenon. It is variable in extent and, when focal, it is indistinguishable on clinical or imaging grounds from some forms of focal cortical dysplasia.

Most forms of lissencephaly occur without other noncerebral malformations (isolated lissencephaly sequence [ILIS]). Isolated lissencephaly is present in 12 in 10^6 live births. Of isolated cases of lissencephaly 60–80% are caused by identifiable mutations in *LIS1*, on 17p13.3, or in X-linked dominant lissencephaly (XLIS) (in *DCX*) on Xq22.3–q24: in 40% the entire gene is deleted. *LIS1* lissencephaly is predominantly posterior in location, and the condition occurs in both sexes and is sporadic. Conversely, XLIS cases occur almost always in boys and the brain anomaly tends to be anterior in location. Genetic testing is available for both forms. Anterior lissencephaly also occurs with abnormalities in the *ARX* gene and a range of phenotypes including West syndrome, dystonia and learning disability. Posterior lissencephaly can be due to abnormalities in the *RELN* gene sometimes associated with cerebellar hypoplasia.

Other forms of lissencephaly have more widespread associations. The best known is the Miller–Dieker syndrome, which is caused by large deletions of *LIS1* and of several other contiguous genes on 17p13.3 (e.g. 14-3-3E). In this syndrome lissencephaly is associated with epilepsy, facial dysmorphism, microcephaly, small mandible, failure to thrive, retarded motor development, dysphagia, and decorticate and decerebrate postures. Other organs, including the kidney and heart, may be affected. Survival varies from months to several decades, and epilepsy is usually profound and intractable. Genetic testing is available. Cobblestone lissencephaly (type II) is also found in some patients with muscular dystrophy and ocular malformations.

Subcortical band heterotopia is caused in about 80% of cases by germline deletions in the *DCX* (XLIS) gene and almost always (but not exclusively) occurs in females. The pachygyria and bands are anteriorly predominant. The genetic anomaly in the other 20% of cases has not been identified. The rare cases of subcortical band heterotopia in boys are probably caused by missense mutations in *DCX* or *LIS1*. Subcortical band heterotopia is a much more benign condition than lissencephaly. It can present in children or in adults, with epilepsy and learning disability. Epilepsy occurs in at least 80% of cases, and 50% of cases present with the Lennox–Gastaut phenotype. However, the manifestations of this anomaly can be slight, and occasional patients present with mild epilepsy and normal intelligence. The clinical severity of the syndrome seems to correlate with the extent of the cerebral anomaly. In two-thirds of those with epilepsy, the seizures are intractable. Similarly, patients with pachygyria or macrogyria also have epilepsy and learning disability of variable severity, depending on the extent and location of the anomaly. The histological changes of lissencephaly, macrogyria, pachygyria and band heterotopia may merge into each other, and in many patients these conditions represent a continuous spectrum rather than distinct entities. The anomalies are caused by abnormal cortical migration, and the factors influencing extent or severity have not been clearly identified. The cytoarchitecture varies, but, in the Miller–Dieker syndrome, for example, the lissencephalic cortex is thickened and has four rather than six layers (type I or classic lissencephaly). The changes can be regional and there may be associated dysplastic lesions.

Drug treatment follows conventional lines. Resective surgical therapy is not indicated, even where the bands or lissencephalic changes seem relatively localized, but callosotomy may help the occasional patients with frequent drop attacks.

Agenesis of the corpus callosum

Agenesis of the corpus callosum is a dysplastic anomaly that occurs in various genetic and congenital disorders. Epilepsy is an invariable association, and often a leading symptom. In Aicardi syndrome, the corpus callosum agenesis is associated with periventricular heterotopia, thin unlayered cortex and diffuse polymicrogyria. It is observed only in females (the only exception being males with two X chromosomes) and is X-linked with male lethality. The causal gene has not yet been identified but linkage to Xp22.3 has been reported. The syndrome may be due to skewed X-chromosome inactivation. Other syndromes with agenesis of the corpus callosum exist, and this anomaly may coexist with other dysplastic features. The L1 syndrome is associated with mutations in the *L1CAM* gene and presents as hydrocephalus, learning disability, spasticity and epilepsy.

Polymicrogyria

The appearance of small and prominent gyri, separated by shallow sulci, is known as polymicrogyria. Polymicrogyria can be diffuse or localized, and varies in severity as well as extent. The underlying cortex is invariably thickened, and can be unlayered or show an abnormal four-layered structure. The former may be a migrational defect in

weeks 13–18 of fetal life, and the latter the result of ischaemia or perfusion failure between weeks 12 and 24 of fetal life. Epilepsy is the leading clinical feature, associated with learning disability and focal neurological signs.

The severity of all of these depends on the extent of the dysplasia. At one extreme the child is severely learning disabled with profound epilepsy and quadraparesis, whereas at the other the epilepsy is mild and presents in adult life. There are various anatomical patterns of distribution of polymicrogyria, which may or may not have clinical specificity. The distribution of the polymicrogyria can be patchy, bifrontal, unilateral, or concentrated in the sylvian or central areas. Polymicrogyria is an invariable association of schizencephaly and is often associated with other cortical dysplasias. Both ischaemic and genetic defects can cause bilateral perisylvian polymicrogyria (Kuzniecky syndrome), a condition in which there is severe upper motor neuron bulbar dysfunction and diplegia as well as severe epilepsy and learning disability. The presenting phenotype is wide, varying from that of the Lennox–Gastaut syndrome to patients with mild adult-onset seizures. In familial cases of polymicrogyria, inheritance conforms to an X-linked or autosomal dominant pattern with reduced penetrance. Some cases are sporadic and in other families individuals have clinical symptoms but no MRI change. There is marked phenotypical heterogeneity. No gene has yet been discovered, but linkage has been reported to *X28p* in 22q11.2. Polymicrogyria can also occur in the presence of chromosomal abnormalities. The medical therapy of polymicrogyria follows conventional lines. Surgical resection is only occasionally possible if the polymicrogyria is well localized.

Periventricular nodular heterotopia

The presence of subependymal nodules of grey matter, located along the supralateral walls of the lateral ventricles, is known as periventricular nodular heterotopia (synonyms: bilateral periventricular nodular heterotopia [BPNH], subependymal nodular heterotopia [SENH]). The heterotopia is usually bilateral, although not always. It is much more common in females and conforms to X-linked dominant transmission. Almost all cases have shown mutations in the *FLN1* (filamin-1) gene. It is the most common, clearly identified form of cortical dysplasia causing epilepsy. At one extreme, the heterotopia can be asymptomatic. It commonly presents in older children or young adults with mild epilepsy, and at the other extreme can account for severe infantile or childhood partial epilepsy. Other features reported include early stroke due to vasculopathy, abnormalities of gastric motility, short digits, strabismus and cardiac anomalies. Depth recordings show that the nodules generate intrinsic epileptiform discharges. Periventricular nodules are found in about 5% of all cases of hippocampal sclerosis. In the presence of heterotopic tissue, temporal lobectomy for hippocampal sclerosis – even with clinical and EEG features typical of mesial temporal epilepsy – will usually fail to control seizures. In patients being assessed for temporal lobectomy it is essential, therefore, to scrutinize preoperative MRI with great care to exclude the presence of these lesions. Treatment is along conventional medical lines, but resective surgery has occasionally been performed in isolated lesions.

Other dysplasias

Various other types of dysplastic lesion exist, including sheets of abnormal neurons forming linear streaks in the white matter, lesions with a 'tail' of abnormal tissue stretching to the ventricular surface, abnormal cortical patterning (including stellate-like gyral formations), isolated clusters of grey matter within white matter and microdysgenesis. The last term refers to abnormally placed microscopic clusters of heterotopic neurons often associated with abnormal lamination of the cortex. Normal brains have occasional heterotopic cells, and distinguishing the truly pathological from the normal is, to an extent, a subjective judgement. As a result of this, widely varying estimates of the frequency of microdysgenesis have been made. At one extreme is a study showing microdysgenesis in 38% of postmortem specimens in epilepsy compared with a frequency of only 6% in control individuals.

Symptomatic epilepsy due to acquired causes

Almost any acquired condition affecting the cerebral grey matter can result in epilepsy, but here only the more common forms of acquired epilepsy are mentioned. Many of the so-called 'acquired' epilepsies have a genetic loading, and in some (e.g. hippocampal sclerosis) the genetic influences may be considerable. The seizures in symptomatic and acquired epilepsy usually take a partial or secondarily generalized form, and there are often no particularly distinctive features associated with any particular cause. The seizures also may have a strongly 'provoked' element, as may those in idiopathic epilepsy.

In acute cerebral conditions, e.g. stroke, head injury or infections, the epilepsies share a number of general features. The epilepsies are often divided into 'early' (i.e. seizures occurring within a week of the insult) and 'late' (i.e. chronic epilepsy developing later). There is often a 'silent period' between the injury and the onset of late epilepsy. Presumably, epileptogenic processes are developing during this period, and this raises the possibility of neuroprotective interventions to inhibit these processes and prevent later epilepsy. To date, however, no effective neuroprotective agent is available, although this is an area of intensive research. Antiepileptic drug therapy will prevent early epilepsy but does not reduce the frequency of late seizures. Early seizures are often not followed by late epilepsy – a fact that is important to emphasize to patients.

The treatment of symptomatic epilepsy due to acquired causes

As the form of epilepsy in different causes is often identical, it is perhaps not surprising (although admittedly rather disappointing) that the antiepileptic drug therapy for most forms of acquired epilepsy follows similar principles whatever the cause. Factors predicting response to therapy are also similar for all conditions. This lack of specificity implies that there are similar underlying processes of epileptogenesis in epilepsies of many different causes. The approach to drug treatment is similar to that of any focal or secondarily generalized epilepsy, and this is described in Chapter 5 of this book. Surgical therapy is appropriate in a number of acquired epilepsies, and the assessment for surgery is described in Chapter 10.

Treatment also needs to be focused on the cause of the epilepsy. Depending on the clinical setting, such therapy will influence the course of the epilepsy, and in some situations effective therapy for the cause will obviate the need for antiepileptic therapy.

Hippocampal sclerosis

Hippocampal sclerosis is the most common cause of temporal lobe epilepsy. It is found in over a third of cases of people with refractory focal epilepsy attending hospital clinics in whom there is no other structural lesion, but is less frequent in population-based cohorts and in patients with mild epilepsy. Hippocampal sclerosis typically causes complex partial seizures, and the highly characteristic clinical features and symptom complex associated with the syndrome of mesial temporal lobe epilepsy and hippocampal sclerosis are described on pp. 8–9.

The principal pathological abnormality is hippocampal neuronal cell loss, which has a characteristic

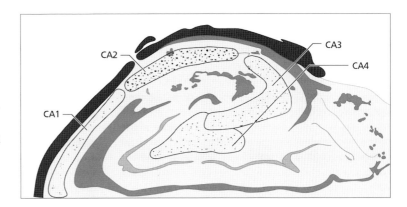

Figure 4.2 The characteristic pattern of hippocampal cell loss in hippocampal sclerosis – note the severe pyramidal cell loss of the CA1, CA3 and CA4 regions, with relative sparing of the CA2 region. Black lines are drawn to outline the boundaries of the regions.

distribution with maximum loss in the CA1 and CA3 regions and in the hilar region of dentate gyrus, and relative sparing of the CA2 region (Figure 4.2). There is also dense fibrous gliosis. The cell loss and gliosis result in atrophy, and the hippocampus is shrunken and hardened. Another common abnormality is an alteration in the laminar arrangement of the dentate gyrus, with dispersal of cells or sometimes duplication of the laminar structure. There is extensive synaptic rearrangement, including recurrent innervation of dentate granule cells by their own neurons, which reinnervate instead of projecting into the hippocampus proper. This aberrant 'mossy fibre' innervation results in alterations in excitatory and inhibitory balance. A large number of neurochemical changes have been documented in the sclerotic hippocampus, although the extent to which these are primary changes or simply consequential to the hippocampal injury is often unclear. There are also pathological changes outside the hippocampus, including widespread subpial fibrillary gliosis (Chaslin gliosis) and nerve cell loss in the neocortex, and gliosis and volume loss in the entorhinal cortex and other mesial structures. Cerebellar atrophy and widespread cerebral atrophy are also not uncommon. In some series, over 70% of patients with hippocampal sclerosis show some evidence of microdysgenesis. MRI morphometry has also recently shown, in cases of unilateral hippocampal sclerosis, a mean 15% reduction of the volume of the rest of the temporal lobe, reductions of similar magnitude in the parahippocampal gyrus and middle and inferior temporal gyri, and a 25% reduction in mean size of the superior temporal gyrus.

The pathogenesis of hippocampal sclerosis is probably multifactorial and the histological changes may be the end-point of a number of different processes. Known causes of hippocampal sclerosis include cerebral trauma, infection (encephalitis or meningitis), vascular damage, toxins (e.g. domoic acid) or raised intracranial pressure. Familial genetic forms exist and, interestingly, in some families, relatives report déjà-vu episodes, which may represent undiagnosed epilepsy.

There is a very clear association with a history of childhood febrile convulsions, and one postulation is that the febrile convulsions, especially if prolonged or complex, damage the hippocampus and result in hippocampal sclerosis. Serial MRI studies have demonstrated that status epilepticus can also result in hippocampal sclerosis and there is clear evidence from animal experimentation that prolonged partial seizures can cause hippocampal damage.

There is also evidence that, in some cases, hippocampal sclerosis may be a congenital lesion, and its frequent association with forms of cortical dysplasia (particularly subependymal heterotopia) adds some strength to the view that hippocampal sclerosis itself may sometimes be a form of cortical dysgenesis.

The medical treatment of hippocampal sclerosis follows conventional lines, similar to that of any focal epilepsy, and the seizures can often be well controlled on medical therapy. Hippocampal sclerosis is also the most common lesion resected in epilepsy surgical practice, and is the most common pathology referred for epilepsy surgery. The surgical therapy of hippocampal sclerosis is dealt with in detail on pp. 320–339.

Prenatal and perinatal injury

Epilepsy has traditionally often been thought to occur owing to perinatal injury, although it is now recognized that in many such cases there are genetic or other prenatal developmental pathologies causing the epilepsy. In most children with epilepsy, minor perinatal problems are quite irrelevant to the subsequent development of epilepsy, or indeed are themselves the result of the underlying defects. In controlled studies only severe perinatal insults, e.g. perinatal haemorrhage and ischaemic–hypoxic encephalopathy, have been found to increase the risk of subsequent epilepsy. Factors such as toxaemia, eclampsia, forceps delivery, being born with the 'cord round the neck', low birthweight and prematurity have only a very modest association, if any, with subsequent epilepsy. Factors reported in some studies are not confirmed in others, but in one large case–control study, early gestational age, vaginal bleeding during pregnancy, birth by caesarean section and socioeconomic factors were found to confer a small risk of subsequent epilepsy.

Cerebral palsy

This term encompasses many pathologies, both prenatal and perinatal, and both genetic and acquired. It therefore has little utility, although it is in widespread use. Whatever the cause, cerebral palsy is indicative of cerebral damage, and thus is strongly associated with epilepsy. In the US National Collaborative Perinatal Project, a prospective cohort study of infants followed to the age of 7 years, epilepsy was found to occur in 34% of children with cerebral palsy, and cerebral palsy was present in 19% of children developing epilepsy. In the same cohort the risk of learning disability (associated with cerebral palsy) was 5.5 times higher among children developing epilepsy after a febrile seizure than in children with a febrile seizure alone. Learning disability (IQ <70) was present in 27% of the children with epilepsy, and seizures were present in about 50% of children with learning disability and cerebral palsy.

Post-vaccination encephalopathy

The possible role of immunization (particularly pertussis – whooping cough – immunization) in causing a childhood encephalopathy and subsequent epilepsy and learning disability has been the subject of intense study, with contradictory claims. There is a fairly general consensus now that the risk of vaccine-induced encephalopathy and/or epilepsy, if it exists at all, is extremely low. Risk estimates in the literature have included: risk of a febrile seizure, 1/19 496 immunizations; risk of an afebrile seizure, 1/76 133 immunizations; risk of encephalopathy after pertussis infection, $0–3/10^6$ immunizations. The situation is complicated by the findings of a recent study which showed that encephalopathy, in 11 of the 14 children studied, although previously attributed to immunization, was in fact due an inherited genetic defect of the *SCN1A* gene, which codes for the voltage-gated neuronal sodium channel. Suggestions that MMR (mumps, measles, rubella) vaccine increases the risks of autism and epilepsy are now thought to be unfounded. Currently conventional medical advice is that the immunization is safer than the disease, although a small number of children do develop an encephalopathic reaction. Quoted figures for a post-measles immunization encephalopathy are $1–2/10^6$, compared with the risk of encephalopathy following the naturally occurring infection of 1–2/1000. Currently, the vaccine with the greatest risk is the smallpox vaccination, with a rate of $10–300/10^6$ of post-vaccination. The vaccines in which there is a possible association with post-vaccination encephalomyelitis are smallpox, measles, DPT (diphtheria, pertussis and tetanus), Japanese B encephalitis and rabies.

Degenerative diseases and dementia

Epilepsy is a common feature of degenerative neurological disease that involves the grey matter, but is seldom a leading symptom in pure leucodystrophy. The most common neurodegenerative disorders are the dementias in late life. Six per cent of those aged over 65 years have dementia, and the rate increases exponentially as a function of age. Alzheimer disease is the most common cause of dementia, and patients with Alzheimer disease are six times more likely to develop epilepsy than age-matched controls. Partial and secondarily generalized seizures occur, and are usually relatively easily treated with conventional antiepileptic therapy. Myoclonus is another common finding in patients with Alzheimer disease, occurring in about 10% of autopsy-verified cases, and is a late manifestation. Non-convulsive status epilepticus can occur, and is often overlooked. An EEG is helpful in diagnosis, and should be considered in any person with dementia whose condition acutely deteriorates. Seizures also occur in the other common dementing illnesses, and are particularly common in cerebrovascular disease (see pp. 64–66). As the population ages, the number of individuals affected by Alzheimer disease and other dementias is going to increase, and so will the number of cases of epilepsy attributed to dementing disorders.

Five per cent of patients with Huntington disease have epilepsy, usually in the later stages. Epilepsy is more common in the juvenile form, and occasionally takes the form of a PME. Epilepsy, and indeed status epilepticus, can be the presenting feature of Creutzfeldt–Jakob disease. Generalized tonic–clonic or partial seizures occur in 10% of established cases, and myoclonus in 80%, and these can be induced by startle or other stimuli. The EEG usually shows the repetitive periodic discharges. In the terminal stages of the condition, the myoclonus and epilepsy usually cease.

Post-traumatic epilepsy

Head trauma is an important cause of epilepsy. Estimates of frequency of injury and of the risk of post-traumatic epilepsy have varied widely in different studies, partly as a result of different definitions and changes in diagnosis and management. The figures given below are best-guess estimates based on modern practice. It is customary to draw a distinction between open head injury, where the dura is breached, and closed head injury, where there is no dural breach. Post-traumatic seizures are traditionally subdivided into immediate, early and late categories. Immediate seizures are defined as those that occur within the first 24 hours after injury, early seizures are those that occur within the first week and late seizures occur after 1 week.

Closed head injuries are most common in civilian practice, usually from road traffic accidents, falls or recreational injuries, and in different series have accounted for between 2 and 12% of all cases of epilepsy. If mild injury is included, the incidence of traumatic brain injury in the USA has been estimated to be as high as 825 cases per 100 000 per year, with about 100–200/100 000 per year admitted to hospital. Early seizures after closed head injury occur in about 2–6% of those admitted to hospital, with a higher frequency in children than in adults. Early seizures indicate a more severe injury, but have not been found generally to be an independent predictive risk factor of late seizures. Approximately 5% of patients – estimates have varied between 2 and 25% – requiring hospitalization for closed head trauma will subsequently develop epilepsy (late post-traumatic seizures). Mild head injury – defined as head injury without skull fracture and with less than 30 min of post-traumatic amnesia – is, in most studies, not associated with any markedly increased risk of epilepsy. Moderate head injury – defined as a head injury complicated by skull fracture or post-traumatic amnesia for more than 30 min – is followed by epilepsy in about 1–4% of cases. Severe head injury – defined as a head injury with post-traumatic amnesia of more than 24 h, intracranial haematoma or cerebral contusion – is followed by epilepsy, in most studies, in about 10–15% of patients. Less than 10% of all head injuries

admitted to hospital are categorized as severe and more than 70% as mild. The extra risk of epilepsy is highest during the first year, with onset of epilepsy peaking 4–8 months post-injury, and diminishes during the ensuing years. After 10 years only severe injuries still exhibit an increased risk of seizures. In one large study the incidence of epilepsy at 1 year post-injury was <1% (but three times the population risk) after mild injury, <1% (but seven times the population risk) after moderate injury and 6% (but 100 times the population risk) after severe injury. The 30-year cumulative incidence of seizures is 2.1% for mild injuries, 4.2% for moderate injuries and 16.7% for severe injuries. In a recent well-conducted study from Denmark, using the National Hospital Register, the risk of epilepsy was increased after a mild brain injury (relative risk [RR] 2.22, 95% confidence interval [CI] 2.07–2.38) and severe brain injury (7.40, 6.16–8.89). The risk was increased more than 10 years after mild brain injury (1.51, 1.24–1.85) and severe brain injury (4.29, 2.04–9.00).

Post-traumatic epilepsy is much more frequent after open head injury. This is particularly so in penetrating wartime injuries with between 30 and 50% of patients developing subsequent epilepsy. Overall, the risk of late epilepsy, if early epilepsy is present, is about 25% compared with 3% in patients who did not have early seizures. The risk of epilepsy after open head injury is greatest if the extent of cerebral damage is large and involves the frontal or temporal regions. About 50–60% of cases have their first (late) seizure within 12 months of the injury, with most cases developing within 4–8 months after the injury and 85% within 2 years.

Calculations of the risk of epilepsy in various circumstances after injury have been made. The presence of a dural breach (e.g. with a depressed fracture), an intracranial haematoma and long post-traumatic amnesia (≥24 h) has been found consistently to increase significantly the risk of subsequent epilepsy. In one series, the risk of seizures by 2 years was 27% in the presence of depressed skull fracture, 24% with subdural haematoma (and 44% if this was severe enough to need surgical evacuation), 23% with intracranial haematoma and 12% with long post-traumatic amnesia. In another study, risks of single and combined factors were calculated. The risk of late epilepsy after an intracranial haematoma alone was 35% and after a depressed fracture alone was 17%. If three factors were combined, the risk of post-traumatic epilepsy exceeded 50%. Conversely, in the absence of a depressed fracture, intracranial haematoma or early seizures, the risk of late epilepsy is less than 2% even if post-traumatic amnesia exceeds 24 h. Other factors found in some studies only to increase the rate of late seizures include the presence of early seizures, prolonged coma, depressed fracture without dural breach and the presence of an unreactive pupil at the time of injury.

The pathophysiology of post-traumatic epilepsy is complex and multifactorial. The kinetic energy imparted to the brain tissue produces pressure waves that disrupt tissue and lead to histopathological changes, including gliosis, axonal damage, wallerian degeneration and cystic white matter lesions. In addition, iron liberated from haemoglobin generates free radicals that disrupt cell membranes and have been implicated in post-traumatic epileptogenesis. Iron and other compounds have also been found to provoke intracellular calcium oscillations. Hippocampal damage after head injury also seems common (>80% in one series), and this may be due to enhanced excitability secondary to the death of inhibitory dentate hilar neurons. Such hyperexcitability can last for months after the trauma with reorganization of excitatory pathways such as mossy fibre sprouting.

Post-traumatic epilepsy can be difficult to treat, and in one series after open head injury 53% of patients still had active epilepsy 15 years after the injury. The risks of epilepsy are increased in those who have a family history of epilepsy, confirming the often multifactorial nature of epilepsy.

Antiepileptic drug therapy reduces the risk of early seizures. However, there has been controversy about the role of longer-term prophylactic antiepileptic drug treatment after head trauma. Early retrospective reports suggested that such prophylactic treatment reduced the incidence of subsequent epilepsy, although none of the subsequent large-scale prospective trials showed any protective effect on late seizures. Nevertheless, in some centres it is still usual to prescribe antiepileptic drugs after severe head injury for a period of 6 months or so.

There is typically a latent period between the head injury and the development of late epilepsy, usually of a few months but sometimes longer. Presumably, during this period, epileptogenic processes are occurring, and thus there is a clear potential for neuroprotective interventions to inhibit or abolish these processes. This is an area in which there is intensive research, but currently no specific therapy has been shown to be effective. Trials of antioxidants, antiperoxidants, steroids and chelating agents have taken place, but none has been shown to have any protective effect.

Epilepsy after neurosurgery

Neurosurgery is in effect a form of cerebral trauma, and not surprisingly can cause epilepsy. It is obviously important to define this risk, because it can influence the indications for surgery, and it is an important topic for preoperative counselling. The risk of late postoperative seizures is greater in patients with younger age, early postoperative seizures and severe neurological deficit. The incidence of seizures varies according to the nature of the underlying disease process, its site and its extent. A large retrospective study found an overall incidence of 17% for postoperative seizures in 877 consecutive patients undergoing supratentorial neurosurgery for non-traumatic conditions. The patients had no prior history of epilepsy and the minimum follow-up was 5 years. The incidence of seizures ranged from 4% in patients undergoing stereotactic procedures and ventricular drainage to 92% for patients being surgically treated for cerebral abscess. The risk of craniotomy for glioma was 19%, for intracranial haemorrhage 21% and for meningioma removal 22%. All these risks were greatly enhanced if seizures occurred preoperatively. Among patients developing postoperative seizures, 37% did so within the first postoperative week, 77% within the first year and 92% within the first 2 years. If early seizures occurred (i.e. those occurring in the first week), 41% of patients developed late recurrent seizures.

Studies after unruptured aneurysm show an overall risk of developing epilepsy of about 14%. The risk of a middle cerebral aneurysm resulting in epilepsy is 19%, and anterior communicating aneurysms and posterior communicating aneurysms carry a risk of about 10%. If the aneurysm has bled, causing an intracranial haematoma, the incidence of epilepsy is much higher, as it is if patients have perioperative complications including hemiparesis or meningitis, implying parenchymal damage. The overall risk of developing epilepsy after shunt procedures is about 10%, although this depends on the site of the shunt insertion. As is the case after cerebral trauma, the risks of epilepsy after neurosurgery are greatest in the first postoperative year, although a substantial proportion of cases (about 25%) experience their first seizures in the second postoperative year.

Whether or not the prophylactic use of anticonvulsants after neurosurgical procedures is worthwhile is highly controversial. The best studies seem to show no effect, although all investigations in this area have been open to criticism. More definitive investigations are required, but currently it is usual to prescribe prophylactic anticonvulsant drugs for several months after major supratentorial neurosurgery and then gradually to withdraw the medication unless seizures have occurred.

Cerebral tumours

Brain tumours are responsible for about 6% of all newly diagnosed cases of epilepsy. The rate is greatest in adults, and about a quarter of adults presenting with newly developing focal epilepsy have an underlying tumour, compared with less than 5% in children. Seizures occur in about 50% of all people with brain tumours. The frequency of seizures is high in tumours in the frontal, central and temporal regions, lower in posterior cortically placed tumours and very low in subcortical tumours. The surgical therapy of tumours is considered on pp. 339–341.

Gliomas

Gliomas are the most common form of brain tumour causing epilepsy. Slow-growing, low-grade, well-differentiated gliomas are the most epileptogenic lesions. In the Montreal series of 230 patients with gliomas, seizures occurred in 92% of those with oligodendrogliomas, 70% of those with astrocytomas and 37% of those with glioblastomas. Overall, slow-growing or benign tumours account for 5–10% of all adult epilepsies, and less in children. The history of epilepsy will often have extended for decades, sometimes even into infancy. In chronic refractory tumoral epilepsy, oligodendrogliomas account for between 10 and 30%, dysembryoplastic neuroepithelial tumours (DNETs or DNTs) for 10–30%, astrocytomas for 10–30%, gangliogliomas for about 10–20% and hamartomas for between 10 and 20%. These tumours are sometimes associated, particularly if situated in the temporal lobe, with hippocampal sclerosis. The generation of epileptic discharges does not take place within the tumoral tissue (the exception is in the DNETs – see below) but in the surrounding tissue, and this has implications for surgical therapy. The mechanisms of epileptogenesis in patients with brain tumours include impaired vascularization of the surrounding cerebral cortex, morphological neuronal alterations, changes in the excitatory and inhibitory synaptic mechanisms, and genetic susceptibility.

Gangliogliomas

These are mixed tumours that are composed of neoplastic glial and neuronal cell types and comprise 10% or more of the neoplasms removed at temporal lobectomy. Seizures are the primary presenting symptom in 80–90% of patients with gangliogliomas, and can develop at any age. These tumours are typically frontal or temporal in location and the outcome for seizure control is good if the tumour can be resected.

Dysembryoplastic neuroepithelial tumours

The DNET is a pathological entity only recently differentiated from other forms of 'benign glioma'. They are in fact a relatively common cause of 'tumoral epilepsy', accounting for 10–30% of resected tumours in the temporal lobe. DNETs are developmental in origin and the tumours coexist with other forms of cortical dysplasia, including focal cortical dysplasia, heterotopias and microdysgenesis. The tumours are most commonly situated in the temporal lobe (two-thirds), but can occur in any cortical region. They are benign tumours with only a slight propensity for growth, and epilepsy is usually the only clinical symptom. The epilepsy can present in children or adults, and the seizures are usually partial in nature and vary considerably in severity. Surgical resection is indicated only if lack of seizure control warrants the risks involved. Surgical resection, or even partial resection, will usually control the seizures and DNETs are thus an important pathology to identify (see pp. 340–341).

Hamartomas

These benign tumours account for 15–20% of tumours removed at temporal lobectomy; they are more common in children. Their pathological features include proliferation of glial and neuronal elements, and they can be associated with other types of cortical dysplasia. Indeed the distinction of cortical dysplasia, hamartomas and relatively indolent neoplasms, such as DNETs, can be blurred. The classic clinicopathological finding in TSC is the periventricular glial nodule or subependymal tuber. Histologically, these lesions are hamartomas and consist of foci of gliosis, which include both glial cells and neurons. Surgical resection of isolated hamartomas is often curative. In tuberous sclerosis complex, however, individual tubers are usually only one part of a wider epileptogenic process, and only rarely can a seizure focus be localized to a single cortical tuber that can be successfully resected.

Hypothalamic hamartomas (and gelastic epilepsy)

Hypothalamic hamartomas are a particular form of hamartoma. These are benign tumours, usually small and sometimes confined to the tuber cinerium. They are present in young children, and characteristically present with gelastic seizures, learning disability and behavioural disturbance, and later with precocious puberty. They are diagnosed by MRI, but the lesions can be very subtle, especially if small, without mass effect, and isodense on both T1- and T2-weighted sequences.

Gelastic seizures are highly characteristic of tumours of the floor of the third ventricle and particularly of hypothalamic hamartomas (although they do occur occasionally in temporal lobe epilepsy). The seizures start before the age of 3 years in most cases, and are often very frequent. The attacks are brief, and take the form of sudden laughter associated with other variable motor features (clonic movements, head and eye deviation). The laughter is 'mirthless', is not associated with any emotional feelings of joy or happiness, and occurs in situations that do not provoke humour. The combination of severe gelastic epilepsy, precocious puberty and intellectual impairment can be a devastating disability. The seizures do not usually respond to conventional drug therapy, but surgical resection of the tumours can be very successful, with complete seizure remission expected in about 50% of cases.

Meningioma

Epilepsy is the first symptom of meningioma in 20–50% of cases. Meningiomas located over the convexity, falx or parasagittal regions or sphenoid ridge are especially likely to cause epilepsy. There is no relationship between the presence of epilepsy and histological type. Surgical resection can be expected to stop seizures in about 30–60% of operated cases.

CNS infection

CNS infections are an important risk factor for epilepsy. Seizures can be the presenting or the only symptom, or one component of a more diffuse cerebral disorder.

Meningitis and encephalitis

The risk of chronic epilepsy after encephalitis or meningitis is almost sevenfold greater than that in the population in general. The increased risk is highest during the first 5 years after infection, but remains elevated for up to 15 years. The risk is much higher after encephalitis (RR 16.2) than bacterial meningitis (RR 4.2) or aseptic meningitis (RR 2.3). The presence of early seizures (i.e. during the acute phase of the infection) greatly influences the risk of subsequent unprovoked seizures. As encephalitis and bacterial meningitis are more prevalent in childhood and early adult life, most cases of postinfectious epilepsy develop in young individuals.

The most common forms of bacterial meningitis are now due to *Streptococcus pneumoniae* (pneumoccal meningitis) and *Neisseria meningitides* (meningococcal meningitis). *Haemophilus influenzae* type b (Hib) used to be a leading cause but new vaccines have virtually eradicated the condition in western countries. Meningococcal meningitis is the most serious common but vaccines are now also available. Its incidence varies, and in Europe, for example, the highest incidence is in Scotland and Iceland. Ninety-five per cent of cases are due to serogroups B and C, and the case fatality rate is between 5 and 10%. Treatment is with penicillin or rifampicin, but antibiotic resistance is growing. Viral meningitis is common but is usually mild and rarely results in epilepsy.

Encephalitis is most commonly due to viral infection, but other infectious agents can cause postencephalitic epilepsy (Table 4.11). The most common serious viral encephalitis is due to herpes simplex virus type 1 (HSV-1). The incidence of severe HSV-1 encephalitis is about $1/10^6$ per year, but it is possible that more minor infection occurs that escapes detection. It has indeed been postulated that many cases of epilepsy, currently considered cryptogenic, are due to occult viral infection – although hard evidence in support of this point of view is entirely lacking. Immunological studies show varicella virus also to be a common cause of CNS infection, but overt varicella encephalitis is less common than HSV-1 encephalitis. In the USA, St Louis virus (a mosquito-borne arbovirus) is common. In Asia, Japanese B viral encephalitis results in up to 15 000 deaths annually. Two recent viral encephalitides that are increasing in frequency are those due to West Nile virus and Nipah virus.

Seizures are a frequent symptom in the acute phase of severe HSV encephalitis, and many survivors are left with neurological sequelae including severe epilepsy. The seizures take partial and secondarily generalized forms, and status epilepticus is common. The prognosis for epilepsy (and other sequelae) is worse in those with delayed antiviral treatment and with a low Glasgow Coma Scale score at the height of the illness. Of the other viral encephalitides, enteroviral encephalitis is usually mild without sequelae and arboviral encephalitis has a variable prognosis (depending on viral type).

The clinical diagnosis can be confirmed by serological tests, from cerebrospinal fluid (CSF) and serum, and by neuroimaging. Viral encephalitis needs to be differentiated from acute disseminated encephalomyelitis (ADEM), which can present with a very similar picture, and other causes of non-infectious encephalopathy. Precise diagnosis of viral encephalitis can be difficult. HSV may be isolated from CSF in up to 50% of cases of neonatal HSV

Table 4.11 Causes of infectious encephalitis.

Causes of infective encephalitis in the immunocompetent patient

Viral: herpes simplex virus (HSV) type 1, other herpes viruses (e.g. varicella, HSV type 2, CMV, EBV, HSV type 6), measles, mumps, rubella, rabies, arbovirus (e.g. Japanese B, St Louis, West Nile, equine and tick-borne viruses), adenovirus, HIV, influenza (A, B), enterovirus, poliovirus

Bacterial and rickettsial (uncommon): *Bartonella* spp., *Borrelia burgdorferi*, *Brucella* spp., *Leptospira interrogans*, *Listeria monocytogenes*, *Mycobacterium tuberculosis*, *Mycoplasma pneumoniae*, *Rickettsia rickettsii*, Q fever and other rickettsial infections, *Treponema pallidum*, leptospirosis, *Nocardia actinomyces*, *Salmonella typhi*, *Legionella*

Protozoal (uncommon): malaria (*Plasmodium falciparum*), *Toxoplasma gondii*, *Naegleria fowleri*, *Acanthamoeba* spp., cysticercosis, *Echinococcus* spp., *Trypanosoma* spp., schistosomiasis

Fungal (uncommon): blastomycosis, coccidioidomycosis, histoplasmosis, cryptococci, aspergillosis, candidiasis

Causes of infectious encephalitis in the immunocompromised patient

Viral: enterovirus, cytomegalovirus, HSV types 1, 2, 6, JC virus, measles, rubella, varicella

Protozoal: amoebic meningoencephalitis, toxoplasmosis

Fungal: *Cryptococcus neoformans*, coccidioidomycosis, blastomycosis, histoplasmosis, *Aspergillus*, *Candida*

CMV, cytomegalovirus; EBV, Epstein–Barr virus.

infection but is rarely found in specimens obtained from older children and adults with HSV encephalitis. Serological testing during the acute and convalescent phases of illness is of little immediate value in the diagnosis of HSV or enteroviral encephalitis. In contrast, the presence of arbovirus-specific immunoglobulin M (IgM) in spinal fluid is diagnostic of arboviral encephalitis. Polymerase chain reaction (PCR) is much more sensitive, with a 95% sensitivity and 100% specificity found in patients with biopsy-proven HSV encephalitis. PCR techniques show excellent specificity and sensitivity in the diagnosis of enteroviral meningitis. MRI may be normal early in the course of HSV encephalitis, but within days focal oedema, typically in the temporal lobes

bilaterally, is evident. EEG is a useful complementary test for the diagnosis of HSV encephalitis, showing focal unilateral or bilateral periodic discharges localized in the temporal lobes. Viral encephalitis should be treated with aciclovir or other antiviral therapies, and the earlier therapy is started the better the outcome. The epilepsy is treated along conventional lines.

Patients with acquired immune deficiency syndrome (AIDS) and other immunocompromised states have a different range of pathogens (see Table 4.11), and cerebral infection is a common feature of the condition; the most common opportunistic CNS infections are cryptococcal meningitis, toxoplasmosis, tuberculosis and cytomegalovirus (CMV) encephalitis. Seizures may also be a sign of progressive multifocal leucoencephalopathy in HIV, although usually it is a minor aspect of the clinical presentation.

Cerebral malaria

Seizures, and typically status epilepticus, are particularly common in the acute phase of cerebral malaria. Convulsive and focal seizures can occur, but in young children in a coma seizures can be subtle, taking minor forms such as eye deviation or changes in respiratory pattern or salivation. Prolonged convulsions are associated with increased mortality and also neurological deficits in survivors, so detection and emergency therapy are important. The benzodiazepines, particularly diazepam, should be used initially, and phenobarbital used as second-line therapy. Artemisinin derivatives should be given as antimalarials in the acute phase, combined with cinchona alkaloids such as mefloquine. Chronic epilepsy is common after cerebral malaria, particularly if seizures occurred in the acute phase, and one study has shown a 9–11 (CI 2–18)-fold increase in risk of epilepsy compared with children without malaria.

Pyogenic cerebral abscess

Pyogenic brain abscess is an uncommon but serious cause of infective epilepsy. Abscesses range in size from microscopic foci of inflammatory cells to major encapsulated necrotic areas of a cerebral hemisphere exerting significant mass effect. Modern imaging has greatly improved the survival rate and management of brain abscesses but the mortality rate of acute cerebral abscess is still 5–10%. The estimated annual incidence of brain abscesses in the USA is 1 in 10 000 hospital admissions, and abscess surgery accounts for 0.7% of all neurosurgery operations. Brain abscesses occur at any age but are most common in young adult life. The abscesses develop in association with a contiguous suppurating process (usually otitis media, sinus disease or mastoiditis; 50%), due to haematogenous spread from a distant focus (25%), as a complication of intracranial surgery (15%) and as a result of trauma (10%). Brain abscesses related to middle-ear infection are the most commonly encountered and are often solitary, developing in the inferior portion of the ipsilateral temporal lobe. Brain abscess is a rare complication of bacterial meningitis in adults; it is, however, more common in infants, particularly those with Gram-negative meningitis. Haematogenous metastatic spread from distant parts of the body frequently leads to the development of brain abscesses. The most common site of origin is a pyogenic lung infection, such as a lung abscess, bronchiectasis, empyema, cystic fibrosis or acute endocarditis. Other potential primary foci include osteomyelitis, wound and skin infections, cholecystitis, pelvic infection and other forms of intra-abdominal sepsis. Brain abscesses from blood-spread infections are most likely to occur in the middle cerebral territory and at the grey–white matter junction, and are frequently multifocal. Brain abscess complicates approximately 3–15% of penetrating craniocerebral injuries, especially those caused by gunshot injuries.

The species of bacterium responsible for brain abscesses depends on the pathogenic mechanism involved. Commonly isolated organisms are streptococci, including aerobic, anaerobic and microaerophilic types. *Strep. pneumoniae* is a rarer cause of brain abscesses, which are often the sequel to occult CSF rhinorrhoea and also to pneumococcal pneumonia in elderly patients. Enteric bacteria and *Bacteroides* spp. are isolated in 20–40% of cases and often in mixed culture. Anaerobic organisms have become increasingly important organisms and in many instances more than a single bacterial species is recovered. Gram-negative bacilli rarely occur alone. Staphylococcal abscesses account for 10–15% of cases and are usually caused by penetrating head injury or bacteraemia secondary to endocarditis. Clostridial infections are most often post-traumatic. Rarely *Actinomyces* or *Nocardia* spp. are the causative agents of a brain abscess.

The diagnosis of brain abscesses has been greatly facilitated by modern imaging, and most cases can now be identified rapidly. Surgical resection (see pp. 343 and 356) is the treatment of choice. The mortality rate is about 10% and up to 50% of patients have permanent neurological deficit after brain abscesses. Epilepsy follows in between 30 and 80% of cases, and can sometimes develop years after the acute infection. All patients with preoperative seizures are likely to continue to have seizures postoperatively, and the risk remains high for several years after the acute infection. Epilepsy is more likely after frontal lobe abscesses. Epilepsy after a cerebral abscess can be very difficult to control. Antiepileptic drug treatment follows the usual principles, but in severe cases resection of the abscess cavity can be considered. Severe secondarily generalized epilepsy following a frontal abscess can respond to corpus callosotomy (see pp. 356–357). Given the high likelihood of developing seizures, all patients with supratentorial brain abscesses should routinely be placed on prophylactic antiepileptic drugs for at least 1–2 years. If no seizures occur at this stage, the drugs can be then withdrawn, but only if the EEG shows no epileptogenic activity.

Neurocysticercosis

Worldwide, neurocysticercosis (NCC) is the most common parasitic disease of the CNS and a major cause of epilepsy in endemic areas such as Mexico, India and China. Epilepsy is the most common clinical manifestation and usual presenting feature of NCC. The condition is a helminthiasis caused by the encysted larval stage, *Cysticercus cellulosae*, of the pork tapeworm *Taenia solium*. In the first stage, the human (definitive) host ingests undercooked diseased pork containing viable cysticerci from within which the scolex (head) of the organism evaginates in the gut and attaches to the intestinal mucosa. Over 3 months, the tapeworm matures to a length of 2–7 m. Gravid segments containing eggs are released into the faeces, often unknown to the host. After ingestion, eggs hatch and activate in the pig (intermediate host) small intestine and develop in the CNS and striated muscle. Humans become intermediate hosts by ingesting infected tissue, and the lifecycle is completed in the human CNS, skin and muscle. Parenchymal cysts usually lie dormant for many years and symptoms usually coincide with larval death and an intense inflammatory response caused by the release of larval antigens. The solitary cerebral parenchymal lesion is a common form of presentation, but lesions are often multiple. Over time, the cysts shrink progressively and then calcify or disappear completely. Seizures are the most common symptom and develop when a cyst is degenerating or around a chronic calcified lesion. In the racemose form of NCC, the cysts can obstruct CSF flow and present with mass effect, hydrocephalus or basal arachnoiditis (the treatment of these cases differs from those presenting simply with epilepsy and is outside the scope of this book).

Diagnosis is made by imaging and by serological tests. CSF and EEG are rather non-specific. Computed tomography (CT) is particularly useful for showing calcified inactive lesions. MRI is superior for demonstrating subarachnoid or intraventricular cysts and for showing inflammation around a cyst. Cysts may be single or multiple and at different pathological stages at any given time. A classification system that corresponds to parasite viability has been proposed, with divisions into active, transitional and inactive forms. In the active stage the CT appearance is that of a rounded, hypodense area or there may be a CSF-like signal on MRI. The 'starry night' effect – the presence of multiple eccentric mural nodules – is characteristic of NCC, although it may also be seen in cases of toxoplasma infection. The transitional stage is due to cystic degeneration. This appears on CT as a diffuse hypodense area with an irregular border which enhances with contrast. They usually appear as high signal areas on T2-weighted MRI. Lastly, when the cyst dies, the lesion either disappears or becomes a calcified inactive nodule of low intensity on proton-weighted MRI or homogeneous high density on CT scan. Standard enzyme-linked immunosorbent assay (ELISA) diagnostic techniques have proved less useful than hoped for because of high false-negative and false-positive rates. Newer enzyme-linked immunoelectron transfer blot (EITB) assays on CSF or serum appear to have higher sensitivity (98%) and specificity (100%) in multiple cysticercosis. Its superiority to ELISA is due to its ability to detect up to seven glycoproteins specific to *T. solium*. It is visualized similarly to a western blot, so that non-specific bands can be ignored, thereby ruling out cross-reactivity. Recently, an antigen detection ('capture') assay specific for viable metacestodes in CSF has been designed. So far, this has proved to be perhaps the most reliable method of detecting active cases of NCC in epidemiological studies. Serology is a sensitive way of detecting exposure, but in endemic areas, where population exposure rates are high, positive serology in any individual does not necessarily imply that NCC is the cause of the symptoms.

Cerebral tuberculoma is the main differential diagnosis, but there are imaging differences. Typically, the lesions of NCC are well circumscribed, discrete, <20 mm in size and superficially located; they enhance relatively little, may have visible scolexes and less perilesional oedema, and only occasionally cause midline shift. Multiple cysts have the characteristic 'starry sky' appearance.

The mainstay of treatment is the control of seizures with antiepileptic drugs. Seizures caused by a single cyst are usually easily controlled. It is not a general policy to use anti-cysticercal drugs, especially with single lesions, because the enhancing cysticerci shown on imaging are by definition dying away and will resolve spontaneously. Multiple lesions are generally treated with anti-parasitic drugs, although these drugs are contraindicated in the presence of cerebral oedema. If needed, two anti-cysticercal drugs are in wide use in endemic areas – albendazole and praziquantel – although there are no controlled trials to establish specific indications, definitive doses and treatment duration. If anti-cysticercal drugs are to be used, steroids need to be given in co-medication to prevent a sudden rise in intracranial pressure and exacerbation of symptoms. The role of surgical biopsy in diagnosis is discussed below.

Tuberculoma

TB remains a major problem in developing countries and the incidence is also rising in industrialized countries with increasing migration and the spread of HIV. The most common form of TB is pulmonary infection, and the incidence of intracranial tuberculoma (tuberculous abscess) has decreased, particularly in western countries, owing to the BCG vaccination programme. In the early twentieth century tuberculomas accounted for about a third of all space-occupying lesions. The incidence fell dramatically throughout the century, although recently it has started rising again, and today tuberculomas account for about 3% of all cerebral mass lesions in India, for example, and 13% of all cerebral lesions in HIV-infected patients. The diagnosis of intracranial tuberculoma depends on neuroimaging. Although both CT and MRI are equally sensitive in visualizing the intracranial tuberculoma, MRI is superior in demonstrating the extent and maturity of the lesion, especially for brain-stem lesions. A 'target lesion' in an enhanced CT scan is considered highly characteristic of tuberculoma, although this sign may also be produced by cerebral toxoplasmosis.

Tuberculomas present particularly with epilepsy, and therapy for the epilepsy follows conventional lines. Surgical resection of the tuberculoma was the usual procedure in the past, but increasingly a conservative approach is now initially taken. Surgery is still indicated in the initial stages in cases of diagnostic uncertainty, and where larger, symptomatic mass lesions cause midline shift and severe intracranial hypertension. In patients presenting simply with epilepsy, it is now usual to treat with anti-tubercular and antiepileptic drugs (with a short course of adjunctive steroids), and to defer surgery. When medical therapy is initiated, without diagnostic confirmation from a biopsy, the patient should be carefully monitored and, if the mass does not decrease in size after 12–16 weeks of therapy, surgical therapy should be considered (the indications for this our outlined on pp. 343–344). With early diagnosis and a balanced combination of surgical and medical management, tuberculomas are now potentially curable.

Acute seizures with CT evidence of a single enhancing lesion

Newly developing seizures associated with a single enhancing lesion on CT are a common clinical problem in endemic areas such as India. The differential diagnosis includes NCC, TB, gliomas and other tumours, toxoplasmosis and other infective lesions. Over 90% of the lesions in India are due to NCC, and currently the usual management strategy is to screen the patient for other signs of TB, and if none is present not to give anti-tubercular therapy. CT is repeated in 12–16 weeks and, if the lesion has not regressed, or has increased, a review of diagnosis including surgical biopsy is the preferred approach (pp. 343–344). Antiepileptic drugs are given.

Cerebrovascular disease

Epilepsy can complicate all forms of cerebrovascular disease. Stroke is the most commonly identified cause of epilepsy in elderly people, and occult stroke also explains the occurrence of many cases of apparently cryptogenic epilepsies in elderly individuals. A history of stroke has been found to be associated with an increased lifetime occurrence of epilepsy (odds ratio [OR] 3.3; 95% CI 1.3–8.5). Among the other vascular determinants, only a history of hypertension was associated with the occurrence of unprovoked seizures (OR 1.6; 95% CI 1.0–2.4). The risk of unprovoked seizures rises to 4.1 (95% CI 1.5–11.0) in individuals with a history of both stroke and hypertension.

Cerebral haemorrhage

The reported risk of chronic epilepsy due to intracranial haemorrhage has varied greatly from series to series, but is generally in the region of 5–10%. The incidence of early epilepsy (seizures in the first week) is higher, up to 30% in some series, with status epilepticus in about 10%. Early seizures do not necessarily lead to chronic epilepsy, although they increase the long-term risk, and about a third of those with early seizures continue to have a liability for epilepsy. Epilepsy is common after large haemorrhages and haemorrhages that involve the cerebral cortex,

less common in deep haematomas and rare after subtentorial haemorrhage. The epilepsy almost always develops within 2 years of the haemorrhage. The risk of seizures after subarachnoid haemorrhage is between 20 and 34%, and the risk of chronic epilepsy among survivors of subarachnoid haemorrhage is highest in those with early seizures, intracerebral haematoma or other persisting neurological sequelae.

Cerebral infarction

After cerebral infarction, epilepsy occurs in about 6% of patients within 12 months and 11% within 5 years of the stroke. Epilepsy is more common in cerebral infarcts located in the anterior hemisphere, and involving the cortex. The standardized mortality ratio (SMR) for epilepsy after infarction has been found to be 5.9 (95% CI 3.5–9.4), and the risk of developing seizures is highest during the first year, and higher if there is a history of recurrent stroke. There is an inverse correlation between age and risk of seizures with a peak in patients younger than 55 years. In a multivariant analysis, early seizures and recurrent strokes were the only clinical factors shown to predict the occurrence of epilepsy after infarction.

Occult degenerative cerebrovascular disease

Epilepsy can also complicate occult cerebrovascular disease. Patients with late-onset epilepsy are significantly more likely to have otherwise asymptomatic ischaemic lesions on CT than age-matched controls, and it has been estimated from such CT-based studies that overt or occult cerebrovascular disease underlies about half of the epilepsies developing after the age of 50 years. Late-onset epilepsy can be the first manifestation of cerebrovascular disease. Between 5 and 10% of patients presenting with stroke have a history of prior epileptic seizures in the recent past, and in the absence of other causes new-onset seizures should prompt a screen for vascular risk factors.

Arteriovenous malformations

An arteriovenous malformation (AVM) is a racemose network of arterial and venous channels that communicate directly, rather than through a capillary bed. Between 17 and 36% of supratentorial AVMs present with seizures, with or without associated neurological deficits, and 40–50% with haemorrhage. Smaller AVMs (<3 cm diameter) are more likely to present with haemorrhage than large ones. Conversely, large and/or superficial malformations are more epileptogenic, as are AVMs in the temporal lobe. About 40% of patients with large AVMs have epilepsy, and epilepsy is the presenting symptom in about 20%. Irrespective of the initial presentation, a significant proportion of patients with cerebral AVMs will develop epilepsy after diagnosis. The risk of seizures seems to be higher the younger the patient at the time of diagnosis. In one study, among patients aged between 10 and 19 years, there was a 44% risk of epilepsy by age 20. This risk declined to 31% for patients aged 20–29 and to 6% for patients aged 30–60. The annual risk of bleeding of an AVM is in the region of 2% per year, irrespective of whether the malformation presented with haemorrhage, and the average mortality rate is about 1% per year. The risk depends on the size of the AVM, its growth, the presence of aneurysms, the type of feeding and draining vessels, and the anatomy. AVMs also show highly characteristic MRI appearances, with high signal on T2-weighted images, often with a notch-like configuration, and areas of decreased signal intensity representing previous intralesional bleeding. The treatment of large lesions is usually carried out with the aim of preventing haemorrhage rather than controlling epilepsy. However, the complete resections of small AVMs will often control seizures.

Cavernous haemangiomas (cavernomas)

Cavernous haemangiomas are well-circumscribed hamartomatous lesions consisting of irregularly walled sinusoidal vascular channels, located within the brain but without intervening neural tissue, with large feeding arteries or draining veins. Pathologically, they consist of endothelium-lined 'caverns' filled with blood and surrounded by a matrix of collagen and fibroblasts. They have the potential to haemorrhage, calcify or thrombose and are multiple in 50% of cases. They account for 5–13% of vascular malformations of the CNS and are present in 0.02–0.13% of postmortem series. Most of these lesions present in the third and fourth decades of life, but 20–30% present earlier in childhood or early adult life. Cavernomas can increase in size and number over time, particularly in genetically determined cases and in those in whom cavernomas have developed after cerebral irradiation. However, in most cases, the factors influencing the development of new lesions or growth of existing lesions is unknown. At least 15–20% of patients remain symptom free throughout their lives. Patients present with seizures (40–70%), focal neurological deficits (35–50%), non-specific headaches (10–30%) and cerebral haemorrhage. The seizures are typically partial in nature and often brief, infrequent and minor in form. Cavernous malformation can lead to death from cerebrovascular accident, but, because of their low flow characteristics, haemorrhage from cavernomas is generally less severe than haemorrhage from AVMs. Retinal, skin and liver lesions have occasionally been reported, presumably on a genetic basis. Familial clustering can be found in 10–30% of cavernous haemangiomas, and familial cases have been found to be linked to genes at three different loci: the *CCM1*, *CCM2* and *CCM3* genes. Forty per cent of familial cases are due to *CCM1*, with higher rates among Hispanic individuals. Genetic testing is available.

The lesions are usually diagnosed on CT or MRI, whereas cerebral angiography often shows no abnormality. Typical CT appearances are those of a well-circumscribed hyperdense area with moderate enhancement and variable mass effect. CT may also show previous bleeding, calcification, oedema or cystic areas associated with the lesion. MRI is the most sensitive investigation. On T2-weighted images the typical appearance of cavernomas is that of a reticulated core of mixed signal representing blood in various states of degradation surrounded by a hypointense haemosiderin halo. T1-weighted images show a similar pattern but they are less sensitive. There is slight contrast enhancement in some cases.

Cavernous malformations are twice as likely to be associated with seizures as other vascular lesions, such as AVMs, or tumours with similar volume and location, and the seizures are probably produced by the deposition of blood breakdown products, notably iron, around the lesions during leaks or small haemorrhages. The risk of overt haemorrhage from a cavernoma is of the order of 0.5–2% per annum.

Medical therapy follows conventional lines, and seizures can often be controlled on relatively simple antiepileptic drug regimens. Surgical therapy is outlined on pp. 342–343, and resection is useful in patients with single lesions and particularly in those with superficial, easily accessible, cortical lesions. Focused beam radiation is an alternative therapy.

Venous malformations

Venous malformations are congenital anomalies of normal venous drainage. They are the most commonly documented intracranial vascular malformation by either brain imaging or postmortem examination, with a prevalence as high as 3%. They can be associated with cavernous malformations or, more rarely, with AVMs. On MRI they appear as a stellate vascular or contrast-enhancing mass. Angiography typically shows a caput medusa appearance in the late venous phase. These lesions are thought neither to have a high risk of haemorrhage nor to cause epilepsy.

Collagen vascular diseases and other cerebral vasculitides

The epilepsy can be due to the primary disease process and also to the secondary complications such as arterial hypertension, infarction, vasculitic changes, immunological reactions, and hepatic or renal failure. Epilepsy is a common symptom of all forms of cerebral vasculitis, and particularly in systemic lupus erythematosus (SLE). In SLE, seizures can be the presenting and only symptom, and occur during the course of the illness in about 25% of cases. Seizures are particularly common in severe or chronic cases and in lupus-induced encephalopathy. Epilepsy can also occur in Behçet disease, Sjögren syndrome, mixed connective tissue disease, Henoch–Schönlein purpura, and other forms of large-, medium- or small-vessel vasculitis, sometimes on the basis of infarction.

Other vascular disorders

Cortical venous infarcts are particularly epileptogenic, at least in the acute phase, and may underlie a significant proportion of apparently spontaneous epileptic seizures complicating other medical conditions and pregnancy. Seizures also occur with cerebrovascular lesions secondary to rheumatic heart disease, endocarditis, mitral valve prolapse, cardiac tumours and cardiac arrhythmia, or after carotid endarterectomy. Infarction is also an important cause of seizures in neonatal epilepsy. Seizures are part of the acute presentation of eclampsia, posterior reversible encephalopathy syndrome (PRES), hypertensive encephalopathy and malignant hypertension, and in the anoxic encephalopathy that follows cardiac arrest or cardiopulmonary surgery. Unruptured aneurysms occasionally present as epilepsy, especially if large and if embedded in the temporal lobe, e.g. a giant middle cerebral or anterior communicating aneurysm.

Other neurological disorders

Demyelinating disorders

Several clinical series have reported an association between epilepsy and multiple sclerosis (MS). In one small population-based study, patients with MS had a threefold but non-significant increase (SMR 3.0; 95% CI 0.6–8.8) in the risk of epilepsy compared with the general population. In another series the cumulative risk of epilepsy in patients with MS was found to be 1.1% at 5 years, 1.8% at 10 years and 3.1% at 15 years. The mean interval until the onset of epilepsy is about 7 years after the onset of MS. Convulsive status epilepticus has been reported more frequently in patients with MS. Epilepsy is more likely to occur in large lesions and lesions that abut the cortex, and occasionally MS presents with an acute mass lesion with seizures. Although in some patients epilepsy precedes MS by years or decades, there is no evidence of an increased risk of epilepsy before the onset of the symptoms due to MS.

ADEM is an acute inflammatory demyelinating disorder that can follow systemic infections, and is immunologically mediated. Epilepsy is a feature of the acute attack, and occurs much more commonly than in an acute attack of MS. ADEM can follow infections with many different viruses (notably measles, mumps, rubella, varicella, HIV, hepatitis A and B, Epstein–Barr virus, CMV) or other infectious agents (notably *Mycoplasma*, *Streptococcus*, *Borrelia*, *Campylobacter* and *Legionella* spp., and *Chlamydia leptospira*). The incidence after measles infection is about 1 in 1000, after varicella infection, about 1 in 10 000 and after rubella infection about 1 in 20 000.

Inflammatory and immunological diseases of the nervous system

Epilepsy can be a complication of many inflammatory and immunological diseases affecting the CNS. The mechanisms of seizures can be due to the direct effect of immunological processes (e.g. in Rasmussen encephalitis) or an indirect effect due to vascular disease and cerebral infarction (e.g. in the cerebral vasculitides). In many conditions the mechanisms are unknown.

Rasmussen encephalitis

This is a rare progressive neurological disorder, of unknown cause, in which severe epilepsy coexists with slowly progressive atrophy of one cerebral hemisphere. The condition usually begins in late childhood, but can start in adults and also in young children. Pathologically, there is severe atrophy of one hemisphere with histological evidence of perivascular lymphocytic infiltration, neuronal loss and microglial nodule formation. The pathological changes are strikingly unilateral, and where changes do occur in the opposite hemisphere they are usually minor. The cause is unclear, although viral and immunological factors have been implicated. The genomes of various viruses have been found in biopsy tissue, including the Epstein–Barr virus and HSV, and IgG, IgA and C3 have been found. Glu-R3 antibodies have been reported in the sera of some patients. None of these findings, however, appears to be consistently present.

Clinically, the condition is highly characteristic, with the slow development of severe epilepsy, a progressive hemiparesis and other signs of unilateral hemisphere dysfunction. The condition usually presents with partial epilepsy. This can take any form and typically progresses and is difficult to control. Episodes of EPC are highly characteristic. Secondarily generalized seizures also occur. As the epilepsy worsens, the patients develop a slowly progressive hemiparesis, which evolves over months or years. Unilateral cognitive dysfunction and other neurological signs, such as aphasia (if the dominant hemisphere is involved), occur. Hemianopia occurs in 50% of cases eventually. Psychiatric disturbances are common. MRI demonstrates progressive cortical atrophy, typically beginning around the sylvian fissure and eventually extending to involve the whole hemisphere. Patchy white matter hyperintensity also occurs involving one hemisphere predominantly, and sometimes the contralateral cerebellum. The CSF is usually normal although it may show oligoclonal bands. The EEG shows multifocal epileptiform discharges predominantly, but not necessarily exclusively, over the affected hemisphere.

Treatment of the epilepsy is difficult. Conventional therapy is frequently ineffective, especially in the case of focal motor seizures or EPC, which can persist in spite of massive antiepileptic therapy. Corticosteroids, plasmapheresis and antiviral agents (ganciclovir, zidovudine) have been given with some success but seem usually not to have major benefit. The best reported results are with high-dose intravenous immunoglobulin, and frequently repeated courses may be required. Hemispherectomy or large multilobar resection is recommended in a proportion of cases and will alleviate the epilepsy in most operated cases. The evaluation for hemispherectomy and its timing can be difficult, and should be carried out by an experienced unit. The condition tends to 'burn out' after a number of years, leaving the patient with permanent and severe unihemispherical dysfunction.

Gastrointestinal inflammatory disorders

Seizures are the most common neurological complication of the inflammatory bowel diseases (ulcerative colitis and Crohn disease), occurring in one series in 6% of cases. The epilepsy may be a direct effect or caused indirectly by dehydration or sepsis. Neurological complications occur in about 10% of patients with Whipple disease, and the condition presents neurologically in 5%. In a series of cases with neurological symptoms, myoclonus occurred in 25% and seizures in 23%. About 10% of patients with coeliac disease have neurological symptoms, and epilepsy is associated with several rather distinctive neurological including seizures with occipital calcification on CT, and

seizures with myoclonus and cerebellar ataxia and sometimes dementia. Coeliac disease may also cause cerebral vasculitis.

Other immune-mediated disorders

Myoclonus and seizures are also a prominent feature of Hashimoto thyroiditis, a relapsing encephalopathy associated with high titres of thyroid antibody. Epilepsy is also a feature, although often not prominent, of the primary granulomatous diseases of the CNS such as sarcoidosis.

Anti-NMDA receptor encephalitis is a common form of acute encephalopathy, usually affecting women of whom 50% will have an ovarian teratoma. It presents with the rapid development of psychiatric symptoms seizures (approx 75%), stupor or coma, characteristic dyskinesias and autonomic instability and respiratory disturbance.

Paraneoplastic disorders can cause seizures. EPC can occur as a paraneoplastic phenomenon. This is usually in the context of a paraneoplastic 'cortical encephalomyelitis' due to various tumours (notably small cell lung cancer and breast carcinoma). The MRI scan can show non-specific T2-weighted signal changes. Seizures also occur in limbic encephalitis of paraneoplastic origin – often associated with memory loss, and psychiatric and behavioural changes.

Limbic encephalitis associated with voltage-gated potassium channel antibodies is another condition presenting acutely with seizures memory disturbance and neuropsychiatric changes. The seizures often take the form of very frequent short complex partial seizures some of which secondarily generalize. The diagnosis is made by measuring levels of the antibody, and treatment is with immunosuppression.

Provoked seizures

One of the worst aspects of having epilepsy is the lack of predictability of seizures. For many people, the fact that a seizure can occur without warning on a more or less random fashion is far more problematic than the actual seizure itself. If there was sufficient advanced notice of seizures, the negative impact of epilepsy would be greatly reduced. Why seizures occur when they do is one of the major unanswered research questions in epilepsy. Of some interest is the tantalizing demonstration that subtle alterations in the EEG occur in the minutes or even hours before a seizure in some patients, without any clinical sign or any conscious awareness. Unfortunately, currently, in spite of considerable research, there seems to be no reliable way of utilizing these changes in a clinical setting to provide advanced warning to a patient, although implanted deep brain stimulators triggered by EEG change and seizure onset are being investigated. An interesting and quirky development has been the claim that dogs can be trained to recognize that a seizure is about to occur. Such 'epilepsy dogs' are now available in a number of countries, but their clinical utility or general applicability has not been subjected to rigorous research.

Provoked seizures can be divided into three categories:

1 Seizure precipitants: factors that do not invariably produce seizures, but that make a seizure more likely to happen. It has been claimed that 50–60% of people with epilepsy report that precipitants can be identified.

2 Metabolic, toxic and drug-induced seizures: acute metabolic or toxic insults do not cause 'brain injury' but can precipitate seizures.

3 Reflex seizures: in a small number of patients, seizures are not unpredictable, but are invariably triggered by an identifiable precipitant – these are the reflex epilepsies (see below).

Seizure precipitants

In many types of epilepsy, both idiopathic and symptomatic, seizures are more likely to occur at times of stress, menstruation, sleep deprivation, fever, alcohol intake/withdrawal, metabolic disturbance, hypoglycaemia, etc. (Table 4.12). These are commonly known as 'seizure precipitants'.

Epilepsy has a multifactorial causation and of course the differentiation of 'underlying cause' from a 'seizure precipitant' is simply one of degree. In a study of 500 drug-resistant patients, published in 1983, it was concluded that in 17% seizure-inducing factors made a significant contribution to the occurrence of seizures, and that manipulating these factors in these cases could greatly improve seizure control. It makes sense therefore to consider seizure precipitants as much a cause as any other. Attention to these factors can improve seizures in susceptible persons, and this is particularly true of avoidance of alcohol, sleep deprivation and stress. Where precipitants are invariable, their avoidance may obviate the need for antiepileptic drug therapy – this is usually only possible in patients with a history of mild epilepsy and infrequent seizures. In most other patients antiepileptic drugs are needed, although

Table 4.12 Seizure precipitants. Factors that commonly influence the precipitation of seizures.

Common factors
Stress
Emotional disturbance
Sleep deprivation and fatigue
Sleep–wake cycle
Alcohol and alcohol withdrawal
Hypoglycaemia
Metabolic disturbances
Toxins and drugs
Menstrual cycle
Fever or ill health
Photic stimulation
Less common factors
Startle
Fright
Dietary changes
Sexual intercourse
Pain
Fasting
Allergy
Hormonal changes

avoiding precipitants will lessen the propensity to seizures.

Stress

Emotional stress is commonly thought to provoke attacks in many individuals, although attempts to define or quantify stress prove highly elusive. Where some measurement is possible, studies usually show a modest association between worsening seizures and stress, although this can be complex and stress reduction in many people has a disappointing lack of effect. A wide variety of often spurious psychic explanations has been made in this difficult area.

Alcohol

In people with pre-existing epilepsy, acute alcohol intoxication and, even more potently, acute alcohol withdrawal can precipitate generalized seizures. A 20-fold increase in the incidence of seizures is found in patients consuming large quantities of alcohol, and avoidance of alcohol is sometimes all that is required to prevent seizures. Antiepileptic drug treatment in patients with alcohol problems is often problematic, owing to interactions, systemic toxicity, poor compliance and psychosocial problems. Where possible the patient should abstain from alcohol, and drug treatment can probably be avoided. Seizures are also common in the 24 hours after acute alcohol withdrawal, taking the form of myoclonus and tonic–clonic convulsions, sometimes with photosensitivity. This period can be covered with benzodiazepine or clomethiazole therapy under medical supervision.

Sleep and fatigue

The timing of seizures in relation to the sleep–wake cycle is intriguing. In the syndrome of IGE, all seizure types (absence, myoclonic and tonic–clonic seizures) are particularly likely to occur within an hour or so of waking or, less commonly, when drifting off to sleep or in the first 2 hours of sleep (most commonly in non-rapid eye movement [REM] stage 2 sleep). About 60% of children with benign rolandic epilepsy have attacks confined to sleep. In autosomal dominant frontal lobe epilepsy, attacks occur only in sleep, and numerous attacks can occur each night without a single event during the day. Some patients with other forms of generalized or partial epilepsy also have attacks only in sleep, and focal EEG disturbances can be activated by light sleep. Seizures of frontal lobe origin have a particular propensity to occur during sleep. The EEG disturbances in electrical status epilepticus during slow-wave sleep (ESES) and in the Landau–Kleffner syndrome are also greatly enhanced by sleep.

Seizures occurring in sleep often have less serious social consequences than daytime attacks. Therapy may not need to be as intensive as in daytime epilepsy, and occasional patients prefer not to have any drug treatment. Drug treatment carries the risk of converting a pattern of regular nocturnal attacks into less frequent daytime seizures with catastrophic social consequences – an important consideration when changing therapy in a patient whose seizures are confined to sleep. It should not be forgotten, however, that nocturnal tonic–clonic seizures carry a particular risk of sudden death, especially if the patient sleeps alone where the seizures are unwitnessed and therefore where emergency attention can not be provided. Advice about treatment should, therefore, be given on an individual basis.

Sleep deprivation and fatigue are undoubted precipitants of seizures in many people, and a few patients have attacks only when in these situations. Young adults with IGE seem particularly liable. EEG abnormalities, and therefore presumably also seizures, are also enhanced by sleep deprivation in many people with partial epilepsy. Fatigue can provoke attacks, although formal studies of why this should be are largely lacking. In susceptible individuals, the avoidance of fatigue or sleep deprivation greatly reduces seizures, and on occasions drug therapy can be averted.

The menstrual cycle and catamenial epilepsy

The occurrence of seizures in females often fluctuates in relation to the menstrual cycle. About 10% of all women with epilepsy note a striking pattern, usually with seizures occurring during or just before menstruation. This may be due to factors such as the high oestrogen levels in the follicular phase of menstruation, premenstrual tension or water retention. Progesterone has a mild antiepileptic effect, and the rapid fall in progesterone levels just before menstruation may be relevant. Fluid retention has also been suggested to have a role, but diuretics are seldom helpful in therapy. Occasionally, seizures occur only around menstruation, and the epilepsy is then referred to as catamenial epilepsy.

Clobazam (10 mg/day; see p. 174) or acetazolamide (250–750 mg/day; see p. 275) can be given intermittently each month around menstruation (usually for periods of 3–5 days), or at other susceptible times during the menstrual cycle, to control catamenial epilepsy. In practice this approach is only occasionally effective, and there are very few women in whom intermittent therapy alone will control seizures, even where there is a striking catamenial pattern.

Perhaps surprisingly, even where the frequency of seizures is clearly related to menstruation, attempts to influence hormonal factors have proved equally ineffective. Trials of contraceptive therapy, progesterone, hormone replacement therapy and even oophorectomy have been reported. None is generally effective.

Fever and general ill-health

Fever, general ill-health and intercurrent illness are potent precipitants of seizures, and effective antipyretic therapy or treatment of intercurrent illness will lower susceptibility to seizures in many people. This relatively non-specific effect, in patients with existing epilepsy, should be differentiated from the phenomenon of childhood 'febrile convulsions' (see pp. 26–28). Many patients consider that seizures are more likely to occur at times of general ill-health, lowered mood or when feeling 'run down'. For these reasons taking vitamins or herbal remedies, regular exercise, adopting healthy lifestyles and measures to improve general health are frequently advised. At an anecdotal level these can greatly improve epilepsy, although rigorous scientific evidence of effectiveness is lacking. Complementary and alternative therapies for epilepsy are outlined on pp. 118–121.

Metabolic, toxic and drug-induced seizures
Metabolic disorders

Many types of metabolic or endocrine disturbances can result in epilepsy. Hyponatraemia is the most common electrolyte disturbance to result in seizures, which typically occur if the serum sodium falls rapidly below 115 mmol/L. Seizures also routinely occur in the presence of hypernatraemia, hypocalcaemia, hypercalcaemia, hypomagnesaemia, hypokalaemia and hyperkalaemia. Ten per cent of patients with severe renal failure have seizures, caused by the metabolic disturbance, renal encephalopathy, dialysis encephalopathy or dialysis disequilibrium syndrome. Asterixis may develop into myoclonus and then epilepsy. The rate of change of the metabolic parameters is an important factor, and acute hyponatremia, for instance, is much more likely to cause seizures than chronic or slowly developing hyponatremia. Seizures are a common occurrence in hepatic failure. Hepatic encephalopathy may be overlooked and routine liver function tests can be relatively normal; hyperammonaemia is sometimes diagnostically helpful. Reye syndrome should be considered in patients with liver failure, especially children, in whom it is associated with intake of aspirin.

Hypoglycaemia is a potent cause of seizures, which can occur if the blood sugar level falls to <2.2 mmol/L. This is commonly due to insulin therapy in patients with diabetes, but can also be due to insulinoma and occasionally to drugs such as quinine and pentamidine. Non-ketotic hyperglycaemia frequently causes seizures. Levels of blood sugar as low as 15–20 mmol/L can cause seizures if there is associated hyperosmolarity. The seizures in nonketotic hyperglycaemia are focal and this implies the presence of cerebral pathology (usually cerebrovascular disease). Diabetic ketoacidosis does not frequently result in seizures.

Thyroid disease can result in seizures that are due either to immunological mechanisms or directly to hormonal change or hormonally induced metabolic change. Twenty per cent of patients with severe myxoedema have seizures. Hashimoto encephalopathy, a steroid-responsive encephalopathy associated with high levels of antithyroid antibody, is an immunologically determined condition that results in altered consciousness, focal signs, and other features of encephalopathy including myoclonus and tonic–clonic seizures.

Alcohol- and toxin-induced seizures

Alcohol abuse is a potent cause of acute symptomatic seizures, and indeed of epilepsy, in many societies. There are various mechanisms. Binge drinking can result in acute cerebral toxicity and seizures. Alcohol withdrawal in an alcohol-dependent person carries an even greater risk of seizures. Withdrawal seizures are typically tonic–clonic in form, occurring 12–24 h after withdrawal, and are associated with photosensitivity. Seizures can also be caused by the metabolic disturbances associated with binge drinking (notably hypoglycaemia, hyponatraemia and hepatic failure), the cerebral damage due to trauma, cerebral infection, subdural haematoma, the chronic neurotoxic effects of chronic alcohol exposure or to acute Wernicke encephalopathy caused by thiamine deficiency. It has been estimated that 6% of patients with alcohol problems investigated for epilepsy have an additional identifiable causative lesion.

The risk of a first generalized tonic–clonic seizure in patients with chronic alcohol problems is sevenfold greater than in non-alcoholic controls, and in the USA, for example, 15% of patients with epilepsy have alcohol problems. The risk of seizures is increased only with a daily alcohol intake of 50 g/day or more, and the higher the intake the higher the risk. Odds ratios according to alcohol intake have been calculated to be 3.0 (95% CI 1.7–5.4) for a daily intake of 51–100 g/day, 7.9 (95% CI 2.9–21.9) for 101–200 g/day and 16.6 (95% CI 1.9–373.4) when the intake is >200 g/day.

Seizures can also be provoked by exposure to many different toxins. Potent causes include heavy metal poisoning and carbon monoxide poisoning (where carboxyhaemoglobin levels are >50%). Although acute toxic exposure causes seizures, these are usually part of an acute encephalopathy. Whether low-level long-term exposure to carbon monoxide or to lead or other heavy metals carries any risk is quite unclear. This is a contentious and murky area in which claims are made without scientific backing, in which science is tangled up with legal processes and in which much nonsense is perpetuated. To what extent organophosphate poisoning can result in seizures is equally contentious, and reliable data seem to be absent.

Drug-induced seizures

A wide range of drugs, toxins and illicit compounds can cause acute symptomatic seizures and epilepsy, although seizures accounted for less than 1% of 32 812 consecutive patients prospectively monitored for drug toxicity. As many as 15% of drug-related seizures present as status epilepticus. In a population-based survey from Richmond, Virginia, drug overdose was the reported cause in 2% of children and 3% of adults with status epilepticus. Drugs can cause seizures due to intrinsic epileptogenicity, patient idiosyncrasy, antiepileptic drug interactions, impairment of the hepatic or renal drug metabolism, drug withdrawal phenomena and direct cerebral toxicity (especially in intentional overdosage).

The drugs most commonly associated with seizures are shown in Table 4.13. Although most psychotropic drugs carry a risk of inducing seizures, the risk seems to be highest with the aliphatic phenothiazines (e.g. chlorpromazine [1–9% risk], promazine, trifluoperazine). The

Table 4.13 Drugs commonly associated with seizures.

Analgesics	**Antipsychotics**
Meperidine	Clozapine
Tramadol	Olanzapine
	Quetapine
Antiepileptic drugs	Phenothiazines (chlorpromazine)
Phenytoin	Lithium
Carbamazepine	
Gabapentin	**Antiviral**
Lamotrigine	Zidovudine
Tiagabine	
Vigabatrin	**Drugs of abuse**
	Cocaine
Anaesthetics	Amphetamines
Lidocaine	Phencyclidine (PCP)
Propofol	MDMA (ecstasy)
Sevoflurane	
	Withdrawal
Antidepressants	Benzodiazepines
Clomipramine	Barbiturates
Amitriptyline (tricyclic	Baclofen
antidepressant)	Alcohol
Imipramine	
Maprotiline	**Chemotherapy/**
Amoxapine	**Immunosuppressants**
Bupropion	Cyclosporin
	Chlorambucil
Respiratory drugs	Ifosfamide
Isoniazid	
Theophylline	**Miscellaneous**
	Busulphan
Antibacterials	Iodinated contrast media
Penicillins (IV)	
Mefloquine	
Imipenem/cilastatin	
Ciprofloxacin	

use of clozapine is associated with a 1–4% risk of seizures and with interictal epileptiform abnormalities. The piperazine phenothiazines (acetophenazine, fluphenazine, perphenazine, prochlorperazine, trifluoperazine), haloperidol, sulpiride, pimozide, thioridazine and risperidone are thought to have the lowest epileptogenic potential, although firm data are lacking. The risk of seizures with antidepressant drugs ranges between <1% and 4%, and varies with the drug category. Agents accompanied by a high risk of seizures include clomipramine and second-generation antidepressants, amoxapine, maprotiline and amfebutamone. The risk of seizures with tricyclic antidepressants (other than clomipramine), citalopram, moclobemide and nefazodone is thought to be lower. The seizure risk with the selective serotonin reuptake inhibitors (fluoxetine, sertraline, paroxetine), monoamine oxidase inhibitors (MAOIs) and trazodone is probably lower, although definitive data are lacking. All these drugs in overdose carry a significant (>10%) risk of seizures. The opiate analgesic meperidine is metabolized in the liver to normaperidine, a potent proconvulsant, which tends to accumulate after prolonged administration and renal failure. The monocyclic antidepressant amfebutamone, which is used to assist the cessation of smoking, provokes seizures in 1 in 1000 patients. Pethidine can also result in seizures, especially in the presence of renal impairment or in combination with MAOIs. Lidocaine-related neurotoxicity is common with intravenous use, especially with advanced age, congestive heart failure, shock, and renal and hepatic failure. The anaesthetics enflurane, propofol and isoflurane can be proconvulsant. Quinine and the other antimalarial drugs, especially mefloquine, can provoke acute seizures, and are relatively contraindicated in epilepsy. Various traditional remedies, including evening primrose oil and some Chinese and Indian herbal medicines, can provoke seizures.

Neurotoxic reactions may occur frequently with β-lactam antibiotics (semi-synthetic penicillins and cephalosporins), probably due to GABA-antagonist action. Benzylpenicillin, cefazolin and imipenem/cilastatin have higher neurotoxic potential, and the risk is increased at higher doses, in the presence of renal failure, blood–brain barrier damage and pre-existing CNS disorders, co-medication with nephrotoxic agents or drugs lowering seizure threshold. Isoniazid can induce seizures by antagonizing pyridoxal phosphate (the active form of pyridoxine), which is involved in GABA biosynthesis. Seizures have also been reported, especially in elderly patients, as a result of aminoglycosides, metronidazole, quinolones and amantadine. Quinolones (nalidixic acid, norfloxacin, ciprofloxacin) probably enhance seizure activity by inhibiting GABA binding to membrane receptors. The tetracyclines seem to be less proconvulsant than these other antibiotics. Zidovudine and other antiviral agents have caused seizures in HIV patients. Seizures (and non-convulsive status epilepticus) have been reported after administration of intravenous contrast media, and the risk is as high as 15% in patients with brain metastases.

The anticancer chemotherapeutic agents can provoke seizures, especially chlorambucil (5%), and ciclosporin (1–3%), asparaginase, tacrolimus and amfebutamone, but also the platin drugs, vinca alkaloids, bleomycin, anthracyclines and azathioprine.

Theophylline is a potent convulsant that can result in seizures or status epilepticus, possibly due to the anti-adenosine action. β Blockers and other antiarrhythmic agents have been reported to precipitate seizures, particularly in overdose. Cimetidine, levodopa, insulin, thiazide diuretics, lidocaine, salicylates, chemotherapeutic agents, L-asparaginase and baclofen have been reported to cause seizures. The non-steroidal analgesics also predispose to seizures, e.g. non-steroidal anti-inflammatory drugs (NSAIDs), tramadol, diamorphine and pethidine.

Seizures may be precipitated after sudden withdrawal of any antiepileptic drug but seem to be a particular problem in benzodiazepine, carbamazepine and barbiturate withdrawal.

Recreational drugs can cause seizures. The greatest risk is with the stimulant drugs such as cocaine, amphetamine and ecstasy (3,4-methylenedioxymethamphetamine, MDMA). The hallucinogens such as phencyclidine ('angel dust') and lysergic acid diethylamide (LSD) less commonly cause seizures. The opiates and the organic solvents are least epileptogenic, although past or present heroin use has been shown to be a risk factor for provoked and unprovoked seizures (OR 2.8; 95% CI 1.5–5.7). Of the performance-enhancing drugs, erythropoietin has strong epileptogenic potential. By contrast, in one study, use of marijuana by men was shown to have a protective action against non-provoked seizures (OR 0.4; 95% CI 0.2–0.8) and provoked seizures (OR 0.2; 95% CI 0.1–0.8).

Reflex epilepsy

The term 'reflex epilepsy' is used to describe cases in which seizures are evoked consistently by a specific environmental trigger. In some cases the stimulus can be highly specific and in others less so. The term is not usually applied to patients whose seizures are precipitated by internal influences such as menstruation, or to situations where the precipitating factors are vague or ill-defined (e.g. fatigue, stress), or to patients with existing epilepsy where seizures are more likely to occur due to specific precipitants (e.g. sleep deprivation, alcohol); transitional cases occur, however, in what can be a nosological grey area. The reflex epilepsies are sometimes subdivided into simple and complex types. In the simple forms the seizures are precipitated by simple sensory stimuli (e.g. flashes of light, startle) and in the complex forms by more elaborate stimuli (e.g. specific pieces of music). The complex forms are much more heterogeneous and the syndromes are less well defined than the simple reflex epilepsies. In hospital practice about 5% of patients show some features of reflex epilepsy. The stimuli most reported to cause seizures include flashing lights and other visual stimuli, startle, eating, bathing in hot water, music, reading and movement.

Visual stimuli, photosensitivity and photosensitive epilepsy

The most common reflex epilepsies are those induced by visual stimuli. Flashing lights, bright lights, moving visual patterns (e.g. escalators), eye closure, moving from dark into bright light, and viewing specific objects or colours have all been reported to induce seizures.

Photosensitive epilepsy is a form of simple reflex epilepsy. The term should be confined to those individuals who show unequivocal EEG evidence of photosensitivity, and differentiated from other, usually more complex, cases in which seizures can apparently be precipitated by visual stimuli but in whom EEG evidence of photosensitivity cannot be demonstrated. Photosensitivity (strictly defined) is present in the general population with a frequency of about 1.1/100 000, and 5.7/100 000 in the age range 7–19, and is very strongly associated with epilepsy. About 3% of people with epilepsy are photosensitive and have seizures induced by photic stimuli (usually viewing flickering or intermittent lights or cathode ray monitors, bright lights or repeating patterns).

The flicker frequency precipitating photosensitivity varies from patient to patient, but is most commonly in the 15–20 Hz range. The peak age of presentation of photosensitive epilepsy is 12 years, the male:female ratio is 2:3, and the propensity to photosensitivity declines with age. Most patients with photosensitivity have the syndrome of IGE, although photosensitivity also occurs in patients with focal epilepsy arising in the occipital region. In IGE, myoclonus, absence and tonic–clonic seizures can be precipitated by photic stimuli, and factors such as sleep deprivation or alcohol intake have additive effects – partying can involve all factors, and seizures are common the morning after the night before. Alternating patterns (such as in some video games, or when looking down large escalators) can precipitate seizures in photosensitive patients, as can disco lights or poorly tuned cathode ray TV screens (which flicker at the mains alternating current frequency of 50 Hz in the UK and Europe, but not in the USA). Other common stimuli include bright light shimmering off moving water, or the flickering of light through trees from a moving vehicle, and the transition from relative darkness into bright light.

Most photosensitive patients have non-photically induced seizures also, but photic seizures can be prevented or reduced by wearing glasses with tinted or polarized lenses, and by avoiding situations known to induce photosensitive responses. Photosensitivity also occurs in some patients with occipital lobe epilepsy and in some of the benign occipital focal epilepsy syndromes.

Television-induced seizures (and, far less common, seizures induced by video games or computer screens) can be reduced by taking the precautions listed in Table 4.14. In photosensitive individuals with occipital lobe epilepsy, seizure discharges may also be caused by fixation-on or fixation-off stimuli.

Treatment with valproate, benzodiazepine drugs or levetiracetam usually completely abolishes photosensitiv-

Table 4.14 Tactics that can reduce the risk of television-induced seizures in susceptible individuals.

Use a small screen, or view screen from a distance, use a remote control for changing channels (thereby reducing the area of screen in the visual field)

View the screen from an angle

Use a 100 Hz television screen, a non-interlaced computer screen with a high refresh rate or a liquid crystal display

Close or cover one eye

Keep the screen contrast and brightness low

Avoid exposure when sleep deprived

Avoid looking at a fixed flickering pattern

Use polarizing glasses

ity, even at doses that do not provide complete seizure control.

Startle-induced epilepsy

Startle can precipitate seizures in susceptible individuals, and occasionally is the only precipitant. Startle-induced seizures usually occur in patients with a frontal or central focus and usually in lesional epilepsy. The seizures usually take a form similar to a tonic seizure, and the EEG is commonly normal or shows rather non-specific changes. A susceptibility to startle is more common in late childhood and adolescence, and may resolve as the patient gets older. The most common stimulus is a loud noise, but touch, sudden movement or fright can also precipitate attacks. Startle-induced epilepsy must be differentiated from hyperekplexia, which has a very similar clinical form, but which is not a form of epilepsy. Treatment can be difficult although carbamazepine and the benzodiazepine drugs have been said, at an anecdotal level, to be most likely to control the attacks.

Primary reading epilepsy

This is a specific rare epilepsy syndrome in which clonic jerking of the jaw or perioral muscles, which can evolve to a generalized convulsion, is precipitated by reading. The age of onset is usually 12–25 years. The condition has various forms. In some patients, the attacks occur only after prolonged reading. In individual cases, different aspects of reading seem to act as precipitating factors – content, comprehension, context, reading difficult or unfamiliar passages, music, nonsense passages and foreign languages. In other patients, reading may precipitate jaw jerking after a few seconds. In some cases, there is evidence of focal onset of the epilepsy and others have features classifiable as a form of 'praxis-induced' juvenile myoclonic epilepsy (JME – see pp. 232–24). The physiological basis of this curious syndrome is unclear, but there is a positive family history in about 25% of cases. The seizures can usually be aborted if reading is terminated as soon as the clonic jerking develops. Conventional antiepileptic drugs have been used with variable success. In the variants that resemble JME, therapeutic approaches are similar to those employed in JME and the prognosis is excellent.

Other forms of reflex epilepsy

Other simple reflex epilepsies include cases with seizures induced by movement, touching or tapping. These should be differentiated from paroxysmal kinesogenic choreoathetosis and stimulus-sensitive myoclonus. Hot-water epilepsy is a remarkable syndrome, common in parts of India but rare elsewhere, in which seizures are induced by pouring hot water over the head or immersion in hot water. The attacks take the form of tonic–clonic or partial seizures. Complex forms of a wide variety of other stimuli have been reported to induce seizures – and among the strangest are: telephones, noise of a vacuum cleaner, specific memories, writing and touch. These conditions are heterogeneous in terms of aetiology, EEG and seizure type. The mechanisms underlying these (and other) reflex epilepsies are uncertain and specific 'reflex arcs' have not been identified. Prevention of the precipitating cause is sometimes helpful, as is drug treatment along conventional lines.

5 Principles of Treatment

Why treat epilepsy? The aims of treatment

All treatment is a balance between risk and benefit. Treatment decisions in epilepsy are sometimes complex and judgements finely balanced. Our Hippocratic promise is 'to abstain from doing harm', and the risks of harm from medical and surgical therapy are seldom far from the surface. Decisions about treatment should, in essence, be made by the patient and/or carer. The role of the treating physician is to assist decision-making by providing information and advice and to provide a sound context.

Seizure control

There is good evidence that antiepileptic drugs substantially reduce seizure recurrence. This of course is a primary goal and the extent to which therapy will control seizures in different clinical settings is discussed below. Complete seizure control is a common aim, but should not be pursued at the cost of severe adverse effects. The art of therapy is to ensure that an appropriate balance between the effectiveness and side effects of therapy is struck. This can be difficult to achieve, and these aspects are discussed further below.

Avoidance of side effects

Side effects are considered in more detail later in this chapter and in the sections related to individual drugs in Chapter 8. Adverse effects can be generally classified as follows.

Idiosyncratic reactions

These include immunologically determined, allergy and hypersensitivity reactions, and are usually rare, but can be severe and occasionally life threatening (see pp. 116–117).

Dose-related reversible side effects

These are common, usually mild, typically central nervous system (CNS) or gastrointestinal in nature, and are reversible when the dose is lowered. The occurrence of these effects depends on dose and also rate of incrementation.

Long-term irreversible side effects

These are not strictly dose related, although they are more common in patients who have taken high-dose therapy for long periods. They are not necessarily reversible, and can affect many body symptoms. They are usually but not always mild in nature.

Teratogenicity

For a discussion of teratogenicity, see pp. 139–141.

Avoidance of social consequences of epilepsy and secondary handicap

Therapeutic endeavours should be also aimed at minimizing the adverse consequences of epilepsy within the broader context of the patient's life and experience. These effects – the effects of 'having epilepsy' – can be far greater than simply having seizures and require a holistic approach to therapy in which drug treatment is often only a small part. The establishment of a good patient–doctor relationship, counselling, psychological therapy and lifestyle advice are all important. The overall aim is to encourage as normal a lifestyle as possible, and to balance risks and benefit.

Suppression of subclinical epileptic activity

Antiepileptic drug therapy, as a rule, should be aimed at suppressing seizures and not at reducing EEG activity. However, in selected situations, therapy can be targeted at EEG disturbances where these are considered to be causing clinical impairment ('subclinical activity'). These particular circumstances include: reduction of 3 Hz spike–wave paroxysms in patients with idiopathic generalized epilepsy; abolition of EEG changes in the

Handbook of Epilepsy Treatment, 3rd Edition. By Simon Shorvon. Published 2010 by Blackwell Publishing Ltd.

Landau–Kleffner syndrome; abolition of photosensitivity; reduction in slow spike–wave paroxysms in patients with Lennox–Gastaut syndrome and other epileptic encephalopathies; and in refractory status epilepticus. In most individuals, it is not appropriate to try to reduce focal interictal epileptic activity by drug therapy, which anyway is often not possible, but there are exceptions and this is a judgement that requires specialist consideration.

Reduction of mortality and morbidity
Epileptic seizures occasionally result in death or accidental injury. The suppression of seizures will reduce this risk.

Prevention of epileptogenesis
It has been postulated that epileptic seizures induce cerebral changes that lead to further seizures. If this is the case, antiepileptic therapy, by controlling seizures, will potentially lessen the chances of this happening. Although a protective effect has been demonstrated in animal experimentation, there is no good evidence for any such action in human epilepsy. It is likely that antiepileptic drugs merely exert a suppressive effect on seizures, and have no influence on the long-term natural course of the disease. Similarly, the use of antiepileptic drugs prophylactically does not seem to prevent epilepsy developing in individuals at high risk, e.g. after head injury, neurosurgery, stroke or tumour. One specific example is after febrile seizures, and it is now generally agreed that continuous pharmacological prophylaxis, in children aged >1 year, after febrile seizures is ineffective. Neuroprotective strategies using other types of drug are in development, and this is an area of intensive research activity, but as yet no effective neuroprotective therapy is available.

Improving quality of life
The efficacy of antiepileptic drugs is conventionally assessed by measuring their impact on seizure frequency but, in recent years, the effect of drug therapy on quality of life has been the subject of intensive study. Not surprisingly, studies have consistently shown that complete seizure freedom is by far the most important predictor of improved quality of life. However, even where seizure freedom is not achieved, drug-induced reductions of seizure frequency or severity can be beneficial, as can the positive psychotropic effects of some drugs. These must be balanced against the side effects, particularly the cognitive and neurological effects, of medication – a balance sometimes difficult to achieve.

Prevention of epilepsy
To date, there is no evidence that antiepileptic drugs prevent the long-term development of the process of epilepsy (epileptogenesis), although they do, at the time of therapy, act to suppress seizures. Thus there is usually little point in prophylactic therapy in patients at risk of epilepsy (e.g. after head injury or stroke) except at times of very high risk.

The risks of epilepsy and its treatment

Active epilepsy is associated with significant risks in terms of both mortality and morbidity and, in making treatment choices, it is obviously important to know the extent of these risks and of risk reduction on therapy. The benefits need also to be set against the risks of the treatment itself.

Risks of epilepsy
The risk of death (mortality) and disability (morbidity) in epilepsy has been extensively studied in recent years.

Mortality in epilepsy
Epilepsy is a potentially life-threatening condition, a fact that is often overlooked. The key question is the extent to which this can be avoided by adequate drug treatment. Deaths associated with epilepsy can be classified into three categories:
1 Those caused directly by the seizures, such as accidental death and sudden unexplained death in epilepsy (SUDEP)
2 Those related indirectly, or only partly, to epilepsy, e.g. suicide
3 Those due to other factors, e.g. the underlying causes of the epilepsy.
   Successful antiepileptic drug therapy should prevent deaths in the first category, may prevent some deaths in the second category, but will have no preventive effect in the third category.
   The risk of death is best expressed as a standardized mortality rate (SMR), which is defined as the ratio of deaths in patients with epilepsy to that of age- and sex-matched control populations.

Newly diagnosed epilepsy
In one study, 161 (29%) of 564 patients with newly diagnosed epilepsy had died within 6 years of the diagnosis. The rate of death was over three times that expected in an age-matched population. However, the

excess mortality was due almost entirely to the underlying disease, and not the epilepsy itself, and AED treatment would be unlikely to have much impact on mortality rates at this stage.

Chronic active epilepsy in adults

In contrast to new-onset epilepsy, much of the excess mortality in patients with chronic active epilepsy is seizure or epilepsy related. Thus, in one study of 601 adult outpatients attending tertiary referral clinics and followed for 3 years, the SMR was 5.1 (95% confidence interval [CI] 2.9–3.1), with 24 deaths being recorded in 1849 patient-years of follow-up. Most patients in this population had long-standing intractable partial or secondarily generalized seizures. Of the 24 deaths, 14 were seizure related, and 11 of these were classified as SUDEP. As risk is much greater in convulsive seizures, and in patients with frequent seizures, successful AED therapy could have an important preventive role.

Chronic active epilepsy in children

In a community-based study in Nova Scotia, mortality rates among 693 children followed up for 14–22 years were 0/97 for absence epilepsy, 12/511 (2%) for partial and primarily generalized seizures, and 9/36 (25%) or 4/49 (8%) for secondarily generalized seizures with onset before or after 1 year of age respectively. Only one patient died as a result of SUDEP. In another paediatric community-based study, mortality rates associated with symptomatic epilepsy were 50-fold higher than in the general population, but there was no increased mortality in idiopathic epilepsy. Thus, in children, the risks of seizure-related deaths are less than in adults, and effective drug treatment will therefore have less impact on mortality.

Causes of seizure-related deaths

There is an obvious potential for AED treatment to reduce the risk of seizure-related death, the main causes of which are as follows.

Sudden explained death in epilepsy

SUDEP is the most common seizure-related cause of death in epilepsy. It almost always occurs after a convulsive seizure, and the risk in other seizure types is very small or negligible. The higher the number of convulsive seizures, the higher the risk – particularly if the seizures are unwitnessed. Thus, patients at high risk are those with a high rate of convulsive seizures, or seizures occurring when asleep and alone. Young adults, and patients with learning disability and structural cerebral lesions, are at

particular risk because of the association with high seizure rates. Drug reduction can be a specific risk and because of this needs to be carried out with extreme caution in patients at risk of generalized convulsions. Suboptimal drug levels are another risk factor in some studies.

SUDEP is usually the result of respiratory arrest in the aftermath of a convulsive seizure, although cardiac arrhythmias may be responsible for a proportion of cases. Respiratory effort after a seizure can be restarted by stimulation and arousal, and this is perhaps why SUDEP is rare in witnessed seizures. For this reason, it is important to come to the assistance of a person in a convulsive seizure and dangerous to leave the person unattended.

In population-based studies, the risk has been found to be about 1 case per 1000–2000 people on treatment for epilepsy per year. The rates of SUDEP in different populations are proportional to the frequency of tonic–clonic convulsions – and in patients with well-controlled epilepsy the risk is very small, whereas in patients with severe intractable epilepsy the risk may be as high as 1–2/100 patients per year. It has been estimated that – as a rough approximation – SUDEP will occur in 1 in every 2000–5000 tonic–clonic convulsions. In the average patient, the risk is therefore small and, as is often worth pointing out, less than the risk of death due to a road traffic accident in many countries.

SUDEP deaths would be potentially preventable if seizures were brought under control. The potential for prevention was demonstrated in a recent sentinel audit carried out by the Department of Health in the UK which found, on the basis of a case-note review, that 39% of deaths in patients with epilepsy might have been prevented with more appropriate drug therapy.

Status epilepticus

About 20% of patients with convulsive status epilepticus admitted to intensive care will not survive. Death is usually due to the underlying cause, which may not be remediable, but some death is iatrogenic. Skilful therapy will lessen both morbidity and mortality rates. Status accounts for less than 2% of deaths among people with epilepsy, and it is comparatively more common in children, especially those with learning disability.

Death in an accident

The SMR for accidental death was found in one study to be 5.6 (95% CI 5.0–6.3). Accidents occur in employment, outside and in the home, and the problem is worse if the seizures involve falls. Common causes of death are falling from heights, road traffic accidents and accidents in domestic settings. Drowning in a bath was a leading cause and, in another study, 58 of 2381 drowning deaths recorded in a 5-year period were seizure related. Effective control of seizures will greatly lessen the risk of accidental death.

Suicide

In a recent Danish study of 21 169 cases of suicide in Denmark between 1981 and 1997, 492 (2.32%) of the suicide cases had epilepsy compared with a rate of epilepsy among a random matched sample of over 400 000 people in the general population of 0.74%. Those with both epilepsy and co-morbid psychiatric disease were almost 14 times more likely to commit suicide, adjusting for socioeconomic factors, than those with neither condition. In cases series, suicide is reported to account for between 2 and 10% of all deaths in epilepsy. The suicide is commonly by drug overdose, and occurs usually in patients with depression and psychosis. In July 2008, the US Food and Drug Administration (FDA) issued a warning, based on placebo-controlled, randomized controlled trials (RCTs) of antiepileptic drugs, that some epilepsy drugs double the risk of suicidal behaviour or thoughts. Whether this is really a drug effect or the psychiatric effects of epilepsy is unclear, and most accept the latter explanation (see pp. 111–112). Effective treatment of the epilepsy and the psychiatric co-morbidities of epilepsy will lessen the risk of suicide.

Morbidity in epilepsy

It is perhaps not surprising that epilepsy results in higher rates of morbidity. It is obvious that seizures with falls carry the risk of accidental injury. There is also often expressed a concern about the risk of seizures to cerebral function, and the psychosocial effects of epilepsy can be profound. These adverse effects are potentially alleviated by reducing seizure frequency or severity.

Accidental injury

Among 100 consecutive epileptic patients attending the author's clinic, 27 patients reported 222 seizure-related injuries. The total number of seizures per year was 4459, of which 1094 were with a fall (24.5%). Soft-tissue injury was the most common (61%), followed by burns (17%), head injury (14%), orthopaedic injury (5%) and injuries in water (3%). The most common site of soft-tissue injury and burns was to the face: 49% and 38% respec-

tively. Burns occurred during cooking in 78% of cases. Two patients had skull fractures. Orthopaedic injuries usually occurred at home (73%). In cases of seizures in water, five of six occurred while swimming. Injury occurred once in every 11 generalized tonic–clonic seizures and every 5 seizures with a fall. The significant risk factors for injury were generalized tonic–clonic seizures, high frequency of seizures and seizures with a fall.

Among 247 consecutive cases of active epilepsy from 3 epilepsy clinics in north-east Thailand, 91 had a seizure-related injury, and the risk is greatest in those with frequent daytime tonic–clonic seizures (a probability estimate can be calculated on the researchers' website – http://sribykku.webs.com).

Fractures of vertebral bodies are common in convulsive seizures (crush fractures), occurring in 15–16% of patients in two series. Neurological deficit due to cervical cord injury in a convulsive seizure is rarer, and only 7 cases of serious paraparesis were observed in about 3500 person-years of follow-up in a residential centre for patients with severe epilepsy, which corresponds to an incidence of about 1 case per 500 person-years.

Head injury is common in severe epilepsy but is usually relatively minor. In a 12-month survey of 255 patients with severe epilepsy in residential care, 27 934 seizures were recorded, of which 12 626 (45.2%) were associated with falls. There were 766 significant head injuries, 422 requiring simple dressing and 341 sutures. There was one recorded skull fracture, and two post-traumatic haematomas, one extradural and one subdural. Thus, 1 in 37 falls resulted in the need for sutures and about 1 in 6000 falls resulted in a potentially life-threatening intracranial haemorrhage. A recent European study found that the hazard ratio for concussion in patients with generalized epilepsy compared with the general population was 6.8 (95% CI 1.1–42.6).

Fractures of facial bones are also common, although there are no authoritative estimates of frequency or severity. In a population-based survey of patients with at least one seizure per year, 24% reported a head injury, 16% a burn, 10% a dental injury and 5% a fracture due to seizures in the previous 12 months. It has been estimated that, in epilepsy, fractures occur at a frequency of about one per person every 14 years, compared with a population risk of one per person every 50 years. Osteoporosis may be more common in patients with epilepsy, possibly as an effect of drug therapy, and this can predispose to fractures. A posterior dislocation of the shoulder is a characteristic injury and said to occur only in major convulsions.

Scalding or burning is also relatively common among people with epilepsy in all societies. The risk depends upon social habits: in some African villages, epilepsy is known as the 'burn disease' because of the frequency of seizure-related burns incurred by falling into open fires. In western societies, burns due to falls against radiators, from hot fluids, during showering or during cooking are common injuries. In one survey of 244 outpatients in the UK, 25 (12%) reported having been burned seriously enough to warrant medical attention and 12 (5%) required hospitalization. Many of these injuries could be prevented by simple advice (such as the use of shielded radiators or using a microwave to cook).

Cerebral damage

One issue that has been the subject of intensive research is the extent to which seizures can result in cerebral damage or changes that render the person more likely to have further seizures or produce motor, sensory or cognitive impairment. The current consensus view is that cerebral damage from short self-limiting seizures is extremely unusual, and furthermore that such seizures do not increase the risk of further seizures. The risk after prolonged seizures (e.g. status epilepticus) is quite a different matter, and severe status can result in significant cerebral damage and consequent cognitive decline, a risk that is probably greatest in children and that increases the longer the seizure persists. A particular question relates to childhood febrile seizures and whether they lead to later epilepsy (see pp. 27–28).

In some of the childhood epilepsy syndromes, there is evidence that ongoing epilepsy results in cerebral damage. The clearest example is the Sturge–Weber syndrome where stepwise deterioration in motor skills follows bouts of seizures. In the severe epileptic encephalopathies of childhood (e.g. West syndrome, the Lennox–Gastaut syndrome, myoclonic–astatic epilepsy, electrical status epilepticus during slow-wave sleep [ESES]), progressive cognitive decline does occur but it is not clear to what extent, if any, this is due to ongoing seizures or to the underlying process.

Psychosocial morbidity of epilepsy

The diagnosis of epilepsy also carries psychosocial morbidity. In all large studies, a high proportion of patients with epilepsy had difficulty accepting the diagnosis, significant fears about the risks of future seizures, anxiety about the effect of stigma and about the effects on employment, self-esteem, relationships, schooling and leisure activities. Patients with epilepsy carry higher rates of anxiety and depression, social isolation, unmarried status and unemployment, and are more likely to be unemployed or registered as permanently sick. These aspects are covered in the following sections. The psychosocial morbidity of epilepsy can be greatly ameliorated if seizures are brought under complete control, although the label of epilepsy (being epileptic) can itself be a cause of morbidity even if seizures are fully controlled.

Psychiatric co-morbidity

Epilepsy is associated with a very significant psychiatric morbidity. This is usually subcategorized into: psychosis, depression, anxiety, personality disorder and organic mental disorders. The relationship is complex, the mechanisms multifactorial and some adverse events are drug induced. These topics are covered in more detail elsewhere (see pp. 107–116). Estimates of the lifetime prevalence for a major depressive episode in the general population ranges from 3.7% to 6.7%. In patients with epilepsy, rates range from 11% (current depression) to 62% (lifetime-to-date depressive disorder), with a mean of 30% across studies. Prevalence is lower (3–9%) in patients with good seizure control. Anxiety disorders are reported in 10–25% of patients and mixed anxiety and depressive disorders in 8.5%. Interictal psychosis is said to be present in about 15% of all patients with epilepsy, although rates have varied considerably.

In patients with epilepsy, the prevalence of axis II personality disorders ranges from 18% to 61% across studies, with a mean of 31%. There has been some debate about the presence of an 'epileptic personality', which comprises features of affective dysphoria, viscosity, hyposexuality, religiosity, hypergraphia, hypoactivity and aggressiveness. It is doubtful whether these personality traits are in reality independently related to epilepsy.

The organic mental disorders classification of Lindqvist and Malmgren (the LM scheme) is a useful classification system of psychiatric disorders in which the organic mental disorder specific to epilepsy (and to epilepsy surgery) are divided into six categories – and this scheme is described further on pp. 114–115.

Antiepileptic drugs are also associated with psychiatric adverse events including, for example:
• barbiturates with depression and attention deficit hyperactivity disorder in children
• phenytoin with toxic schizophreniform psychoses
• valproate with acute and chronic encephalopathies
• vigabatrin, topiramate and other drugs with depression and alternative psychoses
• levetiracetam with irritability, aggressivity and psychosis.

Risks of antiepileptic drug therapy

AED therapy itself carries risks, and these can be summarized as follows.

Life-threatening side effects – AED hypersensitivity

Life-threatening adverse effects are rare with all major antiepileptic drugs, and result from idiosyncratic or hypersensitivity reactions affecting the bone marrow, liver, skin or other organs (these are described further on pp. 116–118).

Other life-threatening side effects

There are not many other life-threatening side effects. Severe bradyarrhythmias have been recorded after intravenous phenytoin, and possibly also after oral lamotrigine. Aspiration pneumonia can occur with nitrazepam in young children, and respiratory arrest can be induced by high-dose intravenous benzodiazepines. Agammaglobulinaemia or hypogammaglobulinaemia has been described due to carbamazepine, lamotrigine, levetiracetam and phenytoin therapy, and can lead to a severe immunodeficient state. The drug–drug interactions of some antiepileptic drugs with antibiotics, immunosuppressants and oncological drugs can also have serious consequences.

Non-life-threatening side effects

There is a large range of side effects, which vary with each individual drug, and are described in Chapter 8. The most significant involve the CNS and include cerebellovestibular and oculomotor symptoms (ataxia, dysarthria, dizziness, tremor, diplopia, blurred vision and nystagmus), drowsiness, fatigue, impairment of cognitive function, and disorders of mood and behaviour. Less commonly, motor disturbances occur including choreoathetosis and tics.

Non-CNS reversible side effects include gatrointestinal, metabolic and endocrine effects. Examples are: the induction of folate deficiency, vitamin D deficiency, disturbances of lipid metabolism, changes in acid–base balance, weight gain, insulin resistance, modification of thyroid levels, alterations in sex hormone levels, dermatological, connective tissue and cosmetic changes, Dupuytren contracture, and changes to hair and gum hypertrophy. There are also occasionally irreversible side effects, including nephrolithiasis with topiramate and visual field restrictions with vigabatrin.

It has been suggested that some of the newer antiepileptic drugs are, overall, better tolerated than older agents, but this claim should be regarded cautiously because, in many comparative studies, the choice of titration schedules or dosing regimens is such that it could bias the findings in favour of the innovative product. Moreover, clinical exposure to the newer drugs is still relatively limited and experience shows that it may take many years for important adverse effects to be discovered (see pp. 84–85). What is clear, however, is that many of the metabolic and endocrine effects are due to metabolic interactions at the hepatic level and in protein binding, and drugs that are free from interactions and not protein bound have significant advantages.

The risks of AED prescribing in co-morbid disease

Prescribing drugs in various conditions is complicated because of interactions with other medication and therapies – this is a major problem in some infections (including HIV), the major psychoses, immunological conditions, transplant practice and dialysis. Prescribing in pregnancy also has specific risks (see pp. 139–144).

Liver disease

Although many antiepileptic drugs undergo hepatic metabolism, their clearance is seldom affected by hepatic disease to an extent that it influences the risk:benefit ratio, except in severe hepatic failure. Similarly, decreased protein binding of phenytoin and valproate has little bearing on risk assessment, even though it is relevant for a correct interpretation of total serum drug concentrations. Valproate should be avoided if possible in patients with liver dysfunction due to its potential hepatotoxic effects. Phenobarbital and benzodiazepines should be avoided in advanced stages of hepatic failure because of the risk of induction or aggravation of hepatic encephalopathy. Theoretically, non-metabolized drugs, such as gabapentin and vigabatrin, are an attractive option for treating patients with hepatic impairment.

Porphyria

Seizures may be a component of an attack of acute intermittent porphyria. Prescribing can be difficult because the enzyme-inducing antiepileptic drugs can precipitate acute attacks (see pp. 40–41).

Renal failure

Renal failure is associated with a decreased protein binding of phenytoin and valproate. The clearance of gabapentin, levetiracetam, pregabalin and vigabatrin will be reduced in severe renal failure, necessitating dose adjustments.

Cardiac disease

Uncontrolled generalized tonic–clonic seizures are likely to be hazardous in patients with severe heart disease. The antiepileptic drugs that act on membrane ion channels can induce cardiac arrhythmias in predisposed patients. Carbamazepine, phenytoin, lamotrigine, oxcarbazepine and possibly topiramate should be generally avoided in patients with pre-existing disturbances in the cardiac conduction system or cardiomyopathies. Routine ECG should be obtained to exclude cardiac disease before starting treatment with these drugs, especially in elderly patients and in those with a history suggestive of heart disease. Intravenous administration of phenytoin should be carried out only with extreme caution in patients with cardiac disturbances.

Choice of antiepileptic drug therapy based on seizure type

Epilepsy can take various forms and can be the result of many different pathological processes. To a large extent, however, individual drugs will have similar antiepileptic effects regardless of the clinical form or cause of the seizures, at least in the non-syndromic epilepsies of adulthood. There are exceptions to this rule, but the remarkable non-specificity of therapy is a striking feature of most partial and tonic–clonic epilepsies of adult life, regardless of cause. This is perhaps because the antiepileptic drugs act mechanistically on the final physiological processes of epilepsy which are similar whatever the cause. Side effects vary, however, more than efficacy, and the choice of drugs is often influenced more by this rather than by any consideration of relative efficacy. It is usual to divide therapy according to seizure type – and the choice of drugs in newly diagnosed epilepsy and in chronic epilepsy (in the author's practice) is shown in Tables 5.1 and 5.2.

The childhood syndromes have much more specificity and drug therapy needs to be chosen only after a syndromic diagnosis has been made. Treatment of

Table 5.1 Newly diagnosed patients: choice of initial monotherapy (based on the author's preferences).

Seizure type	Drug[a]
Partial seizures, secondarily generalized tonic–clonic seizures, primary generalized tonic–clonic seizures	Carbamazepine, lamotrigine, levetiracetam, oxcarbazepine, valproate
Absence seizures (typical absence)	Lamotrigine, levetiracetam, valproate
Myoclonic seizures	Levetiracetam, valproate
Atypical absence, tonic and atonic seizures	Lamotrigine, levetiracetam, topiramate, valproate

[a]Drugs are in alphabetical order.

the major childhood syndromes is considered below (see pp. 89–96).

Generalized tonic–clonic seizures

A wide range of drugs is licensed for use in tonic–clonic seizures whether primarily or secondarily generalized. In almost all RCTs and open studies, the available antiepileptic drugs show similar comparative efficacy.

Newly diagnosed and/or drug-naïve patients

Monotherapy is the rule. The choice of medication is show in Table 5.1. It is currently usual practice to start therapy with carbamazepine (in its slow-release formulation), lamotrigine or valproate. However, there is also sufficient evidence to recommend levetiracetam, phenytoin, oxcarbazepine or topiramate. Choice varies with doctor and patient preference. Other drugs are usually reserved for second-line therapy.

Various comparative studies have been carried out, but no one drug has been found to be consistently superior or inferior in terms of seizure control. The most striking finding from all these studies is the similarity, not the difference, in responder rates among the various drugs.

Patients with chronic epilepsy

Again, there are no antiepileptics that are clearly superior to others in the control of tonic–clonic seizures in chronic epilepsy. Many patients who fail to respond to one drug will, however, respond to another and it is usual (and logical) in this situation to rotate a patient through trials of treatment with all appropriate therapies – and this strategy is discussed on pp. 101–104.

Table 5.2 Choice of medication in different seizure types in chronic epilepsy.

Seizure type	Drugs that show proven efficacy	Drugs that can worsen seizures[a]
Partial seizures, secondarily generalized tonic–clonic seizures, primary generalized tonic–clonic seizures	Acetazolamide, clobazam, clonazepam, carbamazepine, eslicarbazepine, felbamate, gabapentin, lacosamide, lamotrigine, levetiracetam, oxcarbazepine phenobarbital, phenytoin, pregabalin, primidone, tiagabine, topiramate, valproate, vigabatrin, zonisamide	
Absence seizures (typical absence)	Acetazolamide, clobazam, clonazepam, ethosuximide, lamotrigine, levetiracetam, phenobarbital, topiramate, valproate, zonisamide	Carbamazepine, gabapentin, phenytoin, pregabalin, oxcarbazepine, tiagabine, vigabatrin
Myoclonic seizures	Clobazam, clonazepam, lamotrigine, levetiracetam, phenobarbital, piracetam, topiramate, valproate, zonisamide	Carbamazepine, gabapentin, lamotrigine, oxcarbazepine, phenytoin, pregabalin, tiagabine, vigabatrin
Atypical absence, tonic and atonic seizures	Acetazolamide, clobazam, clonazepam, lamotrigine, levetiracetam, phenobarbital, phenytoin, primidone, rufinamide, topiramate, valproate, zonisamide	Carbamazepine, gabapentin, oxcarbazepine, phenytoin, pregabalin, tiagabine, vigabatrin

[a]The drugs listed are those with have a specific worsening effect on seizures. In addition to this list, most drugs worsen seizures in occasional patients.

Idiopathic generalized epilepsy

There is a clinical impression, often voiced, that valproate is a better choice than carbamazepine for first-line therapy of the generalized tonic–clonic seizures in the syndrome of idiopathic generalized epilepsy. However, there is little if any conclusive evidence to support this proposition, and indeed most well-conducted studies show little difference in efficacy between any of the major antiepileptic drugs. However, myoclonus and/or absence seizures often coexist with tonic–clonic seizures in idiopathic generalized epilepsy. These seizures types respond well to valproate or levetiracetam, and are frequently worsened by carbamazepine or oxcarbazepine, so it seems reasonable to start therapy with either valproate or levetiracetam. Lamotrigine or topiramate would be further choices, but these have more variable effects on moyclonus and so are both usually reserved as a second line in idiopathic generalized epilepsy. Other second line drugs are shown in Table 5.2.

Partial-onset seizures

The principles of therapy and the choice of drugs are very similar to those in patients with tonic–clonic seizures.

Newly diagnosed and/or drug-naïve patients

As is the case with tonic–clonic seizures, monotherapy is the rule. The choice of medication is shown in Table 5.1

and is similar (though slightly wider) than that of tonic–clonic epilepsy. As with tonic–clonic seizures, it is currently usual practice to start therapy with carbamazepine (in its slow-release formulation). However, monotherapy with lamotrigine, valproate, levetiracetam, phenytoin, oxcarbazepine or topiramate is also licensed and shown to be equally effective in population terms. As is the case for tonic–clonic seizures, the choice varies with the doctor and the patient.

Various comparative studies have been carried out, but no one drug has been found to be consistently superior or inferior in terms of seizure control. The most striking finding from all these studies is the similarity, not the difference, in responder rates among the various drugs.

Patients with chronic epilepsy

Again, a range of antiepileptic drugs is available (see Table 5.2), without any showing clear superiority in the control of partial-onset seizures in chronic epilepsy. As is the case in tonic–clonic epilepsy, it is usual therefore to recommend sequential trials of treatment of all appropriate therapies in non-responders (see pp. 101–104).

Generalized absence seizures

Generalized absence seizures occur only in the syndrome of idiopathic generalized epilepsy. Valproate is the most common first choice AED. Other drugs that are sometimes used as first-line therapy, but that have less reliable effects, are levetiracetam, lamotrigine, topiramate, zonisamide and the benzodiazepines.

For many years ethosuximide had been the standard drug but it is largely ineffective in controlling generalized tonic–clonic seizures, which often coexist with absence seizures, and has a number of troublesome adverse effects. It still has a role, particularly in children, where there is anxiety about the idiosyncratic effects of valproate.

First-line therapy can be expected to fully control absence seizures in over 90% of patients. In non-responders (or those in whom valproate is inappropriate) trials of alternative first-line monotherapies should be made, and then of second-line therapies (shown in Table 5.2). About 10–20% of absence seizures will be resistant to monotherapy, but only about 10% or so of patients will not gain full control of the seizures on appropriate single or combination drug therapy.

Myoclonic seizures

Myoclonus occurs in various clinical settings (Table 5.3). The myoclonus in idiopathic generalized epilepsy is generally well controlled on single drug therapy with valproate, which is the drug of first choice. Where valproate is inappropriate or ineffective, other agents that are sometimes used are levetiracetam, lamotrigine, topiramate, zonisamide and the benzodiazepines.

The myoclonus in symptomatic, generalized, progressive myoclonic epilepsy or in the focal epilepsies is more difficult to treat, and drug combinations may be necessary.

One second-line agent worth considering is piracetam. This extraordinary compound is the only drug uniquely effective in myoclonus and has no effect in other types of epilepsy. The doses required for myoclonus are extremely high, but the drug is very well tolerated. It is primarily effective in cortical myoclonus, but may also have some value in other myoclonic syndromes, and has most use in the treatment of myoclonus in the progressive myoclonic epilepsy syndromes.

Some drugs exacerbate absence or myoclonic seizures (Table 5.2). The γ-aminoglutamic acid (GABA)-ergic antiepileptic drugs vigabatrin, tiagabine, pregabalin and gabapentin are frequently associated with aggravation of myoclonus, and can indeed precipitate myoclonus for the first time in susceptible patients. Phenytoin has been reported to worsen the myoclonus in Lafora body disease, although the evidence is not conclusive. Both carbamazepine and phenytoin can aggravate myoclonus in juvenile myoclonic epilepsy.

Therapies for specific myoclonic syndromes

Specific therapy has been attempted in a number of the progressive myoclonic epilepsies, although none has an uncontested place in treatment regimens. Antioxidant treatments have been used for some years in the treatment of ceroid lipofuscinosis. N-Acetylcysteine has some advocates in the Unverricht–Lundborg disease; although often prescribed, it is doubtful whether these compounds have any major beneficial effect, and the early claims made for this therapy have been retracted. Alcohol has a beneficial effect on the myoclonus in Unverricht–Lundborg disease, as indeed it does in some forms of subcortical myoclonus.

Myoclonus in focal epilepsy

What is often known as focal myoclonus is equivalent physiologically to a partial motor seizure, and can be treated with any drug used for focal epilepsy. One particularly intractable form of focal myoclonus is epilepsia partialis continua. AED treatment in this situation can be fruitless and difficult, and immunological therapy can be helpful where the myoclonus is the result of an inflammatory disorder.

Atypical absence, atonic and tonic seizures

These seizure types occur largely in the context of the Lennox–Gastaut syndrome or the other severe epileptic encephalopathies. The drug treatment is essentially similar for each, although full control of seizures is usually not possible.

Valproate or lamotrigine is recommended by most as the first choice of drug. Traditional alternatives are the benzodiazepine drugs (e.g. clobazam or clonazepam), acetazolamide, phenobarbital and primidone.

Table 5.3 Epilepsies in which myoclonus is part of the phenotype.

Idiopathic generalized epilepsy
Benign myoclonic epilepsy syndromes of childhood
Severe epilepsy syndromes of childhood
Progressive myoclonic epilepsies
Focal epilepsies in the central region
Symptomatic focal epilepsies due to mitochondrial disease, inherited or acquired metabolic disease, infections, drugs and toxins

Levetiracetam has promise in these types of epilepsy, at an anecdotal level, but formal studies are limited. Phenytoin may be useful for tonic seizures, but may exacerbate atonic seizures. Topiramate (target maintenance dose 6 mg/kg per day) has been shown to be effective in many open and controlled studies. Zonisamide has been shown to be effective in all these seizure types. Felbamate also has a powerful effect in atypical absence, tonic and atonic seizures, and the drug still has a useful place in refractory cases where other medication has failed. Rufinamide is a drug newly licensed specifically for the treatment of these seizure types in the Lennox Gastaut Syndrome.

Drugs that exacerbate seizures

Carbamazepine and oxcarbazepine are frequently reported to exacerbate atypical absence and tonic seizures. Tiagabine can dramatically worsen atypical absence seizures, resulting sometimes in a rather characteristic non-convulsive status epilepticus (see p. 242). It is likely that gabapentin, pregabalin and vigabatrin have similar effects. Benzodiazepine can exacerbate tonic seizures, and occasionally precipitate tonic status epilepticus.

Other factors influencing drug choice
Tailoring drugs to different patient profiles

In spite of the disappointing lack of differentiation between drugs in the regulatory trials, it is absolutely clear that, in routine clinical practice, qualitative differences do exist. The art of therapy is to tailor the drugs to individual patient needs, and the recognition of drug differences is at the heart of skilful prescribing. On an empirical basis, among patients with partial-onset epilepsy, for example, one can discern several distinctive patient profiles, commonly encountered in clinical practice, that require different approaches. Clinical experience suggests that certain drugs convey certain advantages in these groups, either because of a lower risk of side effects in susceptible people or because of particular effectiveness. There are no controlled data on many of these points, and Table 5.4 summarizes the author's own preferences.

There are also other clinical factors that influence drug choice. People differ, for example, in their willingness to risk specific side effects (e.g. weight gain). Preferences will depend on age, gender or co-morbidity, co-medication and dosing frequencies, cost and such factors as risks in pregnancy (Table 5.5).

Prescribing patterns also vary, and are dependent on such factors as prior experience, marketing pressures, the medical system within which they work, and teaching and information sources. There are marked differences

in the use of drugs in different countries, e.g. phenytoin is more widely prescribed in the USA than elsewhere, carbamazepine in northern Europe and valproate in the Francophone world. The pattern of drug usage furthermore varies widely within countries and even within the same institution.

Cost of drugs

The cost of drugs varies considerably, and furthermore differs in different countries and regions. The newer drugs are far more expensive than the older alternatives, and the following are typical UK prices charged to the National Health Service in 2004. The average 28-day cost of prescribing carbamazepine, lamotrigine, phenytoin and valproate is between £2 and £12 (£9 and £15 for the controlled-release formulations). The comparable costs of the newer drugs are: gabapentin 1800 mg – £8; levetiracetam 4 g – £83; oxcarbazepine 1200 mg – £44; tiagabine 30 mg – £76; and topiramate 400 mg – £109.

Licensing of drugs

There has in recent years been a remarkable growth in the number of drugs available for the treatment of epilepsy. Newer drugs have specific licences based on the evidence from clinical trials. Most such clinical trials are carried out first with the drug used as add-on therapy in refractory partial epilepsy. Their licence is then restricted to combination therapy, with no licence for monotherapy (despite the fact that there are no examples of antiepileptic drugs that are effective as add-on therapy but ineffective when used alone). Monotherapy licences have to await monotherapy trials.

Although off-label prescribing is common in epilepsy, in the age of growing litigation and bureaucratic oversight, this carries risks and should be discouraged at least in non-specialist practice or without explicit justification. The current British and European licensed indications of the newer drugs are shown in Table 5.6.

The older drugs – carbamazepine, clobazam, clonazepam, ethosuximide, phenobarbital, primidone, phenytoin and valproate – were all licensed at a time when strict licensing regulations did not exist, and have been permitted to continue to be prescribed on the basis of a 'grandfather clause'. They carry no regulatory age limitations or restrictions to combination therapy or seizure type.

Time it has taken to recognize side effects – the need for caution

Another general point of importance is that it has taken many years for some important side effects to be

Table 5.4 Tailoring antiepileptic drugs in partial-onset epilepsy to patient characteristics (based on preferences from the author's clinical practice).

Patient characteristics	Drugs that are particularly suitable[a]	Drugs that should be particularly avoided
Patients with severe partial-onset seizures	Clobazam, carbamazepine, lacosamide, levetiracetam, oxcarbazepine, phenytoin, topiramate, zonisamide	Gabapentin, lamotrigine, valproate
Patients who wish particularly to avoid cosmetic effects		Phenobarbital, phenytoin, primidone, valproate (for its effects on hair)
Patients with prominent anxiety	Clobazam (and other benzodiazepines), carbamazepine, gabapentin, phenobarbital, pregabalin, valproate	Levetiracetam
Patients with prominent depression	Carbamazepine, lamotrigine, valproate	Levetiracetam, vigabatrin, phenobarbital
Patients with renal stones		Acetazolamide, topiramate, zonisamide,
Patients with migraine	Topiramate, valproate	
Patients with the need to lose weight (or not to gain weight)	Topiramate, zonisamide	Gabapentin, pregabalin, valproate
Patients with hyponatraemia		Carbamazepine, oxcarbazepine
Patients at particular risk from allergy	Clobazam, gabapentin, lacosamide, levetiracetam, pregabalin, topiramate, vigabatrin	Acetazolamide, carbamazepine, felbamate, lamotrigine, oxcarbazepine, phenytoin, zonisamide
Patients at particular risk of heart disease		Carbamazepine, lamotrigine, oxcarbazepine
Patients at risk from osteoporosis	Gabapentin, levetiracetam, pregabalin	Phenobarbital, phenytoin
Patients in whom the risk of hepatic enzyme interactions have to be avoided (e.g. those co-mediated with antibiotics, immunosuppressive drugs, oncological drugs, antipsychotics)	Clobazam, gabapentin, lacosamide, levetiracetam, pregabalin, topiramate, vigabatrin	

[a]First-line drugs.

recognized (Table 5.7). In the light of this experience, it is wise, generally, to exercise caution when using newly licensed drugs, the full side-effect profile of which may not yet be completely apparent.

Evidence for comparative efficacy in chronic epilepsy: meta-analysis of regulatory drug trials

As part of the FDA rules, to be licensed, a new candidate AED is required to show superiority to a comparator, not just simple equivalence. From the clinical (in contrast to the regulatory) perspective, this has had one serious disadvantage – all new drugs have been compared in the RCTs primarily with placebo, rather than with each other. Thus, the trials do not individually give much information to the clinician about the *relative* benefits of individual drugs. One way around this problem has been to perform meta-analyses of trials, and to use meta-analytical statistical methods to compare and contrast the effectiveness of individual drugs undergoing trials against placebo. Such analyses have obvious and

Table 5.5 Factors influencing choice of treatment regimen in epilepsy.

Personal patient-related factors
Age and gender
Co-morbidity (physical and mental)
Social circumstances (employment, education, domestic, etc.)
Emotional circumstances
Attitude to risks of seizures and of medication
Factors related to the epilepsy
Syndrome and seizure type
Severity and chronicity
Aetiology (less important in chronic epilepsy)
Factors related to the drug
Mechanism of action
Strength of therapeutic effects
Severity and nature of side effects
Formulation
Drug interactions and pharmacokinetic properties
Cost

This list illustrates the sort of factors that influence choice of drugs. It is not comprehensive, and the importance of factors will vary from individual to individual.

well-known disadvantages, but currently provide the best information available for making drug choices. The first meta-analysis of antiepileptic drugs was carried out in Liverpool and has become justly influential. In a recent update, 36 randomized clinical trials were analysed in which 1 of 8 new antiepileptic drugs was tested against placebo as add-on treatment in patients with refractory partial epilepsy. The results are shown in Figure 5.1. This shows that the mean odds ratio (OR) with their 95% CIs of responder rates (i.e. having a ≥50% improvement in seizures on therapy compared with a baseline period). In this analysis, all drugs were found to be statistically superior to placebo (i.e. the means and 95% CIs are all >1), and, although there are striking (almost twofold) differences between the mean ORs for different drugs, the CIs are wide and overlap, and thus these differences are not statistically significant.

One criticism of this method of display is that drugs are being compared at the dosages used in the clinical trials, and that higher doses of the seemingly less effective drugs might produce better ORs. Analysis at different doses does certainly produce different mean values, and this effect is most clearly shown for topiramate and levetiracetam.

The rate of premature withdrawal from the RCT is a commonly used measure of tolerability. Similar to all surrogate measures, this measure has limitations and, for example, can be unduly influenced by transient initial side effects and dose escalation regimens. Nevertheless, it is a useful measure of overall tolerability and it is susceptible to meta-analysis using the same statistical treatment as for efficacy comparisons. Figure 5.2 illustrates the results of a meta-analysis of withdrawal rates of the eight antiepileptic drugs. The mean ORs show an almost fourfold difference in tolerability, but again, as the CIs overlap, the differences were not statistically different. It is also noteworthy that the confidence limits for three drugs (lamotrigine, gabapentin and levetiracetam) overlap the placebo response, indicating no significant difference in withdrawal rate between placebo and active therapy.

Other analyses are possible from the same data-set, including a 'number-needed-to-treat' analysis that does show statistical differences between the relatively weaker effectiveness of lamotrigine and gabapentin compared with levetiracetam, topiramate, vigabatrin or oxcarbazepine.

The validity of these meta-analyses has been the subject of wide-ranging criticism. Not least, all studies were on fixed doses, and there is no doubt that there would be different responses at different doses. Nevertheless, the overriding message from the analysis is that none of the newer drugs has any unequivocal superiority in terms of efficacy or tolerability to any of the others.

Evidence for comparative AED efficacy in monotherapy

The landmark monotherapy study for traditional drugs was the double-blind multicentre comparison of phenytoin, carbamazepine, phenobarbital and primidone carried out by the American Veterans' Administration collaborative network. In this study 622 patients were randomized to treatment with 1 of the 4 drugs and followed for 24 months or until toxicity or lack of seizure control required a treatment switch. The patients were adults, and a mixture of newly diagnosed drug-naïve patients and patients who had been previously undertreated. Overall treatment success was highest with carbamazepine or phenytoin, intermediate with phenobarbital and lowest with primidone, but the proportion of patients rendered free of seizures on the four drugs (between 48% and 63%) did not differ greatly. Differences in failure rates were explained primarily by the fact that primidone caused more intolerable acute adverse effects, such as nausea, vomiting, dizziness and sedation (in fact this was perhaps because too high a dose was used

Table 5.6 Licensed indications of the new antiepileptic drugs (in the UK, 2009).

Drug	Licensed indications as adjunctive therapy	Licensed indications for monotherapy
Eslicarbazepine	Partial onset seizures refractory to therapy in adults	Not licensed in monotherapy
Gabapentin	Partial and secondary generalized seizures; ≥6 years	Partial and secondarily generalized seizures ≥12 years
Lacosamide	Partial and secondarily generalized seizures; ≥16 years	Not licensed in monotherapy
Lamotrigine	Partial and generalized seizures and Lennox–Gastaut syndrome; ≥2 years.	Partial and generalized seizures (primarily or secondarily generalized) seizures and Lennox–Gastaut syndrome; ≥13 years. Absence seizures; ≥2 years
Levetiracetam	Partial seizures and secondarily secondary generalization; ≥1 month Myoclonic and tonic–clonic seizures in juvenile myoclonic epilepsy, ≥12 years	Partial and secondarily generalized seizures ≥16 years
Oxcarbazepine	Partial and tonic–clonic seizures (primarily or secondarily generalized) seizures; ≥6 years	Partial and tonic–clonic seizures (primarily or secondarily generalized) seizures; ≥6 years
Piracetam	Myoclonic seizures	Not licensed in monotherapy
Pregabalin	Partial and secondarily generalized tonic–clonic seizures;≥18 years	Not licensed in monotherapy
Rufinamide	Seizures in the Lennox–Gastaut syndrome; ≥4 years	Not licensed in monotherapy
Tiagabine	Second-line therapy in partial and secondarily generalized tonic–clonic seizures; ≥12 years	Not licensed in monotherapy
Topiramate	Partial and tonic–clonic seizures (primarily or secondarily generalized) seizures and the Lennox–Gastaut syndrome; ≥2 years	Partial and tonic–clonic seizures (primarily or secondarily generalized) seizures; ≥6 years
Vigabatrin	Therapy-resistant partial and secondarily generalized tonic–clonic seizures; no age limit specified	Monotherapy in infantile spasms; no age limit specified
Zonisamide	Partial seizures with or without secondary generalization; ≥18 years	Not licensed in monotherapy

Based on guidelines from the summary of product characteristics of the individual medicines in the UK. Indications may vary in other countries.

Table 5.7 Latency between the introduction of antiepileptic drugs to the market and the discovery of important adverse effects.

Drug	Adverse reaction	Incidence of side effects	Year of marketing	Year of discovery of side effects
Phenobarbital	Shoulder–hand syndrome	Up to 12%	1912	1934
Phenytoin	Rickets and osteomalacia	Up to 5%[a]	1938	1967
Trimethadione	Teratogenicity	30–50%	1944	1970
Valproic acid	Hepatotoxicity	1 in 600 to 1 in 50 000	1967	1977
Vigabatrin	Visual field defects	30–40%	1989	1997

[a]Frequency in the 1960s, now lower.

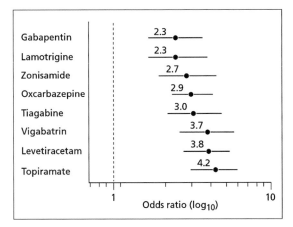

Figure 5.1 Odds ratios for 50% responder rates from placebocontrolled, adjunctive-therapy randomized controlled trials (RCTs) of eight recently introduced antiepileptic drugs. This figure shows the summary odds ratios (overall odds ratio and 95% confidence intervals) of the RCTs of eight newly introduced antiepileptic drugs. Note that the horizontal scale is logarithmic and that there are marked differences between the mean odds ratios. However, as the confidence intervals overlap, there is no statistical difference. Note also that, as the confidence intervals are all to the right of the vertical line, all drugs are significantly more efficacious than placebo.

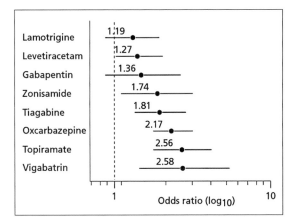

Figure 5.2 Odds ratios for rates of premature withdrawal from published placebo-controlled, adjunctive-therapy RCTs of eight recently introduced antiepileptic drugs. This figure shows the summary odds ratios (overall odds ratio and 95% confidence intervals) of the RCTs of eight newly introduced antiepileptic drugs. Note that the horizontal scale is logarithmic and that there are marked differences between the mean odds ratios. However, as the confidence intervals overlap, there is no statistical difference.

initially). This study confirmed the widely held view that – in terms of antiepileptic efficacy – there was little to choose between the four drugs, and that the main differences relate to their side-effect profiles. A follow-on study comparing carbamazepine and valproate in 480 adult patients showed no differences in the control of secondarily generalized seizures, although carbamazepine was more effective in complex partial seizures.

Two randomized open British studies, on the other hand, found no differences in efficacy when valproate and carbamazepine were compared in adults and children with newly diagnosed partial and/or generalized tonic–clonic seizures. In two additional randomized studies, carbamazepine, valproate, phenytoin and phenobarbital were compared as initial therapy in drug-naïve, newly diagnosed children and adults. No differences in efficacy were noted, but phenobarbital was withdrawn more often in children because of side effects. A similar comparative open monotherapy study in adults found no significant differences among carbamazepine, phenytoin and valproate in efficacy or side effects. Similarly, the efficacy of valproate against absence seizures was found to be similar to that of ethosuximide. Taking these studies together, a few general conclusions can be reached. It seems clear that there are no major differences in efficacy between any of the drugs that are used for the treatment of focal epilepsy. Among these traditional drugs, carbamazepine may have slightly better efficacy in partial seizures than valproate, and both carbamazepine and phenytoin are better tolerated than phenobarbital in newly diagnosed epilepsy in children, but not adults (Table 5.8).

As far as newer drugs are concerned, comparative monotherapy data are also limited. There have been a number of randomized studies in adults comparing lamotrigine with carbamazepine and phenytoin and no major differences in efficacy were found, even though lamotrigine showed some tolerability advantages, particularly in elderly people. Gabapentin has been compared with carbamazepine in one double-blind monotherapy study, which showed no differences in efficacy at higher gabapentin doses. Topiramate has been compared in similar studies with carbamazepine and valproate, and oxcarbazepine with carbamazepine, valproate and phenytoin, and in none of these studies were significant differences in efficacy seen at comparable doses. In newly diagnosed epilepsy, topiramate 100 and 200 mg/day was found to be as effective as carbamazepine 600 mg/day or valproate 1250 mg/day. Oxcarbazepine and topiramate have both been shown to be superior to placebo in monotherapy (using an active control design).

Table 5.8 Comparative monotherapy studies of standard antiepileptic drugs in partial and tonic–clonic seizures.

	No. of studies	Treatment failure	12-month remission	Time to first seizure
Partial epilepsy				
Carbamazepine vs valproate	5	ND	ND	Slight advantage to carbamazepine[a]
Carbamazepine vs phenobarbital	4		ND	ND
Phenytoin vs valproate	4		ND	ND
Phenytoin vs phenobarbital		Slight advantage to phenytoin[b]	ND	ND
Generalized epilepsy				
Carbamazepine vs valproate	4	ND	ND	ND
Carbamazepine vs phenobarbital	3	ND	ND	ND
Phenytoin vs valproate	5	ND	ND	ND
Phenytoin vs phenobarbital		Advantage to phenytoin[c]	ND	ND

The significance was measured by the hazard ratio; ND, no significant difference.
[a]Difference 1.22 (CI 1.04–1.44).
[b]Difference 1.97 (CI 1.09–1.97).
[c]Difference 4.32 (CI 1.77–10.6).

Monotherapy trials, in which vigabatrin and gabapentin were compared with carbamazepine in patients with newly diagnosed epilepsy, also failed to show any advantages in efficacy in favour of the newer drugs and, if anything, there was a trend for rates of freedom from seizures to be higher in the groups assigned to carbamazepine.

The most striking finding from all these studies is the similarity – not the difference – in responder rates among the various drugs in patients with partial-onset epilepsy. As a result of this, choice in these patients will depend to a large extent on tolerability considerations, cost and other factors. The most influential recent investigation was SANAD, a 0 long-term, multicentre, non-blinded, but randomized controlled, trial in the UK. Arm A recruited 1721 mostly newly diagnosed patients, for whom the treating physicians would have given carbamazepine (mostly those with partial epilepsy), and patients were randomised to treatment with carbamazepine, gabapentin, lamotrigine, oxcarbazepine or topiramate was given. The efficacy of all drugs was roughly similar although lamotrigine performed slightly better than the others, largely because of better tolerability. In arm B, 716 patients were recruited, for whom valproate would have been chosen (mostly generalized or unclassified epilepsies), and patients were randomised to treatment with valproate, lamotrigine or topiramate. For those with idiopathic generalized epilepsy, valproate was found to be better tolerated than topiramate and more efficacious than lamotrigine in generalized epilepsies, especially idiopathic generalized epilepsy.

Treatment of specific epilepsy syndromes

There are some specific aspects of therapy of some epilepsy syndromes.

Neonatal seizures

If the seizures are considered non-epileptic, AED treatment is not indicated. Indeed, medication may worsen the phenomenon by decreasing the level of cortical inhibition over subcortical structures. Whether genuine (cortical) but slight (subtle) epileptic seizures require treatment is uncertain, especially in infants who are not paralysed for artificial ventilation. Not uncommonly such seizure manifestations remit spontaneously after days or weeks and the usefulness of treatment in these situations is difficult to assess. Opinions vary about the need to treat infants with EEG evidence of seizure activity without overt clinical signs. There is also disagreement about the duration of therapy, although most would aim for as short a period as possible. Many neonatal seizures are self-limiting and over-long treatment carries its own risks.

For all other neonatal seizures, however, treatment is urgent. Management demands meticulous specialized paediatric care, usually on an intensive care unit, and details are beyond the scope of this book. EEG monitoring is desirable and artificial ventilation often required. The treatment should be directed primarily at the causal disorder where this is possible, and immediate investigation is required to ascertain the cause. Hypoglycaemia requires immediate correction with 2–4 mL/kg of a 20–30% solution of glucose intravenously. Hypocalcaemia requires the slow intravenous injection of 2.5–5% calcium gluconate with ECG monitoring. Hypomagnesaemia requires 2–8 mL of a 2–3% solution of magnesium sulphate intravenously, or 0.2 mL/kg of a 50% solution intramuscularly. Pyridoxine deficiency, although rare, responds dramatically to 50–200 mg pyridoxine. Infections, other metabolic disorders (e.g. hyperammonaemia, organic aciduria) and mass lesions require specific therapy.

Emergency antiepileptic drugs are indicated for all but isolated seizures. Traditional practice is to load the infant with either phenobarbital or phenytoin. Phenobarbital is given to obtain a blood level of 20 mg/mL, which requires a loading dose of 20 mg/kg followed by a maintenance dose of 3–4 mg/kg per day intravenously or intramuscularly. Phenytoin is a second-line drug, with a loading dose of 15–20 mg/kg administered intravenously at a rate not exceeding 1–2 mg/kg per min, and with a maintenance dose of 3–10 mg/kg per day to obtain a plasma level of between 15 and 20 mg/mL. It is mandatory to monitor blood levels in the first 2–3 weeks of life because of abrupt changes in half-lives of the drugs. Others tend to postpone the use of these long-acting antiepileptics until the diagnosis is clarified and/or after shorter-acting agents such as diazepam, lorazepam or clonazepam have failed. The shorter-acting drugs are given for 24–48 h and then withdrawn.

Idiopathic generalized epilepsies

The clinical features of this common and important syndrome (IGE; also known as primary generalized epilepsy) are described on pp. 22–24, and genetic counselling on pp. 123–124. The seizure types in this condition are tonic–clonic, absence and myoclonic seizures. On monotherapy with one of the first-line antiepileptic drugs, complete control of seizures can be expected in at least 75% of patients, whether they have generalized tonic–clonic seizures alone or in combination with absence or myoclonic attacks. The treatment strategy should be to try alternative monotherapies with first-line drugs and lifestyle modification. In the few patients in whom this is ineffective, combination therapy can then be tried, mixing any of the conventional first-line medications. Less than 10% of patients with IGE have seizures that are truly refractory.

Generalized tonic–clonic seizures in idiopathic generalized epilepsy

As most antiepileptic clinical trials have been seizure rather than syndrome oriented, it is at present unclear whether the generalized tonic–clonic seizures of IGE respond to a different AED profile than the generalized tonic–clonic seizures in other types of epilepsy.

There is a clinical suspicion, held by many, that valproate is more effective in the tonic–clonic seizures in IGE than in tonic–clonic seizures of other types, and more effective than any other antiepileptic in this condition, although there is little hard evidence from clinical trials to support this. Nevertheless, valproate is the usual first-line therapy and, if this is ineffective or inappropriate, most would now suggest lamotrigine, levetiracetam or topiramate as alternative monotherapy. Carbamazepine is an effective therapy for tonic–clonic seizures in IGE, but it can exacerbate absence or myoclonus. This restricts its use, but nevertheless it remains a good choice in appropriate cases, and in special situations such as in pregnancy.

These seizures occur predominantly shortly after waking, when drowsy or while asleep, and the timing of some AED therapy can be varied to account for this. Sometimes avoiding sudden waking can prevent tonic–clonic seizures. Waking slowly, and drifting from sleep to wakefulness in a gradual fashion, can be very helpful. Sometimes tonic–clonic seizures occur after a prodromal period of increasing myoclonus. If this prodrome is long enough (>30 min), emergency clobazam or midazolam can prevent the seizure occurring.

Lifestyle advice is very important in avoiding tonic–clonic convulsions, especially those occurring on awakening. The avoidance of sleeplessness, late nights and alcohol will often markedly reduce the occurrence of seizures. The use of prophylactic clobazam or lorazepam at other times of risk (e.g. after a late night, alcohol, fatigue or stress) can be useful.

Absence seizures in idiopathic generalized epilepsy

The absence seizures in IGE are usually well controlled on monotherapy with valproate, ethosuximide, levetiracetam or lamotrigine. These are commonly used drugs of first choice and the benzodiazepines, phenobarbital and topiramate reserved for more resistant cases. The dosage required to obtain full control is usually only moderate.

Myoclonic seizures in idiopathic generalized epilepsy

The myoclonic seizures in IGE are usually treated first with valproate. Alternative therapies of proven efficacy include levetiracetam, topiramate, lamotrigine and benzodiazepine drugs (e.g. clobazam, clonazepam).

Drugs that may exacerbate seizures in idiopathic generalized epilepsy

Vigabatrin and tiagabine can exacerbate primarily generalized tonic–clonic seizures, and have no role in the therapy of IGE.

Gabapentin should also be avoided because it has little effect in generalized tonic–clonic seizures. Vigabatrin, tiagabine, gabapentin, carbamazepine and oxcarbazepine can also exacerbate absence and myoclonus.

Other subcategories of idiopathic generalized epilepsy

The above principles of therapy apply to the various proposed subcategories of IGE, including juvenile myoclonic epilepsy, childhood absence seizures and tonic–clonic seizures on awakening. Eyelid myoclonia can be considered a type of myoclonus, and the syndromes with this as a predominant sign are treated in the same way as other myoclonic epilepsies (albeit accounting for their distinctive prognoses).

Lifestyle measures

Lifestyle manipulation can be very helpful in many cases of IGE, especially in adolescence. The avoidance of sleep deprivation, sleeping late after a late night and excessive alcohol intake can be very beneficial. Many patients learn to recognize dangerous times, and take individual avoidance measures. Alternative or complementary medicine can be a useful adjunct to therapy (see pp. 118–121). Photosensitive patients should be counselled to avoid relevant stimuli (see pp. 72–73). Occasionally, patients with established mild epilepsy can avoid drug treatment altogether with these simple measures. Patients with juvenile myoclonic epilepsy typically also have psychosocial problems that have been attributed to an 'unstable personality' (although this is not a feature of the condition in most patients), and in one series psychiatric difficulties were found in 14%. These should be addressed.

Benign partial epilepsy syndromes of childhood

There is a variety of syndromes of partial epilepsy at various stages of childhood that has an excellent prognosis. The clinical features of these conditions are considered on pp. 24–25 and genetic counselling on p. 124.

Benign epilepsy with centrotemporal spikes

In this common childhood epilepsy syndrome, therapy is usually gratifyingly straightforward and indeed drug treatment is not necessary in all cases. If attacks are infrequent or mild, regular therapy seems inappropriate, especially as some children have only a few attacks before the epilepsy remits. Tonic–clonic seizures carry greater risks than the partial attacks and may tip the balance towards therapy. The partial seizures, when frightening and distressing, can warrant treatment, even if they are infrequent. If treatment is decided upon, over-medication and polypharmacy should be avoided. Both carbamazepine and valproate are highly effective, often at low doses. Other drugs also shown to be effective in open studies (albeit in usually small numbers of patients) include levetiracetam, lamotrigine and topiramate. EEG disturbances in patients without seizures – a very common occurrence – do not require any treatment. Withdrawal of medication should be considered after 1–2 years free of attacks even if the EEG has not normalized. Occasional cases seem to evolve into a more serious form of epilepsy (including into ESES and the Landau–Kleffner syndrome) but, in most, seizures remit without long-term sequelae.

Panayiotopoulos syndrome

In Panayiotopoulos syndrome, the principles of treatment are similar. Over 1000 children have been reported in several large case series. Various drugs have been used without any clear comparative analysis. Therapy has been shown to control seizures immediately in >90% of cases and in all patients seizures remitted within 1–6 years of onset. Long-term treatment is not necessary where seizures are infrequent, a common occurrence because, in most cases, the child may have only one or two seizures in total. An alternative approach is to avoid regular medication and use rescue medication (as for febrile seizures) in prolonged attacks.

Benign occipital lobe partial syndromes

In the occipital lobe partial syndromes, seizures are more frequent and drug therapy is usually required. Valproate may be the drug of choice before carbamazepine, and one has a strong clinical impression that the drug is particularly effective in seizures with occipital foci. In the clinical studies, both result in over 80% control of seizures. Clobazam can be used in seizure clusters. Drug withdrawal should be considered after several years of remission and, in photosensitive forms, photosensitivity on the EEG can be used as a guide to withdrawal.

Febrile seizures

The clinical features of febrile seizures are considered on pp. 26–28 and genetic counselling on pp. 124 and 125.

Emergency antiepileptic treatment

As prolonged febrile seizures carry a risk of causing cerebral damage, urgent therapy is required for any seizure lasting more than a few minutes. The aim of therapy is the rapid termination of the attack and thus the prevention of potential brain damage.

Ninety per cent of seizures are self-limiting, but, if a seizure continues for 5 min or more, emergency therapy is needed. The standard treatment is the administration of diazepam solution at a dose of 0.5–1 mg/kg either by intravenous injection (at a rate not exceeding 2 mg/min) or, as is common in out-of-hospital settings, by rectal instillation. A convenient ready-made proprietary preparation for rectal instillation exists – Stesolid. If there is no rapid effect, the same dose should be repeated. In an out-of-hospital setting, a maximum of two doses can be given. Diazepam should not be given by intramuscular injection or via rectal suppositories as absorption by either method is too slow. Alternatives to diazepam in the out-of-hospital setting include intramuscular or buccal midazolam 0.1–0.2 mg/kg.

In a hospital setting diazepam is given intravenously at 0.2–0.5 mg/kg up to a total (rectal plus intravenous dose) of 2–3 mg/kg over 30 min. A total dose of 20–30 mg diazepam is often required, but higher doses are usually not helpful. An alternative is lorazepam 0.05–0.1 mg/kg. It is rare for these measures not to terminate seizures, but if there is no rapid response an emergency infusion of phenobarbital can be initiated at a dose of 20 mg/kg at a rate no faster than 100 mg/min (with full intensive care unit [ICU] care).

Opinions differ about the value of cooling, but it is often recommended that the child should be cooled immediately using, for example, cold water, cold flannels, tepid sponging and removal of clothes and bedcovers.

Emergency prophylactic treatment

In susceptible children, prophylactic diazepam can be given rectally or orally as soon as a fever develops.

Suitable two- or three-times-daily doses, during the episode of fever, are 0.3–0.5 mg/kg rectally or 5 mg orally for children aged <3 years and 7.5 mg orally for those aged >3 years. One meta-analysis has shown that 11.2% of children treated with diazepam during febrile episodes have a seizure compared with 17.2% treated with placebo. It is also commonly accepted that intermittent diazepam is particularly effective in those at high risk of recurrences.

Intranasal or buccal midazolam (0.2 mg/kg) is an alternative. Measures to lower temperature, including tepid sponging and removal of clothing, should also be taken to prevent a seizure. Administration of paracetamol or ibuprofen has not been shown to prevent febrile seizures. Unfortunately, as the seizure occurs before the fever is apparent in at least a third of cases, prophylaxis is often not feasible.

Any underlying cause must be identified and treated. Blood and urine culture and full haematological and biochemical screening tests should be carried out. Cerebrospinal fluid (CSF) examination should be carried out whenever there is a suspicion of meningitis, in all children aged <18 months at the time of presentation of the first seizure, and in any child with meningism. Computed tomography (CT) should be performed before lumbar puncture in children with focal deficit after a prolonged convulsion or in those who do not recover consciousness. Serological and other investigations depend on clinical circumstances and it is difficult to provide general rules. Antibiotic therapy should be given as appropriate.

Long-term prophylaxis

In the past, antiepileptics were commonly given for long-term prophylaxis in children with a liability to recurrent febrile seizures. However, with increasing concern about the risks to learning and development, long-term therapy is now recommended for a very small number of children who are at a particularly high risk of frequent or complex febrile seizures. An influential meta-analysis of nine placebo-controlled studies reviewed the effect of prophylactic treatment on the recurrence rate of febrile seizures. The risk was significantly lower in children receiving continuous phenobarbital or sodium valproate than in those receiving placebo, but four children would have to be treated with valproate, and eight with phenobarbital, to prevent one recurrence, and typically now treatment is given only to those at risk of recurrent episodes who have had prolonged seizures lasting 30 min or more, and/or who have significant pre-existing neurological disturbance. The antiepileptic drugs used are either phenobarbital 15 mg/kg per day or valproate 20–40 mg/kg per day in two divided doses. Regular pyridoxine or phenytoin was found in the meta-analysis not to prevent recurrences.

Parental counselling

The occurrence of a febrile seizure is a profoundly distressing experience, and almost all parents at the time of a first febrile seizure think that the child is about to die. Parents should be reassured that the risk of brain damage is extremely small, and that febrile seizures are common and harmless and are a presage of epilepsy in only a small percentage of cases. Information about the management of subsequent seizures should be given. The parents should be instructed to stay calm, place the child on his or her side, not to force anything between the teeth and where appropriate to administer emergency therapy (as above). If the seizure lasts more than 5 min, the emergency services should be called and the child brought immediately to the nearest medical facility.

West syndrome

The clinical features of West syndrome are summarized on pp. 28–29. Infantile spasms are among the most serious and resistant of epilepsy syndromes, but opinions about management vary. Adrenocorticotrophic hormone (ACTH) is usually the preferred first-line therapy in the USA and Japan. Vigabatrin is usually given first in most European countries and in Asia and Canada.

ACTH and corticosteroid therapy

ACTH and corticosteroids have for many years been considered the standard therapy, in spite of relatively limited controlled data and serious risks of medium-term toxicity. ACTH is usually preferred to oral corticosteroids. The usual initial recommended daily dose of ACTH is 40 IU (3–6 IU/kg), given for between 1 and 5 months. Seizures remit in 75% of cases, but relapse occurs in about a third of cases after therapy is withdrawn. If seizures relapse either on therapy or after withdrawal, the ACTH should be recommenced immediately and doses of 60–80 IU may be needed. The incidence of adverse events is very high and almost all children develop cushingoid symptoms. Other common adverse effects include infections, increased arterial blood pressure, gastritis and hyperexcitability. These are often severe. The mortality rate of therapy is between 2% and 5%. Lower doses (20 IU) have been used but are less efficacious and higher doses of ACTH (150 IU) have a greater effect initially but do not have greater longer-term efficacy. Long-term

therapy (more than 5 months) at 40 IU/day was shown to be more effective than high-dose short-term therapy.

Oral steroids are less extensively prescribed, although they are better tolerated than ACTH. In one prospective, randomized, blinded study, the efficacy of prednisone (2 mg/kg per day) was inferior to that of high-dose ACTH (150 IU/day) given for 2 weeks, but no differences were found when ACTH was administered at lower doses. Other studies have shown superiority of ACTH over oral steroids, although the reason is not clear. There is also a feeling that the long-term intellectual outcome of patients treated with ACTH is better than that of those treated with oral steroids, although the evidence for this is essentially anecdotal.

Vigabatrin

Vigabatrin is widely used as an alternative to ACTH. It acts extremely rapidly and induces remission in over 50% of cases. Concern about the effects on the retina has tempered its use, not least because visual field testing is not possible in young children. Recently, also, brain vacuolation has been reported in several infants treated with vigabatrin, and if confirmed this too may weigh against the use of this drug. Five randomized studies have been reported comparing vigabatrin and hormonal therapy. Vigabatrin was shown to be superior to ACTH in the treatment of spasms in tuberous sclerosis, but less effective in other aetiologies. In the long term, the efficacy of both ACTH and vigabatrin is maintained in about 75% of cases. In tuberous sclerosis, vigabatrin seems not only more efficacious than hormonal therapy but also to have a better outcome in terms of intellectual function.

There is general agreement that the outcome is better if the spasms are brought urgently under control. Chiron recommends the following treatment schedule: initial therapy should be with vigabatrin 100 mg/kg per day for 1 week or ACTH. If vigabatrin is chosen and there is an incomplete response, the dose should be increased to 150 mg/kg per day. If there is still an incomplete response, hydrocortisone 15 mg/kg per day is added to vigabatrin 100 mg/kg per day for 2 weeks. If there is still an incomplete response, hydrocortisone should be replaced by ACTH. If ACTH is initially chosen, it should be switched to vigabatrin (as above) if ineffective within 4 weeks or increased in dose. The duration of ACTH or vigabatrin treatment in controlled patients will be determined by the balance between the risks of therapy, including visual field defects on vigabatrin, and the risk of relapse of seizures and the effects on cognition. As neither is fully known, decisions are to a large extent empirical.

The persistence of EEG multifocal spikes is the best predictor of relapse of spasms in infants and most paediatricians will discontinue vigabatrin monotherapy at around 2 years of age if the EEG is normal.

Other therapies

The value of antiepileptic therapy in West syndrome is difficult to assess, but most conventional antiepileptic drugs are relatively ineffective. Valproate and clonazepam control 25–30% of cases, but relapse rates are high. Carbamazepine can worsen the spasms. Topiramate, lamotrigine, felbamate and zonisamide have all been reported to help in small open-case series. Nitrazepam has been used but carries life-threatening side effects. High-dose pyridoxine is often given and there are promising reports about intravenous immunoglobulin. The ketogenic diet and thyrotrophin-releasing hormone have been reported to be occasionally helpful in refractory cases.

In the few cases of infantile spasms in which positron emission tomography (PET) shows clear-cut focal abnormalities, surgical resection can be performed with complete abolition of the spasm. The longer-term effects on neurological function of large surgical resection have not been fully established. Equally it is not clear to what extent cognitive development is affected by such radical treatment.

Lennox–Gastaut syndrome

The clinical features of the Lennox–Gastaut syndrome are described on pp. 29–30. It is a severe encephalopathy in which seizures are notoriously resistant to therapy. Complete control of seizures is rare, and almost all patients require polytherapy. A balance has to be drawn between optimum control of seizures and side effects, a compromise that is often difficult to achieve. It is important to resist the tendency – in the face of severe epilepsy – to escalate treatment. Such an escalation is seldom effective, and high-dose polypharmacy may cause drowsiness, which is a potent activator of the atypical absence and tonic seizures and non-convulsive status epilepticus. In addition to control of seizures, some authorities recommend therapy to try to ameliorate interictal EEG disturbances, on the basis that this may improve cognition and responsiveness. To what extent this is a valid approach is unclear.

Antiepileptic drug therapy

There have been five double-blind, placebo-controlled trials in this syndrome, all involving the addition of an AED to existing therapy. In these studies, felbamate, lamotrigine, topiramate and rufinamide have all been shown to be superior to placebo and, although all were maintained in the long-term follow-up, no single drug was highly effective.

As alternative first-line therapies, the usual recommendations are for valproate or lamotrigine. Valproate has a broad-spectrum activity against all the seizure types experienced in the syndrome (notably tonic, atonic, atypical absence, myoclonic, tonic–clonic seizures and status epilepticus). The drug has been reported to control seizures completely in 10% of cases, but this seems optimistic. It should be prescribed with caution in patients aged <3 years in view of the risk of hepatic failure (see pp. 116–118). Lamotrigine is an alternative initial therapy. In one double-blind randomized study of 169 patients, lamotrigine reduced the frequency of all major seizures from a weekly median of 16.4 at baseline to 9.9, and 33% of patients experienced at least a 50% reduction in seizures. It seems particularly effective in preventing falls. Lamotrigine has also been shown to improve cognition and quality-of-life ratings in the syndrome.

Caution needs to be exercised, particularly when used in combination with valproate, in view of their marked pharmacokinetic interaction. Topiramate (at a target maintenance dosage of 6 mg/kg per day) was shown in a double-blind, placebo-controlled trial to result in at least a 50% reduction in the frequency of seizures in 33% of patients, with a median reduction in the frequency of drop attacks of 14.8%. In the open-label extension (with a mean topiramate dosage of 10 mg/kg per day) there was a reduction in drop attacks of at least 50% in 55% of the patients, and 15% of the patients had no drop attacks for at least 6 months.

Other therapies can also be tried. Clobazam, clonazepam and nitrazepam are all widely prescribed. Clobazam probably confers less drowsiness than clonazepam and is often combined with valproate. Small doses of nitrazepam can be helpful. Benzodiazepines can exacerbate tonic seizures. Zonisamide has a broad spectrum of antiepileptic activity, and was reported to reduce seizure frequency by 50% or more in 32% of 132 patients reported in open-label studies from Japan. Levetiracetam in small series has been shown to have similar efficacy. Felbamate has been shown to have a powerful effect in the Lennox–Gastaut syndrome. In a double-blind, placebo-controlled study of 73 patients, felbamate therapy resulted in a 34% decrease in the frequency of atonic seizures and a 19% decrease in the frequency of all seizures. Quality of life was improved and the improvement was maintained for at least 12 months in subsequent open-label follow-up studies. However, the hypersensitivity reactions now limit its use to patients not responding to other appropriate medication.

Phenytoin and carbamazepine are generally of little benefit in the Lennox–Gastaut syndrome, and should generally not be used. Carbamazepine in particular can exacerbate atypical absence and myoclonic seizures. Barbiturates carry the potential for worsening hyperactivity and behavioural disorders, and their sedative effects can exacerbate atypical absence and tonic seizures. Vigabatrin shows some effect in the Lennox–Gastaut syndrome but often exacerbates myoclonic seizures, as can gabapentin and tiagabine. The latter drug in particular has a propensity to induce non-convulsive status in some patients.

A new AED, rufinamide, was licensed in 2007 for use only in the Lennox–Gastaut syndrome – via the fast-track process for 'orphan' diseases. It has proven efficacy in clinical trials (see pp. 235–238), but experience of its long-term clinical use is limited.

Other adjunctive treatments have been tried, in small studies, with very limited success. These include imipramine, amantadine, bromide, allopurinol and flunarizine. ACTH at doses of 30–40 IU/day is reported to be effective if started early but is now seldom used. Steroids can also be given in short courses to tide a patient over a bad patch.

Non-pharmacological therapy

The ketogenic diet has its greatest role in this syndrome. In one study, a significant effect was demonstrated after 3 months of therapy and, when considering all syndromes together, 38% of patients randomized to the ketogenic diet had a >50% reduction in seizures compared with 6% not on the diet.

Resective surgery has an extremely limited role in the Lennox–Gastaut syndrome. Individuals with focal or unihemispherical disease may occasionally be amenable to surgical treatment. Corpus callostomy can be used for the treatment of atonic and tonic drop attacks, but the initially beneficial effects seem to wear off and this operation is now seldom carried out. Vagal nerve stimulation is reported to have led to a >50% decrease in seizures in 37–73% of patients, but the results of these trials are not in accord with clinical experience which shows a much lower response rate.

The underlying cause of the Lennox–Gastaut syndrome should be treated where possible, and this may greatly ameliorate the seizures.

Multidisciplinary approach to therapy

In all the epileptic encephalopathies, AED treatment is a small part of management. A multidisciplinary team approach is vital, needing input from other specialties and disciplines including psychology, psychiatry, education, speech and language therapy, physiotherapy and occupational therapy. Joint neuropsychological and speech and language therapy assessment is particularly important in diagnosis of the Landau–Kleffner syndrome and its subsequent management. All these children will have special educational needs and the choice of appropriate educational settings, in either mainstream or special school settings, will need careful assessment and be tailored to individual need.

Landau–Kleffner syndrome and ESES

The clinical features of these conditions are described on pp. 30–32. In the Landau–Kleffner syndrome control of seizures is often possible with rather modest antiepileptic treatment. Lamotrigine and valproate have been shown to be effective, as have benzodiazepine, sultiame, levetiracetam and topiramate. However, even if the seizures are controlled, the EEG abnormalities may not disappear and the aphasia may not improve. If one accepts that the speech disturbance was caused by the EEG disturbance, then more aggressive antiepileptic therapy to suppress the EEG disturbance is a logical approach, even in the absence of overt seizures. All antiepileptic drugs have been tried in the syndrome, although vigabatrin, oxcarbazepine and carbamazepine may worsen the EEG abnormalities and are therefore sometimes avoided, as should therapy with vigabatrin, gabapentin/pregabalin and tiagabine. ACTH or high-dose corticosteroids are also commonly given for periods of several months. The relative benefits of these approaches are unclear, and no comparative trials have been carried out. Assessment of any therapy is made difficult by the fluctuating course of this curious condition.

There was a fashion for surgical treatment using the technique of multiple subpial transection, although results are very variable and, even if there is improvement, it may be months or years after the operation. It seems quite unclear, to this author at least, whether the operation ever improves the long-term prognosis. All this is unsatisfactory, but, until a better understanding of the underlying pathophysiology and of the prognostic determinants is gained, therapy can be only empirical.

The EEG pattern of ESES does not generally require specific treatment. Indeed, it is often not possible to abolish the spike–wave by oral antiepileptic therapy.

If treatment is decided upon, ethosuximide, benzodiaz-epine drugs, ACTH, corticosteroids, as well as other conventional antiepileptic drugs (phenytoin, phenobarbital and valproate), and also immunoglobulin therapy have been used.

Severe myoclonic epilepsy of infancy (Dravet syndrome)

The conventional antiepileptic drugs that have been shown to have efficacy are valproic acid, benzodiazepines and topiramate. Recently, stiripentol, an inhibitor of cytochrome P450, has been demonstrated to be effective in combination with clobazam in an RCT. Stiripentol increases the concentration of norclobazam, an active metabolite of clobazam, and this undoubtedly explains some of its effect, but it probably also has independent action. Phenytoin, carbamazepine and lamotrigine can worsen seizures in this syndrome. Long-term outcome data are sparse. Mortality rates are around 15% and in survivors seizures persist into adulthood.

Principles of treatment of newly diagnosed patients

The decision to initiate drug therapy has important implications. In addition to its biological effects, therapy confers illness status, confirms the state of 'being epileptic', and can affect self-esteem, social relationships, education and employment. The decision to treat depends essentially on a balance between the benefits and drawbacks of therapy, and should be tailored to the requirements of the individual patient; there are no absolute rules (Table 5.9).

The balance is sometimes difficult to define. The benefits of therapy include the lower risk of recurrence of seizures, and thus of potential injury and even death, and the psychological and social benefits of more security from seizures. The drawbacks of therapy include the potential drug side effects, the psychological and social effects, the cost and the inconvenience. Chronic, long-term or subtle side effects are not easily detected, and weigh heavily on the decision to treat. One example is the potential adverse effect on learning in children, and partly because of this paediatricians initiate therapy less early than neurologists treating adults.

Practice varies in different countries. In the USA, for example, a higher proportion of patients is treated after a single seizure than in the UK and more often too by emergency loading therapy. Practice is also divided in

Table 5.9 Criteria that should be satisfied before initiating drug therapy.

Diagnosis should be certain

Risk of seizure recurrence should be sufficient

Seizures must be sufficiently troublesome (this depends on seizure type, severity, frequency, timing and precipitation)

Adequate compliance should be likely

Patient has been fully counselled about the role of therapy

Other therapy modalities should have been considered (lifestyle changes, avoiding precipitants, etc.)

Patient's wishes have been taken account of fully

Europe. The lack of consensus reflects more the differing social rather than medical contexts of therapy.

One proposition recently researched is that early effective therapy will improve long-term outcome, and thus that early antiepileptic drug therapy will prevent the establishment of chronic epilepsy. There is a striking lack of clear evidence to support this rumour, and there seems to be no reason currently to modify the traditional approach.

Factors influencing the decision to treat
Diagnosis
It is essential generally to establish a firm diagnosis of epilepsy before therapy is started. This is not always easy, particularly in the early stages of epilepsy. There is almost no place at all for a 'trial of treatment' to clarify the diagnosis, as it seldom does. Rarely should treatment be started before a diagnosis is confirmed.

A good first-hand witnessed account is essential, because diagnostic tests are often non-confirmatory. In practice, the misdiagnosis rate is quite high, e.g. about 20% of all patients referred to a tertiary level epilepsy service have psychogenic attacks. The diagnosis is also often delayed. In one study, in over a third of patients, a firm diagnosis could be made only 24 months after the onset of seizures.

The risk of recurrence of seizures
The estimation of the risk of recurrence of seizures is obviously a key factor in deciding whether or not to initiate therapy. Most studied has been the risk of recurrence after a first isolated attack (i.e. the risk of a

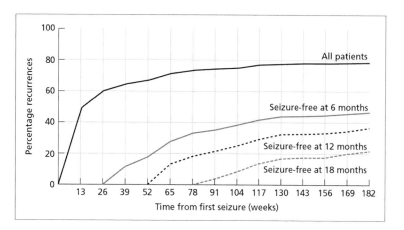

Figure 5.3 National General Practice Study of Epilepsy (NGPSE): actuarial percentage of recurrence after first seizure. A study of 564 patients followed prospectively from the time of diagnosis. Within 3 years of the first seizure, 78% of patients had a recurrence of their attacks. If attacks had not recurred within 6, 12 or 18 months, the chance of recurrence was substantially reduced, falling to 44, 32 and 17%, respectively.

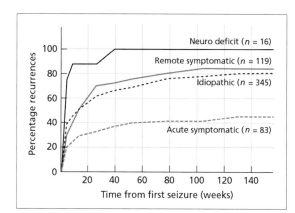

Figure 5.4 Actuarial percentage recurrences after first seizure by aetiological category.

second seizure). Investigations have produced conflicting findings, largely as a result of methodological issues, but most would now accept that between about 50 and 80% of all patients who have a first non-febrile seizure will have further attacks. The risk of recurrence is high initially and then falls over time. In a national UK study, the risk after the first seizure was 44% in the initial 6 months, 32% in the next 6 months and 17% in the second year (Figure 5.3). It follows therefore that the greater the elapsed time since the first attack, the less likely is subsequent recurrence (Figure 5.4).

In many cases, by the time of presentation, seizures will have already recurred. In a hospital-based study from the UK, the median number of tonic–clonic seizures occurring before the diagnosis was made was 4 (range

1–36) and the median number of partial seizures was 6 (range 1–180). If more than one spontaneous seizure has occurred, the risk of further attacks in the future without treatment is, in most clinical circumstances, over 80%, and generally speaking the more seizures that have occurred before therapy, the greater the risk of further attacks.

The risk of recurrence is influenced by the following factors.

Aetiology

This is a most important factor. The risk is greater in those with structural cerebral disease, and least in acute symptomatic seizures provoked by metabolic factors or exposure to drugs or toxins. The risk of recurrence of idiopathic or cryptogenic seizures is approximately 50%, and lower after provoked seizures, provided that the provoking factor is removed. In those with pre-existing learning disability or cerebral damage, the risk approaches 100% (see Figure 5.4).

EEG

Informed opinion concerning the prognostic value of EEG is conflicting. Although there is no doubt that the risk of recurrence is high if the EEG shows spike–wave discharges, the value of a normal EEG or an EEG with other types of abnormality after a single seizure, if there is any value at all, is slight.

Age

The risk of recurrence is somewhat greater in those aged <16 or >60 years, probably because of the confounding effect of aetiology.

Seizure type and syndrome

Partial seizures are more likely to recur than generalized seizures, again because of the confounding effect of aetiology. In most of the childhood epilepsy syndromes, recurrent seizures are almost inevitable. The exceptions are the benign partial syndromes. Many patients with benign partial epilepsy syndromes of childhood or Panayiotopoulos syndrome (see p. 26) often have a single attack only.

The type, timing and frequency of seizures

Some types of epileptic seizure have a minimal impact on the quality of life, e.g. simple partial seizures, absence or sleep attacks. The benefits of treating such seizures, even if they happen frequently, can be outweighed by the disadvantages. If the baseline frequency of seizures is very low, the disadvantages of treatment can be unacceptably high. It would be unusual to treat a person who has fewer than one seizure per year, especially if this was confined to sleep, or it was a minor or partial seizure.

Compliance

Antiepileptic drugs need to be taken reliably and regularly to be effective, and to avoid adverse events or withdrawal seizures. The decision to treat should be reconsidered in all circumstances in which compliance is likely to be poor.

Reflex seizures and provoked seizures

Occasionally, seizures occur only in specific circumstances or with certain precipitants (e.g. photosensitivity, fatigue or alcohol; see pp. 67–74). Avoiding these circumstances may obviate the need for drug treatment.

The risks of mortality and morbidity in early epilepsy

The mortality rate of epilepsy in the early years after diagnosis is two to three times that in the general population. The excess mortality is due almost entirely to the underlying cause of the seizures (e.g. stroke, tumour) and risks from other causes are slight. SUDEP, however, can occur in early epilepsy, and rarely indeed in the first seizure. Opinion is divided about whether a patient should be counselled about this risk on the first consultation – this will depend on clinical circumstances. Certainly, however, SUDEP should be discussed with most patients at some point early after diagnosis, and particularly if therapy is to be withheld.

Accidental injury and the psychosocial and psychiatric morbidity of epilepsy are outlined on pp. 78–79 and 107–116.

The risks of antiepileptic drug treatment

The benefits of treatment need to be balanced against the risk of adverse effects from the antiepileptic drugs.

The patient's wishes

This factor overrides all others. The role of the physician is to explain the relative advantages and disadvantages of therapy; the final decision must be left to the patient. Individuals differ greatly in their views about epilepsy and its treatment, e.g. for some seizure control is paramount – such as for driving or employment. Others have concerns about the concept of long-term medication or specific side effects and would prefer to risk an occasional seizure, particularly if their attacks do not inconvenience them unduly.

The physician must explain the purpose and limitations of antiepileptic drugs. The points covered should include: the likelihood of success of therapy; the suppressant rather than curative role of therapy; the potential side effects; the potential risks of withholding therapy; guidance in the event of idiosyncratic reactions; the need for regular medication; the importance of regular drug taking; guidance when a dose is missed; and the likely duration of therapy.

A protocol for treatment in drug-naïve patients

It will be clear that there can be no absolute rules about when to start therapy and when not to do so. In general terms, if there is a risk of recurrence of convulsive seizures, treatment will be indicated. In other circumstances, however, the requirement to initiate therapy can be quite individual. Where seizures are infrequent and minor, where non-convulsive seizures occur exclusively at night or in the benign syndromes of childhood epilepsy, treatment is often not indicated at all even in established cases. To reiterate, in all situations, the patient should be given advice based on the best available data and be allowed to make the final decision.

A protocol for the initial treatment of newly diagnosed patients is as follows (summarized in Table 5.10; the usual initial and maintenance doses and maximal incremental/decremental rates in routine practice are shown in Table 5.11).

Establish the diagnosis

There is little place for a 'trial of treatment'. Investigation will usually involve EEG, neuroimaging, and other investigations as necessary. Neuroimaging should be with MRI in all patients with partial-onset epilepsy, patients

Table 5.10 Principles of antiepileptic drug prescribing in patients with newly diagnosed epilepsy.

- Aim for complete control without adverse effects
- Diagnosis of epileptic seizures should be unequivocal
- Seizure type, syndrome and aetiology should be established
- Baseline haematological and biochemical investigations should be performed before initiation of drug therapy
- Use one drug at a time (monotherapy) at least initially
- Initial titration should be to low maintenance doses
- Further upward titration will depend on response and side effects
- If first drug fails, alternative monotherapies should be tried
- Upward and downward titration should be in slow, stepped doses
- Polytherapy should be used only if monotherapy with at least the first three drugs chosen has failed to control seizures
- Patients should be fully counselled about goals, role, risk, outcome and logistics of drug treatment

---

with fixed neurological deficit, onset of seizures in the first year of life or after the age of 15 without good explanation.

Identify and counsel about precipitating factors

If these can be avoided, this occasionally obviates the need for drug therapy.

Decide upon the need for AED therapy

If therapy is needed, baseline biochemical and haematological parameters should be measured and an electrocardiogram (ECG) carried out.

Counsel

Counselling should be given about the topics listed in Table 5.12. Patients should be given clear instructions to seek immediate medical attention if signs of hypersensitivity or idiosyncratic drug reactions develop.

Monotherapy

Start monotherapy with the chosen first-choice drug, initially at low doses, and titrate slowly up to a low maintenance dose (see Table 5.11). Emergency drug loading is seldom necessary except where status epilepticus threatens.

If seizures continue, titrate the dose upwards to higher maintenance dose levels (guided, where appropriate, by serum level monitoring). In about 60–90% of patients, these simple steps for initial therapy will result in complete control of seizures. In remaining patients the following applies:

- Failure of first monotherapy: alternative monotherapy should be tried with another appropriate first-choice antiepileptic drug. The second drug should be introduced incrementally at suitable dose intervals, and the first drug then withdrawn in slow decremental steps. The second drug should be titrated first to low maintenance doses and, if seizures continue, the dose increased incrementally to the maximal dose.
- Failure of repeated monotherapies: if the above steps fail, a third alternative monotherapy should be tried in the same manner, or polytherapy used.

If seizures continue, or recur after initial therapy with two to three drugs tried in monotherapy as above, the diagnosis should be reassessed. It is not uncommon in this situation to find that the attacks do not have an epileptic basis. Investigation should be considered to exclude the possibility of a progressive lesion. The possibility of poor compliance should be explored. Alternative monotherapies or polytherapy should be considered. The patient should be referred for specialist advice.

Avoid precipitating factors

Avoiding factors that precipitate seizures can be very important. Excess alcohol intake (or its abrupt withdrawal) was a predominant factor in 6% of first seizures in one UK series, and accounted for 27% of first seizures in those between the ages of 30 and 39 years. Photosensitivity is encountered mainly in adolescents with IGE, and is described on pp. 72–73. Sleep deprivation is also a major precipitating factor for seizures in susceptible individuals, and is often a contributory factor in those abusing alcohol. All these factors seem to be relevant particularly in patients with IGE.

Counselling and information provision

In addition to the topics listed in Table 5.12, it is sometimes important to offer counselling and information on a broader range of topics and lifestyle issues. The need for this will depend on individual circumstances. Most patients with newly diagnosed epilepsy enter rapid remission, and the epilepsy should not pose major problems, a fact that it is important to emphasize. The counselling required is not as intense or comprehensive as for chronic active epilepsy, where seizures are likely to persist. A balance is needed.

Table 5.11 Usual dosing regimens and fastest routine incremental and decremental rates in adults (values in this table are based on the author's own practice, and may vary from those published elsewhere).

Drug	Initial dose (mg/day)	Drug initiation: usual dose increment (mg/day) stepped up every 2 weeks	Usual initial maintenance dose on monotherapy (mg/day)	Usual maximum dose in monotherapy (mg/day)	Dosing intervals (per day)	Drug reduction: usual dose decrement (mg/day) stepped down every 2–4 weeks	Maintenance doses can be different when given as co-medication
Carbamazepine[a]	100–200	200	400–1600	2400	2–3	200	Yes
Clobazam	10	10	10–30	30	1–2	10	No
Clonazepam	0.25	0.25–0.5	0.5–4	4	1–2	0.5	No
Eslicarbazepine	400	200–400	800–1200	1200	1	400	Yes
Ethosuximide	250	250	750–1500	1500	2–3	250	Yes
Gabapentin	300–400	300–400	900–3600	3600	2–3	300–400	No
Lacosamide	50	50	200–400	400	2	50	No
Lamotrigine	12.5–25	50	100–400	600	2	50–100	Yes
Levetiracetam	125–250	250–500	750–4000	4000	2	250–500	No
Oxcarbazepine	300	300	900–2400	3000	2–3	300	Yes
Phenobarbital	30	15–30	30–120	180	1–2	15–30	Yes
Phenytoin	200	25–100	200–450	500	1–2	50	Yes
Pregabalin	50	50	150–400	600	2–3	50	No
Primidone	62.5–125	125–250	250–1000	1500	1–2	125–250	Yes
Rufinamide	400	400	1200–3200	3200	2	400	Yes
Tiagabine	15	4–5	30–45	56–60	2–3	4–5	Yes
Topiramate	25–50	25–50	75–300	600	2	50	Yes
Valproate	200–500	200–500	500–2000	3000	2–3	200–500	Yes
Vigabatrin	500	500	1000–3000	4000	2	500	No
Zonisamide	50	50	200–400	600	1–2	50	Yes

[a]Values are for the slow release formulation, which is the formulation of choice, particularly at high doses.

Table 5.12 Topics for information provision and counselling in newly diagnosed epilepsy.

- Nature of epilepsy
- First aid management of seizures
- Avoidance of precipitating factors, including alcohol and sleep deprivation
- Purpose of medication and likely duration
- Nature of common adverse effects of medication
- Need to take medication regularly
- Risks of seizures (including SUDEP) and advice regarding common hazards
- Legal aspects of driving
- Interaction with other drugs, especially oral contraceptive pill (where relevant)
- Possibility of teratogenicity, where relevant

SUDEP, sudden unexplained death in epilepsy.

Outcome of therapy

The outcome of therapy in newly diagnosed cases is generally good. In about 70% seizures will be brought under rapid control. If long remission occurs (say for 2–5 years), the risk of subsequent recurrence is low (approximately 10%) and most patients are eventually able to discontinue medication. About two-thirds of patients started on therapy will enter a 1-year remission within a year of initiating treatment, and three-quarters will be in 3-year remission at a point 5 years after starting therapy.

The presence of the following factors has been found to lessen the chance of achieving early remission: high frequency of tonic–clonic seizures before therapy; symptomatic epilepsy with structural cerebral disease; childhood epilepsy syndrome; partial or secondarily generalized seizures; and additional neurological handicap or learning disability.

Principles of treatment of patients with established active epilepsy

The goal of drug therapy in newly diagnosed cases is the complete control of seizures, which is attained in about 60–70% of patients within a few years of the onset of the condition. This means that about 30–40% of cases have continuing seizures, and the treatment of this 'chronic active' epilepsy is more complex and more difficult than that of a drug-naïve case. Different issues are raised, and the perspectives of therapy are different.

Complete seizure control in patients with chronic epilepsy can be obtained eventually, even with skilful treatment, in only perhaps 30%, although it should be possible to lessen the frequency or severity of seizures in other cases. There remain a number of patients – perhaps 10% of all those developing epilepsy – whose seizures remain severe, frequent or intractable. Although small in number, these patients require a high level of medical input. The epilepsy often coexists with additional learning disability, psychosocial problems or other neurological handicaps, and these factors complicate medical therapy further.

With active epilepsy there are high rates of morbidity and even mortality. Treatment involves more than antiepileptic drug therapy, but should be targeted at medical co-morbidity, and psychological, psychiatric and social issues. Counselling on a wide range of topics is often required, and is best achieved via a team approach. Issues vary in different individuals and patient groups. A large population-based survey of patients on antiepileptic drugs was carried out in the UK, commissioned by the NHS; the areas in which epilepsy was considered by the respondents to be impacting on their lives are listed in Table 5.13.

Antiepileptic treatment protocol for patients with established active epilepsy

Recent studies have shown that a systematic approach to the antiepileptic drug therapy of chronic patients can result in seizure freedom in about 30% of cases and significant improvement in a further 50%. Taking a nihilistic view (that nothing can be done to improve seizure control in chronic epilepsy) is a common mistake that consigns many patients to lifelong disability.

When first seeing a patient with chronic uncontrolled epilepsy, a two-stage procedure should be adopted:

Table 5.13 Survey of the impact of epilepsy by age group (CSAG survey, 2001).

Mild seizures		Severe seizures	
Impact	Percentage of responders	Impact	Percentage of responders
≤16 years (n = 33; impacts reported, 61)		≤16 years (n = 54; impacts reported, 121)	
School life	36	School life	33
Psychological	27	Psychological	31
Social life	24	Social life	30
Sports	18	Sports	15
Need to take tablets	15	Supervision	11
Sleep	9	Sleep	11
Learning difficulties	9	Play	7
None	9	Need to take tablets	7
17–65 years (n = 568; impacts reported, 140)		17–65 years (n = 347; impacts reported, 842)	
Driving ban	48	Work	51
Work	36	Psychological	35
Social life	19	Social life	32
Psychological	18	Driving ban	28
Loss of confidence	8	Supervision	10
None	11	Independence	9
>65 years (n = 127; impacts reported, 191)		>65 years (n = 28; impacts reported, 57)	
Driving ban	32	Driving ban	39
Psychological	19	Psychological	29
Work	14	Seizures	21
Bad memory	9	Work	21
None	19	Social life	14
		Loss of self-confidence	11
		Mobility	11
		Supervision	11

UK Survey of 3455 unselected people with epilepsy who were taking antiepileptic drugs; 1157 individuals had had a seizure in the past year and a seizure severity score (using the National Hospital Seizures Severity Scale) possible to assess, and completed a questionnaire about the impact of epilepsy on their lives. The results are summarized in this table.

first assessment and second devising a treatment plan (Table 5.14).

The treatment plan can take a number of months to complete, requiring patience and tenacity, and the

Table 5.14 Principles of treatment in chronic active epilepsy.

Assessment
- Review diagnosis and aetiology (history, EEG, imaging)
- Classify seizures and syndrome
- Review compliance
- Review drug history:
- Which drugs were useful in the past?
- Which drugs were not useful in the past?
- Which drugs have not been used in the past? (also dose, length of therapy and reasons for discontinuation)
- Review precipitants and non-pharmacological factors

Treatment plan
- Document proposed sequence of drug 'trials'
- Decide what background medication to continue
- Decide upon the sequence of drug additions and withdrawals
- Decide the duration of drug 'trials'
- Decide when to do serum-level monitoring
- Consider surgical therapy
- Consider non-pharmacological measures (lifestyle, alternative therapy, etc.)
- Recognize the limitations of therapy
- Provide information on above to patient

Table 5.15 Methods for improving compliance with drug therapy.

Information about drug treatment:
- Role
- Limitations
- Expected efficacy
- Potential side effects

Therapeutics:
- Monotherapy if possible
- Minimize dosing frequency where possible (to once or twice a day)
- Introduce drugs in a slow incremental fashion
- Use appropriate formulation (solution, chewtabs, sprinkles where needed)

Aide memoire:
- Drug wallet
- Regular reminders
- Cues, alarm wristwatch

Reinforcement of importance of compliance at clinic visits.

procedure should be explained in advance to the patient to maintain confidence and compliance. This needs the expenditure of time and effort by the doctor, who should be available throughout for guidance and reassurance. Perseverance brings rewards, however, and resolute individuals will, following this protocol, become established on effective long-term therapy.

Assessment
Review the diagnosis of epilepsy
An eye-witnessed account of the attacks should be obtained, and the previous medical records inspected. A series of normal EEG results should alert one to the possibility that the attacks are non-epileptic, although this is not an infallible rule.

Establish aetiology
It is important at this stage to ascertain the cause of the epileptic attacks, and especially to exclude progressive pathology. This will often require EEG and MRI of sufficient quality (see pp. 322–323) and clinical chemistry.

Classify seizure type
This has some value in guiding the choice of medication.

Review previous treatment history
This is an absolutely essential step, often omitted. The response to a drug is generally speaking relatively consistent over time. Find out which antiepileptic drugs have been previously tried, what was the response (effectiveness/side effects), what was the maximum dose and why was the drug withdrawn.

Review compliance
This can be a reason for poor seizure control. A drug wallet, filled up for the whole week, can be of great assistance for patients who often forget to take the medication. Other methods for improving compliance are listed in Table 5.15.

Therapy
A treatment plan (schedule) should be formed on the basis of this assessment, documented in medical records and discussed with the patient.

Treatment plan
Although meta-analysis has shown that none of the currently available first- and second-line drugs is significantly

better than any other in population terms, one thing is clear – individual patients who have failed to respond to one drug may well respond to an alternative. Therefore, it is logical, in any patient in whom improvements in seizure control are desired, to try one suitable drug after another. The treatment plan therefore should comprise, at its heart, a sequence of what are in effect $n = 1$ treatment trials, each to be tried in turn if the previous trial fails to meet the targeted level of seizure control.

The effectiveness of this stepwise approach was shown in one study in which a total of 265 drug additions were studied in 155 adult patients with chronic epilepsy (defined as epilepsy active at least 5 years after initiation of therapy). Other therapy was varied (and some drugs withdrawn) according to normal clinic practice. If one drug addition was ineffective, another would be tried. Of the 155 patients, the study found that, after one, two or three drug additions, 28% overall were rendered seizure free by this protocol of active medication change; 16% of all drug additions resulted in seizure freedom (defined as seizure freedom at last follow-up for 12 months or longer), and a 50–99% seizure reduction occurred in a further 21%.

Ideally, each antiepileptic should be tried in a reasonable dose added to a baseline drug regimen – usually one or two other antiepileptic drugs – and, as the drug is added, withdrawal or change in dose of other drugs may be needed. Thus decisions have to be made about: which drugs to trial and in what sequence, and which drugs to retain as a baseline regimen; which drugs to withdraw; and the duration of each treatment trial.

Choice of drugs to introduce or retain

Generally these should be drugs that are appropriate for the seizure type and that have not been previously used in optimal doses or that have been used and did prove helpful. Rational choices depend on a well-documented history of previous drug therapy. Attention also needs to be paid to drug interactions. The initial dose and maximum incremental increases in dose in routine practice are shown in Table 5.11.

It is usual to maintain therapy with either one or two suitable antiepileptic drugs. If drugs are being withdrawn, it is wise to maintain one drug as an 'anchor' to cover the withdrawal period.

Choice of drugs to withdraw

These should be drugs that have been given an adequate trial at optimal doses and that either were ineffective or

caused unacceptable side effects. There is obviously little point in continuing a drug that has had little effect, yet it is remarkable how often this is done.

Duration of treatment trial

This will depend on the baseline seizure rate. The trial should be long enough to differentiate the effect of therapy from that of chance fluctuations in seizures.

Drug withdrawal

Drug withdrawal needs care. The sudden reduction in dose of an AED can result in a severe worsening of seizures or in status epilepticus, even if the withdrawn drug was apparently not contributing much to seizure control. It is therefore customary, and wise, to withdraw medication slowly, a caution that applies particularly to barbiturate drugs (phenobarbital, primidone), benzodiazepine drugs (clobazam, clonazepam, diazepam) and carbamazepine. Table 5.11 lists the fastest decremental rates that are recommended in normal clinical practice. In many situations even slower rates of withdrawal are safer.

The only advantage of fast withdrawal is better compliance and the faster establishment of new drug regimens. Only one drug should be withdrawn at a time. If the withdrawal period is likely to be difficult, the dangers can be reduced by covering the withdrawal with a benzodiazepine (usually clobazam 10 mg/day), given during the phase of active withdrawal. A benzodiazepine can also be given if clustering of seizures following withdrawal occurs.

It is sometimes difficult to know whether seizures during withdrawal are due to either the withdrawal or simply the background epilepsy, and whenever possible a long-term view should be taken and overreaction in the short term avoided.

Sometimes the simple withdrawal of a drug will result in improved control of seizures by improving well-being, assuring better compliance and reducing interactions.

Drug addition

New drugs added to a regimen should also be introduced slowly, at least in the routine clinical situation. This results in better tolerability, and is particularly important when adding benzodiazepines, carbamazepine, lamotrigine, levetiracetam, primidone or topiramate. Too fast an introduction of these drugs will almost invariably result in side effects. It is usual to aim initially for a low maintenance dose, but in severe epilepsy higher doses are often required.

Concomitant medication

Changing the dose of one antiepileptic (either incremental or decremental) can influence the levels of other drugs, and the changing levels of concomitant medication can contribute to changing side effects or effectiveness.

Limits on therapy

Drug therapy will fail in about 10–20% of patients. In this situation, the epilepsy can be categorized as 'intractable'. Here the aims of therapy change to achieving the best compromise between inadequate seizure control and drug-induced side effects. Individual patients will take very different views about where to strike this balance.

Counselling

Counselling should be offered for chronic patients, as for new patients, on the topics listed in Table 5.12. Those with chronic active epilepsy, however, have additional problems – fears about the risks of future seizures, anxiety about the stigmatizing effects of epilepsy, and its effects on employment, self-esteem, relationships, schooling and leisure activities. The areas on which the condition impacted were demonstrated in one large survey of 3455 people on treatment for epilepsy in the UK, which are summarized in Table 5.13. Many of these could be ameliorated by appropriate counselling and these topics should be addressed. The issues depend on age and the severity of epilepsy.

Monotherapy vs combination therapy

Single-drug therapy will provide optimal seizure control in about 70% of all patients with epilepsy, and should be chosen whenever possible. The advantages of monotherapy are:
- better tolerability and fewer side effects
- simpler and less intrusive regimens
- better compliance
- no potential for pharmacokinetic or pharmacodynamic interactions with other antiepileptic drugs.

Combination therapy is needed in about 30% of all those developing epilepsy, and in a higher proportion of those with epilepsy that has remained uncontrolled in spite of initial monotherapy (chronic active epilepsy). The choice of drugs in combination has not been satisfactorily studied. It has been proposed, but without any substantial supporting evidence, that mixing drugs with differing modes of action has a synergistic effect – a strategy (irrationally) named 'rational polytherapy'. It makes sense too to avoid, where possible, drugs with

potentials for pharmacokinetic interaction because this will only compromise response.

Treatment of patients with epilepsy in remission

Epilepsy can be said to be in remission when seizures have not occurred over long periods of time (conventionally 2 or 5 years). At some point after the initiation of therapy 70–80% of patients will enter a remission. Cases of untreated epilepsy also remit, although exactly how many is not known. In the long term, at least 50% of all patients are in remission and off medication.

The clinical management of ongoing therapy in patients in remission is generally straightforward. In most cases little medical input is required, with appropriate care provided at primary care level and annual visits to the specialist. The seizure type, epilepsy syndrome, aetiology, investigations and previous treatment should be recorded. Routine haematological or biochemical checks are recommended on an annual basis in an asymptomatic individual. Enquiry should be made about long-term side effects (e.g. bone disease in postmenopausal women) and counselling about issues such as pregnancy made where appropriate. At some point, however, the calm of this ideal situation is likely to be disturbed by the question of discontinuation of therapy.

Discontinuation of drug therapy

It is often difficult to decide when (if ever) to discontinue drug treatment. The decision should be made by a specialist who is able to provide an estimate of the risk of re-activation of the epilepsy. This risk is influenced by the factors listed in Table 5.16, but it must be stressed that withdrawal is never entirely risk free. The decision whether or not to withdraw therapy will depend on the level of risk that the patient is prepared to accept.

Probability of remaining free of seizures after drug withdrawal

The best information comes from the Medical Research Council (MRC) AED withdrawal study, which included 1013 patients who had been free of seizures for 2 years or more (Figure 5.5). Within 2 years of starting drug withdrawal 59% remained free of seizures (compared with 79% of those who opted to stay on therapy). Other studies have had essentially similar findings.

Table 5.16 Some factors that increase the risk of seizure recurrence after withdrawal of therapy in patients with epilepsy in remission.

- Short duration of freedom from seizures prior to drug withdrawal
- Age >16 years
- History of myoclonic seizures or secondarily generalized seizures
- History of multiple seizure types
- Certain epilepsy syndromes (e.g. juvenile myoclonic epilepsy, childhood encephalopathies)
- Symptomatic epilepsy
- Progressive aetiology
- History of seizures after treatment was initiated
- Seizure control requiring multiple drug therapy
- Eeg showing generalized spike–wave discharges
- Presence of learning disability or associated neurological handicaps
- Previous attempts to withdraw therapy followed by recurrence

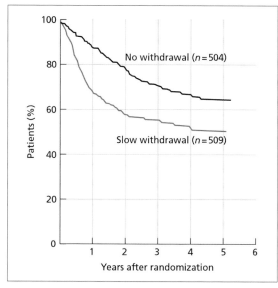

Figure 5.5 Actuarial percentage of patients seizure-free amongst those randomized to continuing or to slow withdrawal of antiepileptic drugs. A study of 1013 patients seizure-free for at least 2 years, randomized to either slow withdrawal of their antiepileptic drug therapy or to continuing drug therapy. Two years after randomization 78% of those who continued treatment and 59% of those who had treatment withdrawn were seizure-free, but thereafter the differences in recurrence rate between the two groups diminished

Period of seizure freedom

The longer the patient is seizure free, the less the chance of relapse, e.g. the overall risk of relapse after drug withdrawal after a 5-year period of freedom from seizures is under 10%.

Duration of active epilepsy

This is probably an under-studied factor. There is a strong impression that the shorter the history of active seizures (i.e. the duration of time from the onset of epilepsy to the onset of remission), the less the risk of relapse.

Type and severity of epilepsy

The type of epilepsy, and its aetiology, is an important influence on prognosis. The presence of symptomatic epilepsy, secondarily generalized or myoclonic seizures, neurological deficit or learning disability greatly lessens the chance of remission, and also increases the chances of recurrence should remission occur. A higher number of seizures before remission, a greater number of drugs being taken to control the seizures, and the presence of two or more seizure types (a surrogate for severity of epilepsy) all increase the risk of relapse.

EEG

The value of EEG in predicting the outcome of patients in remission is controversial, as it is in most other areas of prognostication. The persistence of spike–wave in those with IGE is the most useful prognostic EEG feature, indicating a higher chance of relapse. Other EEG abnormalities have no great prognostic utility, and the presence of focal spikes or changes in EEG background are of little help in estimating the chances of remission or relapse after drug withdrawal. In general, the EEG has more prognostic value in children than in adults.

Age

There is no clear overall relationship between age and the risk of relapse, although there are age-specific syndromes that have specific prognostic patterns. There is a low chance of relapse in the benign epilepsies of childhood or in generalized absence epilepsy. These data simply emphasize the obvious point that the overriding determinant of prognosis is the type and aetiology of epilepsy.

The risk factors are additive and, if two or more adverse factors are present, the risk of recurrence is >70%. On the other hand, if positive factors exist, such as a long duration of remission, a short history of

Table 5.17 Mathematical basis of model predicting risk of recurrence of seizures after drug withdrawal (from MRC drug withdrawal study).

Starting score for all to patients = −175	Factor value added to score	
Age > 16 years	45	
Taking more than 1 AED	50	
Seizures occurring after the start of treatment	35	
History of any tonic–clonic seizure (generalized or partial in onset)	35	
History of myoclonic seizures	50	
EEG while in remission:		
not done	15	
abnormal	20	
Duration of seizure-free period (years), D	$200/D$	
Total score	T	
Exponentiate $T/100$		
($Z = e^{T/100}$)	Z	
Probability of seizure recurrence	**By 1 year**	**By 2 years**
On continued treatment	$1-0.89^Z$	$1-0.79^Z$
On slow withdrawal of treatment	$1-0.69^Z$	$1-0.60^Z$

AED, antiepileptic drug.

epilepsy, mild epilepsy before remission or idiopathic epilepsy with a normal EEG, the risks are lower than the mean relapse rate of 40% found in the MRC study. A predictive model has been developed on the basis of the study, which takes into account some of these features and provides useful estimates of relapse rate (Table 5.17).

How to withdraw therapy – the importance of slow reduction

When a decision to withdraw therapy is made, the drugs should be discontinued one at a time slowly. Of patients who are going to experience a recurrence of seizures on withdrawal 50% do so during the reduction phase and 25% in the first 6 months after withdrawal; this should be explained carefully to the patient. As a result of this, the UK driving licence authority recommends that driving be avoided during drug withdrawal and for 6 months afterwards; this (non-binding) advice should be given to patients.

The fastest recommended rates of withdrawal are given in Table 5.11, although in many instances there is no need to proceed so rapidly. In general terms, the slower the withdrawal, the less likely are seizures to recur. If seizures do recur, the drug should be immediately restarted at the dosage that controlled the attacks.

A further issue, which must be emphasized to a patient before attempting drug withdrawal, concerns the longer-term prognosis if seizure relapse occurs after drug withdrawal. At least 10% of patients will not regain full remission even if the drug is replaced at the dosage that previously resulted in long remission. Why this should be the case is unclear but, in some patients at least, it seems that recurrence alters the risk of subsequent seizures.

Counselling and decision-making

The withdrawal of therapy can have marked psychological benefits. It often removes the stigma of a 'diagnosis' and may ameliorate the sense of 'being ill'.

Side effects, sometimes not recognized on chronic therapy, may also be reversed. On the other hand, the recurrence of seizures can have both psychological and social consequences, and carries a risk of morbidity and even mortality. These issues demand careful consideration and discussion. It must be emphasized to the patient that there is no guarantee that withdrawal of treatment will be successful and that, if seizures do recur, there is no guarantee that a return to therapy will ensure future remission. An estimate of the risks of recurrence on withdrawal from, and of further recurrence on return to, therapy should be given. The benefits of drug withdrawal should also be discussed. The decision to initiate withdrawal must be made by the patient – not the physician – and only after full appreciation of the issues involved. The role of the clinician is to provide information and to respond to queries and concerns; it is never appropriate to insist on drug withdrawal. The personal circumstances of the individual patient can be overriding. In adults, the avoidance of seizures is often of greater importance than in children, e.g. in relation to holding a driving licence or employment. In women, the question of future pregnancy and of a drug-free pregnancy may be uppermost. In children, concerns about the effects of drugs on learning may encourage earlier drug withdrawal. It is not possible to make general recommendations, and the wishes of the individual patient should be paramount. One study has shown how poorly physician expectations are predictive of patients' decisions in this area.

Psychiatric disorders in epilepsy

There is a huge and contradictory literature on the psychiatric risks of epilepsy. Indeed, for many years, epilepsy was considered a 'psychiatric disease' and there is no doubt that there are complex but close relationships with various psychiatric conditions. At a rough approximation, about a third to half of adults with epilepsy have psychiatric difficulties, in a broad sense, and in a population-based study the rate of psychiatric disorders among children with epilepsy was 27%, compared with 7% in the general population. The more chronic or more severe the epilepsy, the higher the rate of psychiatric disorders. The cause of psychiatric disturbances in epilepsy is multifactorial and includes the biological effects of seizures, the genetic and neurological context of the epilepsy, the effects of drugs and social factors. The issue is complicated by the bidirectional nature of the relationship.

Depression and anxiety

Conventional mood disorders are encountered in many patients with epilepsy, and these include anxiety, depression, dysthymia and panic disorders. Intermittent affective–somatoform symptoms are frequently present in chronic epilepsy and include irritability, depressive moods, anergia, insomnia, atypical pains, anxiety, phobic fears and euphoric moods. Some are present continually but others show marked variation in relation to seizure activity. Prodromal dysphoria and peri-ictal dysphoria are common.

Ictal and postictal affective symptoms

Many patients with focal seizures report prodromal states of depression, irritability or anxiety occurring hours to days before a seizure. The symptomatology of simple or complex partial seizures affecting limbic structures includes fear, anger, depression and sexual excitement. These can be severe, and can be confused diagnostically with primary panic attacks, which are also common in patients with epilepsy. Ictal depression may range from mild feelings of sadness to profound hopelessness and despair.

A variety of short-lived (<24 h) postictal affective symptoms can occur after individual seizures or clusters of seizures. In one study of the postictal state, symptoms of depression occurred in 43%, anxiety in 45%, hypomania in 22%, and active and passive suicidal thoughts in 8% and 13%, respectively.

Depression

The main features of a depressive episode include: lowered mood, reduced energy and concentration, diminished capacity for enjoyment or interest, marked tiredness after minimal effort, disturbed sleep (hypersomnia or insomnia), reduced appetite and weight loss, reduced self-esteem and self-confidence, ideas of guilt or worthlessness and 'somatic symptoms' (early morning waking, diurnal variation in mood [worst in morning], psychomotor retardation/agitation and loss of libido). In severe depression there may be recurrent thoughts of death and suicide, delusions, hallucinations and stupor. In epilepsy, it is important to differentiate the effects of medication or cognitive problems, and the Neurological Disorders Depression Inventory for Epilepsy (NDDI-E) is a rating scale specifically designed for patients with epilepsy. The Beck Depression Inventory has also been validated in epilepsy.

Antidepressant drug therapy

The mainstay of treatment of depression is with antidepressant drugs. Many antidepressants are used in epilepsy and citalopram, mirtazepine, normiphensine, amitriptyline and reboxetine have been subjected to clinical trials specifically in patients with epilepsy. The largest clinical antidepressant trial to date, the National Institute of Mental Health (NIMH) STAR-D (sequenced treatment alternatives to relieve depression) trial, was recently completed. The trial protocol consisted of patients sequentially moving through four treatment levels depending on whether or not they responded to a particular antidepressant or combination of antidepressants. The purpose of the trial was to determine the effectiveness of different treatments for people with major depressive disorder who did not respond to the initial antidepressant treatment choice. In treatment level 1, all patients received citalopram. A third entered remission and a further 10–15% showed a clinically significant response. Those who did not respond were switched to treatment level 2, in which the citalopram was either changed to sertraline, venlafaxine or cognitive–behavioural therapy (CBT) or augmented with buspirone or bupropion (both contraindicated in epilepsy) or CBT. Of the patients treated within level 2 25% eventually became symptom free. Level 3 treatment included mirtazepine or nortriptyline and, in level 4, antidepressant drug combinations, such as mirtazepine plus venlafaxine, were used. Although this trial was not carried out in patients with epilepsy (in whom bupropion is contraindicated and nortriptyline best avoided), a simple and evidence-based pathway for the treatment of depression in epilepsy (based on the other factors discussed above) would be to start treatment with citalopram, and then if remission of symptoms is not achieved progress through sertraline, mirtazepine and venlafaxine. Recommended starting doses, usual treatment dose and maximum doses as observed in routine psychiatric practice are outlined in Table 5.18.

On initiation of therapy with antidepressant drugs, common symptoms include a temporary worsening of anxiety and agitation, which usually passes after the first week or two. In very anxious patients, low-dose short-term benzodiazepine cover (e.g. diazepam 2 mg three times a day) may be given, and normal starting doses may be halved. Hyponatraemia, common in patients on oxcarbazepine or carbamazepine, can be exacerbated by most selective serotonin reuptake inhibitors (SSRIs) and is often seen in the older patient group. Mirtazepine is less likely to cause hyponatraemia, or sexual side effects, but often causes sedation and weight gain. The SSRIs and the serotonin–noradrenaline reuptake inhibitor (SNRI) venlafaxine should be taken in the morning because evening use can lead to initial insomnia. Fluoxetine is often said to have an 'activating' effect and may be useful in fatigued or lethargic patients, and those with psycho-motor retardation. It also has the added benefit of being one of the few antidepressants that does not cause signifi-cant weight gain, a particular problem in patients taking antiepileptic drugs that also induce weight gain, such as valproate, gabapentin and pregabalin. In the UK it is the only antidepressant currently licensed for use in children and adolescents aged <18 years. Its other benefit is that the main active metabolite, norfluoxetine, has a half-life of 4–16 days, and in patients who regularly forget to take their medication this can often help to prevent SSRI discontinuation symptoms emerging.

The effects of antidepressants on seizures

One concern is that antidepressants lower the seizure threshold. However, the incidence of seizures in people without epilepsy treated with SSRI, noradrenergic and specific serotoninergic (NaSS) and SNRI antidepressants is actually significantly lower than would be expected in the general population (citalopram <0.3%, sertraline 0%,

fluoxetine 0.2%, duloxetine 0.0%, mirtazepine 0.04%, venlafaxine 0.1%) with the exception of bupropion. Fluoxetine and citalopram have been reported to produce antiepileptic effects in open-label studies of non-depressed epileptic patients, reducing seizure frequency by as much as 35–64%, and it may be that seizures that occur after starting SSRIs merely reflect the increased risk of seizures associated with the depressive disorder. Tricyclic antide-pressants (TCAs, particularly high-dose) and tetracyclic antidepressants are felt to pose a greater level of risk. However, in patients with epilepsy on antiepileptic drugs, the risks of antidepressant-induced seizures seem very low.

Another possible risk is that antidepressant use can 'switch' depressed patients into a manic state in those with hitherto undiagnosed bipolar disorder presenting with depression as the index episode. There are certain features in the history that should act as a red flag for this possibility and would warrant specialist referral before initiating antidepressant therapy:

• Prepubertal, adolescent or postpartum onset
• A hypersomnic/psychomotor retarded or catatonic psychotic episode
• Positive family history for bipolar disorder or consecu-tive generation mood disorder
• An episode of pharmacologically induced hypomania. In general, the risk of switching is thought to be lower with SSRIs than with TCAs.

Drug interactions between antidepressant and antiepileptic drugs

Carbamazepine, phenytoin, primidone and barbiturates are potent inducers of the cytochrome P450 (CYP) enzymes at regular doses, as are oxcarbazepine and topi-ramate at higher doses; these enzymes are involved in the metabolism of TCAs and all SSRIs and SNRIs. The drugs affected include amitriptyline, nortriptyline, doxepine, clomipramine, mianserin, nomifensine, bupropion and, to a lesser extent, citalopram and paroxetine. The doses of these antidepressants will often need to be increased when used alongside these antiepileptic drugs.

Valproate is a broad-spectrum inhibitor of drug metabolism and has been associated with a 50–60% elevation in plasma amitriptyline and nortriptyline concentrations. Valproate also increases concentrations of clomipramine and paroxetine. Certain SSRIs also inhibit CYP enzymes: fluoxetine and fluvoxamine are mild-to-moderate inhibitors of CYP3A4, the primary enzyme involved in carbamazepine metabolism.

Neither paroxetine nor sertraline affects plasma concentrations of carbamazepine or phenytoin, but

Table 5.18 Commonly used antidepressants and antipsychotics: doses, receptor binding and other effects.

Antidepressant/ antipsychotic	Starting dose/timing	Usual treatment dose	Maximum dose	Pharmacology	Adverse/other effects
Citalopram	10–20 mg, morning (use 10 mg if very anxious ± panic)	20–40 mg	60 mg	H_1, inhibits CYP2D6	Inconsistent effect at lower doses Effective in elderly people
Sertraline	50 mg, morning	50–100 mg	200 mg	SRI, DRI, sigma 1 binding	Good for atypical/psychotic (delusional) depression
Fluoxetine	20 mg morning	20–40 mg	60 mg	SRI, NRI, $5HT_{2C}$ antagonist. Inhibits CYP2D6/3A4	Energizing and fatigue-reducing effect
Mirtazepine	15 mg, night	30 mg	45 mg	α_2, H_1, $5HT_{3/2A/2C}$	No significant sexual dysfunction Weight gain Sleep restoring Less nausea/gastrointestinal problems Anxiolytic
Venlafaxine XL	75 mg, morning	150 mg	225 mg	SRI, NRI	Extended-release version reduces side effects, particularly nausea May be linked to more robust and longer remission rates Metabolized by CYP2D6
Risperidone	2 mg	4–6 mg	16 mg (doses >8 mg are rarely used)	$5HT_{2A}$, D_2, α_1, α_2, $5HT_7$	EPSE at higher doses, hyperprolactinaemia, hypertriglyceridaemia, insulin resistance, HONK Less weight gain than olanzapine and clozapine Higher doses may be required due to enzyme induction by carbamazepine/phenytoin (CYP3A4)
Olanzapine	5 mg	5–15 mg	20 mg	mACh, $5HT_{2A}$, D_{1-4}, $\alpha_{1/2}$, H_1, $5HT_{3/6}$, 5HT-C	Weight gain, sedation (less than clozapine) Poses definite cardiometabolic, dyslipidaemia and diabetes risks EPSE not common Enzyme induction possible with carbamazepine (CYP1A2)
Quetiapine	25–100 mg (depending on age)	400–600 mg	750–800 mg	D_2, $5HT_{2A/1A/2C}$, H_1, α_1, α_2, M_1	Virtually no EPSE No hyperprolactinaemia Sedation Intermediate to high risk of dyslipidaemia/insulin resistance

Table 5.18 *Continued*

Antidepressant/ antipsychotic	Starting dose/timing	Usual treatment dose	Maximum dose	Pharmacology	Adverse/other effects
Amisulpiride	200 mg	400–800 mg	1200 mg	D_3. Possible D_2 partial agonist	Low EPSE May cause dose-dependent QTc prolongation Can increase prolactin
Clozapine	12.5 mg	300–700 mg (adjusted according to plasma level and response)	900 mg	D_{1-4}, $5HT_{2A/C}$, $\alpha_{1/2}$, H_1, mACh, $5HT_{3/6/7}$	Weight gain, sedation, hypersalivation, constipation, bowel obstruction, agranulocytosis, myocarditis, seizures Sudden hyperosmolar syndrome/ diabetic ketoacidosis High cardiometabolic risk Reduces suicide risk Cannot be combined with carbamazepine or lamotrigine because of risk of agranulocytosis Needs slow introduction with EEG monitoring Specialist monitoring registration

5HT, serotonin; CYP, cytochrome P450; D, dopamine; DRI, dopamine reuptake inhibition; EPSE, extrapyramidal side effects; H, histamine; HONK, hyperosmotic non-ketotic acidosis; mACh, muscarinic acetylcholine receptor; NRI, noradrenaline reuptake inhibitor; SRI, serotonin reuptake inhibitor.

sertraline doses of between 25 and 100 mg have been associated with both valproate and lamotrigine toxicity. There are several reports of plasma phenytoin concentrations increasing to toxic levels after initiation with fluoxetine, probably due to CYP2C9 inhibition. Phenytoin levels can also rise with co-medication with trazodone, viloxazine and imipramine.

Citalopram, mirtazepine and venlafaxine have the least impact on the CYP enzyme system.

Cognitive–behavioural therapy
It is likely that affective disorders respond better to a combination of pharmacotherapy and psychological therapy than to either modality alone. CBT usually involves 12–16 sessions with a specially trained psychologist or psychiatrist, during which patients' unhelpful beliefs about themselves and the world with which they interact are explored. The behaviours that result from these beliefs act to reinforce the depressed state. In the

therapy these views are challenged, alternative possibilities explored, and a more helpful set of attitudes and beliefs encouraged.

Electroconvulsive therapy
Epilepsy is not a contraindication to electroconvulsive therapy (ECT), and in fact there is good evidence that ECT actually increases seizure threshold. However, the use of ECT has declined significantly in routine clinical psychiatric practice, although it is still employed (albeit rarely) in patients with severe depression, treatment-resistant mania and, on a very occasional basis, in psychosis.

Deep brain stimulation for treatment-resistant depression
Up to 20% of patients with epilepsy and depression fail to respond to pharmacological or psychotherapeutic interventions and may then require a trial of ECT.

Despite this, some patients remain severely depressed. Chronic stimulation to modulate subgenual cingulate grey matter and interconnected frontal and subcortical regions has been tested in experimental situations. Whether these approaches would be beneficial in epilepsy and depression has not been demonstrated.

Atypical affective disorders in epilepsy – the interictal dysphoric syndrome

Many patients with epilepsy have 'atypical affective disorder' (with symptoms that do not conform to the *Diagnostic and Statistical Manual of Mental of Mental Disorders* [DSM] criteria for depression or anxiety). The most common is the 'interictal dysphoric syndrome'. This condition is sometimes intermittent and sometimes chronic, and the symptomatology includes: irritability, low mood, insomnia, anxiety and occasional euphoria, depressive mood, anergia, anhedonia, poor concentration, guilt, recurrent thoughts of death, a sense of worthlessness, weight loss/gain, pain, labile affective symptoms (fear, anxiety), and sometimes paroxysmal irritability and euphoria. Anhedonia can be very prominent

Generalized anxiety disorder

In various studies, the prevalence of anxiety disorders in epilepsy has ranged from 12% to 60%. The main symptoms include persistent nervousness, trembling, muscular tension, sweating, light-headedness, palpitations, dizziness and epigastric discomfort.

Panic disorder

Patients with epilepsy were six times more likely to have panic disorder than the general population, with a prevalence estimated to range from 5% to 30%. The essential features of panic disorder are recurrent attacks of severe anxiety (panic), which are not restricted to any particular situation or set of circumstances and are therefore unpredictable. Episodes of interictal panic are more protracted than those seen in the ictal phase, usually lasting from 5 min to 20 min but sometimes persisting for several hours. The feeling of fear or panic is very intense ('feeling of impending doom') and associated with a range of autonomic symptoms (tachycardia, blood pressure fluctuation, diffuse diaphoresis and shortness of breath). It is important to differentiate true panic attacks from partial seizures, which sometimes can have similar symptoms.

Obsessive–compulsive disorder

The prevalence of obsessive–compulsive disorder is about 15% in patients with temporal lobe epilepsy and less common in other forms. The two key features are:

1 Recurrent obsessional thoughts – ideas, images or impulses that repeatedly enter the patient's mind in a stereotyped form. These are recognized as the patient's own thoughts, but are felt to be distressing and are usually resisted

2 Compulsive acts or rituals that are stereotyped repetitive behaviours, which are not enjoyable and do not result in the completion of useful tasks.

Their function is to prevent some objectively unlikely event, often involving harm to or caused by the patient. Resisting the compulsive act usually leads to an immediate increase in anxiety. Obsessive–compulsive disorder may also follow or be terminated by temporal lobe surgery.

Suicide

Suicide accounts for about 1.5% of deaths worldwide. The suicide rate of epilepsy is estimated to be between 4 and 8%, but two large population studies shown increased standardized incidence ratios of 2.1 and 1.7 for suicide in patients with epilepsy, although the differences were not statistically significant. It has been stated that the lifetime prevalence of suicidal ideation is roughly twice as high among patients with epilepsy as among the general population. The risk of suicide seems greatest in those who are on antipsychotic medication and also those with temporal lobe epilepsy (compared with other types). The risk is also increased after temporal lobe surgery – and of 193 patients followed up after temporal lobectomy for 5–24 years, 9 of 37 deaths were by suicide.

FDA guidance on suicide risk associated with AEDs

One particular rumour that has blighted this area was the suggestion made in 2008 by the FDA that antiepileptic medication increased the risk of suicide. This followed a review of 199 placebo-controlled trials with a total of 27 863 patients in the drug arms and 16 029 patients in the placebo arms. There were four completed suicides in the treatment group, a rate of about 1 in 7000. Suicidal behaviour or ideation occurred in 1 in 270 of the drug-treated group compared with 1 in 416 of the placebo group. The overall number needed to harm was 2 per 1000 and the OR was significant at 1.8. In subanalyses for each individual drug, carbamazepine and valproate appeared to reduce suicidal behaviour and ideation events, although this effect was not significant; nevertheless, the alert currently includes the entire class of antiepileptic drugs. The manufacturers of lamotrigine then submitted three additional placebo-controlled trials, which were not part of the primary analysis. In these three trials there were nine suicidal behaviour or ideation events, only one of which occurred in the drug arm, with the other eight occurring in the placebo arm.

The FDA advice has raised significant concerns that patients might stop their antiepileptic drugs, placing them at a much higher risk of accidental injury and SUDEP. Furthermore, the data on suicide need to be collected in a prospective and systematic way and, in the author's view, given the complexity of the interrelationship of epilepsy, depression and suicide, this meta-analysis is insufficiently robust to be of much value.

Psychosis

Psychosis in epilepsy is usually differentiated into interictal, ictal and postictal categories. However, in practice, these distinctions are not necessarily clear cut and the clinical course of many patients demonstrates a mixed picture. Psychosis can also occur in an 'alternating' pattern and after temporal lobe surgery (see pp. 316–317, 337).

Interictal psychosis

A grumbling chronic interictal psychosis, with occasional exacerbation, is often seen in patients with severe epilepsy. Prevalence rates vary, but a recent review suggested that 15–20% of patients with epilepsy reported psychotic disorders and that these are somewhat more common in temporal lobe epilepsy. The psychosis is similar to that of primary schizophrenia and, although there is a great overlap of symptoms, generally there is, in the interictal psychosis of epilepsy, greater preservation of affect, fewer negative symptoms and arguably greater insight. The positive symptoms are similar, e.g. those of thought disorder, delusions and hallucinations. Psychotic features may be quite mild, and complicated by irritability, anxiety, paranoia and dysphoria. The interictal psychosis of epilepsy almost always develops only after the epilepsy has been present for many years (usually after a decade or so of seizures) and almost always in patients in whom epilepsy control has been poor.

In most cases antipsychotic medication is required. Sulpiride is a good drug for mild psychosis, and its additional anxiolytic effects can be helpful. During acute exacerbations of psychotic behaviour, risperidone, olanzapine or quetiapine may become necessary. The recommended starting, maintenance and maximum doses are given in Table 5.18.

Treatment is complicated by the fact that almost all available antipsychotics are mildly epileptogenic, with seizure incidence rates (in patients who previously had not had seizures) ranging from approximately 0.1% to approximately 1.5% (compared with 0.07–0.09 in the general population). EEG changes seem to occur in about 7% of patients treated with antipsychotic drugs. One study found a risk of 0.3% for risperidone and 0.9% for olanzapine and quetiapine. The risk with clozapine increased in a dose-dependent manner from 1.0% with low doses (<300 mg/day) to 2.7% with moderate doses and 4.4% with high-dose (600–900 mg/day) treatment. The fear of eliciting additional seizures has led to an exaggerated sense of caution in antipsychotic drug use. In patients co-medicated with antiepileptic drugs, the risk of an increase in seizures is lower. The potential risk becomes an issue mainly in those who are seizure free, in whom the recurrence of seizures has a generally greater impact.

The side effects of the antipsychotic drugs are a major problem, in particular sedation, weight gain, worsening of glycaemic control, extrapyramidal effect, haematological toxicity and hepatotoxicity. In addition, pharmacokinetic interactions are common with enzyme-inducing antiepileptics, because the antipsychotics and antiepileptics may share metabolic pathways. Carbamazepine and other enzyme-inducing antiepileptic drugs lower concentrations of haloperidol, chlorpromazine, clozapine, olanzapine, risperidone and quetiapine. These interactions can be very marked (by up to 50% on occasions) and clinically important. Valproate has few interactions, and the antipsychotics do not generally affect AED concentrations.

Sometimes exacerbations of interictal psychosis are prolonged and non-responsive to treatment. In these cases clozapine can be used, but it can precipitate seizures and also carries a significant risk of leucopenia, and close monitoring of blood counts is necessary. ECT has occasionally been used, and is often strikingly effective, but there is a theoretical risk of ECT-induced status epilepticus.

Ictal psychosis

This is the short-term psychosis that occurs in a non-convulsive seizure, and in which the features are due to the epileptic activity itself. It is really an example of complex partial status epilepticus. The seizure symptomatology includes psychiatric features such as inaccessibility, delusions, illusions, visual or auditory hallucinations, ideas of reference, paranoia, thought disorder, and often a rather curious but characteristic perseverative obsessive insistence on oppositions (such as black/white, good/bad, right/left). The hallucinatory experiences often have religious content. The attacks typically last hours, but can be much more prolonged (occasionally continuing for months or years). The attacks are usually self-limiting, and the symptoms frequently fluctuate or 'cycle'.

Postictal psychosis

A postictal psychosis is defined as a psychotic episode occurring within 7 days of the last generalized tonic–clonic seizure or cluster of complex partial seizures. There are a number of common but unusual clinical features:
• A delay between the onset of psychiatric symptoms and the time of the last seizure
• Relatively short duration of psychosis
• Affect-laden symptomatology
• The clustering of symptoms into delusional and affective-like psychoses
• The onset of postictal psychosis after a long duration of epilepsy (for a mean period of >10 years)
• A prompt response to low-dose antipsychotics or benzodiazepines.
Most episodes occur in patients aged between 30 and 40 years, and in 86% they follow a clear increase in generalized seizure frequency. The lucid interval can last between 1 and 6 days (mean 2.5) in 75%, after which hallucinations (mainly auditory) are found in about a third and delusions (mainly persecutory) in a quarter. The psychopathology is similar to that of the primary psychoses, but mood is often markedly abnormal; paranoid delusions and both auditory and visual hallucinations are common, and hypomania and religiosity are common. The mixture of grandiose and religious delusions in the presence of elevated mood and a feeling of mystic fusion of the body with the universe is characteristic. It is likely that at least some cases of apparently 'postictal psychosis' are not in fact 'postictal' at all but result from ongoing seizure activity – and thus can be categorized as cases of non-convulsive status epilepticus. It has been proposed that the psychosis should be subdivided into two types: first, a nuclear type representing the established clinical picture as an indirect after-effect of seizure activity and, second, an atypical peri-ictal type, occurring as a direct manifestation of limbic epileptic discharges (i.e. complex partial status). During the psychotic episode, lorazepam is the drug of choice, and is sometimes sufficient alone. In other cases, antipsychotic drugs are needed, as for the interictal psychosis. Indeed the distinction between the postictal and interictal psychosis of epilepsy is blurred, more so than often appreciated, and the postictal psychosis is sometimes simply an exacerbation of the interictal condition; furthermore, after repeated episodes of postictal psychosis, some individuals develop a clear chronic interictal psychotic state.

Forced normalization (alternating psychosis)

'Forced normalization' is a term coined by Landolt in 1958. He defined this as 'the phenomenon characterized by the fact that, with the recurrence of psychotic states, the EEG becomes more normal, or entirely normal, as compared with previous and subsequent EEG findings'. More recently, the concept has been loosened to refer to almost any psychiatric disorder occurring in patients whose seizure frequency is reduced (disregarding the EEG altogether), and elaborate explanatory theories have been derived from doubtful evidence. One criticism of the original concept, and particularly of the loose extrapolation to include seizures as well as EEG change, is that the reverse situation is much more commonly observed in clinical practice – that psychotic behaviour is increased at times of seizure exacerbation or worsening EEG change. In the eyes of most epileptologists, the concept of forced normalization is of dubious validity and little practical importance, except perhaps in very occasional circumstances. Furthermore, the scalp EEG is a notoriously insensitive tool at detecting epileptic activity in medial limbic structures and a normal scalp EEG is by no means a reliable predictor of quiescent epilepsy.

The exact mechanism of this pattern is unclear. Antipsychotics, antidepressants and anxiolytic drugs, as appropriate, can be used to treat these episodes. In some individuals the psychosis may be at least in part due to the new introduction of an AED (which causes the remission of seizures), and not to the effect on seizure control. In this situation, the correct therapy is the replacement of this drug by others. In exceptional cases it is deemed better to allow seizures to continue rather than risk psychotic breakdown.

Personality disorders

Personality disorders are defined as an 'enduring pattern of inner experience and behaviour that deviates markedly from the expectations of the individual's culture'. These are manifested by abnormalities in:
• the patient's way of seeing him- or herself, other people or events
• the range, intensity, lability and appropriateness of affectivity
• impulse control
• interpersonal functioning.
In patients with epilepsy, the prevalence of personality disorders has been said to range from 18% to 61% (mean 31%).

Much has been written on personality disorders in patients with epilepsy, a lot of which is based on little firm evidence. Furthermore, the biological effects of the epilepsy, the effects of drug treatment, and the secondary handicap of living with epilepsy or growing up with epilepsy may all contribute to personality difficulties. It must also be stressed that most patients with epilepsy have perfectly normal personalities.

Specific patterns of personality disturbance have been postulated. These include five features said to occur more often in temporal lobe epilepsy (Geschwind syndrome): changes in sexual behaviour (usually a decreased interest in sexual matters), hypergraphia (compulsive writing), hyper-religiosity (an expansive interest in religious matters), aggression and viscosity – defined as the tendency to prolong interpersonal encounters, and often associated with circumstantial and pedantic speech. Laterality of the seizure focus is also reported to influence personality difficulties, although evidence here seems especially poor. Those with left-sided epileptogenic foci are said to be more ideative (i.e. to have philosophical interests, sense of personal destiny), with a tendency to have a poor opinion about themselves ('tarnish their own image'), whereas those with right-sided foci have been described as being more emotional, with a tendency to alternate between periods of sadness and periods of elation, and to have a high opinion of themselves ('polish their own image') – this has been referred to as the syndrome of temporal hyperconnection. This contrasts with the Klüver–Bucy syndrome which occurs as a consequence of bilateral anterotemporal destructive lesions and comprises oral exploratory behaviour, hypersexuality and decreased aggression. It may be seen in patients with temporal lobe epilepsy who have had a unilateral temporal lobectomy, and who then undergo compromise of the contralateral temporal lobe due to a brain injury, cerebrovascular disease or other pathology.

It has also been pointed out that some of these personality traits in mild forms have positive implications, in that they make these people honest, reliable, dependable and upstanding members of the community. Patients with juvenile myoclonic epilepsy have been reported as having a tendency to show immaturity and lability of mood and emotion, although, again, evidence to support these propositions is poor.

The treatment of personality problems in epilepsy can be difficult. As in all other personality disorders, the mainstay of therapy is psychological treatments such as CBT, counselling and supportive psychotherapy. These should be aimed at helping the individual and those in his or her environment to identify and to cope with the specific problem areas. A careful choice of AED could prevent or minimize disruption due to intermittent behavioural instability. Some patients require antidepressants or anxiolytic therapy. Antipsychotic agents are helpful in those prone to significant irritability, outbursts of temper and bouts of aggression. A low-potency antipsychotic such as sulpiride, administered continuously, can be a useful adjunctive therapy and prevent adverse behavioural exacerbations in some individuals.

Organic mental disorders

An interesting attempt to classify the personality and other 'organic mental disorders' (OMDs) associated with epilepsy has been made by Lindqvist and Malmgren (the LM scheme). The OMDs are divided into six basic categories:

1 asthenoemotional disorder
2 emotional–motivational blunting disorder (EMD)
3 somnolence–sopor–coma disorder (SSCD)
4 confusional–disorder (CD)
5 hallucination–coenestopathy–depersonalization disorder (HCDD)
6 Korsakoff amnestic disorder (KAD).

Each disorder can occur separately or together with one or more OMDs, and all six disorders may be seen in epilepsy. However, three are more specific to this disorder: the asthenoemotional disorder, the EMD and the HCDD.

In one study, a series of 70 patients, 54 underwent temporal and 16 underwent extratemporal resections. When presurgical evaluation was carried out on all patients, 38.6% of patients were reported to have an OMD, of which asthenoemotional disorder (22.9%) and EMD (15.7%) were the most common. Postoperatively, 60.9% of patients showed an OMD at some time, the most common diagnosis again being the asthenoemotional disorder in both temporal and extratemporal lobe resections (49.1% and 50%, respectively). The frequency of EMD was significantly higher in the extratemporal resection group (37.5% compared with 9.4% in patients with temporal lobe resections). Patients with preoperative anxiety–depressive disorders (ADs) as well as pre- and/or postsurgical asthenoemotional disorder were significantly more likely to develop an AD postoperatively than patients with no such history. This risk was also reported to be higher for patients with a presurgical asthenoemotional disorder than for those who newly developed this disorder after surgery. Laterality or site of resection, histopathology and seizure outcome were not significantly correlated to pre- and/or postsurgical diagnoses of asthenoemotional disorder. One year after the resective surgery, the prevalence of the asthenoemotional disorder was equivalent to the preoperative degree.

Disorders of sexual function

Hyposexuality has been long recognized as a feature of epilepsy in both men and women. Between 30 and 60% of men with epilepsy have reported lack of desire and impotence, and in one study 21% of men with chronic epilepsy had not experienced sexual intercourse. Among women, self-reports of dyspareunia, vaginismus and arousal insufficiency are common, and also dissatisfaction with sexual experience. There are a number of potential mechanisms. Clearly the psychosocial difficulties encountered by people with epilepsy could play a part, including stigmatization, lack of self-esteem, restricted lifestyles, parental overprotection, and depression and anxiety. Biological changes including altered levels of sex hormones (especially free levels) are found in epilepsy, due to seizures and drug therapy; these too could contribute to sexual difficulties. Seizures involving limbic structures might also be expected to alter sexual behaviour, and there is evidence (albeit inconclusive) that those with temporal lobe epilepsy have a greater degree of sexual dysfunction than those with generalized epilepsy. Antiepileptic drugs can alter the metabolism of sex hormones and affect their protein binding. Epilepsy surgery can also profoundly change, usually lowering, sexual drive. Treatment should begin with a careful analysis of potential causes (some of which may, of course, be quite independent of the epilepsy or its treatment). Psychosexual counselling can be very helpful. Control of seizures and reduction of antiepileptic therapy (including the withdrawal of sedative drugs) may improve sexual functioning, as can individual or couple sex therapy.

Acute psychotic or depressive states induced by antiepileptic drugs

Although many antiepileptic drugs have a role in the management of bipolar disorder, virtually all these drugs have also been reported to precipitate severe adverse psychiatric reactions, notably acute psychosis or depression. The risk seems greatest in patients with a previous history of psychiatric disorders. How frequently this occurs is not clearly known, but levetiracetam, phenobarbital, topiramate and vigabatrin carry perhaps the greatest risk. These antiepileptic drugs should be used with caution in patients with concurrent psychosis, and carbamazepine or valproate might be preferred options.

Many of the drugs can also cause mild psychiatric symptoms, particularly feelings of depression, anxiety or irritation. Drugs associated with more severe psychiatric adverse events include: barbiturates with depression and attention deficit hyperactivity disorder in children; phenytoin with toxic schizophreniform psychoses; valproate with acute and chronic encephalopathies; vigabatrin, topiramate and other drugs with depression and alternative psychoses, and agitation; and levetiracetam with irritability, aggressivity and psychosis. The ability of levetiracetam to cause irritability and dysphoria (a 'short fuse') in a small number of patients can be very prominent in occasional patients and have particularly severe consequences. The side effects do not correlate particularly with specific antiepileptic mechanisms of action, and certain individuals seem particularly prone to psychiatric side effects (from any drug) – and predictive factors said to increase the risk of psychiatric adverse effects include a history of drug-resistant epilepsy, a history of febrile convulsions (suggesting that early limbic injury predisposes to psychiatric vulnerability that can be triggered by antiepileptic drugs), and previous and familial psychiatric history.

Psychiatric disturbance and personality change after epilepsy surgery

Epilepsy surgery carries a risk of precipitating psychiatric disturbance. The most common problems are mood swings, anxiety and depression. These are seen in 20–30% of people who undergo surgery for epilepsy. Although distressing, these are generally mild and remit within weeks or months, although some people may need antidepressant medication or counselling.

More severe psychiatric breakdown may also occur. When temporal lobectomy was first introduced in the 1950s, it had been hoped that it would alleviate the psychosis of epilepsy as well as seizures; indeed, psychosis was seen as a positive indication. However, it was rapidly recognized that temporal lobectomy also often made psychosis worse. The literature in this area is extensive but the main themes are as follows: some patients can be cured of their psychosis after surgery (although relapse is common); more commonly, however, the psychosis can be exacerbated by surgery and new psychosis occurs in about 5% of patients after temporal lobectomy. Psychosis is more common if seizures are not controlled by surgery and if bilateral preoperative EEG abnormalities were present. Right-sided resections in some series are associated with an increased vulnerability to developing psychosis postoperatively. In a recent study of individuals who had undergone epilepsy surgery in London, about 10% of patients undergoing temporal lobectomy suffered a depressive or psychotic episode after surgery of a severity that required hospitalization, and many more needed consultation and treatment. Compounding these problems is the fact that no preoperative risk factors have been identified that reliably predict postoperative psychiatric disturbance. The lack of preoperative psychopathology does not seem to protect against postoperative anxiety or depression. There is also no clear relationship between psychiatric disturbance and either the lateralization of the surgery or the nature of the pathological tissue. Postoperative psychosis should be treated in the same fashion as interictal psychosis, and usually responds to therapy, but occasional cases are resistant and permanent psychotic states unfortunately do occur after temporal lobectomy, although the frequency or extent of this risk is not clearly known.

The occurrence of personality change after surgery is a poorly studied subject, but one of great concern. Various changes have been well documented, but their frequency and the factors predicting risk are largely unknown. Well recognized are changes in sexuality (usually hyposexuality), emotionality (flattening of emotional responses), impulsivity and obsessive–compulsive disorders. Anxiety, depression, personality change and psychotic breakdown can also occur after temporal lobe resections. Studies of the effect of epilepsy surgery on OMDs are described above.

Counselling patients in this situation is difficult. In general patients, particular caution must be communicated to patients with a strong past or family history of psychopathology, as they have inherent biological vulnerability. Although it is not clear if co-morbid psychopathology as such increases the risk of postoperative psychopathology, the burden of surgery is likely to be greater in someone who has an ongoing psychiatric illness. Also, candidates for surgery with poor psychosocial support, strained personal and familial circumstances, poor understanding of the process or unreasonable expectations are especially likely to develop postoperative psychopathology.

Life-threatening idiosyncratic reactions due to antiepileptic drug therapy

Life threatening idiosyncratic reactions due to antiepileptic drugs are thankfully rare (Table 5.19).

Haematological reactions

The risk of marrow and/or hepatic failure has been calculated for various drugs. Aplastic anaemia occurs in 2–6 cases per 10^6 of the general population. The risk for carbamazepine, for example, is between 1 in 50 000 and 1 in 200 000 for aplastic anaemia, 1 in 700 000 for agranulocytosis and 1 in 450 000 for death associated with these events. Felbamate is the only antiepileptic drug where the risk of bone marrow suppression is so high as to severely restrict its clinical use, with an incidence of aplastic anaemia estimated to be between 1 in 2000 and 1 in 37 000. Rare cases of aplastic anaemia have also been associated with phenytoin, ethosuximide and valproate. Selective suppression of bone marrow cells may lead to agranulocytosis and pure cell aplasia. Sporadic cases of immune-mediated thrombocytopenia or agranulocytosis have been reported with carbamazepine, lamotrigine, phenytoin, felbamate, primidone and tiagabine; the thrombocytopenia due to valproate is more common and not immune mediated. Pseudolymphoma syndrome, which may be part of the DRESS (drug rash [or reaction] with eosinophilia and systemic symptoms) syndrome spectrum, can be caused by phenytoin and less commonly other antiepileptics with an aromatic structure.

Hepatic failure

The overall incidence of hepatotoxicity has been estimated at 1 in 26 000 to 1 in 34 000. Drug-induced liver toxicity can be due to immune-mediated mechanisms or direct cytotoxic damage. Valproate and felbamate are associated with the greatest risk of potential liver toxicity. The risk of fatal hepatotoxicity with valproate varies with age and clinical context. The highest risk (1 in 600) is found in children aged <2 years with complex neurological disorders receiving polytherapy. In older patients the incidence is no more than 1 in 37 000 for monotherapy and 1 in 12 000 for polytherapy, and fatalities beyond 20 years of age are exceedingly rare (it has been estimated that 132 patients have died of valproate-induced liver failure and/or pancreatitis). The pathogenic mechanism of valproate-induced hepatotoxicity is probably a direct toxic action of valproate and/or its metabolite. There is some evidence that the children at risk may have undiagnosed urea cycle enzyme disorders or mitochondrial disease (and, in particular, Alpers disease). Early recognition of liver failure is important in improving outcome, and blood measurements of liver enzymes, ammonia and prothrombin time are essential if vomiting or somnolence occurs. The risk of hepatic failure on felbamate is between 1 in 26 000 and 1 in 34 000 exposures. The mechanism of felbamate-induced liver toxicity is not clearly understood, but may depend on the formation of reactive toxic metabolites.

Table 5.19 Serious idiosyncratic reactions associated with individual antiepileptic drugs.

	SJS/TEN	Liver toxicity	Pancreatitis	Aplastic anaemia	Agranulocytosis	SLE
Acetazolamide	+	+	−	+	+	−
Carbamazepine	+	+	+	+	+	+
Ethosuximide	+	+	−	+	+	+
Felbamate	+	+	+	+	+	+
Gabapentin	−	−	−	−	−	−
Lamotrigine	+	+	+	+	−	−
Levetiracetam	−	+	+	−	−	−
Oxcarbazepine	+	+	−	−	−	−
Phenobarbital	+	+	−	−	+	+
Phenytoin	+	+	−	+	+	+
Pregabalin	−	−	−	−	−	−
Primidone	+	+	−	−	+	+
Tiagabine	+	−	−	−	−	−
Topiramate	+	+	+	−	−	−
Valproic acid	+	+	+	−	−	+
Zonisamide	+	+	−	+	+	−

Eslicarbazepine, lacosamide and rufinamide – no serious hypersensitivity reported to date, but experience is relatively limited.
Clobazam, clonazepam and piracetam – definitive data not available.
SJS, Stevens–Johnson syndrome; TEN, toxic epidermal necrolysis or Lyell syndrome.

Aromatic antiepileptic drugs have been recognized as a cause of severe immune-mediated hepatitis, as part of the spectrum of DRESS or in isolation. The risk for carbamazepine is 16 cases per 100 000 treatment years. Rare cases of severe lamotrigine-induced liver toxicity have been reported.

Pancreatitis

Pancreatitis occurs with valproate in 1 in 40 000 cases, and most commonly occurs during the first year of treatment or after an increase in dosage. Age <20 years, polytherapy, chronic encephalopathy and haemodialysis are possible risk factors.

Skin reactions and the anticonvulsant hypersensitivity syndrome

The arene oxide-producing drugs – phenytoin, carbamazepine, phenobarbital, primidone and lamotrigine – can all cause acute hypersensitivity. This is a potentially fatal reaction and occurs in about 1 of 1000–10 000 exposures. The main manifestations include fever, rash and lymphadenopathy accompanied by multiorgan system abnormalities. The reaction may be genetically determined and siblings of affected patients may be at increased risk. This severe reaction needs to be differentiated from commonly occurring minor hypersensitivity reactions due to the same drugs (see below).

The DRESS syndrome is a severe form of hypersensitivity characterized by fever, skin eruption, eosinophilia, atypical lymphocytosis, arthralgia, lymphadenopathy and multiorgan involvement. It occurs most frequently with phenytoin (2.3–4.5 cases per 10 000 exposures) and carbamazepine (1.0–4.1 cases per 10 000 exposures). Cases have also been reported with lamotrigine. Pseudolymphoma, sometimes part of the DRESS syndrome, is a rare complication of phenytoin and other antiepileptic drugs with an aromatic structure.

Stevens–Johnson syndrome (SJS) and toxic epidermal necrolysis (TEN; Lyell syndrome) are related severe cutaneous reactions, resulting in bullous reactions accompanied by mucosal involvement and skin detachment. The risk is highest (1 in 50 to 1 in 300) with lamotrigine in paediatric practice, particularly when a high starting dosage is used or when the child is co-medicated with valproate. This limits the use of lamotrigine in young children, and the risk should be clearly mentioned to all patients initiating lamotrigine therapy. In adults, the incidence of lamotrigine-induced SJS is in the order of

1 in 1000, and is again highest with fast escalation, higher initial doses and co-medication with valproate. The risk is between 1 and 10 per 10 000 with carbamazepine, lamotrigine, phenytoin and phenobarbital. The risk of SJS seems to be genetically determined and there is a recently described association in Chinese individuals between carbamazepine-induced SJS and a specific human leucocyte antigen (HLA) type.

Allergic skin rash, without the features of SJS or TEN, is much more common. It typically occurs between days 5 and 60 of therapy, although it can occur at other times and occasionally occurs after months or years of therapy perhaps due to some cross-reactivity. Skin reactions occur in at least 5% of individuals exposed to phenytoin or carbamazepine. A rash can also occur with lamotrigine – with a frequency of about 7% in those not co-medicated with valproate and up to 20% in those co-medicated with high valproate doses. Oxcarbazepine has a somewhat lower rate of skin rash than carbamazepine.

At least for skin reactions, there is considerable cross-reactivity among these drugs. In one study, 20 of 42 patients (48%) who had a rash from phenytoin or carbamazepine also developed a rash after switching to the other drug. Of 51 patients who had a rash from carbamazepine, 14 (27%) also had a rash from oxcarbazepine. It is therefore wise to avoid, if possible, the use of antiepileptic drugs with a potential for cross-reactivity. Valproate or clobazam seem to be safe alternatives in patients who had a rash from aromatic anticonvulsants. Other antiepileptic drugs with a low risk of inducing hypersensitivity reactions include gabapentin, levetiracetam, pregabalin, topiramate, tiagabine and vigabatrin.

The outcome of hypersensitivity reactions depends on rapid recognition and discontinuation of the offending agent. If the drugs are continued, in spite of developing reactions, mortality rates rise steeply. Steroids can be given, and care of conjunctival and skin lesions is important. Immediate hospitalization is recommended, and some patients require intensive care.

Systemic lupus erythematosus

Carbamazepine and, to a lesser extent, phenytoin, ethosuximide, valproate, lamotrigine and other antiepileptic drugs can rarely induce or activate systemic lupus erythematosus. This drug-induced condition is sometimes not easily differentiated from the idiopathic form of the disorder.

Prevention

It is often advised that regular haematological and biochemical screening tests should be carried out in all patients taking potentially allergenic antiepileptic drugs, especially at the start of therapy. However, this strategy has been shown to provide neither advance warning of an idiosyncratic reaction nor sufficient early identification, and the author's view is that regular monitoring is neither necessary nor helpful. However, it seems reasonable to advise that a full haematological and biochemical screen be carried out before starting treatment (or adding any new antiepileptic drug), and regularly in high-risk groups and in patients with impaired ability to communicate.

In selected cases, re-challenge is the only conclusive method to confirm causality. It should not be contemplated after a severe reaction. Skin tests or other biochemical tests are currently not reliable enough to be diagnostically useful.

Treatment

Early identification of idiosyncratic drug reactions is life saving. Patients should be warned to report symptoms or signs. Even with the early signs of an idiosyncratic reaction, the offending drug should be immediately discontinued. In most cases, it is appropriate to substitute another antiepileptic drug considered safe in the specific context. In patients with hypersensitivity reactions to one aromatic antiepileptic drug, other aromatic anticonvulsants should be avoided. Agents with low allergenic potential include benzodiazepines, levetiracetam, gabapentin, pregabalin and topiramate. In patients with early symptoms or the suspicion of an idiosyncratic reaction, baseline and specialized haematological and biochemical tests should be immediately performed. The full gamut of laboratory tests should be carried out to evaluate a possible multiorgan involvement. Treatment with corticosteroids is controversial, although most physicians elect to start prednisone at a dose of 1–2 mg/kg if symptoms are severe. Patients with specific organ involvement need to be managed by the appropriate specialist. Patients with SJS and TEN, in particular, should be admitted to a high dependency unit with adequate supportive management in terms of wound care, hydration, nutritional support, and prevention of infection and other complications.

Complementary and alternative therapy in epilepsy

A definition of complementary therapy is 'treatment that complements mainstream medicine by contributing to a common whole, by satisfying a demand not met by orthodoxy, or by diversifying the conceptual frameworks of medicine'. One recent survey of 228 people with epilepsy found that 39% had used a non-conventional treatment and 25% specifically for epilepsy. There is no doubt that many patients feel dissatisfied by conventional therapy and seek what they consider more natural and gentler treatments. In epilepsy, a wide variety of techniques and therapies has been tried, although it has to be said that few have a scientific basis or have clearly established effectiveness by contemporary scientific standards. Whitmarsh has provided a comprehensive and critical review to which the reader is referred, and this text borrows heavily from this.

Psychological therapies to reduce seizure frequency

These are known as 'countermeasures' and various different approaches have been attempted, including hypnosis, meditation, yoga, biofeedback, operant or classic conditioning, and changing arousal levels. Stress reduction techniques of various types are very commonly employed in epilepsy, and have undoubted benefit, although there are few controlled studies in this important area.

Hypnosis combined with aromatherapy, routinely applied to patients in one epilepsy centre in 100 people, found a helpful and lasting effect. There is a report of hypnosis that reduced jacksonian seizures on one patient from 35 a week to 5 a week.

Meditation (of various forms) and yoga (and similar techniques) are commonly employed by patients with epilepsy, and have an enthusiastic following. There is at least one open study of meditation that showed a moderate benefit in reducing seizures and also changes in EEG parameters. A well-controlled study of Sahaja yoga (included in the Cochrane review) divided 32 patients with uncontrolled epilepsy into three groups. Group I ($n = 10$) was the yoga group, who practised Sahaja yoga meditation under the guidance of an instructor twice daily for 20–30 min for the 6-month duration of the study. Group II ($n = 10$) practised mimicking exercises in the same environment as group I and were provided with the same attention. Group III ($n = 12$) was a control group, just being followed up in outpatients. Four of 10 patients in the active group became seizure free after 6 months of practice, compared with none of 22 in the controls. Nine in the active group had more than a 50% reduction in seizure frequency compared with just 1 among the 22 controls.

Similarly, relaxation methods are widely practised and there are at least four well-controlled studies that show

benefit. In one study a 29% decrease in the frequency of seizures occurred in those trained in progressive muscular relaxation techniques, which was significantly better than in a control group of those treated by 'sitting quietly'. In another study 12 patients who had at least 6 seizures in an 8-week baseline period were trained in the technique of progressive muscular relaxation and followed for 6 months, and a mean reduction in seizures of 54% was observed.

EEG biofeedback has been extensively studied. This is an operant conditioning technique that aims to alter EEG rhythms of impending seizures. There is quite clear experimental evidence in cats, as well as less clear human data, which show positive effects. In one combined analysis of 18 studies, 82% of 174 patients showed seizure reductions of at least 30% when biofeedback was employed; 55 patients became seizure free for at least a year. It has been claimed that most patients with epilepsy who show clinical improvement with EEG biofeedback also show contingency-related EEG changes and a shift towards EEG normalization. However, not all responders show EEG changes, and some patients who do show EEG changes show little clinical response. A few individual patients have been rendered seizure free and have been able to withdraw from AED therapy. A controlled and blinded trial of galvanic biofeedback was also considered in a recent Cochrane review in 18 patients with refractory epilepsy, and 60% showed a 50% or greater reduction of seizure frequency compared with 0% in the sham feedback group. There is general agreement that biofeedback (in its various forms) is a useful therapy for some patients, but it has not been widely applied perhaps because it is time and labour intensive.

Other non-pharmacological therapies

Exercise has been clearly shown to improve the control of seizures in a number of studies, from institutions and outpatient clinics. A mean 40% reduction in seizures was observed in one study of aerobic dancing. The authors of one well-conducted study consider that the effects take months to develop and certainly exercise is no quick fix. Furthermore, some seizures occur during exercise, but the reduction in total number of seizures is much greater than the relatively few seizures induced by hard exercise. Another important effect was 'the normalization of the life situation for severely affected hypoactive and understimulated epileptic patients'.

Acupuncture has been used for thousands of years to treat epilepsy, and there are many anecdotal accounts of long-term reduction of seizures and even status epilepticus – there is a very large Chinese literature on this topic.

One study showed improvement in 89% of 98 cases treated with courses of scalp electro-acupuncture (30 min of electrical stimulation to the scalp at 2–3.5 Hz given daily for 15 days and repeated with a week-long break between courses). There are fewer western studies, and the conventional well-conducted controlled studies have, however, failed to show improvement. A Cochrane review of the effects of acupuncture in epilepsy found no evidence of benefit. There is also some literature on acupuncture in animal experimentation where it is claimed that the technique confers antiepileptic properties.

There are case reports of chiropractic therapy reporting huge improvements in individual patients, e.g. correcting 'upper cervical malalignment' in a 6 year old was reported to reduce the frequency of absence seizures from 25 a day to fewer than 1 a day. Another case report purported to show that chiropractic adjustment at the C6–7 level aborted all seizure activity in a 21-year-old woman who previously had daily convulsive seizures. Other anecdotal reports exist, but there is, however, a complete absence of published investigations with any controlled methodology.

Finally, mention should be made of 'music therapy'. Normalization of the EEG in 23 of 29 patients with epilepsy who listened to a Mozart sonata for two pianos (K448) for 10 min has been clearly demonstrated (the 'Mozart effect'), and there is one case report of an 8-year-old girl with that Lennox–Gastaut syndrome whose seizures were greatly reduced by listening to the sonata for 10 min/hour. Other musical forms have had some success. Another well-documented case report showed a remarkable improvement in the seizure control of a patient with a hypothalamic hamartoma and previously totally resistant gelastic and secondarily generalized epilepsy. 'Medical resonance therapy music' is a commercial product (on CD) of computer-generated contemporary music designed for therapeutic effects rather than listening pleasure, which the manufacturers claim results in a 75% reduction in seizures.

Herbal medicine

Herbal medicine is widely used in epilepsy in many parts of the world. In a recent review, 150 plants were said to be recorded as used in traditional medicines and 10 were thought to warrant further investigation. The Chinese mixture *Saiko-Keishi-To* is made up of nine plants. In one recent open study, when given to 24 patients with frequent seizures, 6 became seizure free and 13 improved in the frequency or severity of seizures, and in another study there was a reduction in seizures of at least 25% in 33%

of patients. Attempts to refine the preparation have so far proved fruitless. Another Chinese traditional herbal mixture has been reported to be very helpful as an adjunct to orthodox antiepileptic therapy, and cannabis has been used quite extensively by patients in Canada – in one survey 48% had tried it and 21% were active users. There is a certain amount of experimental evidence showing that cannabis can improve epileptic discharges.

Homoeopathy

There are no controlled studies of homoeopathic remedies in epilepsy, but open-case series demonstrate some improvements. There are striking individual case reports of improvement on homoeopathic therapy, and one very positive clinical trial in 10 epileptic dogs. However, homoeopathic clinics, in the UK at least, do not on the whole make many claims for efficacious remedies in epilepsy, although moderate improvement is reported.

Special diets and nutritional supplements

The ketogenic diet is widely accepted now as mainline therapy for a few children with severe epilepsy (see pp. 128–129). However, other diets are also increasingly being used as complementary therapy. The Atkins diet (60% fat, 30% protein and 10% carbohydrate) has gained favour, no doubt because of its superficial resemblance to the ketogenic diet (typically 80% fat, 15% protein and 5% carbohydrate). In a small open study of six children and adults, 50% became seizure free. The best results were seen in those who attained ketosis. Fasting also undoubtedly helps epilepsy and, on this basis, low-carbohydrate diets have been attempted and have advocates. Oligoantigenic diets are widely used in paediatric practice, and have been the subject of limited scientific investigation. One interesting double-blind study in a 19-year-old woman with frequent seizures, a history of allergies and eosinophilia was carried out. She was found by an elimination diet to be sensitive to beef. Seizures occurred soon after taking capsules containing beef, but not chicken, and she remained free from seizures long term by avoiding any beef products, having stopped anticonvulsant medication. Diets are also commonly used by patients with adult epilepsy. The author has had one patient who was convinced that eating eggs stopped his seizures. Other patients have tried gluten-free diets with some success.

Nutritional supplements are very commonly used by patients, and all sorts of combinations of vitamins and trace elements are widely sold – and various spurious analytical procedures of hair and other tissue are available to try to ascertain 'deficiencies'. Vitamin E at a dosage of 400 IU/day has been formally studied in one double-blind study in which there was a responder rate of 83%. Vitamin D (at doses of between 4000 and 16 000 IU/day) has in open studies reduced the frequency of seizures by about 30%. However, at an anecdotal level in normal clinical practice, neither vitamin D nor vitamin E has proved at all efficacious. Supplements of fish oils (omega-3 fatty acids), taurine, selenium, zinc, manganese and magnesium have all been reported to improve seizure control in some patients and are widely used. β-Hydroxybutyrate is a food supplement that has been the subject of a number of studies, and can induce ketosis in high doses.

Genetic counselling in epilepsy

Hippocrates recognized over 2000 years ago that epilepsy was a 'genetic disorder', and in recent years the importance of genetic factors has been re-emphasized. Epilepsy, however, is a heterogeneous condition, and genetic influences will vary in different syndromes and aetiologies. Counselling on this topic has become an important part of contemporary practice – for diagnostic and prognostic assessment and also for predictive testing in individuals at risk and assessing risk.

Counselling needs to be carried out by experienced personnel who understand the various difficult aspects relating to:
- analytical validity
- clinical validity
- clinical utility
- ethical and legal aspects.

All these aspects differ, e.g. it is quite possible for clinical validity to be present but not utility, or analytical validity to be good but clinical validity to be poor. However, all are important, and there is absolutely no place for casual or uninformed counselling, however well intentioned.

Single-gene disorders
In Chapter 4, some single-gene disorders underlying epilepsy are described, and counselling in these conditions should always be carried out. The risk of passing on a genetic defect will depend on the mode of inheritance, although variations in penetrance, which may depend on other genes, developmental stage or environmental factors, complicate this. Often the feasibility of predictive

testing will also depend on adequate identification of the familial mutation, and in some conditions (e.g. generalized epilepsy with febrile seizures plus [GEFS+]) a large number of disease-producing mutations at different loci in different genes have been described, rendering genetic analysis difficult in routine clinical practice. Testing can also involve the identification of biochemical or histochemical markers of disease status. In the absence of individual data, genetic counselling will fall back on careful examination of relatives and the pattern of inheritance.

Autosomal dominant inheritance
If there is full penetrance, there is a 50% risk to offspring and siblings. Unaffected members of the family carry no risk of transmission. In conditions that are not fully penetrant, the siblings and offspring have a risk of carrying the gene without expressing the phenotype, the risk depending on the extent of penetrance. Examples of autosomal dominant 'pure epilepsies' are benign familial neonatal seizures (0.85 penetrance), autosomal dominant nocturnal frontal lobe epilepsy (ADNFLE; 0.9 penetrance) and GEFS+ (variable penetrance). Other autosomal dominant conditions with epilepsy include tuberous sclerosis, dentato-rubro-pallido-luysian atrophy (DRPLA), acute intermittent porphyria and neurofibromatosis 1.

Autosomal recessive inheritance
The siblings of probands will have a 25% chance of being affected, a 50% chance of inheriting one disease-causing allele and being a carrier, and a 25% chance of inheriting both normal alleles and being unaffected. The normal siblings of a proband have a two-thirds chance of being a carrier. The offspring of a proband are all obligate heterozygotes. Consanguinity increases the risk. The chance of disease in subsequent generations depends on the frequency of the affected allele in the population and thus the rate of mating between two heterozygotes. Most inherited neurological conditions causing epilepsy are inherited in this manner, including the Unverricht–Lundborg disease, sialidosis, neuronal ceroid lipofuscinosis and many inherited enzyme deficiencies (Table 5.20).

X-linked inheritance
The mutations are usually transmitted from heterozygous healthy females (carriers) to 50% of their offspring. Usually all male offspring will have the disease, because they lack the second normal copy of the gene

Table 5.20 Genetic testing in epilepsy.

Disorder	Gene(s)	Diagnostic validity	Clinical utility
Benign familial neonatal convulsions	KCNQ2 KCNQ3	High in correct clinical context	Limited – KCNQ2/KCNQ3 mutational analysis does not alter management or prognostic implications
Benign familial neonatal–infantile seizures	SCN2A	High in correct clinical context	Limited – SCN2A mutational analysis does not alter management or prognostic implications
Generalized epilepsy with febrile seizures plus	SCN1A, SCN1B, GABRG2	High in correct clinical context	No – variable expressivity of mutations. Mutation does not inform about prognosis or treatment
Severe myoclonic epilepsy of infancy	SCN1A	High in correct clinical context	Yes – early optimization of antiepileptic therapy. Implications for genetic counselling
Autosomal dominant nocturnal frontal lobe epilepsy	CHRNA4, CHRNB2, CHRNA2	High in correct clinical context	Yes – establish aetiology, no need of follow-up imaging. Implications for genetic counselling
Autosomal dominant partial epilepsy with auditory features	LGI1	High in correct clinical context	Yes – establish aetiology, no need of follow-up imaging. Implications for genetic counselling
Unverricht–Lundborg disease	CSTB	High	Yes – inform about prognosis and treatment. Implications for genetic counselling. Detection of at-risk individual
Lafora disease	EPM2A EPM2B	High	Yes – inform about phenotype, prognosis and treatment. Implications for genetic counselling. Detection of at-risk individual
Myoclonus epilepsy and ragged red fibres	tRNA^{lys}	High	Yes – variable expressivity of mutations. Mutation does not inform about prognosis or treatment. Implications for genetic counselling. Detection of at-risk family members
Sialidoses	NEU PPGB	High	Yes – inform about prognosis. Implications for genetic counselling. Detection of at-risk family members
Late infantile neuronal ceroid lipofuscinoses	TPP1	High	Yes – inform about prognosis. Implications for genetic counselling. Detection of at-risk family members
Juvenile neuronal ceroid lipofuscinoses	CLN3		Yes – inform about prognosis. Implications for genetic counselling. Detection of at-risk family members

(hemizygosity). Fifty per cent of female siblings will be carriers and 50% will be normal. Female offspring will be carriers. In most diseases female carriers will be healthy, although in some conditions signs of the disease, usually but not always minor, can be detected owing to inactivation of one X chromosome (a process known as lionization, which is an epigenetic change, in other words a change in gene action without change in DNA). There is no male-to-male transmission of the disease. An example of a typical recessive X-linked condition with epilepsy is Rett syndrome.

Uncommonly, some X-linked genes show a dominant effect and heterozygous females express the full phenotype and males do not survive. *LIS1* lissencephaly and periventricular nodular heterotopia are examples of dominant X-linked conditions.

Mitochondrial inheritance

In human cells, 1% of DNA is carried in the mitochondria. Mitochondrial gene defects are transmitted via the maternal line, and no male-to-male transmission occurs. A characteristic of mitochondrial (mt) disease is marked variation in the severity and manifestations of the condition, because the proportion of mutated mtDNA varies among different cells; in some cells all mitochondria carry the mutated mtDNA (homoplasmy), whereas, in others, only a fraction of the mtDNA is mutated (heteroplasmy). Expression of the disease is strongly influenced by the amount and tissue distribution of mutated mtDNA, and the proportion of offspring with the condition cannot therefore be determined by simple mendelian rules. For the same reason, the offspring or sibling risk of manifesting the disease cannot be predicted. An example of an epilepsy inherited via mtDNA is the progressive myoclonus epilepsy due to myoclonic epilepsy with ragged red fibres (MERRF). To complicate matters, some nuclear genes are also involved in mitochondrial function and, in these conditions, mitochondrial dysfunction has a mendelian pattern (e.g. Alpers disease which is inherited in an autosomal recessive fashion).

Multigenic and complex genetic disorders

Most common disorders show a complex aetiology that includes a variety of genetic and environmental factors – these conditions are said to exhibit 'complex inheritance'. Carrying a genetic defect does not confer disease, but increases the 'susceptibility' and increases the risk of a disease.

In multigenic disorders, the disease develops when several gene-producing mutations coexist. There may be affected family members, but usually not very many. Affected members are more likely to be close relatives. The risk of recurrence for different degree relatives indicates the complexity of the genetic component. The higher the concordance rate among monozygotic twins, the stronger the contribution of genetic factors to the disorder. The lower the risk for relatives of probands, the higher the number of genetic factors involved. In many common diseases with complex inheritance, rare families exist where a single gene carries a major risk and the disease follows a 'mendelian' (single-gene) inheritance pattern. These families are important because they may give a clue to the genes involved in the more common cases with complex patterns of genetic disease. In some conditions, other genetic mechanisms are responsible for causing diseases, including copy number variations and epigenetic factors.

Many forms of epilepsy show a complex inheritance, and recurrence risks can be estimated only from empirical data based on the number of affected members and the degree of relationship. Examples of common epilepsy syndromes showing this pattern are the syndromes of idiopathic generalized epilepsy (IGE), benign epilepsy with centrotemporal spikes (BECTS) and febrile seizures.

Genetic counselling in specific non-mendelian epilepsy syndromes

As an example of the above points, some aspects of risk and counselling for specific syndromes are described here – and the issues involved emphasize the complex nature of counselling in all but the single-gene disorders with high penetrance.

Idiopathic generalized epilepsy

In this condition, there is a strong but complex genetic component. Occasional mendelian families also exist. For most sporadic cases, no diagnostic tests are available.

For sporadic cases, the risk of developing IGE in first-degree relatives is about 5–15%, and the risk to a second-degree or more distant relative is hardly elevated and close to that in the general population. A concordance rate of about 70–80% exists in monozygotic twins, increasing to 90% when EEG changes are considered.

The Rochester study established the following risk estimates. The risk for siblings was 6%, increasing to 8% if photosensitivity was found in the proband or if a parent had epilepsy, to 12% when a parent also showed generalized EEG abnormalities, and to 15% when the sibling showed a generalized EEG trait. The risk to offspring of an affected individual was 4–9% (8.7% in female and 2.5% in male offspring).

An interesting feature of IGE is its clinical variability within a family. In a study of 74 families with at least three affected members, only 25% of the families were concordant for a specific IGE syndrome. In various studies, putative susceptibility loci have been localized on several different chromosomes. So far no genetic mechanism has been found which is responsible for the generality of cases.

The risk of inheritance of EEG patterns (in contrast to epilepsy) is higher, about 25–30% for 3 Hz spike–wave or generalized polyspike–wave patterns.

Occasional mendelian families exist and, in these families, the risks are higher. Genes for rare autosomal dominant families have been mapped or identified for childhood absence epilepsy (CAE) (chromosome 8q) and for juvenile myoclonic epilepsy (JME) (chromosome 6p and the *GABRA1* gene on chromosome 5q).

Benign epilepsy with centrotemporal spikes

The genetics of this condition are complex and ill understood. Concordance in monozygotic twins has varied from 0% to 100% in different studies. For most sporadic cases, the risk of developing epilepsy in first-degree relatives is about 15%, rising to 30% if centrotemporal EEG abnormalities are found. Rolandic epilepsy has also been found to segregate in association with other very rare mendelian neurological conditions such as autosomal dominant rolandic epilepsy with speech dyspraxia, and autosomal recessive rolandic epilepsy with paroxysmal exercise-induced dystonia and writer's cramp.

It is presumed that there is a strong but genetic component in this condition, with multiple genes involved; currently no genetic testing is available.

Severe myoclonic epilepsy of infancy

This sporadic condition is usually caused by mutations in the neuronal sodium channel gene *SCN1A* during gametogenesis. Various mutations and also deletions have been described. Thus, the condition has a genetic basis, but is usually not 'inherited'. Genetic analysis of the *SCN1A* gene is possible, and can help refine diagnosis, but, when the mutations are sporadic and during gametogenesis, there is no increased risk to relatives.

However, in a few cases, there is a positive family history; in these cases, a germline mutation is probably responsible, and counselling may be required to assist relatives in determining risk.

Febrile seizures

In monozygotic twins 35–70% clinical concordance has been found. Population-based studies have shown an increased risk for first-degree relatives ranging from 8% in white people to up to 20% in Japanese individuals. In most cases, inheritance seems likely to be polygenic, although there are a few reported large families with dominant inheritance. From the counselling point of view, it is therefore important to gain a detailed family history before estimating risk rates. There is also a two- to tenfold increased risk of developing later afebrile seizures, but the later epilepsy probably has a major environmental as well as a genetic basis (see pp. 26–28).

Affected individuals in GEFS+ families have mutations on *SCN1A*, *SCN2A*, *SCN1B* and *GABRG2* genes, but these are not common in sporadic cases. One locus on chromosome 19p has also been found in a single family with apparently autosomal dominantly inherited febrile seizures.

Genetic counselling has currently to be based on the empirical risks outlined above, except where there is familial clustering. No genetic testing is available in sporadic cases.

Genetic counselling in specific mendelian epilepsy syndromes

Counselling for mendelian epilepsies is less empirical but can still be complicated. There are over 100 single-gene neurological conditions with epilepsy as part of the phenotype (Table 5.20 shows the more common examples) and the reader is referred to texts on these conditions for advice about counselling.

Benign familial neonatal convulsions

Genetic testing for benign familial neonatal convulsions includes the mutational screening of *KCNQ2* and *KCNQ3* using genomic DNA from patients. This is expensive and should be reserved for cases in which the clinical diagnosis is highly likely. For genetic counselling, the risk estimate is typical of any autosomal dominant single-gene disorder with high penetrance, with a 50% risk of transmission for offspring or siblings of affected individuals.

Benign familial neonatal–infantile seizures

Benign familial neonatal–infantile seizures (BFNIS) is due to mutations affecting *SCN2A*, the gene encoding the α_2-subunit of the neuronal voltage-gated sodium channel. So far, only a few families with BFNIS have been reported and mutational screening of *SCN2A* can help confirm the diagnosis in highly suggestive families but has no other particular clinical utility.

Benign familial infantile seizures

The mode of inheritance of benign familial infantile seizures (BFIS) is typically autosomal dominant, although occasionally the disease is transmitted from apparently healthy individuals. It is not clear whether this is due to incomplete penetrance or difficulties in collecting a reliable history from adults. Furthermore, non-familial cases with idiopathic seizures with onset within the first year of age, spontaneously remitting and showing overlapping clinical features with BFIS, have been described. Two different BFIS loci have been identified on chromosomes 19q and 2q. Other families exist without linkage to either focus. Other cases exist with overlap with the syndrome of familial infantile seizures and paroxysmal choreoathetosis (ISCA syndrome). Some cases of BFIS have shown *SCN2A* mutations, but screening of this gene is usually negative and should not be routinely requested.

Generalized epilepsy with febrile seizures plus

This condition has an autosomal dominant mode of transmission, and three major causal genes have been identified: voltage-gated sodium channel subunits α_1 and β_1 genes (*SCN1A* and *SCN1B*, respectively) and the GABA$_A$-receptor subunit γ gene (*GABRG2*). Incomplete penetrance and variable expression of the disease suggest that minor alleles might influence the phenotype. Genetic counselling should take into account the variability of the disease, which may manifest with severe or mild phenotypes and incomplete penetrance (about 80%) lowers the risk for relatives of probands. The three genes so far identified account for only about 20% of the GEFS+ phenotypes and, although screening is possible, it is expensive and the current advice is that it should be undertaken only to confirm diagnosis when febrile plus seizures are consistently found in different family members.

Autosomal dominant nocturnal frontal lobe epilepsy

Autosomal dominant nocturnal frontal lobe epilepsy (ADNFLE) is an inherited autosomal dominant condition with 80% penetrance. The condition is due to mutations in the neuronal acetylcholine receptor α_4- and β_2-subunit genes (*CHRNA4* and *CHRNB2)* or the α_2-subunit of the acetylcholine receptor – *CHRNA6*. Analysis of the condition is complicated by clinical as well as genetic heterogeneity, and seizures may be subtle and are frequently misdiagnosed as sleep disorders such as nightmares, hysteria and paroxysmal dystonia. Genetic screening of *CHRNA4* and *CHRNB2* is available, and may be attempted when the transmission pattern supports autosomal dominant inheritance. *CHRNA6* mutations have been identified in only a single family so far and routine screening is not available.

Autosomal dominant partial epilepsy with auditory features

This rare condition is due to mutations in the *LGI1* gene. It is almost invariably present in families although one sporadic case has been described. Mutations in this gene

are not present in patients with common forms of temporal lobe epilepsy. It is inherited in an autosomal dominant fashion, and screening of *LGI1* is recommended in suggestive families for diagnosis confirmation. However, there is variable expression and limited prognostic value in genetic tests.

Benign familial adult myoclonic epilepsy

Benign familial adult myoclonic epilepsy is inherited in an autosomal dominant fashion with high/complete penetrance and genetic heterogeneity. Linkage has been identified to chromosome 8q24 and chromosome 2p11.1–q12.2. Sporadic cases are occasionally found, and may be due to new mutations. Genetic tests are not available.

Genetic counselling in the progressive myoclonic epilepsy syndromes

Unverricht–Lundborg disease, Lafora body disease, MERRF, sialidoses and neuronal ceroid lipofuscinoses are the most common forms. All are inherited in an autosomal recessive manner except MERRF, which has a mitochondrial pattern of inheritance, and some cases of adult-onset neuronal ceroid lipofuscinosis, which seem to have dominant inheritance.

Unverricht–Lundborg disease (Baltic myoclonus)

This condition is due to a mutation in the gene encoding cystatin B (*CSTB*). The most common mutation is an expansion of an unstable dodecamer repeat in the 5′-untranslated region, which suppresses transcription. In the general population, 2 or 3 repeats usually occur, whereas up to 100 repeats are found in patients. There is no correlation between clinical severity or age at onset and size of expansion. Genetic testing is available.

Lafora body disease

Lafora body disease results from mutations in either the *EPM2A* or the *EPM2B* gene. Lafora bodies detected in skin biopsies are a useful clinical marker, but genetic testing based on mutational screening of *EPM2A* and *EPM2B* has a high sensitivity and is now the preferred diagnostic tool, and it can be used for risk assessment.

Myoclonus epilepsy and ragged red fibres

MERRF is inherited mitochondrially as a missense mutation (*A8344G*) affecting tRNA[lys]. Genetic analysis of *A8344G* mutations is sensitive and genetic testing can be used for diagnosis, prenatal diagnosis and to identify at-risk individuals.

Sialidoses

The sialidoses are very rare autosomal recessive lyso-somal disorders characterized by complex phenotypes subgrouped into sialidosis types I and II. Clinical diagnosis can be confirmed by documenting elevated urinary sialylyloligosaccharides and a deficiency of α-N-acetylneuraminidase in leucocytes and cultured skin fibroblasts. Mutations can be detected in the neuraminidase gene (*NEU*) on chromosome 6p and in cathepsin A gene on chromosome 20q encoding a 32-kDa protein (protective protein for β-galactosidase or PPGB). Biochemical assays focus on measuring the activity levels of neuraminidase and β-galactosidase. Mutational screening of the *NEU* and *PPGB* genes is a powerful tool for confirming the clinical diagnosis in probands and can be utilized in prenatal diagnosis and carrier identification.

Neuronal ceroid lipofuscinoses

This disease complex has a variety of forms. The late infantile neuronal ceroid lipfuscinosis (NCL) is due to mutations of a gene identified as encoding tripeptidyl peptidase 1 (TPP1). Diagnosis can be by electron microscopic detection of typical curvilinear lipidic inclusions, and genetic testing is also now available. The juvenile type (Batten disease – *CLN3*) is caused by mutations in the gene that encodes for an integral membrane protein (*CLN3*). More than 20 different mutations have been observed so far but a 1-kb deletion is found in 70% of disease chromosomes, suggesting a strong founder effect. Diagnosis is by electron or mutational screening of *CLN3*. The genetic basis of the adult form (Kufs disease) has not been identified, and electron microscopic examination of muscle biopsies to detect curvilinear bodies is the only diagnostic test available.

Dentato-rubral-pallido-luysian atrophy (DRPLA)

This condition (p. 44) is caused by a CAG trinucleotide expansion in the *ATN1* gene. The disease is particularly common in Japanese populations (with a prevalence of 0.2–0.7 in 100 000), but occurs less frequently in other ethnic groups. The normal allele contains 6–35 repeats, and the disease has been found to be caused when the repeat number exceeds 47. The highest number of repeats recorded in any case to date is 93. There is a tendency to genetic anticipation, with younger age of onset in succeeding generations, and an inverse correlation between the age at onset and the size of the expanded CAG repeat. Targeted mutation analysis by PCR amplification of the trinucleotide repeat region, followed by gel electrophoresis, is now a reliable and widely available diagnostic test.

6 Treatment of Epilepsy in Specific Groups

Treatment of epilepsy in children

General considerations

The treatment of epilepsy in infancy and early childhood differs in a number of ways from that in late childhood or adult life.

Clinical context

The aetiologies, clinical features and response to treatment of epilepsy are very different. Both seizures and antiepileptic drugs can affect behaviour, learning, schooling, and social and emotional development. Special attention is needed to overall mental and neurological development. Approximately 20–30% of children with epilepsy have learning disabilities and, in many cases, attention to intellectual impairment takes precedence over epilepsy. Careful psychological and educational assessment is needed to identify problems and tailor treatment and educational programmes.

Social impact of epilepsy

The impact of epilepsy on the life of children can be very different from that in adults (see Table 5.13 in Chapter 5). Growing up with seizures affects the development of personality and can interfere with many aspects of everyday life, schooling and choice of career. Support for the child and his or her family is an important part of management. It is essential to spend time providing information and advice, and there are few areas where counselling is so important. Children with epilepsy should have a lifestyle that is as normal as possible, and the common tendency to over-protect ('cocoon') children should be discussed with parents and consciously avoided. Small increases in risk are to be preferred to extensive prohibitions.

Handbook of Epilepsy Treatment, 3rd Edition. By Simon Shorvon. Published 2010 by Blackwell Publishing Ltd.

Epilepsy with falls

Where epilepsy occurs with falls (e.g. drop attacks in the Lennox–Gastaut syndrome), special precautions are necessary. These epilepsies inevitably interfere with daily activities, and special schooling measures and protection of the head and face by wearing an adequate helmet is often required.

Treatment of different epilepsy syndromes

The categorization of an epilepsy syndrome is far more important in children than in adults. The type of treatment, the effect of treatment and the prognosis vary considerably between different syndromes, and epilepsy is much more heterogeneous in children than in adults. The specific therapies of the common syndromes are outlined on pp. 89–95.

Specific therapies of different aetiology

There are a number of specific medical therapies for several of the inherited metabolic disorders that cause childhood epilepsies, which should not be overlooked. Table 6.1 lists some of these.

Antiepileptic drug treatment

Antiepileptic drug regimens in young patients are often different from those in adults and also change with age through childhood. Absorption of antiepileptic drugs is usually faster in infants and young children than in adults. The half-lives of most antiepileptic drugs are prolonged in the first 1–3 weeks of life and shorten thereafter. The metabolism of antiepileptic drugs is faster during childhood and slows to adult rates during adolescence. Thus, higher doses per unit of weight are required by children, and dosage requirements can change over time.

The pharmacodynamic effects of antiepileptic drugs may also differ. The paradoxical effect of barbiturates and benzodiazepines causing excitation in children and sedation in adults is an example.

Table 6.1 Disorders presenting in infancy with epileptic seizures for which there is a specific non-AED treatment.

Disorder	Diagnostic test	Treatment
Glucose transporter deficiency type 1 (Glut-1)	CSF:plasma glucose ratio <0.5 Mutation in *Glut1* gene	Ketogenic diet
Biotinidase deficiency	Biotinidase assay – blood	Biotin
Pyridoxine deficiency	Trial of treatment Urinary α-aminoadipic semialdehyde dehydrogenase Mutation in antiquitin gene	Pyridoxine
Pyridoxal 5′-phosphate deficiency	Trial of treatment CSF neurotransmitters	Pyridoxal phosphate
Serine biosynthesis disorders	Low CSF serine levels Enzyme activity in fibroblasts	Serine
Fatty acid oxidation disorders	Urine organic acids Blood acylcarnitines	Diet
Creatinine synthesis disorders	MRS Urine guanidinoacetic acid	Creatinine

AED, antiepileptic drug; CSF, cerebrospinal fluid; MRS, magnetic resonance spectroscopy.

Side effects are difficult to recognize in infants and in those with learning disability, and children may not be able to communicate their symptoms. These groups therefore require extra surveillance for side effects.

In school-aged children, three-times-daily regimens (requiring dosing at school) should be avoided, because the middle dose is easily overlooked and can embarrass the child. Slow-release preparations of carbamazepine and sodium valproate have made it possible to maintain adequate plasma levels with twice-daily dosing.

The use of the newly marketed antiepileptic drugs in paediatrics has not been as extensively studied as in adults, and these drugs should generally not be used as first-line therapy except for special situations (e.g. vigabatrin in West syndrome associated with tuberous sclerosis). Details of studies of individual drugs in children are found in Chapter 8.

The ketogenic diet

The ketogenic diet is a high-fat, low-carbohydrate diet that was introduced into epilepsy therapy in the 1920s, and which in recent times has been the subject of a resurgence of interest. Its use is confined to the treatment of severe childhood epilepsy that has proved resistant to more conventional therapy. It has no role in adult epilepsy, where its use has proved difficult and dangerous.

The diet is high in fat and low in carbohydrate, with adequate protein, and provides nutrition with 1 g/kg of protein and 5–10 g of carbohydrate per day, the remainder of the calories (usually 75% of the recommended daily allowance) being in the form of long-chain triglycerides. The diet must be followed strictly, an arduous and difficult task for the child and parent(s) alike.

Exactly how the diet exerts its undoubted antiepileptic effect is unknown. It mimics the biochemical changes of starvation (low carbohydrate intake) and this results in a switch from aerobic to ketogenic metabolism and the production of ketone bodies in the liver. These are transported into the brain by a monocarboxylic acid transporter, where they are utilized instead of glucose for energy production. This metabolic change has marked antiepileptic effects, as demonstrated in animal and human studies. To alter metabolism, however, requires dedication to a diet that is difficult to maintain and often unpalatable.

The diet is usually reserved for children with West syndrome, the Lennox–Gastaut syndrome or other less-specific forms of severe epilepsy. A special indication is in children with glucose transporter protein (GLUT-1) deficiency and pyruvate dehydrogenase deficiency, where the diet is first-line therapy and can be life-saving. Patients with gastrostomy tubes in place may be ideal candidates. The diet is potentially dangerous, and should be avoided, in pyruvate carboxylase deficiency, porphyria, carnitine deficiency, fatty acid oxidation defects and mitochondrial disorders (Table 6.2).

The exact constitution of the diet must be calculated individually for each patient. The ratio of fats to carbohydrates and protein is based on the age, size, weight and

Table 6.2 Indications and contraindications of the ketogenic diet.

Indications

Refractory epilepsy in children

Glucose transporter protein deficiency (GLUT-1)

Pyruvate decarboxylase deficiency

Epilepsy with encephalopathy (e.g. West syndrome, Lennox–Gastaut syndrome)

Tuberous sclerosis complex and other severe epilepsies with cortical dysplasia

Rett syndrome and other severe epilepsies of metabolic origin

Severe myoclonic epilepsy of infancy (SMEI, Dravet syndrome)

Formula-fed infants

Gastrostomy tube-fed children

Certain mitochondrial disorders

Contraindications

Pyruvate carboxylase deficiency

Porphyria

Carnitine deficiency (primary)

Fatty acid oxidation defects

Table 6.3 Side effects of the ketogenic diet.

Constipation
Exacerbation of gastro-oesophageal reflux
Water-soluble vitamin deficiency (if unsupplemented)
Elevated serum cholesterol, triglycerides, and low-density lipoprotein-cholesterol
Renal stones
Growth inhibition
Weight loss
Worsening of acidosis with illnesses
Bone fractures
Vitamin D and selenium deficiency
Cardiomyopathy

activity level of the patient. A young child or infant is often prescribed a 3:1 diet to provide additional protein and older children a 4:1 diet. Obese children and adolescents are usually given a 3:1 diet. Calorie intake is generally about 75% of the recommended daily intake for age. Fluid intake must be rigorously maintained, and supplementation with magnesium, zinc, vitamin D, vitamin C, vitamin B complex and calcium is recommended.

The effects on epilepsy can be dramatic. Early studies in the 1920s and 1930s consistently showed impressive results, and these have been largely confirmed in more recent investigations carried out to modern standards. A recent study from Johns Hopkins University showed, at 1 year, a reduction in seizures of more than 50% in 50% of 150 treated children, and a reduction of more than 90% in 27%. At 3–6 years, 44% maintained the improvement. The use of the diet allows a reduction of adjunctive

drug therapy, which is an added benefit. Other benefits of the diet include improvement in behaviour in those with and without autism. The diet can be given for months or years. A typical period of treatment is 1–2 years, if the diet proves initially successful. About 10% of children maintain the diet for 4 or more years, and one patient is reported who has maintained the diet for 15 years with no major side effects. Discontinuation of the diet should take place gradually over 3–6 months.

Side effects are not uncommon (Table 6.3). Vomiting, dehydration and food refusal are common initially but are transitory. Other minor side effects include constipation, oesophageal reflux and acidosis. The effect of the diet on growth is a problem. A recent review of the diet in 237 children showed that the rate of weight gain decreased at 3 months but then remained constant for up to 3 years. There is also an effect on height. Renal stones occur in 5–8% of patients. Hypercholesterolaemia is common. Rare side effects that have been reported include cardiomyopathy, pancreatitis, bruising, vitamin deficiency, hypoproteinaemia, Fanconi renal tubular acidosis and prolonged Q–T interval. In adults, for whom the diet is not normally recommended, coronary heart disease and myocardial infarction have occurred, associated with hypercholesterolaemia.

Treatment of epilepsy in patients with additional handicaps

The treatment of people with learning disabilities is complicated by a number of different issues (Table 6.4).

Table 6.4 Specific problems of diagnosis and management in handicapped patients.

Problems of diagnosis
- Communication
- Difficulty in recall
- Unusual forms that the epilepsy can take
- Distinguishing between epileptic seizures and psychogenic attacks
- Distinguishing between epilepsy and mannerisms and stereotypies
- Identifying neuroleptic- and other drug-induced symptoms
- Co-morbid psychiatric and other conditions

Problems of treatment
- Communication and 'management by proxy'
- Interictal disturbances
- Difficulties in recognizing side effects (e.g. sedation, behavioural change)
- Unusual forms of side effects
- Seizure exacerbations caused by antiepileptic drugs
- Brittle epilepsy and tendency to status epilepticus
- Avoiding seizure-induced brain damage
- Treating co-morbidities and 'diagnostic overshadowing'
- Attitude of family and carers
- Risks of over-medication
- Unusual choice of drugs and drug formulations

These include difficulties in recall and communication, the coexistence of mental illness, the fact that decisions on therapy are often made on the basis of carers or family ('management by proxy'), the unusual form that epilepsy may take, the poorer adaptive and social skills and additional speech difficulties of the individual, and sometimes challenging behaviour. There is, furthermore, a rather nihilistic tendency to under-investigate epilepsy, which should be resisted.

Antiepileptic drug treatment

Between 25 and 50% of those with severe learning disability have epilepsy, often associated with other physical and behavioural co-morbidities that influence antiepileptic drug therapy. The epilepsy in patients with learning difficulty is furthermore often severe and resistant to drug therapy. The usual principles of antiepileptic drug therapy apply, although certain points need specific emphasis:

Overlooking epileptic phenomenon and the role of interictal disturbance

Brief non-epileptic seizures can be overlooked. Behavioural problems can be a manifestation of seizure activity or interictal activity. Autistic behaviour in particular can be correlated with epileptic activity. Occasionally drug therapy based on the EEG can be justified. In the Landau–Kleffner syndrome, autistic features can be a manifestation of EEG activity even in the absence of clinical 'seizures'. In the Lennox–Gastaut and other syndromes, uncontrolled evidence suggests that behavioural disturbances may be improved if interictal EEG disturbances are reduced by antiepileptic therapy.

Overlooking side effects

Vigilance for side effects is particularly important. In the presence of cerebral damage, drug side effects tend to be more frequent, occur at lower serum levels and take unusual forms. This is particularly the case with cognitive, neurological or behavioural effects. Examples are confusion, neurological side effects, behavioural changes and mental deterioration, encephalopathy and weight gain that may be attributed to neuroleptics or inactivity. Hypotonic children are hypersensitive to the muscle-relaxing effects of benzodiazepines, and dystonia and ataxia may occur in patients with pre-existent motor deficits.

The lack of ability to communicate means that side effects of drugs are not reported and may be overlooked, and indeed the frustration of being unable to communicate may itself enhance behavioural disorder. It is an essential duty of the prescribing physician to maintain vigilance for side effects, to prevent distress or harm.

Misdiagnosis of epilepsy

Various repetitive mannerisms, bruxism, head-rocking and other stereotypies, common in learning disability, may be misdiagnosed as epileptic. In Rett syndrome, various non-epileptic phenomenon such as hyperventilation, Valsalva manoeuvres, syncopes and stereotypies are common and can be mistaken for epilepsy.

Seizure exacerbation caused by antiepileptic drugs

Many drugs will cause an increase in seizure activity in the occasional individual with learning disability, and this can sometimes be severe. This is an under-recognized problem particularly in patients with learning disability. Sedative drugs exacerbate seizures in many individuals and should generally be avoided. Drowsiness commonly worsens seizures and doses of any drug inducing somnolence should be reduced.

Carbamazepine and oxcarbazepine may exacerbate 'minor' generalized seizures, atypical absences and myoclonic or atonic seizures. Benzodiazepines can cause or exacerbate tonic seizures, and vigabatrin and tiagabine can cause serious exacerbation in absence, tonic and myoclonic seizures, and cause non-convulsive status epilepticus. Lamotrigine has been shown to exacerbate seizures in severe myoclonic epilepsy of infancy and levetiracetam has been reported to cause new generalized tonic–clonic seizures in patients with learning disabilities. Phenytoin can worsen seizures and function of patients with the Unverricht–Lundborg disease. In patients with myoclonic epilepsies (including the Lennox–Gastaut syndrome) carbamazepine, oxcarbazepine, tiagabine and vigabatrin can exacerbate seizures.

Serial seizures, clusters and episodes of status

These are common in patients with severe epilepsy and learning difficulty. They can be precipitated by seemingly minor problems such as intercurrent infections or trivial environmental changes. Emergency therapy (see pp. 287–288) is often needed earlier and more frequently than in a non-handicapped population. Drug regimens may need to be modified as handicapped individuals often show special sensitivities to the usual drugs. Tailored regimens for emergency intervention need to be defined for each individual, based on previous experience. It is helpful to document these in writing, and to have them available to all carers and emergency medical services.

Over-medication

Over-medication in the face of intractable epilepsy is a particular problem in handicapped individuals. The reasons are complex and include the severity of the epilepsy, the need for a third party to decide upon treatment on behalf of the individual, the difficulty in communicating side effects and the carer's tendency to over-protect. It is vital to resist this tendency. Great benefits (without loss of seizure control) are often gained by reducing the overall antiepileptic drug load.

Prevention of seizure-induced brain damage

There is some evidence that seizures may damage the developing brain in some epilepsy conditions. The best example is the stepwise motor deterioration that may result from episodes of severe seizures in the Sturge–Weber syndrome, and thus status epilepticus and prolonged seizures in this condition should be treated very aggressively. Early control of epilepsy in Down syndrome also improves prognosis. The early surgical resection of focal lesions, especially cortical dysplasias, if successful in controlling seizures, will sometimes greatly improve developmental progress.

Psychiatric considerations

Affective disorder and other mental health problems are twice as likely in those with learning disorder and epilepsy. Depression can be overlooked and attributed to the learning disability ('diagnostic overshadowing'), and needs to be treated as in a patient without handicap. Non-epileptic attack disorders are more common in people with intellectual handicap, perhaps partly because of the limited communication skills with which to express emotional conflicts.

Surgical therapy

Surgery can benefit a small number of individuals with epilepsy. The presence of handicap is not itself a bar to considering this. However, assessment should be carried out in experienced centres, and other issues such as quality-of-life gain and informed consent are often problematic.

Choice of drugs

In general, broad-spectrum antiepileptic drugs should be used and monotherapy should be the aim where possible. The non-sedative drugs are preferred. In many patients with learning disability, there is a preference for drugs such as lamotrigine, valproate, topiramate and zonisamide, and the avoidance of phenytoin, barbiturates and pregabalin. Levetiracetam can be helpful, but great care needs to be taken in view of its strong tendency to worsen behaviour and especially cause aggressive behaviours. Carbamazepine is an excellent drug in focal epilepsy in patients with learning disability but should be avoided in generalized seizure disorders due to its tendency to exacerbate atypical absence or myoclonic seizures.

However, drugs can have specific effects in patients with learning disability. Lamotrigine has mood-stabilizing effects, and beneficial effects on behaviour social engagement in patients with the Lennox–Gastaut syndrome and other conditions with learning disability. It can increase attention and alertness. Conversely, hyperactivity and irritability, exacerbation of myoclonic seizures blepharospasm, tics and Gilles de la Tourette syndrome-like symptoms can occur. Severe valproate toxicity is a greater risk in patients with developmental delay and inborn errors of metabolism, particularly mitochondrial disorders, which can go unrecognized. It should be used with caution in infants with learning disability. Gabapentin has been associated with aggression, myoclonus, hyperexcitability, temper tantrums and involuntary choreiform in patients with learning disability.

Drug formulation is also an issue in some situations, and especially in those unable to swallow pills or with parenteral feeding.

Institutional care

Overall, among individuals requiring long-term institutional care, between 30 and 50% have epilepsy. Epilepsy has been found to occur in 50% of those with IQ levels <20, and in 35% of those with IQ levels in the 35–50 range. Seizures are particularly common in those with postnatal cerebral damage. The frequency of handicap among those with epilepsy is difficult to ascertain. In a 1983 study of 223 adults with epilepsy in Finland, 30% had an IQ of <50, 20% were institutionalized and 15% were completely dependent. A more recent study, also from Finland, found handicap in 20% of children with epilepsy compared with 1% of controls.

The needs of individuals with multiple handicaps are often complex, and care is difficult to organize. In patients with severe epilepsy, the seizures usually pose the major problem but, in others, the problems of epilepsy are secondary to the other handicaps. Epilepsy adds a dimension that care providers often find difficult to deal with. The responsibility of dealing with potentially life-threatening seizures is felt to be too great by many otherwise competent authorities. It is therefore often difficult to find suitable residential, daytime or vocational placements for people with epilepsy. A few specialized institutions provide expert epilepsy care and, although these provide a secure environment from the epilepsy point of view, they may be geographically distant, risking family estrangement. All institutions dealing with epilepsy require specialist medical input, and a failure to monitor the epilepsy is a dereliction of care. Teamwork is needed, with facilities for outpatient and inpatient treatment and good communication between the different professional groups and also the family. Care can be shared between an institution and the family, and in both settings a balance has to be set between over-protection and neglect. This balance can be very difficult to define or achieve, and there is no one single correct position. Individuals deserve

an individually tailored solution, and the issues involved (and the risks taken) should be explicitly agreed with the individual, the family and professional carers.

Epilepsy in elderly people

Epilepsy is a frequent and generally under-recognized problem in elderly people. Annual incidence rates in a recent study were 87 per 100 000 in the 65–69 age group, 147 per 100 000 of people in their 70s, and 159 per 100 000 of people in their 80s, and about 30% of new cases now occur in people aged >65 years. The prevalence rate of treated epilepsy in those aged >70 years is almost double that in children. Currently, about 0.7% of the elderly population are treated for epilepsy, and epilepsy in elderly people is now the third most common neurological condition after dementia and stroke. As the number of elderly people in the population is rising, the number of elderly people requiring treatment for epilepsy is also greatly increasing. The medical services must catch up to make adequate provision.

Cerebrovascular disease accounts for between 30 and 50% of cases, but this can be occult. Epilepsy is the first manifestation of previously silent cerebrovascular disease, and imaging evidence of cerebrovascular disease is found in about 15% of those presenting with apparently idiopathic late-onset epilepsy. The onset of seizures in elderly people can be a harbinger of future stroke and, in a recent study of 4709 individuals with seizures starting after the age of 60 years, there was a 2.89-fold (95% confidence interval [CI] 2.45–3.41) increased incidence of subsequent stroke. In fact, the onset of seizures was a greater risk factor for stroke than either elevated cholesterol level or hypertension. Seizures also follow stroke, with a frequency of about 6% in the acute phase after stroke and 11% in the first 5 years after ischaemic stroke. Subdural haematoma is another underdiagnosed cause of epilepsy in elderly people, and cerebral tumours account for between 5 and 15% of all late-onset epilepsies. Ten per cent of the late-onset epilepsies are due to metabolic causes, such as alcohol, pyrexia, dehydration, infections, and renal or hepatic dysfunction. Drug-induced epilepsy is common in elderly people both because drugs are given more frequently and because of the complex pharmacokinetics in elderly people.

Diagnosis

It can be difficult to differentiate seizures from the abundance of other causes of 'funny turns' in elderly people.

Syncope, hypoglycaemia, transient ischaemic attacks, transient global amnesia, vertigo and non-specific dizziness afflict up to 10% of the older population. Syncope can have cardiac causes or it may be due to blood pressure changes or impairment of the vascular reflexes linked to posture, and carotid sinus hypersensitivity is also common. Acute confusional states or fluctuating mental impairment can be ictal, postictal or result from non-convulsive status, but are frequently misdiagnosed as manifestations of functional psychiatric illness, dementia or vascular disease. The history may be less well defined, and the differentiating features less clear cut than in younger patients, and pathologies may coexist.

There are furthermore various EEG changes that are easily mistaken for epileptogenic patterns. Brief runs of temporal slow activity, especially on the left, become increasingly evident after the age of 50 years and should be considered a normal variant. Small sharp spikes during sleep and drowsiness also increase in frequency with age. Runs of temporal–parietal activity can occur in individuals over the age of 50 years (the subclinical rhythmic electrographic discharge in adults [SREDA] pattern) and are not associated with epilepsy. Cerebrovascular disease produces focal and bilateral temporal changes that are also commonly mistaken for epilepsy, and yet do not provide any assistance in determining which patients with vascular disease will or will not develop overt epileptic seizures.

General aspects of management

Seizures in elderly people have a serious impact. Postictal states can be prolonged. A confusional state lasting more than 24 hours has been found to occur in the wake of 14% of seizures in elderly people, and in some cases confusion lasted over a week. Postictal Todd paresis is also more common than in young people, and seizures are commonly misdiagnosed as a stroke. Fractures and head injuries are a potential risk. Falling in a seizure can mark a watershed in an older person's life, after which there is a sharp decline in functional independence. The loss of confidence and fear of further falls can render the person electively housebound. This loss of confidence can be compounded by other factors including the stigmatization of epilepsy, the assumption of impending death, the reaction of family and friends, the exclusion from activities, marginalization, loss of a driving licence, disempowerment and a perception of a shrinkage of life space.

Reassurance that seizures do not usually indicate cerebral tumour, psychiatric disorder or dementia, and that they can usually be controlled on medication, is of overriding importance.

Management often involves other professionals. Confidence needs to be rebuilt, mobility restored and the home circumstances reviewed. Advice and input from social services, remedial and occupational therapists are often needed. A home visit to identify sources of potential danger is helpful. A personal alarm can be very useful, as can counselling and written advice for friends and relatives. Factors known to precipitate seizures should be avoided, such as inadequate sleep, excess alcohol or hypoglycaemia.

Uncontrolled seizures are likely to be more hazardous in an elderly patient. Convulsive attacks carry greater risks in patients with cardiorespiratory disorders, and the elderly, fragile patient is more susceptible to fractures as a consequence of seizure-induced falls.

Principles of antiepileptic drug therapy

The general principles of drug treatment in elderly people are generally similar to those in other adults. However, there are some aspects that deserve special mention.

Pharmacokinetic differences

The relationship between dose and serum level can be much more variable in elderly people than in young adults, and published pharmacokinetic values are often expressed as mean values that do not necessarily take into account the wide range in elderly people. Protein binding may be reduced as albumin concentrations are lower in elderly people. Clearance is often lower in elderly people due to reduced hepatic capacity and lower glomerular filtration rates (Table 6.5), and the volume of distribution for lipid-soluble drugs is often increased. For all these reasons, the half-life of many drugs is longer than in young adults. The interaction of the many medicaments taken by elderly people can greatly complicate the handling of drugs, by competition for absorption, protein binding, hepatic metabolism and renal clearance. In the USA people aged >65 years comprise 13% of the population and yet receive 32% of prescribed medications and, in one study of epilepsy patients aged 75, a mean of three medications per patient were being taken in addition to the prescribed antiepileptic drugs.

Pharmacodynamic differences

There are pharmacodynamic differences between elderly people and young adults. Anecdotal evidence suggests that elderly people are more sensitive to the neurological side effects of drugs, and also that lower drug doses are

Table 6.5 Average changes in apparent oral clearance of older and newer antiepileptic drugs in elderly patients.

Antiepileptic drug	Decrease in drug clearance in elderly people compared with young adults (%)
Carbamazepine	25–40
Felbamate	10–20
Gabapentin	~30–50
Lacosamide	~10–35
Lamotrigine	~35
Levetiracetam	~20–40
Oxcarbazepine	~25–35[a]
Phenobarbital	~20
Phenytoin	~25[b]
Tiagabine	~30
Topiramate	~20
Valproic acid	~40[c]
Vigabatrin	~50–85[d]

Acetazolamide, clobazam, clonazepam – clearance reduced but extent not clear.

Eslicarbazepine, ethosuximide, pregabalin, zonisamide – no definitive data

Primidone (derived phenobarbital) – as per phenobarbital.

Piracetam, rufinamide – no change in clearance in elderly people (in the absence of hepatic/renal dysfunction).

[a]MHD, the active metabolite of oxcarbazepine.
[b]Decrease in clearance of unbound drug may be greater.
[c]Decrease in unbound drug clearance. Clearance of total (unbound + protein bound drug) may not change.
[d]These patients, who had various pathologies, were preselected to cover a wide range of impaired renal function.

sufficient to control seizures in elderly people compared with younger adults. The adverse effects of drugs in elderly people may take unfamiliar forms. Confusion, general ill-health, affective change, or uncharacteristic motor or behavioural disturbances can occur with many antiepileptic drugs. Thus, the 'therapeutic ranges' defined in younger age groups do not necessarily apply to elderly people, and should be generally adjusted downwards. It is important to be vigilant for unusual side effects – both neurological and metabolic.

Systemic side effects

Membrane-stabilizing drugs (e.g. phenytoin, carbamazepine, lamotrigine) carry a risk of promoting arrhythmia and hypotension, which is increased in elderly people, although the extent of this risk is unknown. Other side effects in elderly people include the dangers of loss of bone mass due to enzyme-inducing drugs such as phenytoin, carbamazepine or phenobarbital, a particular risk in postmenopausal women. Phenytoin and carbamazepine also pose potential problems and should be used cautiously in individuals with autonomic dysfunction, e.g. in diabetes. Carbamazepine has an anticholinergic effect that can precipitate urinary retention.

Compliance

Compliance with medication can be poor owing to memory lapses, failing intellect or confusion. In these situations, drug administration should be supervised. The provision of a weekly drug wallet can also be worthwhile. Other methods of improving compliance include using simple drug regimens, providing clear written instructions and clearly labelled medication, avoiding childproof bottles and blister packs, employing assistance from carers, relatives and others, and home visits or telephone contact by a specialist nurse.

Drug dosing and regimens

For all the above reasons, therapy should generally be initiated with lower doses than in the young adult. Renal and hepatic function and plasma protein concentrations should be measured before therapy is started. Blood level measurements should be made at regular intervals, for relevant drugs, at least until stable regimens have been achieved. Drug combinations should be avoided where possible, and the advantages of monotherapy over polytherapy are greater in elderly people than in young adults.

Antiepileptic drugs in elderly people

Annoyingly, most drugs have not been subjected to rigorous trials in elderly people, and as a result data on the use of antiepileptic drugs in this group are generally sparse. This is an area where studies are needed.

Carbamazepine

Carbamazepine is the drug usually given initially in partial epilepsy. This preference is supported to a certain extent by evidence from a meta-analysis of individual data from 1265 elderly patients from 5 trials, in which carbamazepine showed a non-significant trend towards superior control of seizures when compared with valproate. There is little information about age-related changes in the pharmacokinetics of carbamazepine – surprisingly, in view of its widespread use. One study of a small number of patients showed a 40% reduction in clearance in elderly people, and a longer half-life, compared with young adults, whereas a study in normal volunteers showed no age-specific changes in the area under the concentration–time curve, in the elimination rate constants or in carbamazepine 10,11-epoxide concentrations. Side effects that are more common or more troublesome in elderly people include hyponatraemia and a small risk of drug-induced osteoporosis. Elderly patients are more vulnerable to antiepileptic drug-induced impairment of gait, as well as action and postural tremor, and possibly other subtle adverse neurological effects.

It is usual to initiate carbamazepine therapy slowly in individuals aged >65 years, and only cautiously to increment the dosage. The slow-release formulation should always be used, because this causes fewer side effects. A reasonable regimen would be to initiate therapy on 100 mg/ day, and to increase the dose by 100 mg increments every 2 weeks, to an initial maintenance dose of 400 mg/day. This can be then be increased as clinically indicated.

Gabapentin

Gabapentin is absorbed by a saturatable transport mechanism, and it is not known if this is affected by age. As it is not metabolized, and there is minimal protein binding, age-related changes in distribution or metabolism should not be expected. Age-related decreases in renal function significantly increase the renal clearance of gabapentin, so the dose should be reduced in elderly people if renal function is impaired (see p. 187, 189). For all these reasons, one would not expect age to modify gabapentin usage, provided that renal function is unimpaired, and it should be a particularly safe drug in elderly people. Its effectiveness has been demonstrated in one of the few randomized clinical trials designed for elderly people, and its generally mild action is well suited to the often mild epilepsy in this age group.

Lamotrigine

Lamotrigine has been studied relatively extensively in elderly people. A double-blind randomized monotherapy comparison in elderly patients with new-onset epilepsy found lower rates of drop-out due to adverse events on lamotrigine (18%) compared with carbamazepine (42%). No difference in efficacy was found. There are pharmacokinetic differences in the disposition of lamotrigine in elderly people. The plasma clearance of lamotrigine is reduced by about a third when compared with young adults. The drug is about 55% bound to plasma proteins and undergoes extensive hepatic metabolism, and also interacts with other antiepileptic drugs, all of which can result in age-related irregularities.

It is wise to initiate therapy at lower doses than in young adults. Recommended maintenance doses are 100 mg in monotherapy, 50–100 mg when co-medicated with valproate alone, or 200 mg in patients co-medicated with other enzyme-inducing antiepileptic drugs. Drug-level measurements should be made regularly until a stable regimen is established.

Levetiracetam

The lack of drug interactions, and the simple pharmacokinetics, of levetiracetam are advantages in elderly people, although detailed studies of its usefulness in this group have not been carried out. Anecdotal evidence suggests, however, that levetiracetam is useful and safe although surveillance is needed for behavioural side effects. Age-related changes in renal function can greatly affect the clearance of the drug, and doses should be reduced accordingly (see pp. 201–202). An initial dose of 125 mg is recommended, with incremental steps of 125–250 mg until an initial maintenance dosage of 750–1500 mg/day is reached.

Phenobarbital

Phenobarbital was once widely used in elderly people, but in recent years it has fallen from fashion, in recognition of the risk of adverse neurological and psychiatric effects. It is partly eliminated by the kidneys and, as renal excretion declines with age, one might expect concentrations of phenobarbital to be higher per milligram per kilogram dosage. There have been surprisingly few comprehensive studies of metabolism or of absorption, metabolic or elimination parameters, and no studies of interactions, in elderly individuals. This is a galling omission because phenobarbital has been widely used for many years, and there are intensive pharmacokinetic studies in other age groups. Anecdotal experience suggests that elderly people are more sensitive to the sedative side effects of phenobarbital, especially when co-medicated with benzodiazepine.

It would seem reasonable to use lower dosage than in young adults. The usual starting dose is 30–60 mg at night. Because older persons are more sensitive to the neurological side effects of phenobarbital, dosage increments should be cautious and carefully monitored.

Phenytoin

Phenytoin is commonly prescribed to elderly people, in spite of its complex pharmacokinetics; indeed it is probably the most prescribed antiepileptic drug in the USA despite the view of clinical authorities that it should be not be recommended as either a first-line or even a side-line medicine. As it is metabolized by saturatable processes, age-related declines in hepatic size and function could be expected to be of real significance. However, published studies are inadequate, and results have been conflicting. Early reports suggested that free phenytoin concentrations do indeed increase with age, although others showed increased clearance, partly attributable to the decreased albumin concentrations, and others showed no difference in the various elimination parameters between young and elderly people. The metabolism of phenytoin can be saturated at lower levels than in younger people. The picture is therefore rather confusing and advice is difficult to give. It would be wise to initiate therapy with phenytoin cautiously, at a relatively low dose (initial maintenance of 200 mg/day) followed by small dose increments (50 mg steps) as clinically indicated. Frequent measurements of phenytoin serum levels are essential. The measurement of free phenytoin concentrations is worthwhile in special circumstances (but not routinely), especially in ill or debilitated patients where serum albumin concentrations are low.

Topiramate

Studies of topiramate in elderly people are very limited, but it has good efficacy and can be safely used. Clearance is reduced in the presence of hepatic or renal impairment. The incidence of central nervous system side effects can be reduced with a slow-dose titration. For these reasons, dosage should be lower than in young adults. A recommended initial dose is 25 mg at night and dosage increments can be made in 25 mg steps to an initial maintenance dosage of between 50 and 100 mg/day in monotherapy.

Valproate

Valproate is widely used in elderly people, particularly to control generalized tonic–clonic seizures. It is as effective as carbamazepine in this indication. There are pharmacokinetic differences in elderly people compared with young adults. Free valproate concentrations are increased and in one study the percentage of unbound valproate was found to be 10.7% in elderly people compared with 6.4% in younger people. A 65% decrease in valproate clearance and a 67% increase in free valproate concentrations in old age were found in one study, and the half-life of valproate can be doubled in elderly people. Other studies have found lesser effects, and there is clear variability between patients. Valproate generally has few interactions at the hepatic level, and this is an advantage over other conventional antiepileptic drugs in older patients, who are often taking a cocktail of other drugs for various conditions. The drug should not be used if there is evidence of hepatic disease. There is an impression that encephalopathic side effects of valproate are more common in elderly people and these should be carefully monitored.

For all these reasons, valproate should be initiated in elderly people at lower doses than those used in younger adults. A recommended starting dosage is 200 mg/day, and this should be increased in 200 mg increments to an initial maintenance dose of 600 mg. Whether the slow-release ('chrono') formulation has any real advantage is unclear.

Treatment of epilepsy in women

There are aspects of therapy specific to women with epilepsy that are dealt with here.

Fertility and endocrine effects
Fertility
Fertility rates have been shown to be lower in women with treated epilepsy than in an age-matched control population. In one study of a general population of 2052922 people in England and Wales, the overall fertility rate was 47.1 (95% CI 42.3–52.2) live births per 1000 women with epilepsy per year compared with a national rate of 62.6. The difference in rates was found in all age ranges between 20 and 39 years (Figure 6.1). The reasons for these lower rates are probably complex. There are undoubtedly social effects: women with epilepsy have low rates of marriage, marry later, and suffer social isolation and stigmatization. Some avoid having children because of the risk of epilepsy in the offspring, and some because of the teratogenic potential of antiepileptic drugs. Other patients have impaired personality or cognitive development. However,

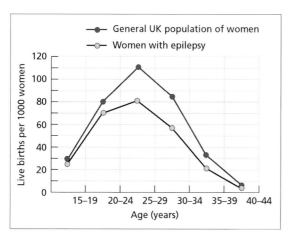

Figure 6.1 Live birth rates in mothers with epilepsy on treatment compared with general population (study of a UK population of over 2 million persons).

there are other biological factors that could lead to reduced fecundity, and smaller studies have shown that, when women with such severe co-morbidities were excluded, fertility rates approach those of the general population.

Endocrine dysfunction and also antiepileptic drugs can affect fertility and this is discussed below. The lowering of fertility is a worrying finding which is another important source of disadvantage for women with epilepsy. If there are potentially preventable causes, these should be sought.

Fertility in men due to epilepsy or drug therapy is a poorly studied area. It has been suggested that there is reduced sperm motility or morphology in patients with epilepsy on long-term antiepileptic drug treatment and that this may be due to a direct effect of phenytoin, carbamazepine and valproic acid on sperm membrane function.

Polycystic ovarian syndrome and endocrine function

Among the known endocrine problems in epilepsy are anovulatory cycles, hypothalamic amenorrhoea, polycystic ovary syndrome (PCOS), hyperprolactinaemia, premature menopause, and changes in androgen and other sex hormones.

It has been estimated, in different studies, that between a third and two-thirds of menstrual cycles in women with epilepsy are anovulatory, compared with 8–14% in controls. The causes are complex, and having seizures may

in itself influence fertility and ovulation, presumably mediated via hypothalamic mechanisms. It is known in animal experimentation, for example, that limbic (and particularly amygdaloid) seizures can cause anovulation, elevated serum testosterone levels and the accumulation of follicular cysts in the ovaries. Similarly, a recent study of 50 women with temporolimbic epilepsy found that 28 patients had menstrual irregularities; 10 with PCOS and amenorrhoea, oligoamenorrhoea, or abnormally long or short menstrual cycle intervals; 19 of the 28 women with epilepsy and menstrual disorders had readily identifiable reproductive endocrine disorders including PCOS, hypothalamic amenorrhoea and hyperprolactinaemia. There was no relationship with antiepileptic drug usage and the authors concluded that the endocrine problems were related to the epilepsy itself.

Limbic seizures have also been associated with lack of libido, anorgasmia, dyspareunia, vaginismus, or insufficient vaginal lubrication and reduced genital blood flow during erotic stimulation. Similarly, sexual interest and activity can change after epilepsy surgery.

The effects of antiepileptic drugs on sex hormone levels has been the subject of study. There is no doubt that the hepatic enzyme-inducing antiepileptics (e.g. phenytoin, carbamazepine, phenobarbital, lamotrigine) can influence hormone levels, possibly particularly by action on the cytochrome P450 enzymes CYP19. Changes include elevated levels of sex hormone-binding globulin concentrations, lowered androgen, changes in testosterone and oestrogen levels, increased cortisol and prolactin levels, and an exaggerated luteinizing hormone (LH) response to the gonadotrophin and thyrotrophin-releasing hormone (TRH) stimulation. The causes may, however, be complex and the clinical relevance is not clear.

The main focus on the reproductive effects of antiepileptic drugs has been on the possibility that antiepileptic drugs can induce PCOS. PCOS is defined as ovulatory dysfunction with clinical evidence of hyperandrogenism and/or hyperandrogenaemia in the absence of identifiable adrenal or pituitary pathology. This should be differentiated from the simple finding of polycystic ovaries which occur in up to 80% of some female populations (depending on age and other factors), and which do not have any significant pathological significance. PCOS has both genetic and environmental causes and has a prevalence ranging from about 4% up to 18% in the general female population, and from 10% to 20% in populations of women with epilepsy. The question of antiepileptic drug-induced PCOS has been the topic of considerable controversy. Initial studies from Finland suggested that valproate therapy in particular induces PCOS. In one study, 30–40% of patients taking valproate therapy had polycystic ovaries and hyperandrogenism, compared with 5–15% of those taking carbamazepine or lamotrigine. However, no difference between valproate- and carbamazepine-treated patients was found in other studies. In one randomized open-label study, hyperandrogenism and ovulatory dysfunction developed in 44% of those randomized to valproic acid compared with 23% of those on lamotrigine if treatment was initiated before age 26 years, whereas the rates were similar (24% vs 22%) if treatment was started after age 26 years. Furthermore, studies have shown the reversal of the syndrome on switching from valproate to lamotrigine therapy or withdrawal of valproate therapy. Valproate can induce obesity and this, in turn, can lead to peripheral insulin resistance, hyperandrogenism and hyperinsulinaemia, and on theoretical grounds these could contribute to the induction of polycystic ovaries. How valproate does induce obesity is also unclear, but this may be due to increased leptin levels.

Endocrine function in general has been poorly studied. In young female patients one small cross-sectional investigation failed to find any differences in those treated with valproate or carbamazepine when compared with healthy controls in terms of linear growth, polycystic ovaries and sexual maturation. However, long-term follow-up showed normal endocrine function in those who had come off medication but an increased prevalence of endocrine disorders including PCOS among those remaining on antiepileptic therapy. Withdrawal of carbamazepine in seizure-free male and female patients has also been shown to result in an increase in serum testosterone and free androgen index.

Contraception
The combined oral contraceptive

There is no reason why women with epilepsy should not take the combined oral contraceptive. However, drugs that induce hepatic enzyme activity (particularly the CYP3A family enzymes – barbiturates, phenytoin, primidone, oxcarbazepine and carbamazepine) increase the metabolism of the oestrogen and progesterone components of the pill (sometimes by 50%), thereby reducing its efficacy. Topiramate lowers the level of oestrogen by 30% by a different mechanism. Patients co-medicated with these drugs therefore need higher doses of the pill to achieve contraceptive effect, and a preparation with at least 50 μg estradiol should be safe in most women, but not all. Breakthrough bleeding (midcycle bleeding) is a useful sign of inadequate oestrogenic effect, but it is not infallible, and contraceptive failure can occur without midcycle bleeding. Occasionally, 80 or even 100 μg estradiol is needed for contraceptive effect. In addition, 'tricycling' a 50 μg oestrogen preparation can be employed, which entails taking 3-monthly packets of the contraceptive without a break, followed by an interval of 4 days rather than the usual 7. Women should be advised that, even using higher-dose preparations, there is a higher risk of contraceptive failure, and figures of 3 failures per 1000 women-years are quoted compared with the 0.3/1000 rate in the general population, although the rates are probably lower with tricycling. It is also worth pointing out that the higher-dose contraceptives that are prescribed undergo rapid metabolism, and the oestrogen levels attained are equivalent to those provided by lower-dose contraceptives in non-epileptic women, and so there is no excess risk of oestrogen-induced complications such as thrombosis.

There is no risk of such interactions with non-CYP3A enzyme-inducing drugs (e.g. vigabatrin, valproate, clobazam, gabapentin, lamotrigine, levetiracetam, pregabalin, valproate or vigabatrin). These drugs do not affect the metabolism of the combined pill and so a 30 μg estradiol compound can be safely taken. However, the combined contraceptive pill tends to lower lamotrigine levels by 40–60%, so starting the pill in patients co-medicated with lamotrigine can result in poorer control, and higher lamotrigine dosage may be required. Furthermore, lamotrigine levels can rise quickly in the pill-free week and result in side effects and, for these reasons, lamotrigine is not a good choice in patients on the contraceptive pill.

In spite of the well-known risks of drug interaction, the inappropriate prescribing of low-dose contraceptives with enzyme-inducing drugs is widespread. In a large UK general practice survey, 17% (390/2341) of all women with epilepsy were on an oral contraceptive. Of these, 200 were co-medicated with an enzyme-inducing antiepileptic drug, and 44% (87 of the 200) were taking a contraceptive pill with less than 50 μg estradiol. That this is a real problem is shown in one study that reported that 8.5% of pregnant women with epilepsy reported oral contraceptive failure.

Progesterone-only preparation

The progesterone-only pill (the 'mini-pill') is affected in a similar manner, and patients should take at least double the usual dose or use alternative forms of contraception.

Injectable contraceptives

Medroxyprogesterone acetate (Depo-Provera®) has no interactions with antiepileptics, because there is virtual 100% clearance on first pass through the liver, and enzyme induction should have no effect. The progestogen implant Implanon® is affected by enzyme-inducing drugs, and so should not be used in women with epilepsy.

Postcoital contraception (the morning-after pill)

The efficacy of this contraceptive is also affected by enzyme-inducing antiepileptic drugs, and so the first dose should be doubled and a second single dose given 12 h later.

Intrauterine contraception (coils)

Coils are not affected by enzyme-inducing drugs.

Menstruation and catamenial epilepsy

There is no doubt that, in a sizeable proportion of women with active epilepsy, the pattern of seizures is related to the menstrual cycle. Oestrogen is mildly epileptogenic, and the high oestrogen concentration in the follicular phase of the menstrual cycle is a possible underlying cause for the greater propensity to seizures at this time. Premenstrual tension and water retention are other possible contributory factors.

Epilepsy in which the seizure pattern has a strong relationship to the menstrual cycle is referred to as catamenial epilepsy. There have been attempts to devise special treatment approaches to patients with catamenial seizures. Hormonal manipulation has been attempted with oral progesterone or norethisterone, with only marginal benefit. Attempts to abolish the menstrual cycle by hormonal means or even oophorectomy have had surprisingly disappointing results. In most patients seizures tend to continue at much the same frequency, albeit with some loss of pattern regularity. Intermittent antiepileptic therapy, taken around the risk period each month, has also been widely tried. Therapy with diuretics or acetazolamide for 5–7 days has not proved generally successful. Clobazam, taken in the same manner, has shown more promise, with improvement noted in one study in 78% of women. This approach in routine clinical practice, however, produces a worthwhile effect in only a small number of women. Reasons for these disappointing results include irregularities of the cycle, the fact that the catamenial exacerbation is seldom reliably linked to any particular day of the cycle and tolerance to the effects of clobazam.

Teratogenicity of antiepileptic drugs

In clinical practice, it is this topic that raises the greatest concern among women with epilepsy, and the issues must be fully discussed.

The first report of an antiepileptic drug-induced malformation was in 1963 (due to methphenytoin). In 1968, Meadows conducted a pioneering enquiry and concluded that congenital malformations were twice as common in children exposed *in utero* to antiepileptic drugs as would be expected in unexposed populations, and this has set the scene for numerous subsequent investigations, which have demonstrated conclusively that antiepileptics do increase the rate of malformations. Evidence includes: animal testing showing patterns of malformation similar to those seen clinically; drug-specific effects; malformation rates in the offspring of mothers with epilepsy on treatment higher than those off treatment; mean antiepileptic drug levels higher in the mothers of infants with malformations than in those without; and infants of mothers on polytherapy with higher malformation rates than those exposed to single-drug treatment. Factors complicating studies in this area are, however, the potential for seizures themselves to cause malformations, although this effect is probably small, social, dietary and socioeconomic factors, resulting in greater maternal ill-health, and maternal genetic factors that increase the risk of both epilepsy and malformations (particularly in idiopathic or cryptogenic epilepsy). Much of the evidence is highly contradictory, and this area is a minefield in which accurate clinical advice is difficult to give. However, carbamazepine and lamotrigine are considered by many to be the least teratogenic of the commonly used antiepileptic drugs.

It is worth remembering too that when advising on this matter in relation to newer antiepileptic drugs: first, even today, the full range of the teratogenicity has not been not established, as the number of pregnancies studied is small; second, the risk of even major malformations was not noticed until the traditional drugs had been in extensive use for decades; and third, negative animal results are not a reliable indicator of safety. Any claims for safety for newer drugs should be taken in this context. Currently the advice from the package inserts is to avoid the use of any of these drugs in pregnancy until more definitive advice can be given.

Major malformations associated with antiepileptic drugs

The most common major malformations associated with traditional antiepileptic drug therapy (phenytoin, phenobarbital, primidone, benzodiazepine, valproate, carbamazepine) are cleft palate and cleft lip, cardiac malformations, midline defects, neural tube defects, hypospadias and skeletal abnormalities. Unfortunately, because most studies have been of women on multiple drug therapy, the risks of individual drugs are not fully established.

The risk of spina bifida has been particularly well studied. The background population risk of spina bifida is approximately 0.2–0.5% with geographical variation. Valproate is associated with a 1–2% risk of spina bifida aperta, a risk that is dose related. Carbamazepine carries a risk of spina bifida aperta of about 0.5–1%. It is instructive to note that the induction of neural tube defects by valproate (and to a lesser extent carbamazepine) was not noticed in animal toxicology. The mechanism of production of drug-induced spina bifida may be different from that in unexposed populations, which could reduce the protective action of folate.

The overall risk of malformations due to exposure to phenytoin was thought at one time to be particularly high, but recent studies of phenytoin monotherapy have shown a very low incidence of major defects. It may be that the previously high rates were attributable to polytherapy and exposure to high levels of phenytoin at a time when blood level control was not possible.

One study purported to demonstrate smaller head circumference in babies of mothers on carbamazepine, but the statistical basis of this observation was not well founded. Small increases in rates of pre- and postnatal growth retardation have been found in controlled studies of mothers taking antiepileptics, but the growth differences had disappeared by the time the offspring were 5 years old.

It is not clear whether or not the benzodiazepines have any teratogenic potential, although there are case reports of facial clefts, and cardiac and skeletal abnormalities.

Although the patterns of malformations associated with all epilepsy drugs seem to overlap, there are some specific features. In addition to the malformations mentioned above, valproate is also particularly associated with skeletal and midline abnormalities, lamotrigine and phenytoin with oral clefts, and carbamazepine with congenital heart defects. Both carbamazepine and valproate have been associated also with hypospadias. Infants, born to mothers taking vigabatrin, with spina bifida, cleft palate, absent diaphragm and conjoined twins have been reported. Topiramate, in animal models, causes right-sided ectrodactyly and rib and vertebral abnormalities, a pattern similar to that observed with acetazolamide, also a carbonic anhydrase inhibitor. No similar abnormalities

have been reported in humans on carbonic anhydrase inhibitors, but there have now been reported a number of malformations associated with topiramate usage, in a relatively small denominator, and this drug should be avoided in pregnancy. Gabapentin causes hydroureter and hydronephrosis in rabbits, but there have been no reported human pregnancy abnormalities. Uniquely, phenytoin therapy has been clearly associated with an increased risk of neuroblastoma, although the absolute risk is very small. Various recent data has been presented giving a malformation rate for first trimester exposure to levetiracetam of between 0–3.1%.

Drug dosage has also been shown to be relevant in the case of valproate – with higher rates of malformations linked to dosages >1000 mg/day, and also lamotrigine with dosages >200 mg/day. In fact, in one study, the rate of malformations associated with valproate at doses <1000 mg/day were less than the rate associated with lamotrigine at doses >200 mg/day.

More minor developmental abnormalities

In addition to the major malformations, less severe dysmorphic changes ('fetal syndromes') have been postulated, although there is little agreement about their frequency or indeed in some instances even their existence. The problem is further complicated by the confounding influences of socioeconomic and genetic factors. The fetal phenytoin syndrome was the first to be described, and is said to comprise a characteristic pattern of facial and limb disturbances (Table 6.6). Most of these features are, however, minor and overlap with the normal variation seen in children born to healthy mothers. Recent prospective and blinded studies have shown that only hypertelorism and distal digital hypoplasia occurred with any greater frequency, and even these associations are weak. Furthermore, the nail hypoplasia tends to disappear during childhood. Cases of a 'carbamazepine syndrome' are reported with craniofacial abnormalities, growth retardation, neural tube defects and fingernail hypoplasia. Reports of barbiturate 'syndromes' have been published, comprising facial changes and developmental delay. The complexity of the subject is shown by one report of four siblings with the classic 'hydantoin syndrome' born to a mother taking phenytoin and primidone for the first three pregnancies but only primidone during the fourth. A 'carbamazepine syndrome' has been claimed on the basis of a few case reports that are unconvincing. Finally, recent interest has focused on a 'valproate syndrome' said to occur in up to 50% of infants born to mothers on valproate; again no blinded studies have been carried out and the true status of this syndrome is

Table 6.6 Some features reported to occur in fetal anticonvulsant syndromes.

Growth
- Pre- and postnatal growth deficiencies
- Microcephaly

Craniofacial
- Short nose, low cranial bridge
- Hypertelorism
- Epicanthic fold
- Strabismus and other ocular abnormalities
- Low-set ears and other aural abnormalities
- Wide mouth, and prominent lips
- Wide fontanelles
- Cleft palate and cleft lip

Limbs
- Hypoplasia of nails
- Transverse planar crease
- Short fingers
- Extra digits

Cerebral
- Learning disability
- Developmental delay

General
- Short neck, low hairline
- Rib, sternal and spinal anomalies
- Widely spaced hypoplastic nipples
- Hernias
- Undescended testicles
- Neuroblastoma and neural ridge tumours
- Cardiac and renal abnormalities
- Hypospadias
- Neural tube defects

This is a list of reported abnormalities, although many are uncontrolled observations and the frequency of the anomalies is unclear. The contribution of antiepileptic drugs is unclear, and genetic, environmental and socioeconomic factors may also have a role in their development.

quite unclear. There are also reports of alcohol and benzodiazepine 'syndromes'.

Cognitive disability as a teratogenic risk

Even greater controversy exists in relation to the question of whether maternal drug usage results in developmental delay, and cognitive and learning disability. Although there is no doubt that these occur at a higher frequency among infants born to women with epilepsy (between a two- and sevenfold increase), the association could be attributed at least in part to genetic, environmental or socioeconomic factors. A recent study showed that 41 children exposed to valproate monotherapy had, when measured at school age, significantly lower verbal IQ (VIQ) scores when compared with 52 children exposed to carbamazepine and 21 to phenytoin monotherapy, and the rates were highest after fetal exposure to valproate doses >800 mg/day. Low VIQ was also associated with the occurrence of five or more tonic–clonic seizures during pregnancy in a regression analysis.

There were higher rates of dysmorphic features in the children exposed to valproate, and these were most common in those with low VIQ scores. Some caution needs to be exercised in interpreting these results. The study was a retrospective survey, the mothers were not randomized to different monotherapies, there was only a 40% response rate, and there are some inconsistencies, e.g. the fact that significant differences in VIQ rates were not found in fetuses exposed to valproate polytherapy, nor was there a significant dose response. Other smaller studies have not consistently confirmed these results. This is of course an extremely important issue, but one where the quality of evidence is not strong and further study is needed, although really no major randomized prospective study is now either feasible or ethically justified given these potential purported risks.

Pregnancy

There are a number of other issues, in addition to teratogenesis, that need to be considered when considering the issues of epilepsy and pregnancy.

Effects of epilepsy on pregnancy and delivery

About 3–4 live births per 1000 women of child-bearing age with epilepsy occur each year. Epilepsy has been reported in retrospective (and therefore selected) series to increase by up to threefold the risks of various common complications (Table 6.7). The perinatal mortality rate has been found to be twice that of the general population. No large-scale prospective investigation has been carried out, but there seems little doubt that these pregnancies require special consideration. The obstetrician may be more likely to recommend intervention and to manage the case in a distinctive manner. About 1–2% of all women with epilepsy will have tonic–clonic seizures during delivery and this can clearly complicate labour, and occasional maternal and fetal fatalities have been reported. The fetal heart rate can be dramatically slowed

Table 6.7 Complications of pregnancy that occur with increased frequency in women with epilepsy.

- Bleeding *in utero*
- Premature separation of the placenta
- Toxaemia of pregnancy and pre-eclampsia
- Miscarriage and stillbirth
- Intrauterine growth retardation, low birthweight
- Perinatal mortality
- Premature labour
- Breech and other abnormal presentations
- Forceps delivery, induced labour, caesarean section
- Precipitant labour
- Psychiatric disorders
- Seizures and status epilepticus

by a seizure, and fetal monitoring is recommended during vaginal delivery. Home birth should not generally be contemplated.

Effect of pregnancy on the rate of seizures

Pregnancy has an unpredictable effect on the frequency of seizures. In a recent large study, 59% of seizure-free patients remained seizure free during pregnancy. Traditionally it has been said that seizure control improves in a third of patients during pregnancy and worsens in a third. Recent evidence suggests, however, that seizure control deteriorates only in a relatively small proportion of patients on modern therapy, although one consistent observation is that the more severe the pre-pregnancy epilepsy, the more likely are seizure exacerbations. There are a number of potential causes for increased seizures including hormonal effects, non-compliance with medication, inappropriate dose reductions, changing drug disposition and serum levels, fluid retention, vomiting, stress, anxiety and sleep deprivation. Seizures are particularly likely around the time of labour and delivery – about 1–2% of all susceptible. 3 patients will have a tonic–clonic seizure at this time, and for this reason the author's practice is to recommend clobazam 10 mg to be taken at the onset of the second stage of labour.

The effect of seizures on the fetus

This is a controversial area. Clearly, in the later stages of pregnancy, a convulsion carries the risk of trauma to the placenta or fetus, especially if the woman falls, and convulsive seizures can also precipitate premature labour.

However, most debate has revolved around the postulation that tonic–clonic seizures damage the fetus through lactic acidosis or hypoxia. The hypoxia is usually very short-lived and the placenta is a well-buffered system, and these risks seem intuitively likely to be small. Fetal asphyxia manifested by prolonged bradycardia has been recorded after a maternal seizure, and one case of postictal fetal intracranial haemorrhage has been recorded. However, these are probably exceptional, and in most situations isolated seizures are harmless. One study suggested that first-trimester seizures are accompanied by a higher risk of fetal malformation than seizures at other times, although methodological issues cloud the reliability of the conclusions. Stillbirth has been recorded after a single seizure or series of seizures, but this must be very rare.

Partial absence or myoclonic seizures have no known effects upon a fetus.

Status epilepticus during pregnancy results in greater risks, both of fetal morbidity and mortality and of maternal mortality. A 50% infant mortality rate and 30% maternal mortality rate were reported in one early study, although more recently there was only 1 case of status-induced fetal death in 36 episodes and no maternal deaths.

Pharmacokinetics of antiepileptic drugs during pregnancy

Pregnancy, particularly in the last trimester, can exert marked effects on the pharmacokinetics of antiepileptic drugs. Serum levels of phenobarbital and phenytoin can fall by up to 40% during pregnancy, and rise to pre-pregnancy levels in the first month after delivery. Similar falls in the active metabolites of oxcarbazepine and levetiracetam are reported. Carbamazepine levels decline less in general and this is another reason for choosing this drug in pregnancy. The greatest problems seem to arise with lamotrigine, with levels falling in some patients by 60% and, if there is a fall, this is reversed in the few days postpartum.

Drug dosage may need modification. In all patients, it is good practice to measure baseline levels and then to check levels with at least one measurement made in the first and second trimesters and more frequently in the third trimester. Weekly levels are required in some patients on lamotrigine in whom seizure control is critically linked to serum level.

Screening for fetal malformations

Some malformations can be detected in the prenatal phase. If therapeutic termination of pregnancy is acceptable, screening procedures should include, where appropriate, a high-quality ultrasound scan at 10, 18 and 24 weeks, measurement of α-fetoprotein levels and amniocentesis. About 95% of significant neural tube defects can be detected prenatally in this manner, as well as cleft palate, major cardiac kidney and midline defects, and thus ultrasound protocols such as these can almost (but not completely) eliminate the risk of a live birth with these malformations.

Folic acid supplementation

The fetus of a woman with epilepsy is at a greater than expected risk of a neural tube defect, particularly if the mother is taking valproate, but an association is also noted with exposure during pregnancy to other antiepileptics. It has been said that the pathological mechanism of antiepileptic drug-induced neural tube defects differs from the naturally occurring form. A recent Medical Research Council (MRC) trial of folic acid supplementation during pregnancy showed a 72% protective effect against neural tube defects in women who had conceived a fetus previously with neural tube defects, and a positive primary preventive action has also been demonstrated. Although there has been no specific study in epilepsy, and despite the fact that the pathophysiology may differ, it would seem reasonable for all women with epilepsy to be given folic acid supplementation during pregnancy, especially as many patients with epilepsy have low serum and tissue folate levels owing to enhanced drug-induced hepatic metabolism. This advice is given notwithstanding the weak evidence that folic acid may predispose to increased seizures (an effect not seen in clinical practice). A dosage of at least 4 mg/day is recommended on an empirical basis, because lower dosage may not fully restore folate levels.

Vitamin K

When the mother is taking enzyme-inducing antiepileptic drugs, the infant may be born with a relative deficiency of vitamin K-dependent clotting factors (factors II, VII, IX and X) and proteins C and S. This predisposes to infantile haemorrhage, including cerebral haemorrhage. The neonate should therefore receive 1 mg vitamin K i.m. at birth and at 28 days of life. Previous concern that intramuscular vitamin K increased the risk of neuroblastoma has been dismissed, but there is possibly a slight increase in the rate of later acute lymphoblastic leukaemia. If any two of the clotting factors fall below 50% of their normal values, intramuscular vitamin K will be insufficient to protect against haemorrhage and fresh frozen plasma should be given intravenously. Similarly, if there is evidence of neonatal bleeding, or if concentrations of factors II, VII, IX or X fall below 25% of normal, an emergency infusion of fresh frozen plasma is required. It was also previously recommended that the mother take oral vitamin K (20 mg/day) in the last trimester, although the evidence that this improves neonatal clotting is rather contradictory and this practice has been largely abandoned.

New-onset epilepsy during pregnancy

The incidence of new-onset epilepsy in women at child-bearing age is about 20–30 cases per 100 000 women, and so epilepsy occurring by chance during pregnancy is not uncommon. Occasionally, epileptic seizures occur only during pregnancy (gestational epilepsy) but this is a rare pattern. Certain underlying conditions have a propensity to present during pregnancy. Some meningiomas grow in size faster during pregnancy as a result of oestrogenic stimulation. Arteriovenous malformations are also said to present more commonly in pregnancy although evidence for this is weak. The risk of ischaemic stroke increases 10-fold in pregnancy, underlying causes including arteriosclerosis, cerebral angiitis, moya-moya disease, Takayasu arteritis, embolic disease from a cardiac or infective source, and primary cardiac disease. Haematological diseases can also present as stroke, including sickle cell disease, antiphospholipid antibody syndrome, thrombotic throbocytopenic purpura, and deficiencies in antithrombin, proteins C and S, and factor V Leiden. There is also a higher incidence of subarachnoid haemorrhage and cerebral venous thrombosis. Pregnancy can predispose to cerebral infections due to bacteria (including *Listeria* spp.), fungi (*Coccidioides* spp.), protozoa (*Toxoplasma* spp.), viruses and HIV infection, which can compromise fetal development. Epilepsy can be the presenting symptom, or occur, in all these conditions.

The extent of the investigation will depend on the clinical setting. Radiation with X-rays (including computed tomography) should be avoided wherever possible. The risks of magnetic resonance imaging (MRI) to the developing fetus are unknown; nevertheless, MRI is the imaging modality of choice if urgent imaging is required. In the non-urgent situation, investigation should be deferred until the pregnancy is completed.

The treatment of new-onset epilepsy follows the same principles in the pregnant as in the non-pregnant woman. The underlying cause may also need specific therapy.

Eclampsia and pre-eclampsia

Most new-onset seizures in the late stages of pregnancy (after 20 weeks) are caused by eclampsia. Pre-eclampsia is characterized by hypertension, proteinuria, oedema, and abnormalities of hepatic function, platelets and clotting parameters. About 1–4% of cases progress to eclampsia. The eclamptic encephalopathy results in confusion, stupor, focal neurological signs and cerebral haemorrhage as well as seizures. The epilepsy can be severe and progress rapidly to status. The incidence of eclampsia in western Europe is about 1 in 2000 pregnancies, but it is more common in some developing countries with rates as high as 1 in 100. It carries a maternal mortality rate of between 2 and 5% and significant infantile morbidity and mortality.

Traditionally, obstetricians have used magnesium sulphate for the treatment of seizures in eclampsia, and the superiority of magnesium over phenytoin and/or diazepam has been clearly demonstrated in recent randomized controlled studies. Not only does magnesium confer better control of seizures, but there are also fewer complications of pregnancy, and infant survival is better. Magnesium also seems to lessen the chance of cerebral palsy in low birth weight babies and has been shown to decrease secondary neuronal damage after experimental traumatic brain injury. The mechanism by which magnesium sulphate acts in eclampsia is unclear; it may do so via its influence on N-methyl-D-aspartate (NMDA) receptors or on free radicals, prostacyclin, other neurochemical pathways or, more likely, by reversing the intense eclamptic cerebral vasospasm. It is possible that patients would benefit from magnesium and a conventional antiepileptic, but this has not been investigated. Magnesium sulphate is given intravenously as a loading dose of 4.6 g over 20 min followed by a maintenance dose of 1–2 g/h as a continuous intravenous infusion. In about 10% of cases, seizures will recur, and in this situation a further 2 g bolus of magnesium is given.

Labour and the puerperium
Management of labour

Regular antiepileptic drugs should be continued during labour. If oral feeding is not possible, intravenous replacement therapy can be given for at least some drugs. Tonic–clonic seizures occur in about 1–2% of susceptible mothers, and in patients at risk oral clobazam (10–20 mg) is useful when given at the onset of labour as additional seizure prophylaxis. Fetal monitoring is advisable. Most women have a normal vaginal delivery, but sleep deprivation, overbreathing, pain and emotional stress can greatly increase the risk of seizures. Elective caesarean section should be considered in patients at particular risk. A history of status or life-threatening tonic–clonic seizures is an indication for a caesarean section and, if convulsive seizures or status occur during delivery, an emergency caesarean section should be performed. Intravenous lorazepam or phenytoin should be given during labour if severe seizures occur and the patient should be prepared for a caesarean section.

There is a maternal as well as an infant mortality associated with severe seizures during delivery. The hypoxia consequent on a seizure may be more profound in gravid women. Resuscitation facilities should be immediately at hand in the delivery suite.

Puerperium

There is still an increased risk of seizures in the puerperium, and precautions may be necessary. It is sometimes helpful to continue clobazam for a few days after delivery to cover this period. If antiepileptic drug dosage had been increased due to the fall of levels during pregnancy, the dosage should be returned during the first week to its previous level; this is necessary because the pharmacokinetic changes of pregnancy are rapidly reversed in the puerperium and if dosages are not lowered acute antiepileptic drug toxicity will result. Drugs circulating in the mother's serum cross the placenta. If maternal antiepileptic drug levels were high, the infant may experience withdrawal symptoms (tremor, irritability, agitation and even seizures) and neonatal serum levels should be measured in cases at risk.

Breast-feeding

The concentration of most antiepileptic drugs in breast milk is less than 30% that of plasma; exceptions are concentrations of ethosuximide, gabapentin, lamotrigine, levetiracetam, phenobarbital and topiramate. Furthermore, even if a drug is present in significant concentrations in breast milk, the amount ingested by the infant is usually much less than would normally be considered necessary for clinical effects. Only in the case of ethosuximide, lamotrigine and phenobarbital (including from primidone) are significant doses absorbed. Thus, only with these drugs – and possibly levetiracetam, although data are sparse – are precautions necessary at least at normal doses. The problem of lamotrigine is compounded if co-medication with valproate, which prolongs the half-life of the drug, is given. Particular

Table 6.8 Pharmacokinetic parameters of antiepileptic drugs transmitted to the fetus in breast milk.

	Dose of antiepileptic drug acquired from breast milk (%)[a]	Breast milk:plasma concentration ratio	Elimination half-life (h)	
			Adult	Neonate
Carbamazepine	<5	0.3–0.4	5–26	8–28
Ethosuximide	>50	0.9	30–60	40
Lamotrigine	>50	0.6	12–60	n/k
Phenobarbital	>50	0.4–0.6	75–120	45–300
Phenytoin	<5	0.2–0.4	7–42	15–100
Valproate	<5	0.01	12–17	30–60

[a]Amount of drug received in a fully breast-fed infant, expressed as a percentage of the lowest recommended daily therapeutic dose for an infant (Dr M O'Brien, personal communication).
n/k, not known.

caution is advised in the case of maternal phenobarbital ingestion, as in neonates the half-life of phenobarbital is long (up to 300 h) and the free fraction is higher than in adults; neonatal levels can therefore sometimes exceed maternal levels. The neonatal half-lives of phenytoin and valproate are also increased (Table 6.8). The long-half life of *N*-desmethylclobazam also means that caution should be observed in relation to this drug, although adequate data are not available. It seems sensible to watch for neonatal lethargy, irritability and feeding difficulties as signs that the infant is affected by maternal antiepileptic drug intake. Serum levels of the antiepileptics can also be measured in the infant, and indeed perhaps should always be measured.

Maternal epilepsy

Maternal epilepsy carries other risks for the infant. There is a danger of dropping the child or leaving the child unattended during a seizure and sensible precautions should be taken, such as avoiding carrying the child unaccompanied, changing and feeding the infant at floor level, and bathing the infant only when someone else is present.

Preconception counselling and therapy review
Counselling

The mother's antiepileptic drug regimen should be reviewed before conception; the counselling should include the following:

• Genetic counselling in relation to both the risks of epilepsy and any underlying cause
• Risks of teratogenicity due to drugs
• Risks of seizures in pregnancy
• Prenatal diagnosis and, where appropriate, therapeutic termination
• Folate and vitamin K
• Lifestyle issues
• The principles of antiepileptic drug therapy and the optimization of therapy, and compliance
• Issues in relation to delivery, labour and obstetric issues
• The chances of changes in seizure frequency
• Measuring blood levels
• Breast-feeding.

Therapy review

As most of the major malformations are established within the first trimester, many within the first 8 weeks, optimization of therapy should be carried out before conception. This is a counsel of perfection often not realized, yet it is of great importance. Referral of a woman for a review of drug therapy when she is 10 weeks' pregnant is too late to make changes that will minimize the teratogenic risks.

It is important to establish whether antiepileptic therapy is needed at all. This will be an individual decision, based on the estimated risk of exacerbation of seizures and their danger (remembering that tonic–clonic seizures can result in injury and occasionally death to both mother and fetus). The decision will balance the risks of teratogenicity against the risks of worsening epilepsy. Some women with partial or non-convulsive seizures will elect to withdraw therapy even if seizures are active or likely to become more frequent. Conversely, some women who are free of seizures will wish to continue therapy because of the social and physical risks of a recurrence of seizures.

In many patients it is reasonable to withdraw therapy for the first half of pregnancy and then to reinstate the drugs; this approach is based on the fact that the teratogenic risk is greatest in the first trimester and the physical risk of seizures greatest in the later stages of pregnancy. The relative risks need to carefully assessed, however, and a specialist review is needed before embarking on this course.

If the woman elects to continue therapy, the appropriate regimen in most cases is the minimally effective dose of the single antiepileptic that best controls the epilepsy. A few women with severe epilepsy will need combination therapy, but this should be avoided wherever possible. It is useful to measure the serum drug concentrations that give optimal control of the epilepsy before contraception. These values form a starting point on which to base subsequent drug dosage adjustments.

The use of valproate and prescribing in idiopathic generalized epilepsy

A particular issue relates to the use of valproate which now, particularly because of the teratogenic risks and the possibility of a risk of later cognitive impairment in the offspring, should be avoided wherever possible, if other equally effective treatment options are available. The main problems arise in patients with idiopathic generalized epilepsy (IGE; including juvenile myoclonic epilepsy) in which valproate is undoubtedly the most effective therapy. There are no universally applicable guidelines and decisions about therapy need to be individually decided and will depend on such factors as seizure frequency, prior experience with other drugs, outcome of previous pregnancy, maternal preferences and the clinical and social context. Lamotrigine is an alternative but often less effective and its prescription in pregnancy is associated with pharmacokinetic and other problems. The handling of levetiracetam may be less problematic in pregnancy but data on pregnancy outcomes are insufficient at present to guarantee safety and lack of teratogenicity. In the author's own practice, carbamazepine is often recommended which controls tonic–clonic seizures to the same extent as valproate in cases of IGE but can aggravate myoclonic seizures.

7

Pharmacokinetic Principles of Antiepileptic Drug Treatment

To use drugs effectively, the reader should be aware of certain pharmacokinetic principles, some of which are enumerated here (see also pharmacopoeia, pp. 365–377); ignorance of these aspects of simple pharmacology will expose a patient to risks and inefficiencies.

Drug absorption

Oral absorption

This process depends on both the physical and the pharmacological properties of the drug and the biological properties of the person ingesting it. Physical properties include the formulation of the tablets, the lipid solubility, the binding and the degree of ionization at the pH levels in the gastrointestinal (GI) tract. Solutions are usually rather more quickly absorbed than tablets or capsules.

The movement from the GI tract to plasma for most drugs is a passive process which depends on factors including the following:
- The concentration gradient across the gut membrane
- The lipid solubility of the drug: as the non-ionized form of the drug is generally the most lipid soluble, absorption is quickest of drugs that are not ionized at physiological pH level
- The absorption area and time in contact with the absorption surface: although acidic drugs are less ionized in the stomach than the small intestine, most orally administered drugs, whether acidic or basic, depend largely on the small intestine for absorption because of its large absorptive area.

Several antiepileptics are absorbed by an active transport system (e.g. gabapentin, pregabalin and possibly phenytoin). The gabapentin absorption mechanism has a limited capacity, and higher doses may saturate the system. At saturated levels, increases in dosage do not

greatly increase drug uptake. P-glycoprotein (see below) is widely distributed in the GI tract and it could have a role in the absorption of antiepileptic drugs. The expression of the drug can be induced and inhibited by other drugs, many of which are also inhibitors or inducers of the cytochrome P450 enzyme CYP3A4, and some of the so-called hepatic enzyme effects may in fact be due to alterations of oral absorption.

The following parameters are important to know for any drug being administered orally.

pK_a

The pK_a is the pH at which there is maximum ionization. The equation $pH = pK_a + \log[\text{ionized drug/total drug}]$ will provide the concentration of drug available for absorption in the GI tract environment with its varying pH levels. Some drugs have different structural properties at different pH levels and may have different pK_a values for each structural subtype (e.g. clonazepam, gabapentin).

Oral bioavailability

This is the proportion of the oral dose that is absorbed and therefore available for use by the body. It is important to know to what extent such factors as age, gender or food taken with the drug alter its bioavailability. For drugs requiring an active system for absorption, the bioavailability may be reduced at higher doses as the system becomes saturated (e.g. as for gabapentin). As a result of the dependence of absorption on gut motility, drugs with a low bioavailability tend to show high dose-to-dose variability of absorption. Motility is also reduced in some gastrointestinal diseases and in acute illness. Certain drugs interact with antiepileptics to reduce absorption, an example being the interaction of antacids and phenytoin. If possible, several hours should elapse between dosing with individual drugs that have the potential to interact at the level of absorption. Food has an effect on the absorption of a number of antiepileptic drugs, but is only clinically important routinely in the case of tiagabine (which should always be taken at the

Handbook of Epilepsy Treatment, 3rd Edition. By Simon Shorvon. Published 2010 by Blackwell Publishing Ltd.

end of a meal – it is important to advise patients about this; if taken without food, high levels rapidly occur, and cause transient side effects).

The oral bioavailability of most antiepileptics approaches 100%. The exceptions are carbamazepine (75–85%), clonazepam (80%) and gabapentin (dependent on saturation and sometimes below 60%). These drugs are particularly subject to variable absorption. Different formulations of phenytoin have slightly different bioavailability and this too is occasionally clinically important.

T_{max}

The time taken for peak serum levels to be reached following oral ingestion is known as T_{max}. This reflects a balance of absorption, distribution and elimination, and is in effect the beginning of the time when elimination exceeds absorption. For practical purposes, for most drugs the rate of absorption is, however, the major factor. At steady state, for drugs that are subject to autoinduction, T_{max} is reached earlier than after the initial phase of drug therapy. The importance of this is shown in the case of carbamazepine, where initial T_{max} can be 4–8 h and the T_{max} at steady state 1–3 h.

Modified-release formulations

The absorption of the standard preparation of many antiepileptics is relatively fast. Modified-release formulations can be used to slow down absorption for more prolonged effect or to produce less fluctuation in serum levels. The slow (or controlled)-release formulations are modified by such devices as coating the tablets in an acid-insoluble covering, increasing the size of the drug particles or embedding the drug in a matrix. The bioavailability of such preparations can differ from that of the unmodified parent. The slow-release formulation of carbamazepine, for example, can have lower bioavailability than the standard preparation.

Generic formulations

Generic formulations of a compound are required to have a bioavailability that is approximately similar to the proprietary compound. Rates of absorption do, however, vary somewhat, even if the extent of absorption does not. For most drugs, in all but the occasional patient, generic formulations are probably acceptable. However, for some drugs, in susceptible patients and particularly those who are seizure free, switching from one formulation to another risks changes in pharmacokinetics and seizure recurrence.

Rectal administration

Some drugs are readily absorbed by the rectal mucosa. This is an important mode of administration in emergency practice, because the rate of absorption is often very rapid. Solutions are better absorbed than lipid-based suppositories. The conveniently packaged Stesolid preparation of diazepam is a good example of a valuable liquid formulation that has greatly improved the therapy of febrile seizures, in contrast to the wax-based diazepam suppository, which is absorbed rectally much more slowly.

Parenteral administration

Parenteral formulations are needed in acute situations (e.g. status, acute seizures) and for temporary substitution of oral administration (e.g. in acute illness or peroperatively). Most antiepileptics cannot be given by intramuscular administration, as the extent and rate of absorption are inadequate. Only phenobarbital or midazolam – for emergency therapy – can usefully be given intramuscularly. Phenytoin, which crystallizes at tissue pH, can result in muscle necrosis. Intravenous administration is possible for many antiepileptics and special formulations are available to minimize thrombophlebitis and other local complications (e.g. the Diazemuls® formulation of diazepam and the fosphenytoin formulation of phenytoin).

Buccal and intranasal administration and inhalation

There has been recent interest in these forms of administration for acute seizures. Midazolam has been assessed rigorously by buccal and intranasal instillation, and absorption is excellent. The inhalation of antiepileptic drugs to obtain immediate effect in acute situations is also under investigation.

Drug distribution

Once in the plasma, drug molecules are available for transfer to other body areas (compartments); the resulting drug concentrations at different sites are determined by the process of distribution. Drug distribution is complex, depending on diverse factors, some of which differ over time in the same individual. Distribution to most sites is by concentration-driven passive transfer across lipid membranes. Lipid solubility is an important determinant of this. The more lipid soluble the drug, the greater its penetration into tissue. The blood–brain barrier has particularly tight intercellular junctions and only lipid-soluble drugs are able to cross it to enter the brain.

Drug transport systems across the blood–brain barrier – 'drug resistance' proteins

Many drugs have been shown to be actively removed from the brain by transport systems (some referred to as 'drug resistance' systems), and the relevant genes and transporter proteins have been identified. Genes for the latter include *MDR1* (P-glycoprotein; multiple drug-resistance protein) and *MRP1*. Their importance has long been known in cancer therapy, but recent interest has focused on antiepileptic drugs. P-glycoprotein mediates the absorption of drugs such as phenytoin, phenobarbital, lamotrigine and felbamate across the blood–brain barrier, and over-expression may be one mechanism of drug resistance. Although this is an obviously attractive idea, there is little evidence currently to support it, and it is also quite obvious that there must be many factors influencing 'drug resistance'. Some are related to: the drug – mode of action, dose, pharmakokinetics; the patient – receptor status, enzyme induction, lifestyle (alcohol, stress, lack of sleep); the epilepsy – aetiology, syndrome, extent/position of lesion, severity. Genetic variations in drug-resistance proteins probably play a minor role in most patients, and indeed the idea that drug resistance is a unitary concept is inherently unlikely.

Other factors influencing drug distribution

Other lipid tissues (e.g. muscle and fat) compete with brain for lipid-soluble drugs, and the concentration of a drug in any one compartment will depend on equilibrium with the others. The distribution of less lipid-soluble drugs may depend on blood flow through an organ (e.g. intravenous phenobarbital into brain during status epilepticus). Mathematical modelling of drug concentrations in the various compartments is possible in chronic oral and acute intravenous therapy, and an appreciation of intravenous drug distribution is necessary in the emergency therapy of status epilepticus (see pp. 288–289). The amount of drug available for distribution is the free fraction in the plasma, which is considerably lower than total plasma concentrations for protein-bound drugs (e.g. valproate, phenytoin).

Apparent volume of distribution

The apparent volume of distribution (V_d) is a proportionality constant that provides an estimate of the extent of distribution of the drug in tissues (Table 7.1). It is defined as the volume of fluid that would be required to contain the drug if a single compartment were assumed. The larger the volume of distribution, the greater the distribution in tissues (and the greater the risk of accumulation).

Table 7.1 Volume of distribution (V_d) of common antiepileptic drugs.

Drugs with very low V_d (<0.15 L/kg)
Nil

Drugs with low V_d (0.15–<0.5 L/kg)
Valproate

Drugs with moderate V_d (0.5–0.8 L/kg)
Ethosuximide
Felbamate
Lacosamide
Levetiracetam
Oxcarbazepine
Phenobarbital
Phenytoin
Pregabalin

Drugs with a high V_d (>0.8 L/kg)
Carbamazepine
Clobazam
Clonazepam
Eslicarbazepine
Gabapentin
Lamotrigine
Primidone
Rufinamide
Tiagabine
Topiramate
Vigabatrin
Zonisamide

Thus, if V_d is approximately 0.05 L/kg (5% of body volume) the drug is confined to the vascular compartment, if it is 0.15 L/kg the drug is confined to the extracellular water, and if it is 0.5 L/kg the drug is distributed throughout the total body water. Higher values indicate that the drug is concentrated in tissue. V_d can also be used to make a rough estimate of peak plasma level after the initial dose (very approximately equal to dose/V_d).

Protein binding

The protein binding of a drug is expressed as a percentage, denoting the proportion of the total plasma concentration that is bound chemically to plasma proteins. The bound portion is not available for distribution. Plasma protein binding may alter in disease states (e.g. hepatic or renal disease), and tends to fall with age. There can be competition for binding sites between drugs. The effects of mild alterations in protein binding are often complex, but usually have few practical clinical implications.

The most important in epilepsy is the displacement of bound phenytoin by valproate, and this can account for the signs of phenytoin toxicity on co-medication with valproate, with 'normal' total phenytoin blood levels. Tiagabine is also displaced by valproate, and this may also be an important effect.

Total and free antiepileptic serum level

The total serum level refers to the total plasma concentration of a drug, i.e. both its bound and its unbound fractions. The free serum level is the amount of unbound drug, i.e. that available for distribution. The clinical utility of 'free blood level' measurements is outlined on p. 156.

Drug elimination (metabolism and excretion)

A drug is cleared (eliminated) from the body by the processes of metabolism and excretion.

Table 7.2 Some of the known interactions of antiepileptic drugs with hepatic enzyme systems.

Enzyme	Antiepileptic drugs metabolized by enzyme	Antiepileptic drugs that induce enzyme	Antiepileptic drugs that inhibit enzyme	Other drugs that induce enzyme[a]	Other drugs that inhibit enzyme[a]
CYP3A4	Carbamazepine	Carbamazepine	Stiripentol	Glucocorticoids	Many others including:
	Clobazam	Felbamate		Rifampicin	Cimetidine
	Clonazepam	Oxcarbazepine			Ciclosporin
	Ethosuximide	Phenobarbital			Diltiazem
	Midazolam	Phenytoin			Erythromycin
	Phenytoin	Primidone			Fluconazole
	Tiagabine	Rufinamide			Fluvoxamine
	Zonisamide	Topiramate			Verapamil
					Grapefruit juice
CYP2C9	Phenytoin	Carbamazepine	Eslicarbazepine	Rifampicin	Amiodarone
	Phenobarbital	Phenytoin	Valproate		Chloramphenicol
	Valproate	Phenobarbital			Fluoxetine
		Primidone			Fluoxamine
					Miconazole
CYP2C19	Diazepam	Carbamazepine	Felbamate	Rifampicin	Cimetidine
	Lacosamide	Phenytoin	Lacosamide		Fluoxamine
	Phenytoin	Phenobarbital	Oxcarbazepine (weak)		
	Phenobarbital	Primidone	Stiripentol		
	Valproate		Topiramate (weak)		
CYP2E1	Felbamate			Alcohol	
	Phenobarbital			Isoniazid	
UGT1A4	Lamotrigine	Carbamazepine	Valproate		
	Oxcarbazepine (MHD derivative)	Lamotrigine			
	Phenobarbital	Oxcarbazepine			
	Valproate	Phenytoin			
		Phenobarbital			

[a]A selection of drugs known to interact commonly with the antiepileptic drugs.

Table 7.3 Metabolic pathways of antiepileptic drugs.

Drug	Phase 1 reactions	Phase 2 reactions[a]	Percentage of drug eliminated by phase 1 reaction	P450 enzymes identified in the phase 1 reactions[b]
Carbamazepine	Epoxidation, hydroxylation	Conjugation	75	CYP3A4 CYP2C8 CYP1A2
Clobazam	Demethylation, hydroxylation	Conjugation		CYP3A4
Clonazepam	Reduction, hydroxylation	Acetylation		CYP3A4
Eslicarbazepine	Hydrolysis	Conjugation		
Ethosuximide	Oxidation	Conjugation	70	CYP3A4
Gabapentin	Renal excretion without metabolism		0	
Lacosamide	O-Desmethylation		30	CYP2C19
Lamotrigine	No phase 1 reaction	Conjugation (UGT1A4)	0	
Levetiracetam	Hydrolysis by non-hepatic enzymes		0	
Oxcarbazepine	Reduction	Conjugation	<5	
Phenobarbital	Oxidation, glucosidation, hydroxylation	Conjugation	30	CYP2C9 CYP2C19 CYP2E1
Phenytoin	Oxidation, glucosidation, hydroxylation	Conjugation	90	CYP2C9 CYP2C19 CYP3A4
Pregabalin	Renal excretion without metabolism		0	
Primidone	Transformation to phenobarbital and a phenylethyl derivative, then metabolized as per phenobarbital			
Rufinamide	Hydrolysis by hepatic carboxylesterases			
Tiagabine	Oxidation	Conjugation	90	CYP3A4
Topiramate[c]	Hydroxylation, hydrolysis	Conjugation	<25	
Valproate	Oxidation, hydroxylation, epoxidation, reduction[d]	Conjugation	10	CYP4B1 CYP2C9 CYP2A6 CYP2B6 CYP2C19
Vigabatrin	Renal excretion without metabolism		0	
Zonisamide	Acetylation, reduction	Conjugation	20 (acetylation)	CYP3A4

[a]Conjugation (phase 2) is always by glucuronidation involving the UDPGT (uridine diphosphate glucuronosyl transferase) family of enzymes.
[b]This lists known enzymes. Other enzymes, not yet fully characterized, play a part in the metabolism of many of these drugs.
[c]In non-induced patients, most topiramate is excreted renally without metabolism.
[d]Some of the biotransformation of valproate is via non-P450 enzyme systems.

Drug metabolism (biotransformation)

Most antiepileptics are metabolized in the liver by hepatocyte microsomal enzymes. Metabolism is frequently in two phases (Tables 7.2 and 7.3). The metabolites are usually less biologically active, although this is not always the case (e.g. phenobarbital from primidone, desmethyl-clobazam from clobazam). Most oxidation process are carried out by the cytochrome microsomal P450 enzyme system, although there are exceptions, e.g. the oxidation of valproate via a non-microsomal branched-chain fatty acid enzyme system involving monoamine oxidase, and the hydrolysis of levetiracetam by enzymes in red blood cells and other tissues. In phase 2 reactions the resulting metabolites are conjugated, usually by glucuronidation. The conjugates are almost always biologically inert and more polar (therefore more easily excreted) than the parent drugs. Biotransformation rather than renal excretion of unchanged drug is the main route of elimination for most antiepileptics (see drug excretion section below).

Drug interactions due to induction/inhibition of hepatic enzymes

The most important antiepileptic drug interactions are those mediated by changes in the cytochrome P450 enzyme system. These metabolic processes can be induced or inhibited by antiepileptic drugs, and also autoinduced (induction of the drug's own metabolism). In fact carbamazepine, phenytoin and phenobarbital are among the most potent enzyme inducers in the pharmacopoeia. Pharmacokinetic interactions between antiepileptics (and other drugs) are therefore very common and can have a serious impact on clinical therapeutics. In recent years the characterization of the isoenzymes involved in antiepileptic drug metabolism has greatly improved our understanding of drug interactions.

There are two main families of enzymes. The cytochrome P450 enzyme system is involved in the phase 1 metabolism of a number of antiepileptic drugs (see Table 2.4 in Chapter 2). Five of the isoenzymes (CYP3A4, CYP2C9, CYP2C19, CYP2E1 and CYP1A2) are the most important from the point of view of the antiepileptic drugs. Phase 2 reactions (conjugation) are usually mediated by the uridine glucuronyl transferase enzyme families (UGTs), of which 16 subtypes are recognized.

Examples of the most common and important interactions between antiepileptic drugs in routine epilepsy practice are as follows:
• The inducing effects of carbamazepine, phenytoin, phenobarbital and primidone on cytochrome P450 and UGT enzymes, which commonly result in clinically significant reductions in levels of carbamazepine, ethosuximide, lamotrigine, oxcarbazepine, tiagabine, topiramate, valproate and zonisamide, e.g. in one study, valproate concentrations were reduced by 76%, 49% and 66% by co-medication with phenobarbital, phenytoin and carbamazepine, respectively.
• The inhibiting effects of valproate on CYP2C9, CYP2C19 and UGT1A4 can elevate levels of phenobarbital and lamotrigine, sometimes by as much as 80%, and almost always necessitate dosage modification. Lesser effects of valproate occur on phenytoin and carbamazepine epoxide concentrations.
• Other inhibiting effects occur, but are generally less important. These include the effects of phenytoin and phenobarbital on the metabolism of each other, and the inhibiting effects of carbamazepine and oxcarbazepine on phenytoin metabolism. Felbamate is by far the strongest inhibitor of CYP enzyme activity and has been shown to result in clinically significant elevations of the levels of phenytoin, valproate, phenobarbital, carbamazepine epoxide and N-desmethylclobazam.

Other non-antiepileptic drugs are also involved in interactions at the level of hepatic enzymes, including: many antipsychotic drugs, many antidepressants, many oncological and immunosuppressant drugs, many antibiotics (including rifampicin, erythromycin, clarithromycin), theophylline, warfarin, antifungal drugs, antihypertensive drugs (e.g. verapamil, diltiazem) and many cardiovascular drugs. The list of known interactions is very long, and before any co-medication is considered the potential for drug interaction should be checked.

Drug excretion

Most drugs and their metabolites are excreted via the kidney. Nearly all the various processes of renal excretion are mediated by concentration-dependent passive transfer, although acidic molecules, including the glucuronide conjugates, are also actively pumped into the proximal renal tubules. The more polar the molecule, the less resorption occurs in the distal tubule. Severe renal disease affects this process and can result in impaired excretion and greater drug accumulation. Mild renal disease rarely has any practically important effects on antiepileptic drug handling. Some antiepileptics are excreted without prior hepatic metabolism (e.g. gabapentin, piracetam, pregabalin and vigabatrin) and doses have to be reduced in severe renal disease. Alkalinization of the urine will reduce the absorption of acidic drugs from the renal tubules and this is an interaction that can affect the blood levels of phenobarbital (and is used therapeutically in barbiturate overdose).

Drugs can also be excreted through the lungs, sweat, tears and maternal milk, but, with the exception of the pulmonary excretion of gaseous anaesthetics used in status, these routes of excretion are generally of no importance with regard to the antiepileptic drugs, although excretion in maternal milk does have implications for prescribing in breast-feeding women (see pp. 144–145).

Elimination half-life

This is the period of time after absorption over which half the drug is eliminated from the body. For most drugs this depends primarily on their metabolism. There can be marked interindividual variation as well as intra-individual changes over time. Drug interactions can also have marked effects on elimination half-life. Three-quarters of a drug is eliminated within two half-lives, and approximately 93% within four half-lives. Once a steady state has been reached, at a very rough approximation, dosing a drug at intervals at least as frequently as one half-life will keep trough levels within 50% of peak concentrations.

Fraction (of dose) excreted unchanged in urine ($Fu_{(x)}$)

After a drug is given intravenously and the patient's urine is collected for seven half-lives, the proportion of the drug present in an unchanged form ($Fu_{(x)}$) measures the contribution of renal excretion to total drug elimination (the rest being eliminated by metabolism). If this fraction ($Fu_{(x)}$) is high, renal impairment may require drug doses to be lowered; if it is low, renal impairment is unlikely to seriously affect drug kinetics. Similarly, high values of $Fu_{(x)}$ imply that modification of drug dosage will be unnecessary in hepatic disease, and low $Fu_{(x)}$ values that such modification may be necessary. In elderly people, as renal excretory capacity falls, it is wise to consider lower than average doses of drugs with high $Fu_{(x)}$ values. Antiepileptic drugs with a high $Fu_{(x)}$ value include gabapentin, levetiracetam, piracetam, pregabalin and vigabatrin.

Clearance

This is defined as the amount of drug excreted over a unit of time. Plasma clearance is a measure of the amount of drug removed from the plasma. Renal clearance is a measure of the amount of drug removed by the kidneys. As a general rule, if $Fu_{(x)}$ is low, then clearance is largely dependent on hepatic metabolism; conversely, if $Fu_{(x)}$ is high, clearance is largely dependent on renal excretion. When drugs are avidly metabolized in by the liver, clearance values can be as high as 1.4 L/kg per h (i.e. the rate of hepatic blood flow).

Kinetics of biotransformation

Metabolism is an enzyme-catalysed process that is potentially saturatable, described by the Michaelis–Menten equation:

$$V = V'_{max}C/(K_m + C)$$

where V is the velocity of the process, V_{max} the maximum velocity possible, K_m the Michaelis–Menten constant and C the concentration of the drug. For most drugs, the required serum concentrations are well below their K_m values, and in these circumstances V is virtually equal to V_{max} (i.e. metabolism is not saturated). These drugs have a linear relationship between drug dose and serum level in the ranges that are clinically useful, so-called 'first-order kinetics'. A few antiepileptic drugs, however, have levels close to saturation (e.g. phenytoin, thiopental). When concentrations reach levels that overwhelm the capacity of the system (i.e. where V is close to V_{max}), the velocity of metabolism cannot be increased. In this situation, small increases in dose may result in large and unpredictable rises in the level in the blood.

Steady-state values

Steady-state values are those that are achieved when, for any particular drug dose, the pharmacokinetic processes reach equilibrium. The time to steady state (T_{ss}) is dependent on many factors, but as a rule of thumb it is equal to five times the elimination half-life of the drug. In long-term treatment, steady-state values (e.g. for serum levels, clearance, V_d, half-life, T_{max}) are generally of greater use to clinicians than values at initial dosing.

Blood level measurements

When a steady state has been reached, there is a fairly consistent relationship between plasma concentration of any drug and the concentration in brain or other tissues. It should therefore be possible to define those plasma levels that are associated with optimal clinical effects (i.e. an optimal balance between effectiveness and side effects). As a result of biological variation, such levels vary from individual to individual (Table 7.4), but nevertheless a range can be developed that is based on statistical or population parameters. This is the 'target range' (also known as the 'therapeutic range' or the 'optimal range').

In practice, skill is needed to interpret serum drug concentrations wisely. The clinician should know when to ignore as well as when to heed blood level information.

Table 7.4 Factors influencing levels of antiepileptic drugs.

Drug factors
Formulation
Interactions

Patient factors
Genetic/constitutional factors affecting pharmacokinetics (absorption, metabolism, excretion)
Disease states affecting pharmacokinetics (renal, hepatic, changes in plasma proteins, gastrointestinal disturbance)
Pregnancy, nutritional status, body weight changes

Timing of blood samples

Generally, blood samples should be taken at steady state, i.e. at a period after any dose change that is greater than fives times the drug elimination half-life. Steady-state serum levels of drugs with short half-lives fluctuate through the day in patients on oral medication, and thus blood sampling should be taken at a similar time (the trough level – that taken before the morning dosing – is a conventional preference) to assess blood level changes. For drugs with a long half-life (e.g. phenobarbital), there is little diurnal fluctuation and timing is unimportant.

Rapid assay

Technology exists for the rapid assay of the commonly used drugs. It can be extremely helpful to have blood level data available before a consultation and in large clinics it is cost-effective to offer an immediate assay service (equivalent to having the blood sugar results during a diabetes clinic).

Salivary vs serum concentrations

The salivary concentration of certain drugs (e.g. ethosuximide, carbamazepine, phenytoin) correlates well with the unbound (free) serum concentration. Salivary measurements avoid the need for venepuncture and so are particularly acceptable in children. However, measurement is more difficult and more prone to error than serum measurements, and can be complicated by gingivitis and dose residues in the mouth, and so have not been widely adopted and have fallen from favour. It should also be noted that the relationship between unbound drug concentration in plasma and drug concentration in saliva is not the same for all drugs. The

salivary concentration of phenobarbital, for example, varies with salivary pH, and meaningful results must account for this. Similarly, valproate salivary concentrations, for various pharmacological reasons, have no consistent relationship with plasma concentrations.

Target range

The target range is an estimate derived largely from hospital studies with a bias towards relatively severe cases. In fact there are many individuals whose epilepsy is well controlled at 'suboptimal' levels – for instance, at least a third of patients treated with phenytoin. There are also others whose seizures are only controlled, without side effects, at 'supraoptimal' levels. Drug response varies a lot in epilepsy, but generally speaking the more severe the epilepsy, the higher the required blood levels. Thus, patients with frequent seizures or those with partial epilepsy often have higher 'therapeutic ranges' than those with less severe forms of epilepsy. The effectiveness and side effects will vary in individuals due to genetic, constitutional and exogenous factors, which may not correlate well with blood levels. For all these reasons, too rigid an adherence to the 'range' is totally inappropriate, and in all cases treatment must be tailored to individual requirements; the patient should be treated, not his or her blood level.

The concept of a 'target range' has most utility in the case of drugs that have a moment-by-moment action on cellular membrane function; phenytoin, carbamazepine, ethosuximide and lamotrigine, drugs acting at membrane ion channels, are the best examples of this (Table 7.5). Where drugs have more indirect antiepileptic actions, or multiple actions, blood level may be less well correlated with effect, e.g. in the case of gabapentin, vigabatrin and topiramate. Also, the concept of a therapeutic range is undermined where pharmacological tolerance develops as, for example, with barbiturates or benzodiazepines.

The 'individualized' therapeutic range

It is sometimes feasible to establish empirically a plasma concentration range for an individual patient in which the best therapeutic response is obtained. The measurement of blood levels during periods of optimal response will provide a useful reference. As emphasized above, the individualized therapeutic ranges can differ markedly from the published population-based ranges.

Table 7.5 Value of measurement of blood levels of antiepileptic drugs.

Drug	Target level (mmol/L)	Value of blood level measurements in routine practice	Comments
Carbamazepine	20–50	+++	Measurements useful because response is closely linked to blood level, although kinetics are linear and often dose change can be made simply on a clinical basis. Measurements useful also to monitor the effects of drug interactions and because both the parent drug and the active metabolite contribute to clinical effect
Ethosuximide	300–700	+++	Measurements useful because response is closely linked to blood level, although kinetics are linear and often dose change can be made simply on a clinical basis
Lamotrigine	10–60	++	Response is only partially correlated with blood level. However, measurement is useful where lamotrigine levels are affected by antiepileptic drug interactions, interactions with the contraceptive pill and pregnancy
Oxcarbazepine	50–140[a]	+	Measurements of limited usefulness only as response is not broadly linked to blood level. However, as parent drug and active metabolite contribute to clinical effect, it is sometimes useful to monitor changes
Phenobarbital	50–130	++	Measurements have moderate utility, but tolerance complicates assessment, and the upper limit is imprecise because of the sedative effects
Phenytoin	40–80	+++	Measurements useful because response is closely linked to blood level, and because it is hazardous to alter dose without measurements owing to non-linear kinetics
Primidone	25–50[b]	++	Measurement of the derived phenobarbital levels of moderate utility (see above) but measurement of primidone level is of only limited usefulness
Topiramate	10–60	+	Measurements of limited usefulness only as response is not broadly linked to blood level. However, serum level measurement useful to monitor effects of drug interactions
Valproate	300–700	++	Measurement is of only limited usefulness, as response is only partially correlated to blood level and this varies widely through the day. However, serum level measurement is useful to monitor effects of drug interactions
Zonisamide	30–140	+	Measurements of limited usefulness only as response is not broadly linked to blood level. More experience with blood level monitoring in this drug may lead to reassessment of value
Benzodiazepines (e.g. clobazam and clonazepam)		0	There is no consistent relationship between blood levels and clinical response
Eslicarbazepine, lacosamide, rufinamide		0	The usefulness of routine measurements of these drugs has not been established

Table 7.5 *Continued*

Drug	Target level (mmol/L)	Value of blood level measurements in routine practice	Comments
Felbamate, gabapentin, levetiracetam, pregabalin tiagabine		0	Target blood levels have been quoted, but their usefulness in routine practice is doubtful. The measurements are required only in exceptional circumstances or to check compliance
Vigabatrin		0	Blood level not correlated with pharmacological effect (irreversible enzyme inhibition

+++ Useful, measurements required often.
++ Useful, measurements used in routine practice.
+ Limited usefulness, measurements occasionally required.
0, no general utility, measurement only required in exceptional circumstances (or to check compliance).
[a]MHD derivative.
[b]Primidone levels – measurement of derived phenobarbital levels is more useful.

Total vs free serum drug concentrations

Routine analytical methods measure the total drug concentration (i.e. the protein-bound and unbound [free] fractions), whereas it is actually the free fraction that is available for biological action. Measurement of the total level is satisfactory as there is usually a consistent relationship between the free and the total levels. However, in certain states this relationship can be altered, e.g. in low protein states, severe renal disease, severe hepatic disease, pregnancy, old age and the neonatal period. In these situations the free levels may be higher than would be predicted from the total concentration, and reliance on total concentration may be misleading. Some advocate the routine direct measurement of free levels in all these situations. However, assay techniques are difficult and the results less accurate, and in routine practice free level estimations are rarely required.

Active metabolites

Some drugs are converted into active metabolites (see pharmacopoeia, pp. 374–375), and interpretation of parent drug level measurements without accounting for the potential contribution of the active metabolite can lead to therapeutic errors. Carbamazepine is metabolized to a 10,11-epoxide which can cause side effects similar to those of the parent drug. Measurement of the concentra-

tion of the parent drug alone may be misleading, especially as the proportion of carbamazepine converted to carbamazepine 10,11-epoxide can vary markedly (e.g. in the presence of enzyme-inducing co-medication). In the case of clobazam and primidone, the concentrations of the active metabolites at steady state are much higher than those of the parent drug, and in this situation measurements of the level of the metabolites are more informative.

When is blood level measurement required?

There is no doubt that the practice of monitoring plasma drug concentrations has improved the quality of epilepsy care. It has led to an appreciation of the variability of drug levels, kinetic principles and drug interactions, and the value of tailoring doses to individual patient needs.

Feedback from blood level measurement has improved clinical experience and clinical acumen and, as a result, effective therapy can often be chosen now on purely clinical grounds, as shown in a recent study in which there were no differences in outcome between patients randomized to have their regimens adjusted empirically and those in whom dosage was tailored based on drug concentration measurements.

Table 7.6 Indications for blood level monitoring.

- To identify a pharmacokinetic cause for poor therapeutic response in spite of adequate dosage. The measurement of levels of the parent drug and active metabolites may be necessary
- To identify the cause of adverse effects where these might be drug induced. The measurement of levels of the parent drug and active metabolites may be necessary
- To monitor phenytoin dose changes in view of the non-linear kinetics and lack of predictability of the phenytoin dose–blood level relationship
- To measure pharmacokinetic changes in the presence of physiological or pathological conditions known to alter drug disposition (e.g. pregnancy, liver disease, renal failure, gastrointestinal disease, hypoalbuminaemic states)
- To identify and minimize the consequences of adverse drug interactions in patients receiving multiple drug therapy
- To identify which drugs require dosage changes to optimize therapy in patients on antiepileptic drug polytherapy
- To assess changes in bioavailability when a drug formulation has been changed
- To identify poor compliance

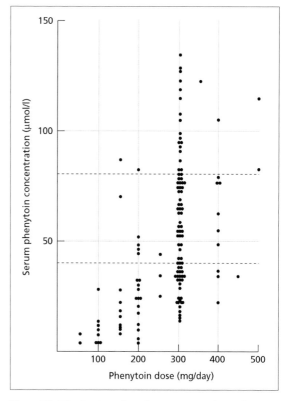

Figure 7.1 Distribution of steady-state serum phenytoin concentrations in 131 adult epileptic patients on admission to a residential centre. Note the large variability observed in patients receiving the same dosage.

The situations in which blood level measurements are most often required are shown in Table 7.6, and it will be apparent that these are relatively restricted; the variability of phenytoin levels is one example (Figure 7.1).

In many clinical situations drug-level monitoring is wrongly relied upon, and measurements made unnecessarily or interpreted incorrectly. The most common mistake is to adhere too closely to the 'therapeutic range', and it is incorrect, for example, to:

- increase drug doses in patients fully controlled, simply because the serum level is below the therapeutic range
- lower drug doses in patients without side effects because the serum level is above the therapeutic range
- ignore adverse effects because the levels are within the therapeutic range.

The importance of 'treating the patient, not the serum level' cannot be overstated.

8 The Antiepileptic Drugs

Carbamazepine

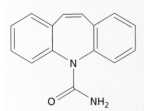

Proprietary name: Tegretol[a]

Primary indications
Monotherapy and adjunctive therapy in partial and generalized seizures (excluding absence, tonic and myoclonic seizures) and in childhood epilepsy syndromes. Adults and children

Commonly used as first-line drug
Yes

Usual preparations
Tablets: 100, 200, 400 mg; chewtabs: 100, 200 mg; modified-release formulations: 200, 400 mg; liquid: 100 mg/5 mL; suppositories: 125, 250 mg

Usual dosage – adults
Initial: 100–200 mg at night; increased by increments of 200 mg every 2 weeks
Maintenance: 400–1600 mg/day (maximum 2400 mg)
(modified-release formulations – require 15–35% higher doses for same bioavailability)

Usual dosage – children
<1 year, 100–200 mg/day (initial dose 50 mg/day)
1–5 years, 200–400 mg/day (initial dose 100 mg/day)
5–10 years, 400–600 mg/day (initial dose 200 mg/day)
10–15 years, 600–1000 mg/day (initial dose 200 mg/day)
(higher for modified-release formulation)

Dosing intervals
2–3 times/day (2–4 times/day at higher doses or in children)

Is dose commonly affected by co-medication?
Yes

Is dose affected by renal/hepatic disease?
Severe hepatic disease

Does it affect dose of other drugs?
Yes

Handbook of Epilepsy Treatment, 3rd Edition. By Simon Shorvon.
Published 2010 by Blackwell Publishing Ltd.

Does it affect the contraceptive pill?
Yes

Serum level monitoring
Very useful

Target range
Carbamazepine 20–50 μmol/L, 4–12 μg/mL
Carbamazepine 10,11-epoxide – <9 μmol/L

Common/important adverse events
Drowsiness, fatigue, dizziness, ataxia, diplopia, blurring of vision, sedation, headache, insomnia, gastrointestinal disturbance, tremor, weight gain, impotence, effects on behaviour and mood, hepatic disturbance, rash and other skin reactions, bone marrow dyscrasia, leucopenia, hyponatraemia, water retention, endocrine effects, effects on cardiac conduction, effects on immunoglobulins

Risk of hypersensitivity
Yes

Major mechanism of action
Inhibition of sodium channel conductance. Also action on monoamine, acetylcholine and NMDA (N-methyl-D-aspartate) receptors

Main advantages
Highly effective, extensively studied and usually well-tolerated therapy; proven relative safety in pregnancy

Main disadvantages
Minor adverse effects especially on initiating therapy; occasional severe hypersensitivity and other toxicity; variable absorption; potential for drug interaction; active metabolite

Comment
Drug of first choice in adults and children in partial seizures, tonic-clonic seizures and some childhood epilepsy syndromes

aName of proprietary brand available in the UK.

Carbamazepine: pharmacokinetics – average adult values

Oral bioavailability	75–85%
Time to peak levels	4–8 h
Volume of distribution	0.8–2 L/kg
Biotransformation	Hepatic epoxidation and hydroxylation, and then conjugation
Elimination half-life	5–26 h (varies with co-medication)
Plasma clearance	0.133 L/kg per h (varies with co-medication)
Protein binding	75%
Active metabolite	Carbamazepine epoxide
Metabolism by hepatic enzymes	Yes – CYP3A4, CYP2C8, CYP1A2 and then UGT (15%)
Inhibition or induction of hepatic enzymes	Yes – induces of CYP2B6, CYP2C, CYP2C19, CYP3A, CYP1A2, UGT1A4
Drug interactions	Common

CYP, cytochrome P450 enzyme; UGT, uridine glucuronyl transferase.

Carbamazepine (CBZ) is the veritable workhorse of the antiepileptic drugs. Initial open clinical trials were carried out in the early 1960s, and the first controlled trial in 1966. It was licensed in Britain in 1965, then in Europe and finally in the USA in 1974. It rapidly became established as the major first-line antiepileptic drug for partial and secondarily generalized seizures, a position that it retains in spite of the many antiepileptic drugs licensed since. It is the most commonly prescribed drug in Europe for epilepsy, and is very widely used worldwide.

It was originally developed in the search for new antipsychotic compounds as an alternative to chlorpromazine. Disappointingly, no strong effect against psychosis was noticed, and then, as has been the case for many antiepileptics, its value in epilepsy was discovered largely by chance. Its first clinical licence was for its analgesic effect in trigeminal neuralgia, and it remains a drug of choice in trigeminal neuralgia and other neuralgic pain.

It is a tricyclic compound, related chemically to chlorpromazine and the tricyclic antidepressants, and is now widely used for the treatment of epilepsy, bipolar disorder and other psychiatric syndromes, neuropathic pain syndromes and trigeminal neuralgia.

Physical and chemical characteristics

Carbamazepine (5H-dibenzyl[b,f]azepine-5-carboxamide, molecular weight 236.3) is a crystalline substance, which is virtually insoluble in water, but highly soluble in lipid and organic solvents. It is stable at room temperatures, but its bioavailability can be reduced by up to 50% by hot or humid conditions or when there has been absorption of moisture, and so care is needed in storage.

Mode of action

Carbamazepine binds to the neuronal sodium channel, pre- and postsynaptically, and this binding results in a use- and frequency-dependent blockade of the channel and thus the inhibition of high-frequency repetitive firing and excitatory neurotransmission. This is its main mode of action (an action shared by phenytoin and also, among other actions, by lamotrigine, felbamate, topiramate and zonisamide). It also affects various protein and signalling pathways. It has also been proposed that carbamazepine acts on other receptors including the purine, monoamine and acetylcholine receptors.

Pharmacokinetics

Absorption

The gastrointestinal absorption of carbamazepine is rather slow and variable, and this is a disadvantage of the drug. Between 75 and 85% of the drug is absorbed after oral ingestion of the immediate-release or chewable formulations, and 10–35% lower for the slow-release formulations. Absorption can, however, be erratic and change over time, with marked intraindividual variation, and different formulations have different absorption characteristics. It does not appear to make any difference whether the drug is taken before or after food. The bioavailability of modified-release formulations is 15–35% lower, but these formulations produce smoother serum level profiles and are generally preferred in all clinical situations. Peak levels are reached between 4 and 8 h after absorption.

Preparations of carbamazepine in sorbitol do exist for rectal administration, but are not used in routine clinical practice. There is no parenteral preparation of carbamazepine currently marketed, although intravenous formulations are under development.

Distribution

Approximately 75–80% of the drug is bound to plasma proteins. The free fraction of carbamazepine ranges from 20% to 24% of the total plasma concentration, and cerebrospinal fluid (CSF) carbamazepine levels vary in a range from 17% to 31%. The relationship between dose and plasma concentrations, in the normal clinical range, is linear, but there is a large inter- and intraindividual variability in the protein binding and the ratio of bound to unbound drug. Salivary levels bear a constant relationship to free blood levels, and can be a useful method of assaying drug concentrations. Hair concentrations are also reliably related to dose, and can be used to monitor compliance.

The protein binding of the 10,11-epoxide is 50%. The apparent volume of distribution of carbamazepine is between 0.8 and 2.0 L/kg in adults, and of the 10, 11-epoxide it is 0.59–1.5 L/kg. Brain levels are somewhat higher than plasma levels, for both carbamazepine epoxide and the parent drug, and there appears to be rather non-specific binding of carbamazepine to brain tissue, uninfluenced by gliosis.

Biotransformation and excretion

Carbamazepine is extensively metabolized in the liver. The major pathway is first epoxidation to carbamazepine 10,11-epoxide (CBZ epoxide) and then hydrolysis to carbamazepine 10,11-trans-dihydrodiol, followed by glucuronidation and sulphuration, and less than 1% of the drug is excreted unchanged in the urine. The main pathway is epoxidation via the cytochrome P450 CYP3A4 enzyme system. The drug induces its own metabolism and there is a marked increase in clearance and a fall of about 50% in serum half-life during the first few weeks of carbamazepine therapy. This autoinduction is usually completed within a month. Carbamazepine is also subject to heteroinduction by other enzyme-inducing antiepileptic drugs.

After a single dose, the elimination half-life is between 20 and 65 h but, because of autoinduction, on chronic therapy the half-life is usually between 5 and 26 h (and 3–23 h for the 10,11-epoxide), although there is marked individual variation. In the post-induced state, a new steady state after changes in drug dosage will be achieved within 3 days. Autoinduction is complete within 2–30 days of initiation of therapy.

CBZ epoxide levels are generally about 50% of carbamazepine plasma levels, although the ratio is subject to marked variation. The rate of metabolism varies both within and between individuals, and is affected by age, co-medication and dosing schedules. There is a relatively low extraction ratio (<10%), which reflects the limited ability of the liver to handle the plasma carbamazepine load. As a result of the low intrinsic clearance and low extraction ratio, changes in hepatic blood flow do not alter carbamazepine clearance to any great extent.

The mean clearance of carbamazepine is 0.133 L/kg per h but individual values are very variable.

Greater variations in serum levels are found during once-daily, rather than two- or three-times-a-day, dosing regimens. One study showed a mean 79% change between peak and trough levels on twice-daily dosing, which was reduced to 40% on four-times-a day dosing. Peak-level side effects are common in clinical practice, and these can be avoided by flattening out the diurnal blood level swings, which can be achieved by more frequent dosing or the use of the controlled-release formulation of carbamazepine. There are no significant differences in the absorption and steady-state concentrations, efficacy or tolerability between conventional and chewable tablets, or suspension and syrup.

There are no major differences between children and adults in the absorption, protein binding or distribution of carbamazepine or CBZ epoxide. The volume of distribution in infants is, however, one to one and a half times that of the adult level. The clearance of carbamazepine is higher in infants and young children, and the ratio of CBZ epoxide:carbamazepine levels ranges from 16% to 66%. In older children, absorption, half-life and clearance show marked intraindividual variations, although the mean population values are similar to those in adults. The diurnal variation in levels in children is greater than in adults, and to avoid peak dose side effects it is often necessary to use two- or three-times-a day dosing and the slow-release formulation. In gastrointestinal disease, the absorption of carbamazepine can be quite severely reduced, and drug levels require careful monitoring.

In the presence of severe liver disease, carbamazepine pharmacokinetics may be disordered and dose reductions needed, but moderate disease has little effect. Renal disease has no effect on carbamazepine kinetics, and dialysis does not have a marked effect on carbamazepine plasma levels. Severe congestive cardiac failure has been shown to result in abnormally slow absorption, and the drug is also cleared and metabolized at a slower rate. The water and sodium retention induced by the antidiuretic action of carbamazepine can also aggravate cardiac failure.

The absorption of carbamazepine is not modified during the first two trimesters of pregnancy. In the last trimester, the unbound levels of carbamazepine and CBZ epoxide are not changed (nor is their ratio), but total levels fall as maternal plasma protein concentrations decline towards the end of pregnancy. These effects are relatively minor, and dose adjustments are only occasionally needed. If clinically indicated, measurement of free levels can be useful. Breast milk concentrations of carbamazepine are about 20–70% of those of maternal plasma.

As a result of the wide variation in the dose–serum level relationship, at both an inter- and an intraindividual level, carbamazepine (and CBZ epoxide) levels are commonly measured. There is a relationship between carbamazepine level and therapeutic effectiveness, but no invariable 'therapeutic range'. Thus, although levels are useful as a guide, particularly in long-term therapy, there is little point in adhering to any predetermined target range, and daily dosage should be tailored to individual need. Having said this, the maximum effect is usually observed between 10 and 50 μmol/L. The CBZ epoxide has antiepileptic action and also contributes to the side effects of carbamazepine, and for this reason it is often useful to measure the serum levels of both carbamazepine and CBZ epoxide. The target range for the CBZ epoxide is up to 9 μmol/L.

Drug interactions

Drug interactions involving carbamazepine are common and often clinically important. The drug is a potent hepatic enzyme inducer of CYP3A4 in particular and this is the major source of interaction. However, interactions

Table 8.1 Effects of carbamazepine on the serum concentrations of other antiepileptic drugs.

Increased concentration	Decreased concentration	Variable (increase, decrease or no change)	No effect
Phenobarbital metabolically derived from primidone	Clobazam Clonazepam Diazepam Ethosuximide Felbamate Lamotrigine Levetiracetam Midazolam Oxcarbazepine[a] Primidone Rufinamide Stiripentol Tiagabine Topiramate Valproic acid Zonisamide	Phenytoin Phenobarbital	Gabapentin Pregabalin Vigabatrin

[a]Monohydroxymetabolite.

Table 8.2 Effect of other antiepileptic drugs on serum concentrations of carbamazepine.

Increased concentration	Decreased concentration	No effect
Stiripentol Valproic acid[a] Valpromide[a]	Felbamate[b] Phenobarbital Phenytoin Primidone Oxcarbazepine Rufinamide (minor effect)	Ethosuximide Gabapentin Lamotrigine[c] Levetiracetam Pregabalin Topiramate Tiagabine Vigabatrin[d] Zonisamide[d]

[a]Little effect on serum carbamazepine concentration, but marked increase in serum carbamazepine-10,11-epoxide, particularly with valpromide.
[b]The decrease in serum carbamazepine concentration is associated with an increase in serum carbamazepine-10,11-epoxide.
[c]Possible appearance of neurotoxic effects may be related to a pharmacodynamic interaction.
[d]Variable effects have been reported in some studies.

with CYP2C9, CYP2C19 and CYP1A2 also occur. In addition it is itself highly susceptible to enzyme induction (including autoinduction), and any drug that influences CYP3A4 (of which there are many) can have a marked effect on carbamazepine levels. The first metabolite of carbamazepine (carbamazepine 10,11-epoxide) itself has antiepileptic action and a toxic profile, which complicates the prediction of the clinical consequences of carbamazepine interactions.

The effect of other drugs on carbamazepine levels
The interactions with antiepileptic drugs are listed in Tables 8.1 and 8.2. The effects can be due to induction or competitive or non-competitive inhibition of both carbamazepine and CBZ epoxide metabolism.

Antiepileptic drugs
Among the antiepileptic drugs, one of the most important interactions is the lowering of carbamazepine levels due to phenytoin (Figure 8.1), which can be so marked that carbamazepine concentrations cannot be raised to therapeutic levels without causing intoxication – presumably as a result of high CBZ epoxide levels. Less

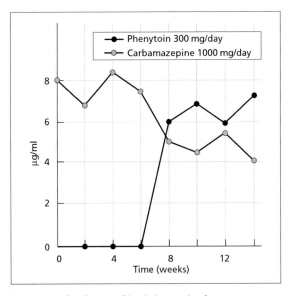

Figure 8.1 The pharmacokinetic interaction between carbamazepine and phenytoin: 50% fall in plasma carbamazepine level following the addition of phenytoin as co-medication.

commonly, similar effects can be due to felbamate, lamotrigine and phenobarbital.

The effects of valproate depend on a balance of induction, inhibition and protein displacement. Even where carbamazepine levels are unchanged on valproate co-medication, CBZ epoxide levels may be increased by as much as four times, an interaction resulting form valproate-induced inhibition of the enzyme epoxide hydrolase. The valproic acid prodrug, valpromide, is associated with an even greater inhibition, with up to eightfold increases in CBZ epoxide levels. Co-medication with stiripentol can double carbamazepine levels. Carbamazepine levels are not affected by gabapentin, levetiracetam, pregabalin, tiagabine, topiramate or vigabatrin.

Serum carbamazepine levels in monotherapy have been shown to fluctuate by between 23 and 45% diurnally; this fluctuation will be greater in the presence of combination therapy, and the use of the slow-release formulation is advised in any patient on moderate doses of carbamazepine in combination with other drugs.

Non-antiepileptic drugs

Various drugs and classes of drug inhibit the metabolism of carbamazepine, and this can result in marked increases in carbamazepine serum levels (Table 8.3). These include: the macrolide antibiotics such as erythromycin, which can increase levels two- to threefold; the calcium channel blockers diltiazem and verapamil, which can double levels (nifedipine has no effect); cimetidine, which can cause a 20–30% increase in carbamazepine levels (ranitidine has no effect); imidazole drugs such as nifimidone; propoxyphene, which increases concentrations by 30–60%; and antidepressants and antipsychotics such as fluoxetine, respiridone, fluvoxamine and viloxazine. Other drugs that increase carbamazepine levels markedly include danazol and the experimental antiepileptic denzimol.

The effect of carbamazepine on levels of other drugs
Antiepileptic drugs

Carbamazepine itself induces the metabolism and hence lowers the concentration of a wide variety of concurrently administered drugs, including phenytoin, ethosuximide, felbamate, lamotrigine, rufinamide, tiagabine, topiramate and valproate, although this is not usually a very marked effect. Dose adjustments are most often needed for lamotrigine and valproate. The effects of carbamazepine on levels of phenobarbital and phenytoin are complex and variable.

Table 8.3 Effect of other drugs on serum concentrations of carbamazepine.

A Drugs causing an increase in serum carbamazepine concentration

Antidepressants
Fluoxetine
Fluvoxamine
Nefazodone
Trazodone
Viloxazine

Antimicrobials
Clarithromycin
Erythromycin
Fluconazole
Isoniazid
Ketoconazole
Metronidazole
Ritonavir
Troleandomycin

Miscellaneous
Cimetidine
Danazol
Dextropropoxyphene
Diltiazem
Risperidone
Quetiapine
Ticlopidine
Verapamil

B Drugs causing a decrease in serum carbamazepine concentration

Probenecid
St John's wort

Non-antiepileptic drugs

Carbamazepine co-medication can compromise clinical effects of antidepressants, antipsychotic drugs, oral anticoagulants, β blockers, chemotherapeutic agents and theophylline (and others) by lowering their serum levels (Table 8.4). Carbamazepine also induces the metabolism of the oestrogen content of the oral contraceptive, carrying the risk of contraceptive failure (see pp. 138–139). The levels of the common tricyclic antidepressants, clozepine, haloperidol, olanzapine, ciclosporin, nimodipine, doxycycline, vincristine and oral anticoagulants have been shown to be routinely reduced by as much as 30–60%

Table 8.4 Effects of carbamazepine on the serum concentrations of other drugs.

Decreased concentration		
Antidepressants	*Antimicrobials*	*Antipsychotic drugs*
Amitriptyline	Albendazole	Chlorpromazine
Bupropion	Doxycycline	Clozapine
Citalopram	Indinavir	Haloperidol
Clomipramine	Itraconazole	Mesoridazine
Desipramine	Metronidazole	Olanzapine
Desmethylclomi-pramine	Praziquantel	Quetipine
Doxepin		Risperidone
Imipramine		Ziprasidone
Mianserin		
Mirtazepine		
Nefazodone		
Nortriptyline		
Paroxitine		
Protriptyline		
Immunosupressants	*Steroids*	*Miscellaneous*
Ciclosporin A	Dexamethasone	Fentanyl
Sirolimus	Hormonal contraceptives	Meperidine
Tacrolimus	Hydrocortisone	Methadone
Oral anticoagulants	Methylprednisolone	Metyrapone
Dicoumarol	Prednisone	Misonidazole
Warfarin	Prednisolone	Paracetamol
		Theophylline
		Thyroxine
		Vecuronium

Table 8.5 Frequency of adverse effects of carbamazepine monotherapy (VA study) therapy.

Effect	Percentage of patients[a] ($n = 231$)	Percentage at 12-month visit[b] ($n = 130$)
Sedation	42	8
Weight gain large	32	9
weight gain	8	3
Nystagmus	30	6
Gastrointestinal symptoms	29	6
Gait problems	25	4
Change in affect or mood	24	4
Tremor	22	5
Cognitive disturbances	18	3
Rash	11	1
Diplopia	10	0
Impotence	7	2

[a]Percentage of patients in whom each type of adverse effect occurred at any time during the trial (mean follow-up, 36 months);
[b]Percentage of patients in whom each type of adverse effect was noted at the 12-month visit.

when carbamazepine co-medication is prescribed; these are significant interactions that may have clinical effects. Carbamazepine can also increase the serum levels of other drugs by competing with or inhibiting their metabolism; the most common examples are listed in Table 8.4.

Adverse effects

The reported frequency of side effects in different studies has varied greatly, but overall between 30 and 50% of individuals taking carbamazepine will experience some, albeit usually mild, side effects especially on initiation of therapy (Table 8.5). These are not only usually mild but also often transient. Less than 5% of patients will need to withdraw the medication because of side effects.

The dose-related side effects are often exacerbated by fluctuations in serum level, and the use of the slow-release formulation of carbamazepine will greatly reduce these. There are few antiepileptic drugs where a slow-release formulation has such clear-cut advantages, and in clinical practice it has become common to recommend the slow-release formulation routinely in all patients on twice-daily dosage or in patients on co-medication. Most clinical studies of the drug were conducted using normal formulations, and this may explain why side effects were more commonly reported than is the experience in routine clinical practice.

Neurological and gastrointestinal side effects

These are common on initiating treatment with carbamazepine or when the dose becomes too high. Once a stable regimen has been established, however, adverse neurological effects are uncommon or mild. The most common side effects (especially when initiating therapy) are sedation, fatigue, diplopia, headache, depression, dizziness, nausea and ataxia. Weight gain is occasionally reported.

These can be largely avoided by starting treatment at a low dose and incrementing the dose slowly.

When the drug level is too high, a highly characteristic side-effect pattern occurs with visual blurring or diplopia and unsteadiness (described often as if being on a boat), and sometimes dizziness. These side effects tend to be manifest a few hours after dosing, and are due to peak blood levels either of the carbamazepine itself or of its 10,11-epoxide. Peak level side effects can be reduced in frequency and intensity by switching to the slow-release formulation of the drug, or by increasing the frequency of dosing. These reversible transient neurotoxic side effects are more common in patients taking combination therapy and also in elderly people.

The carbamazepine 10,11-epoxide:carbamazepine ratio is particularly high in infants and children, and this metabolite can contribute to adverse effects. For the same reason, carbamazepine intoxication in children is commonly caused by metabolic interactions with frequently prescribed co-medication, particularly macrolide antibiotics. Carbamazepine-induced intermittent ataxia can occur in infants after the intake of syrup formulations, which produce high post-absorptive peaks in serum drug concentrations, especially when high doses are ingested to compensate for the high drug clearance in this age group.

The only other common neurological side effects due to carbamazepine are drowsiness, cognitive slowing and memory disturbance. Although these are frequently complained about in the clinic and blamed on drug therapy (including carbamazepine), a causative association can often not be established with certainty. Furthermore, formal testing of the drug in normal doses in normal volunteers has failed to show any marked sedative effect or change in cognitive ability.

Other rarer central nervous system (CNS) side effects include asterixis, dystonia, insomnia and tremor. Sporadic psychiatric disturbances have occurred in relation to carbamazepine therapy, but these are generally rare, and are less prominent with carbamazepine than with most of the other older or newer antiepileptic drugs. At very high levels, coma can occur, and sometimes seizures. It was claimed when the drug was first introduced that the drug had a 'positive psychotropic action' owing putatively to its tricyclic structure (such claims are now not made and, interestingly, similar claims were made for phenytoin, phenobarbital, lamotrigine and levetiracetam when they were introduced – reflecting over-ambitious marketing, placebo effect or simply over-optimism on the part of the doctor or patient).

Carbamazepine can markedly exacerbate atypical absence, tonic and myoclonic seizures, and has been said to worsen the aphasia in occasional patients with the Landau–Kleffner syndrome.

Hypersensitivity, dermatological, hepatic and haematological side effects

Carbamazepine may cause acute hypersensitivity. This most commonly affects the skin and bone marrow, although hepatic and renal hypersensitivity can very rarely occur.

When carbamazepine was first introduced, a number of serious skin reactions were recorded. These included fatal cases of Stevens–Johnson syndrome, Lyell syndrome, DRESS (drug-related rash eosinophilia and systemic symptoms) and exfoliative dermatitis. It has been suggested that the rashes were due to the carbamazepine incipient in the early formulations, although there seems no doubt that carbamazepine itself can cause severe skin reactions. It has also been postulated that the lack of serious recent problems is due to the slow incrementation of dosage now recommended. Although the rate of severe skin reactions on carbamazepine has fallen, carbamazepine is still the third most common drug to cause Stevens–Johnson syndrome (14 cases per 100 000).

Among Han Chinese people in Taiwan, an exceptionally strong association has been noted with HLA-B*1502 allele and the occurrence of a Stevens–Johnson syndrome reaction. This allele occurs in 8% of Han Chinese people and in 1–2% of Caucasians, and is in linkage disequilibrium with a causative polymorphism that has not been identified. It has been recommended that genetic testing for this polymorphism should be carried out in susceptible populations before initiating therapy.

Although a Stevens–Johnson syndrome or other severe skin reactions are rare, minor skin rash is common – occurring in about 5–10% of people in whom carbamazepine therapy is initiated. When a rash appears, it is often difficult to distinguish between the beginnings of severe hypersensitivity and a benign rash, and so discontinuation of therapy is usually recommended. However, some paediatricians particularly give a short course of steroids when a rash appears. The rash fades with the steroids and, if it does not recur on steroid withdrawal, the drug is continued. The rash is mediated by activation of the suppressor-cytotoxic subset of T cells, and successful desensitization by the reintroduction of the drug at very low doses has been carried out without complications.

Systemic lupus erythematosus has very rarely been induced by carbamazepine, although less often than with phenytoin. Isolated renal effects have occasionally been reported.

About 20 cases of carbamazepine hepatotoxicity had been reported by the 1980s, with a mortality rate of about 25%. The risk is now cited to be about 16 cases per 100 000 treatment years. It usually occurs within 3–4 months of initiation of therapy. This takes the form of either a hypersensitivity-induced granulomatous hepatitis or acute hepatitis with hepatic necrosis. The hepatic disturbance is often associated with other signs of hypersensitivity.

Severe haematological complications have also been recorded. During the first 25 years of clinical usage of carbamazepine, 31 cases of thrombocytopenia, 27 cases of aplastic anaemia, 10 cases of agranulocytosis and 8 cases of pancytopenia were reported. The prevalence of aplastic anaemia is now estimated to be between 0.5 and 2 cases per million and the prevalence of agranulocytosis 1.4 cases per million. The overall risk of death due to marrow suppression is 2.2 cases per million. These hypersensitivity reactions usually develop in the first few months of therapy, and carry an appreciable mortality rate. They seem to be more common in elderly people.

In contrast to the rarity of severe hypersensitivity, carbamazepine frequently results in lowered total white blood cell and neutrophil counts. This is usually of no clinical significance. A white cell count <5000 cells/mm^3 is encountered in between 10 and 30% of adults or children treated with carbamazepine, and does not seem to be dose related. If the neutrophil count is <1200 cells/mm^3, the patient should be monitored carefully but dose reduction is not necessary if the neutropenia is asymptomatic. If the neutrophil count falls to <900 cells/mm^3 the drug dosage should be reduced. In this situation restitution of the white count usually occurs within a few days. If red blood cell counts are also reduced in the presence of normal iron and low reticulocyte counts, the drug should be stopped.

Hyponatraemia and other endocrine and biochemical changes

Carbamazepine has a dose-related antidiuretic effect, resulting in low serum sodium and water retention. This effect is very common, and is especially frequent in elderly people. The mechanism is obscure, and evidence has been adduced for both a renal and a pituitary effect. Usually, the mild hyponatraemia and water retention are asymptomatic, and require no correction. Occasionally, a large fluid load (typically, pints of beer) will cause symptomatic hyponatraemia with nausea, weakness and dizziness. Caution is needed when prescribing carbamazepine to elderly people on low-sodium diets, and all patients should be monitored for symptoms of hyponatraemia. As a general rule, if the serum sodium is >125 mmol/L in the absence of symptoms, no action is needed. If hyponatraemia becomes symptomatic, or where levels are repeatedly <120 mmol/L, even in the absence of symptoms, the carbamazepine dosage should be reduced.

Elevated hepatic enzymes are found in up to 5–10% of patients taking carbamazepine, owing to induction of the hepatic enzyme systems, but these changes are without clinical significance.

Carbamazepine can induce a variety of changes in circulating pituitary and sex hormones, but the clinical significance of these effects is quite unclear. Carbamazepine can have, usually minor, effects on testosterone (free, albumin bound and sex hormone-binding globulin [SHBG] bound), luteinizing hormone and prolactin. Hyposexuality, effects on menstruation and reproductive function have been attributed, on rather shaky evidence, to carbamazepine therapy. Free cortisol levels can be increased. Complex effects on the biochemistry of thyroid function occur, but frank hypothyroidism is rare (although it can occur in those with a predisposition or pre-existing hypothyroid state). Thyroxine (T$_4$) levels can be reduced without hypothyroidism, owing to effects on binding, and the measurement of thyroid-stimulating hormone concentrations is a reliable way of assessing thyroid status.

Mild hypocalcaemia and lowered vitamin D levels have been recorded, but frank osteomalacia has not. Although it has been suggested that antiepileptic drugs can contribute to osteoporosis, there is no conclusive evidence that carbamazepine can cause significant bone disease.

Carbamazepine may alter cholesterol metabolism, leading to elevations of the low-density lipoprotein (LDL):total cholesterol ratio, apparently in women and children in particular. The higher LDL:cholesterol ratio and low apolipoprotein A-I levels theoretically could increase the risk of atherosclerosis. Interestingly, elevated cholesterol concentrations also significantly decrease plasma carbamazepine concentrations by enhancing total body clearance.

Levels of immunoglobulins have been shown to be decreased in some patients on carbamazepine. Occasionally a severe and irreversible deficiency state can develop.

Cardiac effects

Carbamazepine can rarely cause bradycardia, Adams–Stokes attacks, aggravation of sick sinus syndrome, tachyarrhythmias and development of congestive heart failure. Very occasionally these are potentially life threatening and this is a risk in those with underlying cardiac disease and particularly in elderly people. Heart block has, however, been reported in otherwise healthy children and in patients with tuberous sclerosis. Caution should therefore be employed, or the drug avoided, in those with pre-existing heart disease and especially in those with atrioventricular conduction defects. Very rarely, there is cardiac involvement in acute hypersensitivity.

Teratogenicity

Large-scale prospective studies show a rate of major congenital malformations of 2–3% in association with carbamazepine monotherapy, a risk that is only 1–2% greater than in the general untreated population. This is a lower risk with valproic acid or higher doses of lamotrigine. The risk of neural tube defects is 0.5–1%. In a case–control study based on 8005 cases of malformations in an international registry, 299 infants had been exposed *in utero* to carbamazepine. Among these infants, the only significant malformations were hypertelorism and localized skull defects, spina bifida on monotherapy and cardiac malformations on polytherapy.

Prospective population-based studies do not suggest any adverse effects on postnatal cognitive development in children exposed to carbamazepine *in utero*. In contrast to earlier reports, there is no real evidence of a risk of reduced head circumference or other body measures in infants exposed to carbamazepine *in utero*.

Other side effects

About 5–10% of individuals develop mild gastrointestinal side effects such as nausea, vomiting or diarrhoea. Other rare side effects that have been reported include colitis and stomatitis, and renal failure (usually in the context of acute hypersensitivity). A retinopathy and effects on the retinal pigment epithelium can occur as a result of carbamazepine (as with other tricyclic compounds), usually causing asymptomatic alterations in colour vision. Very occasional renal effects including proteinuria, haematuria, nephrotic syndrome and renal failure have been recorded in patients on carbamazepine therapy.

Overdose

Death can occur when very large quantities of carbamazepine are taken. The lowest known lethal dose is 60 g. In one series, 2 of 23 cases died. The highest serum level reported was 65 µg/L and the patient survived, as did one patient taking 400 200-mg tablets. At levels above 170 µmol/L, coma and seizures occur. Overdose can also be complicated by cardiac arrhythmia, respiratory depression, seizures, hallucinations, anticholinergic effects, chorea, ataxia and gastrointestinal effects.

Gastric lavage is useful, because gastric emptying is delayed by the drug, as is haemoperfusion. Forced diuresis, peritoneal dialysis and plasmapheresis are now considered to be contraindicated. Seizures should be treated with benzodiazepines.

Antiepileptic effect

The drug was introduced on the basis of a number of open clinical studies before the introduction of current regulatory licensing regulations, which require strictly monitored randomized controlled studies. The open studies have, however, uniformly shown great effectiveness in adults and children, and in monotherapy and combination therapy. These studies were followed, after years of licensed experience, by a series of large-scale comparative studies, in which some element of randomization and control was introduced, and these too consistently showed superiority over placebo and valproate in partial epilepsy, and usually equal effectiveness when compared with phenytoin, valproate, phenobarbital, primidone, lamotrigine and clonazepam in generalized convulsive epilepsy. In some studies, carbamazepine was found to be more effective than phenobarbital.

In the large comparative veterans' study, for example, 1-year remission rates were recorded in 58% and 44%, respectively, of patients with generalized and/or partial seizures. Complete freedom from seizures occurred with carbamazepine more frequently than with phenobarbital at 1, 2 and 3 years of follow-up (Figure 8.2). A second prospective randomized comparative study of 243 adults with previously untreated tonic–clonic or partial epilepsy, with or without secondary generalized seizures, compared patients randomized to phenobarbital, phenytoin, carbamazepine or sodium valproate monotherapy. Complete seizure control was achieved in 27% and 1-year remission after 3 years of follow-up in 75%, with no difference between drugs. Adverse effects necessitating withdrawal were more common in phenobarbital-treated patients (22%) than in patients treated with

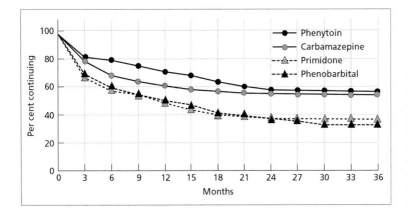

Figure 8.2 The proportion of patients continuing on therapy with carbamazepine, phenobarbital, phenytoin and primidone. Patients were randomized to one of the four drugs and followed for 36 months. More than 50% of patients randomized to phenytoin or carbamazepine remained on therapy, significantly more than those on phenobarbital or primidone.

carbamazepine (11%), valproate (5%) or phenytoin (3%). A double-blind randomized trial compared carbamazepine and vigabatrin in 459 patients, finding higher seizure-free rates with carbamazepine (58%) than with vigabatrin (38%). In a recent double-blind study in newly diagnosed partial-onset or generalized tonic–clonic seizures, patients were randomized to controlled-release carbamazepine (400–1200 mg/day, $n = 285$) or levetiracetam (1000–3000 mg/day, $n = 291$), and each drug was equally effective with 73% seizure free for at least 6 months at the last evaluated dose. Of those achieving remission on carbamazepine, 85% did so at the lowest dose level (400 mg/day). The rates of seizure freedom and the time to first seizure were similar for carbamazepine (immediate-release tablets) and lamotrigine in a double-blind randomized trial including 260 newly diagnosed adult patients with partial-onset or generalized tonic–clonic seizures. In another randomized controlled trial (RCT), topiramate 100 mg/day or 200 mg/day was compared with carbamazepine 600 mg/day, and no significant difference was observed. Carbamazepine has also been compared with oxcarbazepine in a double-blind randomized study of 235 patients with newly diagnosed partial-onset or generalized tonic–clonic seizures, with no differences found.

A randomized comparison of carbamazepine and valproate in 300 adults with newly diagnosed generalized epilepsy was made in the open, multicentre EPITEG study. Overall control of primary and secondary generalized seizures was similar on both drugs, but adverse effects were more common with carbamazepine. In the SANAD (Standard and New Antiepileptic Drugs) study,

1721 patients with epilepsy, for whom carbamazepine was deemed to be preferable to valproate as an initial treatment choice, were randomized to carbamazepine, gabapentin, lamotrigine, oxcarbazepine or topiramate. Carbamazepine had significantly higher 12-month remission rates than gabapentin, and non-significantly higher rates than lamotrigine, topiramate and oxcarbazepine.

Children
There are no class I or II RCTs on partial epilepsy in children. However, a double-blind randomized trial compared carbamazepine 600 mg/day with valproate 1250 mg/day or topiramate 100 or 200 mg/day in children with newly diagnosed epilepsy (partial-onset seizures in most cases), and the time to exit (primary outcome measure) was similar for the different treatment arms. In an open study in newly diagnosed children, patients were randomized to valproate ($n = 130$) or carbamazepine ($n = 130$) and followed for 3 years with similar results in both primary generalized seizures and partial-onset seizures. In another study, 167 children aged 3–16 years, with tonic–clonic or partial seizures, were randomly allocated to treatment with phenobarbital, phenytoin, valproate or carbamazepine; 73% of patients achieved 1-year remission by 3 years of follow-up, with minor differences between the three assessed drugs (the phenobarbital arm was terminated prematurely because of side effects).

Carbamazepine is generally considered to be the drug of choice for complex partial and secondarily generalized seizures in adults and children, and to be superior to other drugs in these patients. Carbamazepine is also considered by many to be the drug of choice in benign childhood epilepsy with centrotemporal spikes (benign rolandic epilepsy), and other benign partial epilepsy syndromes.

Generalized seizures

The use of carbamazepine in the generalized epilepsy syndromes is more controversial.

In adults with idiopathic generalized epilepsy, carbamazepine will, according to most studies and analyses, control tonic–clonic seizures with the same efficacy as valproate or other antiepileptics, but it can exacerbate absence or myoclonic seizures. It is probably more efficacious than valproate in the secondarily generalized seizures (seizures with partial onset and secondary generalization). In the generalized seizure syndromes of childhood, however, its value is less clearcut. In idiopathic generalized epilepsy, it is usually avoided because of its adverse effects on absence seizures or myoclonus, but it nevertheless is as effective in controlling tonic-clonic seizures as valproate or other drugs. Some authors have reported benefit in the Lennox–Gastaut syndrome, but most consider carbamazepine to be contraindicated, and it can certainly exacerbate myoclonus and the nonconvulsive generalized seizures in this syndrome, even when controlling the convulsive attacks. Infantile spasms and febrile convulsions are also generally resistant to carbamazepine therapy.

Clinical use in epilepsy

Carbamazepine is one of the most widely used antiepileptic drugs in the world, and certainly one of the most widely studied. It is the drug of first choice for the entire range of partial seizure types (simple partial, complex partial and secondarily generalised seizures), and in the cryptogenic and symptomatic partial seizure syndromes. It is often the first drug tried in these patients in routine practice.

Carbamazepine is also useful in generalized tonic–clonic seizures associated with idiopathic generalized epilepsy, but usually has little value against other forms of generalized seizure types or generalized epilepsy syndromes. It may exacerbate myoclonus, generalized absence seizures and other non-convulsive types.

It is usual in adults to start at 100 mg/day (or, in induced patients, 200 mg/day) and to double this dose every 2 weeks to a level of 400–800 mg/day in two divided doses. In adults, maintenance doses of between 400 and 1600 mg are commonly used, although higher doses (up to 2800 mg) are occasionally required and tolerated. Starting at a higher initial dose often results in

acute nausea, diplopia, dizziness and drowsiness, and slow introduction at a low dose reduces the risk of this reaction. The slow-release formulation should be prescribed if the drug is poorly tolerated, and this formulation should be used anyway if the drug is taken at a dose of 800 mg/day or higher. It is usual to give the drug at a twice-a-day regimen, and the use of the slow-release formulation on a twice-daily basis (equivalent to four-times-a-day dosing of the conventional formulation in terms of blood level fluctuations) is a far better option than a higher dosing frequency in most situations.

Measurements of plasma concentrations are advisable at the early stages of medication to establish baseline measures, when changes of seizure control or medication occur, or where toxic side effects are suspected. The tolerability of carbamazepine is generally good, but side effects can occur and elderly people, in particular, tolerate carbamazepine (and other antiepileptic drugs) less well. Blood count and serum sodium levels should be checked regularly (annually in patients on stable doses). Plasma carbamazepine and CBZ epoxide measurements are moderately helpful in choosing regimens, but are only poorly correlated with clinical effects. Diurnal interindividual and intraindividual variation, variability in plasma protein binding and co-medication affect plasma concentrations of carbamazepine and CBZ epoxide. Therefore, there is no universal 'therapeutic' level, although plasma concentrations are usually kept between 20 and 50 μmol/L. Having said this, low doses and low blood levels will completely control seizures in many cases, and some patients do not experience side effects when the range is exceeded.

In children the same therapeutic principles apply. Children aged <1 year require a maintenance dose of 100–200 mg, between 1 and 5 years a maintenance dose of 200–400 mg, between 5 and 10 years 400–600 mg, and between 10 and 15 years 400–1000 mg. As the clearance of carbamazepine in children is faster, three-times-daily dosing is often required.

In combination therapy, drug interactions are sometimes problematic. These can be complex and interactions of both carbamazepine and CBZ epoxide metabolism can complicate their interpretation. In combination therapy, the blood levels are even more difficult to interpret.

Of the antiepileptic drugs for which there is sufficient information, carbamazepine is considered to be the safest antiepileptic drugs for use in pregnancy (but is classified as a category C teratogen by the US Food and Drug Administration [FDA]).

Clobazam

Clobazam

Proprietary name: Frisium[a]

Primary indications
Adjunctive and monotherapy in epilepsy. Also for intermittent therapy, one-off prophylactic therapy. Adults and children

Commonly used as first-line drug
No

Usual preparations
Tablet, capsule: 10 mg

Usual dosage – adults
Initial: 10 mg/day; increase by increments of 10 mg/day; maintenance 10–30 mg/day

Usual dosage – children
3–12 years: initial dose 0.25 mg/kg per day; maintenance dose 0.25–1.5 mg/kg per day

Dosing intervals
Once or twice a day

Is dose commonly affected by co-medication?
No

Is dose affected by renal/hepatic disease?
Severe hepatic disease

Does it affect dose of other drugs?
Yes – usually slight effect, occasionally clinically significant

Does it affect the contraceptive pill?
No

Serum level monitoring
Not useful

Common/important adverse events
Drowsiness, sedation, asthenia, ataxia, weakness and hypotonia, diplopia, mood and behavioural change, dependency, withdrawal symptoms

Risk of hypersensitivity
Yes – but slight

Major mechanism of action
$GABA_A$-receptor agonist

Main advantages
Highly effective in some patients with epilepsy resistant to first-line therapy; fewer side effects than with other benzodiazepines

Main disadvantages
Development of tolerance in up to 50% of patients

Comment
Drug of second choice in patients with partial and generalized epilepsy

[a]Name of proprietary brand available in the UK.
GABA, γ-aminobutyric acid.

Clobazam: pharmacokinetics – average adult values

Oral bioavailability	90%
Time to peak levels	1–4 h
Volume of distribution	0.9–1.8 L/kg
Biotransformation	Hepatic demethylation and hydroxylation and then conjugation
Elimination half-life	10–30 h (clobazam); 50 h (N-desmethylclobazam)
Plasma clearance	0.021–0.038 L/h per kg (N-desmethylclobazam)
Protein binding	83%
Active metabolite	N-Desmethylclobazam
Metabolism by hepatic enzymes	CYP3A4
Inhibition or induction of hepatic enzymes	Generally slight effects only
Drug interactions	Usually minor only

Clobazam is a remarkable drug, the role of which in epilepsy is often underestimated. This is partly because it is a benzodiazepine, with all the encumbrance of this drug class, but there has also been a surprising lack of promotion by its manufacturers, in a market place not generally characterized by reticence. The drug has a 1,5-substitution instead of the usual 1,4-benzodiazepine structure. It is unique in this regard, and this structural change results in an 80% reduction in its anxiolytic activity and a 10-fold reduction in its sedative effects, when compared with diazepam in animal studies. The drug was introduced as an anxiolytic and its potent antiepileptic effects were demonstrated later. Its human antiepileptic effect was first reported a decade after its introduction. It has been licensed in Europe since 1975 and in Canada since 1988, but it is unavailable in the USA. It is widely used in specialist epilepsy clinics, where this underdog of a drug has many champions.

Physical and chemical characteristics

Clobazam (molecular weight 300.73) is a crystalline powder, relatively insoluble in water throughout the range of physiological pH, and therefore cannot be given by intravenous or intramuscular injection. It is a weak organic acid. It is also relatively insoluble in lipids, with lipid solubility about 40% of that of diazepam.

Mode of action

Clobazam acts at the benzodiazepine-binding site of the γ-aminobutyric acid A (GABA$_A$)-receptor complex, thus enhancing the inhibitory neurotransmitter action of GABA at the ligand-gated chloride ion channel. It enhances the conductance of the channel up to a concentration of 3 μmol. Quite why its action is distinct from

that of other benzodiazepine drugs is not clearly known, but this could reflect differential binding to the various GABA$_A$-receptor subunits (at least 16 have already been identified). The drug may also exert an action away from the GABA receptor, affecting voltage-sensitive calcium ion conductance and sodium channel function. Studies to investigate whether common genetic variations in the channel correlate with effects have proved negative.

Pharmacokinetics
Absorption

Clobazam has an oral bioavailability of about 90%. It is absorbed rapidly and the time to peak plasma concentrations (T_{max}) after oral dosing is 1–4 h. Absorption is relatively unaffected by age or gender. The rate of absorption is reduced when the drug is taken with or after meals, but the extent of absorption is unaffected. For the patient with epilepsy the timing of ingestion is seldom critical. It could be given rectally, and is rapidly absorbed, but this method of administration has not been adopted in clinical practice.

Distribution

The plasma protein binding of clobazam has been found to be 83%, and the proportion of bound to unbound drug is independent of clobazam concentrations. There is a higher free (unbound) proportion, however, in situations where plasma protein concentrations are greatly lowered, e.g. in advanced hepatic or renal disease, and dosage should be reduced in these situations. Clobazam is distributed widely, but the concentration in brain is proportional to the concentration of the unbound drug in the serum, as is the drug concentration in saliva. There is a good correlation between plasma concentration and dose in an individual patient, but there are large interindividual variations. The drug does enter breast milk to some extent, and the potential for side effects should be considered in breast-fed infants.

Biotransformation and excretion

Clobazam is metabolized in the liver to *N*-desmethylclobazam (otherwise known as norclobazam). This is an important fact, because *N*-desmethylclobazam could be responsible for much of the antiepileptic effect of the drug (Figure 8.3). Arguing against this proposition is the fact that the lipid solubility of the metabolite is lower than that of the parent drug, and that its affinity for the benzodiazepine receptor is at least 10-fold less than that of clobazam. However, the half-life of norclobazam is very much longer, about 50 h or so in healthy volunteers, but less in patients on other enzyme-inducing drugs, and its plasma concentration is considerably higher than that of the parent drug. This is swings and roundabouts, and the exact role of the metabolite has not been fully established. The elimination half-life of clobazam is variable, usually from 10 h to 30 h, with the longest half-lives being in elderly people, and the shortest in patients receiving other antiepileptic drugs. Desmethylclobazam is itself conjugated in the liver and excreted in the bile as the glucuronide and in the urine as a sulphate. At normal clinical doses the plasma concentration of the metabolite is between 300 and 3500 ng/mL, about 10 times higher than the usual clobazam concentrations (20–350 ng/mL).

Drug interactions

Clobazam has a potential for complex interactions, although usually these are clinically insignificant. It can cause either elevation or reduction in phenytoin, phenobarbital or carbamazepine drug levels. However, some patients with high phenytoin levels develop phenytoin toxicity when clobazam is added. Carbamazepine epoxidation can also be enhanced by clobazam co-medication. A rare but unpredictable increase in sodium valproate levels has also been reported, resulting in a confusional state, and clobazam and valproate combinations should be carefully observed. Desmethylclobazam levels can be raised and clobazam levels lowered in patients on combination therapy with phenobarbital, phenytoin or carbamazepine. In the great majority of patients, however, the clinical effects of these interactions are slight and in normal practice problems are rare. However, the adverse effects occasionally observed when clobazam is added to polytherapy regimens can be caused by occult drug interactions.

Adverse effects
Central nervous system and other effects

As clobazam has been so widely used in psychiatric practice as an antianxiolytic, its side-effect profile is well known. The side effects are essentially similar to those of other benzodiazepines, although sedation is much less common than in other drugs (Table 8.6). The frequency

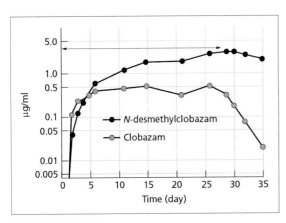

Figure 8.3 Plasma concentrations of clobazam and *N*-desmethylclobazam after 28 days of therapy with clobazam 20 mg/day. Note that the *N*-desmethylclobazam levels at steady state are 10 times greater than those of clobazam. This explains why the active metabolite may be responsible for much of the pharmacological action of clobazam.

Table 8.6 Summary of the reported side effects of clobazam, diazepam and placebo from 70 double-blind studies of the anxiolytic effects of clobazam.

	Clobazam ($n = 1690$)	Diazepam ($n = 1084$)	Placebo ($n = 889$)
Drowsiness	25.8	45.5	9.9
Dizziness	7.0	12.0	2.8
Headache	2.1	3.2	2.9
Nausea	1.6	1.5	2.1
Dry mouth	3.0	2.3	0.9
Constipation	2.1	3.4	0.3
Depression	1.7	2.2	0.3

Table shows the percentage of patients reporting side effects.

in clinical trials of its anxiolytic effect has been reported to lie between 20 and 85%. In clinical trials, the most common side effects reported were sedation and drowsiness, a feeling of dissociation, dizziness, dry mouth, nausea, headache and depression. Amnestic effects are reported. Occasionally, behavioural disturbances, insomnia, irritability and disinhibition are reported, especially in institutionalized populations. Muscle fatigue and weakness occur and it should not be used in patients with severe respiratory disease. As with other benzodiazepines, because it can cause disorderly recruitment of motor units, the drug should not be given to patients with myasthenia gravis. In clinical trials, the side effects were of a severity sufficient to change dose or terminate treatment in 5–15% of patients. In clinical practice it must be said that side effects are seemingly less common, possibly reflecting the different patient group. Of all these side effects, sedation is the most important, but the measured effects of normal dosages of clobazam on cognitive tests have been shown to be very slight. There is a slight risk of dependency, as with all benzodiazepines, although in epilepsy patients this is not common. There are no definitive data on teratogenicity.

Tolerance and symptoms on withdrawal

Undoubtedly, clinically the most problematic phenomenon is the tendency for clobazam to lose its beneficial effect (the development of tolerance). This is a property shared by all benzodiazepines, but in animal studies tolerance developed more frequently with clobazam than with clonazepam. It is traditionally claimed that 30–50% of patients prescribed clobazam can expect to develop tolerance, although more recent studies show lower proportions, and this problem, in routine clinical practice, may have been exaggerated. Despite the importance of tolerance, the mechanisms are unknown, and the frequently quoted 'downregulation of the GABA$_A$ receptor' is descriptive rather than explanatory. Better news is that tolerance to the sedative effects is much more prominent than tolerance to the antiepileptic effects and, if a patient develops sedation on starting treatment, it is well worth while persisting with therapy, because the sedation usually wears off within a week or so. Tolerance is more common at higher doses and with continuous rather than intermittent therapy.

Withdrawal symptoms (irritability, restlessness or difficulties in concentrating) are noticeable in about 5–10% of patients during the first few weeks after withdrawal. Idiosyncratic allergic reactions are very rare and, as far as this author is aware, no fatal side effects have been reported.

Antiepileptic effect

The drug was introduced before double-blind placebo-controlled clinical trials had become a fundamental requirement. The first report was an open study by Gastaut in 1977, who became a great enthusiast of the drug, noting positive results in 76% of 140 patients with severe epilepsy, an effect maintained, however, in only 53% after a few months. Many other trials have followed. There have more recently been nine double-blind trials in refractory partial epilepsy, and all demonstrated striking benefit. In one study, over 50% of patients showed a greater than 50% reduction of seizures, and in another the mean reduction was 30%. The largest of the clobazam double-blind cross-over trials involved 129 adults, mainly with resistant partial-onset seizures, and involved 12 weeks on active medication and 12 weeks on placebo. Fifteen per cent of patients achieved seizure freedom. As the trials were all carried out in patients with longstanding chronic and previously refractory epilepsy, this is an impressive result – and certainly better than observed with many other currently available drugs. A recent Cochrane review concluded that 'clobazam as an add-on treatment may reduce seizure frequency and may be most effective in partial-onset seizures. However, it is not clear who will best benefit and over what timeframe'.

The drug has also been the subject of numerous open studies, often with a wider range of patients, and some reported quite remarkable effects. The biggest study is a retrospective survey from Canada of 877 patients, which showed a greater than 50% response in more than 40% of patients, and 10–30% became seizure free; at 4 years 40–50% of patients continued the drug. The seizure frequency for each seizure type, except tonic seizures, was reduced by more than 50% in 40–50% of patients. Twenty per cent of patients stopped clobazam because of poor efficacy, 4% stopped for safety-related reasons including drug interactions and 8% stopped for both reasons. Possible side effects (predominantly somnolence) were reported by 32%; however, in only 11% were the side effects sufficiently severe to cause discontinuation of medication. Tolerance leading to discontinuation of clobazam was reported in 9%.

It has been claimed, on an anecdotal basis, that patients with partial seizures but no widespread cerebral impairment obtain the most worthwhile benefit. Patients with secondarily generalized seizures also respond, however, as do those with absence seizures, myoclonus, the Lennox–Gastaut syndrome, startle epilepsy, non-convulsive status epilepticus, electrical status during slow-wave sleep (ESES), reflex epilepsies, alcohol withdrawal seizures and seizures that accompany the benign childhood partial epilepsies.

There have been no large-scale trials of clobazam in monotherapy in adults, but a recent multicentre Canadian study in 235 drug-naïve children with recent-onset partial, secondarily generalized and generalized tonic–clonic seizures found the drug as effective as monotherapy with phenytoin or carbamazepine.

No clear relationship has been found between serum level and seizure control, but it is complicated by the development of tolerance. An optimum range of serum levels in chronic epilepsy has not been established.

Other studies in specific circumstances include a comparison with phenytoin in cysticercosis in which clobazam provided superior efficacy, a prophylactic study of the prevention of febrile seizures in which intermittent clobazam reduced the risk of recurrent seizures from 12.0% on placebo to 1.7% on clobazam, and studies in catamenial epilepsy and non-convulsive status. In each of these indications, the drug showed marked efficacy

Clinical use in epilepsy

Clobazam should be considered as adjunctive therapy whenever treatment with a single first-line antiepileptic drug has proved ineffective. In the author's own practice, clobazam is often the first adjunctive drug to be tried. It is effective in a wide range of epilepsies, although perhaps best in those with partial seizures alone. It can be used in patients with Lennox–Gastaut syndrome and other primarily and secondarily generalized epilepsies. It is effective in a broad spectrum of other types of epilepsy and non-convulsive status syndromes. It is, in routine practice, very well tolerated, with few side effects. Its mild anxiolytic effect is also useful in some patients with epilepsy. The development of tolerance is the most prominent clinical problem. Manoeuvres such as drug holidays, initiation at very low doses or the use of very high doses have all failed to circumvent this problem.

In Canada, clobazam is particularly popular where, in children, clobazam monotherapy is used as first-line treatment for many epilepsy syndromes, including benign myoclonic epilepsy of infancy, most unspecified cryptogenic and symptomatic generalized epilepsies, and idiopathic, symptomatic and cryptogenic partial epilepsies. It is relatively contraindicated in children with abnormal behaviour.

Clobazam also has a particularly useful role in other situations. It is helpful as a temporary therapy to cover drug withdrawal or a period during which other major medication changes are under way. It is also useful as one-off prophylactic therapy on special occasions when it is particularly important to prevent a seizure (e.g. on days of travel, interviews, examinations). Although there are no formal studies of the drug used in this way, the effect is often rapid and reliable, and the low incidence of side effects makes it an ideal choice for such therapy.

Clobazam can also be used in intermittent therapy for fever to prevent febrile seizures and in catamenial epilepsy (see p. 139), and is the best available drug for these purposes. It can be used to prevent clusters of seizures developing (with 10 mg given after the first seizure) and in non-convulsive status epilepticus.

In children, the usual starting dose is about 0.25 mg/kg per day and this is increased over a few weeks to 0.5 mg/kg per day. The maximum dose is usually 1.5 mg/kg per day. In adults it is administered orally at a dose of 10–20 mg/day (occasionally 30 mg/day), usually taken at night or in a twice-daily regimen. The only available preparation is as 10 mg tablets. Higher dosages are seldom effective and should be avoided. The rectal administration of the drug has been explored experimentally, but is not used in clinical practice. There are no parenteral formulations. Blood level monitoring is not commonly performed. It should not be used in patients with myasthenia or severe respiratory disease, or in those with severe hepatic disease. Withdrawal should be gradual (routinely, 10 mg every 1–2 months). It is advisable to observe the same precautions with clobazam as with other benzodiazepine drugs in relation to the risk of dependency.

Clonazepam

Clonazepam was one of the earliest benzodiazepine drugs used for epilepsy. It was licensed in Europe in 1975 and then in North America and throughout the world. It is a 1,4-substituted benzodiazepine, a structure shared with diazepam and all the other antiepileptic drugs of this class, with the notable exception of clobazam. It has in the past been widely used, although now it has largely been superseded by other drugs with fewer side effects.

Physical and chemical characteristics

Clonazepam is a crystalline powder (5-(2-chlorophenol)-1,3-dihydro-7-nitro-2H-1,4-benzodiazepin-2-one;

Clonazepam

Proprietary name: Rivotril[a]

Primary indications

Monotherapy and adjunctive therapy in partial and generalized seizures (including absence and myoclonus) and also the Lennox–Gastaut syndrome, neonatal seizures, infantile spasms and status epilepticus. Adults and children

Commonly used as first-line drug

No

Usual preparations

Tablets: 0.5, 1, 2 mg; liquid: 1 mg and 2.5 mg in 1 mL diluent

Usual dosage – adults

Initial: 0.25 mg at night; increments of 0.25–0.5 mg/day every 2 weeks
Maintenance: 0.5–4 mg/day

Usual dosage – children

Initial: <1 year: 0.25 mg/day
1–5 years: 0.25 mg/day
5–12 years: 0.25 mg/day
Maintenance:
<1 year: 1 mg/day
1–5 years: 1–2 mg/day
5–12 years: 1–3 mg/day

Dosing intervals

Once or twice a day

Is dose commonly affected by co-medication?

No

Is dose affected by renal/hepatic disease?

Severe hepatic disease

Does it affect dose of other drugs?

No

Does it affect the contraceptive pill?

No

Serum level monitoring

Not useful

Common/important adverse events

Drowsiness, sedation, asthenia, ataxia, weakness and hypotonia, diplopia, mood and behavioural change, drooling and hypersalivation, dependency, withdrawal symptoms

Risk of hypersensitivity

Yes – but slight

Major mechanism of action

$GABA_A$-receptor agonist

Main advantages

Useful action especially in children; wide spectrum of activity

Main disadvantages

Side effects, particularly sedation; tolerance; withdrawal syndrome

Comment

Second-choice antiepileptic drug, with wide spectrum of activity, used particularly in children. Use limited by side effects

[a]Name of proprietary brand available in the UK.

Clonazepam: pharmacokinetics – average adult values

Oral bioavailability	80%
Time to peak levels	1–4 h
Volume of distribution	3 L/kg
Biotransformation	Hepatic reduction, hydroxylation and acetylation
Elimination half-life	20–55 h (mean 30)
Plasma clearance	0.09 L/kg per h
Protein binding	86%
Active metabolite	None
Metabolism by hepatic enzymes	CYO3A4
Inhibition or induction of hepatic enzymes	Generally slight effects only
Drug interactions	Usually minor only

molecular weight 315.7) with pK_a values of 1.5 and 10.5, and is virtually undissociated throughout the physiological pH range. It is highly lipid soluble.

Mode of action

Clonazepam, similar to all other benzodiazepines, is an agonist at the $GABA_A$ receptor. The benzodiazepines increase channel opening frequency at the $GABA_A$ receptor, resulting in enhanced chloride conductance and neuronal hyperpolarization. Clonazepam has higher affinity binding to the benzodiazepine receptor than diazepam or other benzodiazepines, and furthermore clonazepam binds to subgroups of the $GABA_A$ receptor that do not bind the other benzodiazepine drugs. In the rat, clonazepam alone binds in the spinal cord and striation and has a high concentration in the cerebellum. The drug also has some action on sodium channel conductance.

Pharmacokinetics

Absorption

Clonazepam is well and reliably absorbed, with an oral bioavailability of 80% or more. It reaches a peak plasma level within 1–4 h of oral administration in most people, although this may be delayed up to 8 h. Intravenous preparations are widely used for emergency therapy. Buccal or intranasal administration of a solution has been explored, but is not in common clinical usage.

Distribution

Clonazepam is 86% bound to plasma proteins, with a volume distribution of between 1.5 and 4.4 L/kg, reflecting its high lipid solubility. It rapidly crosses into the brain, where it is passively absorbed with a linear brain:plasma concentration ratio.

Biotransformation and excretion

Clonazepam is metabolized in the liver first by nitro-reduction and then by acetylation and hydroxylation, and the metabolic processes are greatly influenced by genetic factors (especially acetylator status). There are various metabolites, none of which has clinically important pharmacological activity. The clearance of clonazepam is slow, in adults approximately 0.09 L/kg per h. Less than 0.5% of the parent drug is recovered unchanged in the urine. As metabolism is influenced by individual genetic variation, the half-life of clonazepam is very variable, falling in most patients between 20 and 55 h. In studies in neonates half-lives have been recorded of 20–43 h and in children of 22–33 h. There seems to be no correlation between antiepileptic efficacy and plasma level.

Drug interactions

It is rare for clonazepam to alter levels of other drugs in any clinically relevant manner, although minor effects are common. Clonazepam levels are lowered by co-administration with carbamazepine or phenobarbital and presumably other enzyme-inducing drugs. Lamotrigine can raise clonazepam levels. However, these effects are seldom of clinical importance.

Adverse effects

Neurological effects

The most common important side effect of clonazepam is sedation. There is no doubt that, even at low doses, a significant number of patients experience unacceptable levels of drowsiness and this limits the value of the drug in normal clinical practice. This adverse effect seems to be less marked in children than in adults, which might explain the greater popularity of clonazepam among paediatricians than among neurologists treating adults. Other side effects are much less troublesome and are typical of those of other benzodiazepine drugs. These include incoordination, hypotonia, blurred vision, hyperactivity, restlessness, irritability, short attention span, behavioural change, psychosis, depression and other neuropsychiatric effects. This list may be long, but the side effects are not commonly dose limiting. Behavioural changes seem to be more prominent in patients with psychiatric problems. The mixture of hypotonia, hypersecretion, somnolence and ataxia is characteristic and can be troublesome, especially in young children.

Other side effects

Hypersecretion and hypersalivation may be troublesome in infants and children. In infants, too, cardiovascular depression and respiratory depression have been observed. Similar to other benzodiazepines, clonazepam may occasionally increase the frequency of certain seizure types (e.g. tonic seizures). Occasional idiosyncratic allergic reactions including marked leucopenia have been observed. As with other benzodiazepines, because of an effect on motor unit recruitment, it should not be used in myasthenia gravis. The teratogenicity of clonazepam has not been well studied, although an increased risk of major malformations has been reported in individual cases, as have growth retardation and dysmorphism.

Tolerance and symptoms on withdrawal

Tolerance to the antiepileptic effects has been well described, and is common (although possibly less common than with clobazam) and troublesome. Cross-tolerance between benzodiazepine drugs is observed. Withdrawal symptoms can be prominent, and in one study in children symptoms occurred in over 50%. The symptoms most commonly reported on withdrawal include seizures, increased anxiety, insomnia, restlessness, confusion and occasionally catatonia, and these are most marked in patients with psychiatric co-morbidity. Sudden withdrawal carries a serious risk of seizure exacerbation and status epilepticus. Gradual withdrawal minimizes these problems and, in routine practice, withdrawal at a decremental rate not exceeding 0.5 mg/month is strongly advised.

Overdose

Benzodiazepine overdose produces respiratory depression and coma, and death is common if untreated. Supportive therapy is effective, and activated charcoal, exchange transfusions and flumazenil infusion can be used.

Antiepileptic effect

Clonazepam is a potent antiepileptic drug, and is effective against most types of seizures and in most syndromes. However, because of its potential to cause sedation and other side effects, and the problem of tolerance, it is now not commonly used in routine practice, but is reserved as second-line adjunctive therapy in severe epilepsy.

Although it has a wide spectrum of activity, its main role nowadays is in the treatment of the generalized epilepsies, and especially those with a myoclonic element, and is indeed one of the drugs of choice for this indication in the progressive myoclonic epilepsies, primary generalized epilepsy and also the symptomatic secondary myoclonic epilepsies. It can be useful against all the seizure types in the Lennox–Gastaut syndrome. It is frequently used by specialists in movement disorders for subcortical myoclonus. It is also undoubtedly effective in absence epilepsy, and may work where other drugs have failed, and has a useful effect against tonic–clonic seizures whatever their cause. Early reports suggested that it was useful in partial seizures, although a recent literature review concluded that its effect is relatively modest. However, it is occasionally used in benign rolandic epilepsy and epilepsia partialis continua. Clonazepam has also been shown to be relatively safe in acute intermittent porphyria, and intravenous clonazepam is effective in controlling neonatal convulsions.

Clonazepam is still used widely in the treatment of various forms of status epilepticus. Its indications are exactly the same as those for diazepam, and its effectiveness is similar. It can be given intravenously or rectally in the emergency setting (see pp. 307–308). In status epilepticus, clonazepam has a longer duration of action (about 24h) than diazepam (about 2h).

Clinical use in epilepsy

Clonazepam is used less often than clobazam in most countries (France may be an exception). The reason is its greater propensity to cause side effects, including behavioural problems in children, somnolence and ataxia. It should be considered when myoclonus or other generalized seizures have failed to respond to other first-line medications. Clonazepam is usually introduced very slowly, starting in children with approximately 0.025 mg/kg per day and gradually increasing the dose to 0.1 mg/kg per day. The initial dosage in adults is usually 0.25 mg and this is increased slowly to between 0.5 and 4 mg/day in a once- or twice-daily regimen. It is more widely used in status epilepticus as a perfectly reasonable alternative to diazepam.

Eslicarbazepine acetate

Eslicarbazepine acetate (Zebinex®; known previously as BIA 2-093) is a voltage-gated sodium channel blocker

Eslicarbazepine acetate

Proprietary name: Zebinix[a]

Primary indications
Adjunctive therapy in refractory partial-onset seizures. Adults only

Commonly used as first-line drug
No

Usual preparations
Tablets: 400 mg, 600 mg, 800 mg; suspension: 50 mg/mL

Usual dosage – adults
Initial: 200–400 mg at night; increments of 400 mg every 2 weeks
Maintenance 800–1200 mg/day

Dosing intervals
Once a day

Is dose commonly affected by co-medication?
Yes

Is dose affected by renal/hepatic disease?
Dose adjustments needed in moderate renal disease

Does it affect dose of other drugs?
Yes

Does it affect the contraceptive pill?
Yes

Serum level monitoring
Utility not established

Common/important adverse events
Headache, dizziness, somnolence, nausea, diplopia, vomiting, blurred vision, vertigo, fatigue, constipation and diarrhoea others as with oxcarbazepine but probably less hyponatremia

Risk of hypersensitivity
None to date

Major mechanism of action
Inhibition of voltage-dependent sodium conductance.

Main advantages
It is not metabolized by CYP enzymes; properties similar to oxcarbazepine but may cause less hyonatraemia; once daily dosing

Main disadvantages
New antiepileptic drug with limited clinical experience. Properties similar to oxcarbazepine

Comment
Drug of second choice for partial seizures. Its pharmacological and clinical properties are similar to those of oxcarbazepine

[a]Name of proprietary brand available in the UK.

Eslicarbazepine: pharmacokinetics – average adult values	
Oral bioavailability	<100%
Time to peak levels	2–3 h[a]
Volume of distribution	2.7 L/kg[a]
Biotransformation	Hydrolysis to eslicarbazepine, and then glucuronidation (33%), with 67% excreted unchanged
Elimination half-life	13–20 h[a]
Plasma clearance	0.055 L/kg per h[a]
Protein binding	30%[a]
Active metabolite	Eslicarbazepine
Metabolism by hepatic enzymes	Non-CYP enzymes: hydrolysis and conjugation
Inhibition or induction of hepatic enzymes	Inhibits CYP2C9
Drug interactions	Common

[a]Refers to eslicarbazepine, the active metabolite.

that was identified for clinical development in the mid-1990s by Bial. It is related to carbamazepine, but unlike carbamazepine is not metabolized to carbamazepine 10,11-epoxide. Eslicarbazepine acetate is metabolized to eslicarbazepine, which is responsible for its activity. Oxcarbazepine is also a prodrug of eslicarbazepine, but is metabolized into the *R*-isomer (*R*-licarbazepine) as well as the *S*-isomer (*S*-licarbazepine) (Figure 8.4). Differences between eslicarbazepine acetate and oxcarbazepine are presumably largely due to this metabolic distinction. Eslicarbazepine acetate was licensed in 2009 for use in Europe.

Physical and chemical characteristics
Eslicarbazepine acetate is the *S*-isomer (*S*)-10-acetoxy-10,11-dihydro-5*H*-dibenz[*b,f*]azepine-5-carboxamide and has a molecular weight of 296.32. It is a neutral compound, insoluble in water but freely soluble in organic solvent.

Mode of action
Eslicarbazepine is, similar to carbamazepine and oxcarbazepine, a sodium channel blocker, with a similar profile to oxcarbazepine.

Pharmacokinetics
The pharmacokinetics have been studied in patients and healthy volunteers.

Absorption
Absorption is virtually complete with peak levels 2–3 h after dosing and unaffected by food.

Distribution
About 30% of eslicarbazepine is bound to plasma protein. The volume of distribution is 2.7 L/kg. Data on distribution in the CSF and brain in routine practice are not yet available.

Biotransformation and excretion
Eslicarbazepine acetate is rapidly hydrolysed with peak levels of eslicarbazepine reached within 2–3 h of dosing. Eslicarbazepine is glucuronidated (about 30% of the total dose) but not metabolized by the CYP enzymes, and is then excreted by the kidneys (two-thirds unchanged and one-third as the glucuronide). Formal studies have shown few differences between kinetic parameters in healthy young adults and elderly people, and the clearance in young adults with epilepsy is similar to that in elderly people with epilepsy. In those with renal impairment, where the creatinine clearance is <30–60 mL/min, the dose should be halved, but there are no data on people with creatinine clearance levels <30 mL/min. Haemodialysis removes eslicarbazepine completely. Moderate liver impairment has no effect on the kinetics of eslicarbazepine and there are no data in severe hepatic failure. There are also no data in pregnancy.

Drug interactions
Eslicarbazepine inhibits CYP2C9 but none of the other P450 enzymes. Eslicarbazepine acetate has no effect on carbamazepine, lamotrigine levetiracetam or valproate. Phenytoin levels may rise in co-medication. Eslicarbazepine acetate decreases the plasma levels of steroid oral contraceptives, and may reduce contraceptive

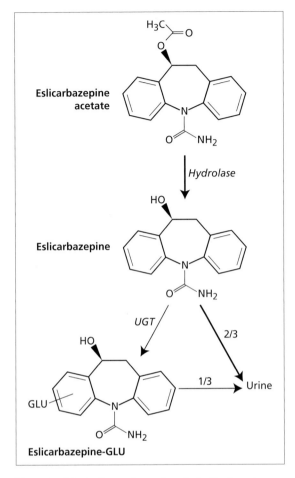

Figure 8.4 Metabolism and excretion of of eslicarbazepine acetate.

vomiting, blurred vision, vertigo, fatigue, constipation and diarrhoea (Table 8.6). These were generally dose related. At 1200 mg/day, 19% of patients discontinued the clinical trial because of side effects (compared with 4.5% in the placebo group). Most side effects were mild to moderate and less than 5% of patients had side effects rated as severe. Hyponatraemia was recorded in only four patients in the clinical trials, which is a much lower rate than with oxcarbazepine, but patient selection in the trials would have acted to avoid hyponatremia. There are no post-marketing data as yet and very limited long-term data, and no data on teratogenicity.

Antiepileptic effect

Efficacy data are based on several phase 2 and three phase 3 studies. The latter were multicentre, double-blind, randomized, placebo-controlled studies in 1049 adult refractory patients enrolled by 125 sites in 23 countries. In the pooled analysis of the intention-to-treat findings, the 50% responder rates were on 21% for placebo and for eslicarbazepine acetate 23% at 400 mg/day, 36% at 800 mg/day and 43% at 1200 mg/day, with significant differences between placebo and eslicarbazepine acetate at doses of 800 and 1200 mg/day. The relative reduction in seizure frequency on eslicarbazepine was 18% on 400 mg/day, 29% on 800 mg/day and 31% on 1200 mg/day compared with 9% on placebo. Of the 857 patients who completed the double-blind phase, 833 (97%) entered the long-term extension phase and 612 completed 1 year of treatment, a retention rate of 73.5%.

Clinical use in epilepsy

Eslicarbazepine acetate is a recently licensed antiepileptic drug, with, at the time of writing, very limited experience in routine clinical practice. It is very similar to oxcarbazepine, and in fact oxcarbazepine is a prodrug of eslicarbazepine. Whether it will prove in the longer run to have any advantage over oxcarbazepine, a much more established compound, remains to be seen. The main difference is that oxcarbazepine is also metabolized to the *R*-isomer of licarbazepine and differences between the drugs are presumably largely related to this aspect of metabolism. There are a number of favourable features to eslicarbazepine that are worth emphasizing. The drug is hydrolysed and then undergoes glucuronidation without significant involvement of CYP-mediated metabolism, which is an advantage over carbamazepine, for example. It seems to have efficacy in combination with other sodium channel-blocking drugs and can, it is

effectiveness. Carbamazepine, phenobarbital and phenytoin decrease plasma eslicarbazepine levels, but valproate, lamotrigine, gabapentin, clobazam, levetiracetam and topiramate have no effect on eslicarbazepine levels. Eslicarbazepine acetate 1200 mg, when given once daily to females co-medicated with the combined oral contraceptive, resulted in a mean decrease of 37% and 42% in systemic exposure to levonorgestrel and ethinylestradiol, respectively, caused presumably by an induction of CYP3A4.

Adverse effects

In the clinical trials, the most frequent adverse effects were headache, dizziness, somnolence, nausea, diplopia, claimed, be used in combination with carbamazepine. It seems relatively well tolerated (at least from data from the clinical trials) with discontinuation rates similar to other major antiepileptic drugs, including pregabalin and levetiracetam. The lack of hyponatremia (if confirmed in less selected populations) and better tolerability at higher dose would be advantages. No idiosyncratic reactions have been reported and relatively little weight gain. It seems reasonable to give the compound in once-a-day dosing which is also a relative advantage over some other antiepileptic drugs. On the less positive side are its interaction with the contraceptive pill, which may reduce its effectiveness, its other drug interactions and dosing that has to be modified in those with renal impairment. In summary, eslicarbazepine acetate seems a promising new antiepileptic drug.

Ethosuximide

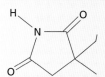

Proprietary names: Zarontin,[a] Emeside[a]

Primary indications
Monotherapy or adjunctive therapy for generalized absence seizures. Adults and children

Commonly used as first-line drug
No

Usual preparations
Capsules: 250 mg; syrup: 250 mg/5 mL

Usual dosage – adults
Initial: 250 mg; then increased by increments of 250 mg/day every 2 weeks
Maintenance: 750–1500 mg/day

Usual dosage – children
Initial: 10–15 mg/kg per day
Maintenance: 20–40 mg/kg per day

Dosing intervals
2–3 times/day

Is dose commonly affected by co-medication?
Yes

Is dose affected by renal/hepatic disease?
Hepatic disease and severe renal disease

Does it affect dose of other drugs?
No

Does it affect the contraceptive pill?
No

Serum level monitoring
Very useful

Target range
300–700 μmol/L

Common/important adverse events
Gastrointestinal symptoms, drowsiness, ataxia, diplopia, headache, dizziness, hiccups, sedation, behavioural disturbances, acute psychotic reactions, extrapyramidal symptoms, blood dyscrasia, rash, lupus-like syndrome, severe hypersensitivity

Risk of hypersensitivity
Yes – marked risk

Major mechanism of action
Inhibition of calcium T-channel conductance

Main advantages
Well-established treatment for generalized absence seizures; less risk of hepatic toxicity than valproate in young children

Main disadvantages
Side effects common; risk of hypersensitivity; no effect against tonic–clonic seizures

Comment
Drug now usually of second choice for typical generalized absence seizures (petit mal)

[a]Name of proprietary brand available in the UK.

Ethosuximide: pharmacokinetics – average adult values	
Oral bioavailability	<100%
Time to peak levels	<4 h
Volume of distribution	0.65 L/kg
Biotransformation	Hepatic oxidation then conjugation
Elimination half-life	40–70 h (adults; varies with co-medication) 30–40 h (children; varies with co-medication)
Plasma clearance	0.010–0.015 L/kg per h
Protein binding	<10%
Active metabolite	None
Metabolism by hepatic enzymes	CYP3A4, CYP2E1 and then conjugation
Inhibition or induction of hepatic enzymes	No
Drug interactions	Common

In the 1950s and 1960s a series of succinimide drugs were widely prescribed for the treatment of all types of epilepsy. Their toxicity limited their utility, however, and today only ethosuximide is in general use. Ethosuximide, introduced into clinical practice in 1958, has only one indication – the treatment of generalized absence seizures (petit-mal seizures). Its usage has largely ended with the introduction of newer drugs, but some paediatricians still occasionally consider this drug as first-line therapy for absence seizures, although this role has been largely superseded by valproate, levetiracetam, lamotrigine and topiramate, or more often now for patients resistant to these newer first-line therapies.

Physical and chemical properties

Ethosuximide (molecular weight 141.2) is a white crystalline racemate, freely soluble in water and alcohol, and it has a pK_a of 9.3. It is a racemate mixture, but with no stereoselectivity.

Mode of action

The drug exerts a voltage-dependent blockade of low-threshold T-type calcium currents in the thalamus and this is almost certainly the mechanism of its effect against absence seizures. The drug also enhances postsynaptic GABA action and affects ATPase and membrane transport processes, but these effects are thought not to contribute to its antiepileptic properties.

Pharmacokinetics
Absorption

Ethosuximide is rapidly absorbed, with an oral bioavailability of over 90%. Peak plasma levels are probably mostly reached within 4 h of administration, although some studies have shown some delay with peak levels in some patients reached only after 7 h. The syrup formulation tends to be more rapidly absorbed than the capsules, but both formulations are bioequivalent.

Distribution

Ethosuximide is widely distributed. Concentrations in saliva, CSF and tears are similar to those in plasma. The apparent volume of distribution after oral administration is 0.62–0.65 L/kg body weight in adults and 0.69 L/kg in children. There is negligible plasma protein binding. The drug readily crosses the placenta and also readily crosses into breast milk (with a breast milk:serum ratio of 0.8–0.9) and the serum levels of a breast-feeding infant are approximately 30–50% of those of the mother.

Biotransformation and elimination

Ethosuximide shows linear kinetics over the usual dosage ranges. The drug is extensively metabolized in the liver, first by oxidation and then by conjunction. The major enzymes involved are the CYP3A subgroup of the hepatic cytochrome P450 system, with some contribution from CYP2E1. The metabolites have no significant antiepileptic action. About 10–20% of the drug is excreted unchanged in the urine. Ethosuximide is cleared slowly, with a mean half-life in adults of 40–70 h and 30–40 h in children and neonates. The steady state is reached in 12 days in adults and 6 days in children. There is considerable interindividual variability, but the elimination half-life is unaffected by drug dosage. The total body clearance is 0.010–0.015 L/kg per h and may be slightly lower in women. Ethosuximide does not induce hepatic microsomal enzymes, nor is there autoinduction.

Renal disease, unless very severe, does not affect ethosuximide concentrations; 50% of the drug is removed by 6 h of dialysis. The effect of hepatic disease has not been formally studied, but, as ethosuximide is heavily metabolized, one would expect severe hepatic disease to alter its pharmacokinetics. Haemodialysis and peritoneal dialysis readily remove ethosuximide from the plasma.

Drug interactions

Ethosuximide does not generally affect serum levels of other antiepileptic or non-antiepileptic drugs.

However, co-medication can affect ethosuximide levels. Sodium valproate has variable and complex effects, but can result in an increase of up to 50% in ethosuximide levels owing to valproate-induced inhibition of ethosuximide metabolism. Co-medication with carbamazepine can result in a significant decrease (up to 50%) in ethosuximide plasma concentrations, as a result of the hepatic enzyme-inducing properties of carbamazepine. Co-medication with phenytoin and phenobarbital also lowers ethosuximide levels. The potential for interactions with the newer antiepileptic drugs has not been studied. Rifampicin, a classic inducer of CYP3A, has been shown to increase the clearance of ethosuximide by 90%. Other drugs acting on this enzyme system would also be expected to have a similar effect.

Adverse effects
Idiosyncratic reactions

Ethosuximide has the potential to cause severe idiosyncratic reactions. The skin is most commonly affected, followed by the formed elements of the blood and the liver, and to a lesser extent the nervous system and kidneys. These reactions range from non-specific symptoms such as lymphadenopathy, arthralgias, eosinophilia and fever to more severe allergic dermatitis, rash, erythema multiforme, Stevens–Johnson syndrome, autoimmune thyroiditis, myocarditis, pericarditis and systemic lupus erythematosus. Blood dyscrasias have occurred but are rare, and include aplastic anaemia and agranulocytosis. In the early years of therapy, severe haematological effects were thought to be relatively common. However, only eight cases of ethosuximide-associated aplastic anaemia were reported between 1958 and 1994, all with onset 6 weeks to 8 months after initiation of ethosuximide therapy. Most patients were on polypharmacy, and five of the eight patients died.

Other side effects

The side effects in 12 clinical trials published between 1958 and 1966 are summarized in Table 8.7. The overall incidence of adverse effects ranged from 26% to 46%. The most common adverse effects involve the gastrointestinal system, and include nausea, abdominal discomfort, anorexia, vomiting and diarrhoea. These are dose dependent but occasionally are severe enough to preclude therapy. Ethosuximide can also cause a wide range of dose-dependent CNS effects. The most common are

Table 8.7 Summary of the adverse effects due to ethosuximide; data from 12 early studies, published between 1958 and 1966, each involving 50 or more subjects receiving ethosuximide.

Adverse effect	Range (median), %
Any adverse effect	26–46 (37)
Gastrointestinal disturbances (nausea, abdominal discomfort, anorexia, vomiting and diarrhoea)	4–29 (13)
Drowsiness	0–16 (7)
Rash	0–6 (0)
Ataxia	0–1 (0)
Dizziness	0–4 (1)
Hiccups	0–5 (0)

insomnia, nervousness, dizziness, hiccups, lethargy, fatigue, ataxia, and behavioural changes such as aggression, euphoria, irritability and hyperactivity. Headache is a particular problem, occurring in one in eight treated children and is often not dose dependent. The effect of ethosuximide on cognition is unclear.

There are some reports of memory, speech and emotional disturbances, and ethosuximide can certainly occasionally cause severe behavioural changes, particularly irritability, depression and anxiety, delirium, hallucinations and occasionally a psychotic reaction. The psychotic reaction has been attributed to 'forced normalization', but seems to occur with a higher frequency with ethosuximide than with other anti-absence drugs. For this reason, the drug should be used with caution in patients with a history of psychiatric disturbance. However, other reports show striking cognitive improvement on ethosuximide therapy, possibly related to the better control of spike–wave discharges. Other rarer neurological side effects include bradykinesia, parkinsonism and other extrapyramidal symptoms. Sedation can be a problem and is not uncommon after the increase in plasma level of ethosuximide in patients in whom valproate has been added. Occasionally, a severe encephalopathy can be induced by ethosuximide, as it can by other succinimide drugs.

The incidence of ethosuximide-related granulocytopenia ranged from 0% to 7% in early studies, and is dose dependent. This is of no concern, but must be distinguished from the severe marrow depression in ethosuximide hypersensitivity. Some teratogenic effects have been reported, but the incidence of these is quite unknown.

Overdose

Cases of ethosuximide overdose have been reported. Coma and respiratory depression occur and treatment is by supportive measures. Additional recommended measures include the use of activated charcoal, gastric lavage and haemodialysis. Exchange transfusion and forced diuresis have no value.

Antiepileptic effect

Ethosuximide, like valproate, is highly effective in controlling generalized absence seizures. Although it was introduced before the current vogue for randomized controlled trials, well-conducted open studies in the 1970s demonstrated a clear and powerful effect in often previously resistant patients. In one study of 37 patients, 19% were rendered free from seizures, and 49% had a >90% reduction and 95% a >50% reduction in seizures.

In another study complete control of seizures was obtained in 47% of patients, an effect closely correlated to plasma level.

The effectiveness of the drug has been shown to be equal to that of valproate in five controlled trials, and furthermore the drugs in combination can have a synergistic effect in patients who have not responded adequately to either drug alone. Tolerance does not develop with ethosuximide. Although ethosuximide does not generally control tonic–clonic seizures, a gratifying effect is occasionally encountered in resistant idiopathic generalized epilepsy. This lack of effect in tonic–clonic seizures is a disadvantage compared with valproate, which has a much broader spectrum of action.

Ethosuximide has a moderate effect in atypical absence seizures (in the Lennox–Gastaut syndrome), and is reported to be helpful in absence status epilepticus, severe myoclonic epilepsy in infancy, juvenile myoclonic epilepsy, epilepsy with myoclonic absences, eyelid myoclonia with absences, epilepsy with continuous spike and wave during slow-wave sleep, photosensitive seizures, the Landau–Kleffner syndrome, Angelman syndrome and gelastic seizures.

It probably has little or no effect in simple partial, complex partial or partial secondarily generalized tonic–clonic seizures.

Plasma level measurements of ethosuximide are useful in defining dosage, and there is a clear relationship between plasma level and clinical effectiveness. The target range of drug levels is between 300 and 700 µmol/L.

Clinical use in epilepsy

Ethosuximide remains a useful drug in the treatment of childhood absence seizures, although its first-line use has been largely supplanted, particularly in older children or young adults, by other drugs and especially by valproate because of the latter's superior action in tonic–clonic seizures. It still has a place in the treatment of young children where there is a risk of valproate-induced hepatotoxicity. It may be usefully added to valproate in patients whose absence seizures are not controlled on valproic acid monotherapy, and also in a number of childhood syndromes (see above). In addition, it has a limited role in other seizure types where more conventional therapy has failed.

A common starting dose for children is 10–15 mg/kg per day, with subsequent titration according to the patient's clinical response. Older children and adults often initiate ethosuximide at 250 mg/day and increase by 250 mg increments until the desired clinical response is reached. Ethosuximide can be administered as once-, twice- or even three-times-daily dosing, with meals to maximize seizure control while minimizing adverse effects. In younger children, maintenance dosages are usually between 15 and 40 mg/kg per day. In older children and adults, common maintenance doses are 750–1500 mg/day. Ethosuximide withdrawal should be carried out at a decremental rate not exceeding 250 mg every 2 weeks.

Serum level monitoring of ethosuximide is more useful than of any other antiepileptic drug with the exception of phenytoin, and effectiveness and toxicity are closely correlated with serum levels. Nevertheless, the dose should still be escalated according to clinical response rather than serum level. The therapeutic range is generally between 300 and 700 μmol/L (40–100 μg/mL), although patients with refractory seizures may need a serum concentration of up to 1000 μmol/L. Routine laboratory monitoring of blood count is not useful in preventing idiosyncratic haematological reactions. However, if the total white blood cell count falls to <3500 or the proportion of granulocytes to <25% of the total white blood cell count, the dose should be reduced or the drug withdrawn.

Gabapentin

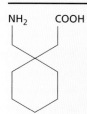

Proprietary name: Neurontin[a]

Primary indications
Partial or secondarily generalized epilepsy: adjunctive therapy in adults and children ≥6 years. Monotherapy in adults and children ≥12 years (Europe; not licensed for monotherapy in the USA)

Commonly used as first-line drug
No

Usual preparations
Capsules: 100, 300, 400. 600, 800 mg
250 mg/5 mL oral solution

Usual dosage – adults
Initial: 300–400 mg/day; increased by increments of 300–400 mg/day (600–800 mg/day at higher doses) every 2 weeks
Maintenance: 900–3600 mg/day

Usual dosage – children
Initial: 10–15 mg/kg per day
Maintenance 40 mg/kg per day age 3 and 4 years; 25–35 mg/kg per day age 5–12 years

Dosing intervals
2–3 times/day

Is dose commonly affected by co-medication?
No

Is dose affected by renal/hepatic disease?
Severe renal disease

Does it affect dose of other drugs?
No

Does it affect the contraceptive pill?
No

Serum level monitoring
Not useful

Common/important adverse events
Drowsiness, dizziness, ataxia, headache, tremor fatigue, weight gain, exacerbation of non-convulsive generalized seizures

Risk of hypersensitivity
No

Major mechanism of action
Action on α_2–δ-subunit of the voltage-gated calcium channel.

Main advantages
Lack of side effects, especially at low doses; good pharmacokinetic profile

Main disadvantages
Lack of therapeutic effect in severe cases; absorption variable, especially at high doses; seizure exacerbation in some cases

Comment
Effective second-choice antiepileptic drug for partial epilepsy, particularly in mild cases. Easy to use and few side effects at low doses

[a]Name of proprietary brand available in the UK.

Gabapentin: pharmacokinetics – average adult values

Oral bioavailability	<65% (dose dependent)
Time to peak levels	2–3 h
Volume of distribution	0.65–1.04 L/kg
Biotransformation	Not metabolized
Elimination half-life	5–9 h
Plasma clearance	0.120–0.130 L/kg per h
Protein binding	None
Active metabolite	None
Metabolism by hepatic enzymes	No
Inhibition or induction of hepatic enzymes	No
Drug interactions	None

Gabapentin, although only recently introduced, has had a colourful history. The drug was designed as a GABA agonist, with a close structural relationship to GABA, although subsequent clinical and experimental evidence has shown little or no action at the GABA receptor. It was first studied as an antispastic drug and an analgesic, but early clinical trials of its antispastic action proved disappointing. Attention then turned to its antiepileptic action, although this was not a priority with the manufacturers who considered that they had more efficacious alternatives. However, an antiepileptic drug action was shown on the basis of a series of clinical trials, and it became licensed widely in the USA, Britain, Europe and other countries for this indication. Initial clinical experience in routine practice in epilepsy was, however, rather disappointing, although its off-label effects on neurogenic pain were generally considered stronger and, in their enthusiasm to pursue these indications, the manufacturers were then heavily fined for improper marketing of off-label

indications. The drug then underwent trials in 8 non-epilepsy indications, including neuralgic pain, and was licensed for use in pain and other indications, and by 2003 gabapentin was one of the 50 most prescribed drugs in the USA with almost US$2.7 billion of sales in 2003. The sales in non-epilepsy indications accounted for up to 90% of all sales according to some estimates. Meanwhile, in epilepsy, it was soon realized that greater effectiveness was possible with higher doses than those used in the clinical trials, and this has revived interest in the drug.

Gabapentin has now achieved a solid place as second-line treatment in partial epilepsy, with moderate effect and certain advantages over other, possibly stronger, therapies. It is currently approved for adjunctive therapy in partial epilepsy in many countries and for monotherapy for epilepsy in 30 countries (but not the USA). It has larger use in other indications and the Cochrane group has found efficacy in pain from cancer and in diabetic neuropathy, postherpetic neuralgia, migraine and perioperative pain, and there are reports of effectiveness in movement disorders and cocaine dependence.

Physical and chemical characteristics
Gabapentin is a highly soluble crystalline substance (molecular weight 172.24), with two pK_a values, 3.7 and 10.7, and at physiological pH it is a zwitterion, an electrically neutral compound carrying both positive and negative charges. It has a chemical structure that is very similar to that of GABA, with the same four-carbon chain but with an additional cyclohexyl ring incorporated.

Mode of action
Gabapentin does not act at the GABA$_A$ receptor, in spite of its close structural similarity. Similar to pregabalin, gabapentin binds to the α_2–δ protein associated with the

voltage-gated calcium channel. It is thought that the drug may act by influencing the trafficking of the calcium channels to the membrane. Other actions may include subtle effects on a wide variety of neurotransmitters including noradrenaline, glutamate, acetylcholine, substance P and calcitonin gene-related peptide.

Pharmacokinetics
Absorption
The bioavailability of gabapentin is only about 60% at doses of 1800 mg/day or less and 35% or less for doses >3600 mg/day, even when given in a three-times-daily regimen. This is because gabapentin is actively transported across the gut wall by an L-amino acid transporter that is saturatable. Absorption varies considerably between individuals. What few data there are suggest that age has little effect on absorption; nor does food, although food rich in neutral amino acids or monosaccharides may enhance absorption. As absorption is incomplete and relies on an active transport system, caution should be exercised when gabapentin is used in those clinical circumstances in which absorption might be expected to be compromised. Peak serum levels are achieved within 2–4 h of oral dosing.

Distribution
The volume of distribution of the drug is 0.65–1.04 L/kg at steady state. Gabapentin is not bound to plasma proteins at all. The drug readily crosses the blood–brain barrier, utilizing the L-amino acid transport system, which is saturatable, and plasma:brain concentrations fall at higher plasma concentrations. Two clearance mechanisms, active transport and passive diffusion, limit its accumulation. The CSF concentration is 7–35% of the plasma concentration and rises for hours after the peak concentration.

Biotransformation and elimination
The drug is not metabolized at all and is completely excreted in an unchanged form. This lack of hepatic metabolism is of course a great advantage, and there are no pharmacokinetic drug interactions.

Gabapentin is eliminated unchanged entirely by renal excretion with an elimination half-life of 5–9 h. The renal clearance is 0.120–0.13 L/kg per h and is linearly correlated with creatinine clearance. Gabapentin clearance varies with age-related changes in creatinine clearance and glomerular filtration rate. Clearance is highest in young children, and children between the ages of 1 month and 5 years require approximately 30% higher doses to achieve a given plasma concentration than children aged 5–12 years. Age-related and disease-related decreases in renal function significantly reduce gabapentin clearance, and the dose needs to be lower in patients with creatinine clearance levels <60 mL/min. In haemodialysis, the dosing should be related to creatinine clearance, with small supplemental doses given immediately after each 4 h of dialysis.

Steady-state levels are achieved within a few days, however, and the half-life does not change on chronic administration nor is it influenced by co-medication. Serum levels of gabapentin are not routinely measured and there are few data on the correlation between serum level and effectiveness.

Drug interactions
Gabapentin has no known pharmacokinetic drug interactions owing to its lack of protein binding and hepatic metabolism. There is potential for interaction at the renal level, but no specific effects have been reported.

Adverse effects
Gabapentin has the reputation of having very few side effects, with only sedation and fatigue, dizziness, weight gain, ataxia, headache, tremor, nausea and diplopia being at all prominent in the clinical trials and usually only of mild intensity. However, experience shows that some individuals develop pronounced drowsiness even at low doses. Weight gain is often a significant clinical problem.

In the early double-blind studies, 44% of patients reported adverse effects on gabapentin 900 mg. Similar levels of side effects were recorded in later studies on 1200 mg. The pooled data from all the studies are shown in Table 8.8. Most of the adverse effects were mild and, overall, only 7.4% of 1748 patients who received gabapentin in any clinical study have been withdrawn from the study owing to adverse events.

The effect of gabapentin on mood is unpredictable. It has been variously reported to improve, have no effect on and adversely affect mood, and there are reports of aggressive behaviour, hyperactivity and irritability in patients with learning disability. In formal studies of cognition, no adverse effects have been reported on attention, psychomotor speed, language and speech in healthy volunteers or in patients with complex partial seizures.

Worsening of seizures is a particularly marked phenomenon in some patients treated with gabapentin. In the US study, 19% of patients treated with gabapentin 1800 mg/day, and in the UK study 20% treated with 1200 mg/day, experienced a worsening of seizure

Table 8.8 The 10 most common adverse effects of gabapentin reported in clinical trials; number (percent) of patients with adverse effects.

	Controlled studies		All studies
	Placebo ($n = 307$)	Gabapentin ($n = 485$)	Gabapentin ($n = 1160$)
	56.7	76.1	81.4
Adverse events			
Somnolence	9.8	20.2	24.4
Dizziness	7.8	17.9	20.3
Ataxia	5.2	13.2	17.4
Fatigue	4.9	11.1	14.7
Nystagmus	4.9	9.3	15.0
Headache	9.1	8.7	15.2
Tremor	3.9	7.2	15.0
Diplopia	2.0	6.4	10.7
Nausea and/or vomiting	7.5	6.0	9.3
Rhinitis	3.9	4.5	8.7

frequency. Gabapentin can also specifically worsen myoclonus and absence seizures.

Gabapentin has been given to over 10 million patients, for various indications, and remarkably few potentially serious side effects have been reported. The incidence of rash is 0.5% and that of neutropenia 0.2%. ECG changes and/or angina was reported in 0.05% of cases. There are extremely rare reports of Stevens–Johnson syndrome and hepatotoxicity. There are no consistent changes in any other clinical or laboratory measure, and no serious idiosyncratic or hypersensitivity reactions. Pancreatic carcinoma was reported in the animal toxicology studies, but there have been no clinical reports of pancreatic disease. Three cases of massive gabapentin overdose have been reported without serious effects.

The abrupt withdrawal of gabapentin has been associated with a range of symptoms, many related to sympathetic overactivity, and as with all other antiepileptics in routine practice the drug should be withdrawn gradually.

Antiepileptic effects

Gabapentin has been studied in a series of open and double-blind, randomized controlled investigations in partial epilepsy, and a consistent picture has emerged. The large multicentre study carried out in the UK randomized patients to add-on therapy with either gabapentin 1200 mg

or placebo. Twenty-five per cent of the gabapentin patients showed a reduction in partial seizures of at least 50% compared with 9.8% of those taking placebo. In a similar study from the USA, patients were randomized to 600, 1200 or 1800 mg/day of gabapentin or placebo. The percentage of patients with a reduction in seizures of at least 50% ranged from 18% to 26% with gabapentin and 8% with placebo. These trials showed that the drug has antiepileptic action in partial epilepsy; however, the number of responders is disappointingly low and, at the doses tried, the drug seems rather weak.

Since licensing, it has become customary to prescribe much higher doses and, although these doses have not been studied in double-blind controlled trials, there is a universal clinical impression that higher doses are more effective, at least in some patients. The side effects at higher doses are also more prominent.

Gabapentin has a narrow spectrum of activity and is not effective in primarily generalized seizures, absence seizures and myoclonus (and indeed absence seizures and myoclonus are frequently worsened by the drug).

In newly diagnosed patients, gabapentin has shown similar or less efficacy than carbamazepine or lamotrigine in open and controlled studies. In the SANAD study, gabapentin was significantly less efficacious than lamotrigine in terms of time to treatment failure and to carbamazepine in terms of time to 12-month remission.

Long-term follow-up studies have demonstrated sustained benefit without the emergence of longer-term toxicity or new toxicity. However, in long-term retention studies, fewer than 40% of patients taking gabapentin remained on the drug for 6 years and fewer than 4% became free from seizures.

A double-blind trial of gabapentin for benign rolandic epilepsy (with centrotemporal spikes) demonstrated statistically significant superiority of gabapentin over placebo.

Clinical use in epilepsy

Gabapentin is a useful drug in the treatment of partial and secondarily generalized tonic–clonic seizures. It has an excellent pharmacological profile, and its lack of protein binding, metabolism and drug interactions is an attractive property. It has particular value in renal or hepatic disease and in patients on complicated drug regimens. It can be rapidly titrated, which is an advantage in some settings. Also, it is relatively well tolerated although side effects do occur, particularly at higher doses. The severe behavioural or psychiatric disturbances found with other drugs do not occur with gabapentin nor do idiosyncratic or serious systemic side effects.

There are, however, disadvantages. The drug appears to have only a rather modest efficacy, and most patients with severe epilepsy derive little benefit. Furthermore, a substantial minority of patients treated with gabapentin have a worsening of seizure frequency and occasionally this deterioration can be marked. In addition the drug is ineffective in most generalized seizure types including tonic–clonic and absence seizures, and in myoclonus. Although its pharmacokinetic profile is generally good, its absorption is erratic, particularly at higher doses, and this can be problematic.

Its main role is therefore in mild epilepsy, in elderly people and in patients in whom dose-limiting side effects are commonly experienced on other drugs.

It is common practice to titrate this dose up at weekly intervals to a maximum of 3600 mg/day. The usual initial maintenance doses are between 900 and 2400 mg/day. In children aged 3–12 years, the usual starting dose is 10–15 mg/kg per day, and this can be increased within a week or so to the usual maintenance dose of 40 mg/kg per day in children aged 3 and 4 years, and 25–35 mg/kg per day in children aged 5–12 years. Dosages up to 50 mg/kg per day have been well tolerated.

Although all the trials used three-times-a-day dosing, a twice-a-day regimen seems equally effective. However, at high doses, dosing three or four times daily will probably avoid saturation of the processes of absorption. In routine practice withdrawal can be carried out at weekly decremental rates of 400 mg. Serum antiepileptic drug levels can be helpful to assess absorption, particularly where higher doses are contemplated, but serum level is not closely related to effectiveness. The dose should be halved in patients with creatinine clearance values between 30 and 59 mL/min, reduced by a further half where creatinine clearance is between 15 and 29 mL/min, and reduced further at lower levels.

Lacosamide

Proprietary name: Vimpat[a]

Primary indications
Adjunctive therapy of partial-onset seizures. Adults only

Commonly used as first-line drug
No

Usual preparations
Tablets: 50, 100, 150, 200 mg tablets; intravenous solution 10 mg/mL; syrup 15 mg/mL

Usual dosage – adults
Initial: 50 mg/day; increased by increments of 50 mg/day every 2 weeks
Maintenance: 200–400 mg/day

Dosing intervals
Twice a day

Is dose commonly affected by co-medication?
No

Is dose affected by renal/hepatic disease?
No

Does it affect dose of other drugs?
No

Interactions with the contraceptive pill
No

Serum level monitoring
Utility not established

Common/important adverse events
Dizziness, headache, nausea, diplopia ataxia, memory impairment, somnolence, tremor, vertigo, constipation, pruritus, asthenia, fatigue

Risk of hypersensitivity
None to date

Major mechanism of action
Inhibition of sodium channel conductance

Main advantages
Well-documented efficacy, seemingly well tolerated

Main disadvantages
Limited clinical experience, nervous system and gastrointestinal adverse effects

Comment
Newly licensed antiepileptic drug

ᵃName of proprietary brand available in the UK.

Lacosamide: pharmacokinetics – average adult values	
Oral bioavailability	<100%
Time to peak levels	0.5–4 h
Volume of distribution	0.5–0.8 L/kg
Biotransformation	O-Desmethylation
Elimination half-life	12–16 h
Plasma clearance	No published data
Protein binding	<15%
Active metabolite	None
Metabolism by hepatic enzymes	CYP2C19
Inhibition or induction of hepatic enzymes	Inhibits CYP2C19
Drug interactions	Some drug interactions

Lacosamide (Vimpat® [SPM 927], formerly known as harkoseride) was initially synthesized as an intravenous antiepileptic for status epilepticus. Studies have been conducted in parallel in patients with epilepsy and neuropathic pain. The drug was licensed in 2009 as adjunctive therapy for refractory partial epilepsy, but its range of effects has not yet been fully explored.

Chemistry

Lacosamide, (R)-2-acetamido-N-benzyl-3-methoxypropionamide, is an amino acid with a chemical formula $C_{13}H_{18}N_2O_3$ (molecular weight 250.30). It is a soluble crystalline powder.

Mode of action

Lacosamide selectively enhances slow inactivation of voltage-gated sodium channels without affecting fast inactivation, which is an action not shared by other sodium channel blockers. Another mechanism that may or may not contribute to its efficacy in epilepsy and neuropathic pain is an effect on the collapsin response mediator protein 2 (CRMP-2).

Pharmacokinetics
Absorption

Lacosamide is rapidly and completely absorbed after oral administration. The oral bioavailability is approximately 100%. Peak plasma concentrations occur between 0.5 and 4 h after the dose. The pharmacokinetics are linear. Food intake has no influence on absorption.

Distribution

Lacosamide is <15% bound to plasma proteins and is distributed in total body water, with an apparent volume of distribution of about 0.5–0.8 L/kg.

Metabolism and elimination

The plasma half-life of lacosamide is approximately 12–16 h. Steady-state plasma concentrations are achieved after 3 days. Approximately 40% of orally administered lacosamide are excreted unchanged in the urine, and another 30% are recovered in the form of the inactive O-desmethyl metabolite SPM 12809. The cytochrome P450 isoenzyme CYP2C19 is involved in the formation of SPM 12809, but the variations in CYP2C19 genotype seems to have no major influence on plasma lacosamide concentrations.

Preliminary data suggest that, in elderly people, steady-state plasma lacosamide concentrations are 10–35%

higher than those recorded in non-elderly adults (which may reflect decreased renal function).

In individuals with mild or moderate renal impairment, the lacosamide area under the curve (AUC) is increased by approximately 30% compared with healthy individuals and in those with severe renal impairment (creatinine clearance <30 mL/min) by approximately 60%, and dosage should be reduced.

Individuals with hepatic impairment (Child–Pugh score B) showed approximately 50% higher AUC compared with healthy people, which was attributed, in part, to reduced renal function in these patients. No dosage adjustment is thought to be needed in patients with mild-to-moderate hepatic insufficiency.

Drug interactions

Overall, lacosamide exhibits a low drug–drug interaction potential, and no dose adjustment is necessary when lacosamide is co-administered with other drugs.

Effects of other drugs on lacosamide concentrations

In a population pharmacokinetic study, co-medication with enzyme-inducing antiepileptic drugs (carbamazepine, phenytoin, phenobarbital) reduced lacosamide exposure by 25%. Digoxin, metformin, omeprazole and a combined oral contraceptive do not influence the pharmacokinetics of lacosamide.

Effect of lacosamide on other drugs

In clinical studies, plasma concentrations of concomitant antiepileptic drugs were unaffected by concomitant intake of lacosamide at any dose. Lacosamide has no effect on the pharmacokinetics or hormonal effects of an oral contraceptive containing 0.03 mg ethinylestradiol and 0.15 mg levonorgestrel in healthy individuals.

Serum level monitoring

There is insufficient information on the value of monitoring lacosamide plasma concentrations.

Adverse effects

Adverse events (Table 8.9) observed during the lacosamide clinical trials included dose-related CNS and gastrointestinal system adverse effects. Dizziness, diplopia, headaches, nausea and vomiting are the most common events. Other side effects include ataxia, memory impairment, somnolence, tremor, vertigo, constipation, pruritus, asthenia and fatigue.

In the three pivotal, double-blind controlled trials, overall discontinuation rates during the treatment period were 18%, 23% and 38% in the groups assigned to lacosamide doses of 200 mg/day, 400 mg/day and 600 mg/day, compared with 13% among patients randomized to placebo. Dizziness was the most common adverse event leading to premature withdrawal, especially in the 600 mg/day group. A small, dose-related increase in P–R interval was observed with lacosamide treatment, with a mean increase from baseline to the end of the maintenance phase of 1.4 ms, 4.4 ms and 6.6 ms for 200, 400 and 600 mg/day lacosamide, compared with a 0.3 ms decrease for placebo. The incidence of treatment-emergent first-degree atrioventricular (AV) block was

Table 8.9 Incidences of treatment emergent adverse events reported by ≥10% of subjects in any lacosamide treatment group, based on a pooled analysis of the three double-blind pivotal lacosamide trials in patients with refractory partial-onset seizures.

Side effect	Placebo, % ($n = 364$)	Lacosamide 200 mg/day, % ($n = 270$)	Lacosamide 400 mg/day, % ($n = 471$)	Lacosamide 600 mg/day, % ($n = 203$)	Lacosamide total, % ($n = 944$)
Dizziness	8	16	30	53	31
Headache	9	11	14	12	13
Abnormal co-ordination	2	4	7	15	8
Tremor	4	4	6	12	7
Nystagmus	4	2	5	10	5
Diplopia	2	6	10	16	10
Vision blurred	2	2	8	16	8
Nausea	4	7	11	17	11
Vomiting	3	6	9	16	9
Fatigue	6	7	7	15	9

0.4% for lacosamide and 0% for placebo. It is too early to say whether the full range of lacosamide side effects has been recognized.

Efficacy

Adjunctive treatment with lacosamide was evaluated in a number of phase 2 and 3 trials in adults with simple partial-onset seizures and/or complex partial-onset seizures, with or without secondary generalization. Both the oral and parenteral formulations were tested in clinical trials, although the intravenous formulation was studied for safety only. Lacosamide also underwent a parallel clinical development in patients with diabetic neuropathic pain.

The three pivotal, randomized placebo-controlled, clinical trials in epilepsy patients titrated lacosamide up to the target dose of 200 mg/day, 400 mg/day and 600 mg/day administered as adjunctive therapy in adults with uncontrolled partial-onset seizures. In the first trial, the median percentage reduction in seizure frequency, from baseline to maintenance, was 10% in the placebo group and 26%, 39% and 40% in the lacosamide 200 mg/day, 400 mg/day and 600 mg/day groups, respectively. Reductions in seizure frequency over placebo were significant for the lacosamide 400 mg/day (28.4%) and 600 mg/day (21.3) groups. In the second placebo-controlled trial, there was a median percentage reduction in seizure frequency of 35% and 36% for lacosamide 200 mg/day and 400 mg/day, respectively, compared with 21% for placebo. The proportion of patients showing at least a 50% reduction in seizure frequency was 26% in the placebo group, 35% in the 200 mg/day group and 41% in the 400 mg/day group (these results were all significantly different on statistical testing). In the third trial, a reduction in seizure frequency of at least 50% was recorded in 38.3% of patients treated with 400 mg/day and in 41.2% of patients treated with 600 mg/day lacosamide, compared with 18.3% of patients allocated to placebo. The difference versus placebo was statistically significant at both doses. Among the patients who completed the pivotal trials, 3.3% and 4.8% of those taking lacosamide 400 mg/day and 600 mg/day, respectively, were seizure free compared with 0.9% of the patients in the placebo arm. There is very little post-marketing experience.

Place in current therapy

Lacosamide is a new antiepileptic drug with a novel mode of action. It is licensed as adjunctive therapy for the treatment of partial-onset seizures in individuals aged 16 years or more in Europe and in those aged 17 years or more in the USA. It has a number of advantageous features, including good pharmacokinetics and a low potential for drug–drug interactions. The efficacy data show potential utility in partial epilepsy. There is little experience in other epilepsy types. The usual effective dose range appears to be 200–400 mg/day, to be achieved after gradual titration. It is too early to predict the value of this drug, but the initial experience is promising.

Lamotrigine

Proprietary name: Lamictal[a]

Primary indications
Adjunctive or monotherapy of partial seizures and generalized seizures, and seizures associated with the Lennox–Gastaut syndrome in those aged ≥13 years. Adjunctive therapy of partial seizures and generalized seizures, and monotherapy of typical absence seizures in those aged 2–12 years

Commonly used as first-line drug
Yes

Usual preparations
Tablets: 25, 50, 100, 200 mg; dispersible chewtabs: 2, 5, 25, 100 mg

Usual dosage – adults
Initial: 12.5–25 mg/day; increased by increments of 50–100 mg/day every 2 weeks
Maintenance: 200–600 mg/day (depends on co-medication – see text and Tables 8.13 and 8.14).

Usual dosage – children
Depends on co-medication; see Tables 8.13 and 8.14

Dosing intervals
Twice a day

Is dose commonly affected by co-medication?
Yes

Is dose affected by renal/hepatic disease?
Avoid in hepatic disease

Does it affect doses of other drugs?
No

Does it affect the contraceptive pill?
No (although contraceptive may lower doses of lamotrigine)

Serum level monitoring
Useful

Target range
2–20 mg/L

Common/important adverse events
Rash (sometimes severe), blood dyscrasia, headache, ataxia, asthenia, diplopia, nausea, vomiting, dizziness, somnolence, insomnia, depression, behavioral effects, psychosis, tremor

Risk of hypersensitivity
Marked risk

Major mechanism of action
Inhibition of sodium channel conductance

Main advantages
Moderate effectiveness, generally well tolerated
Main disadvantages
High instance of rash (occasionally severe) and other side effects, complicated pharmacokinetics
Comment
A useful antiepileptic, especially in generalized epilepsies

[a]Name of proprietary brand available in the UK.

The history of epilepsy has seen many drugs developed on incorrect premises, and lamotrigine is a recent example. In the 1960s it was postulated – wrongly – that the antiepileptic effects of phenytoin and phenobarbital could be mediated through their antifolate properties. Lamotrigine was then developed as an antifolate drug. However, as it turns out, lamotrigine does not have a marked antifolate action and there is, anyway, no correlation between an anti-folate action and antiepileptic effects. Such is fortune, however – lamotrigine was then found to have a pronounced antiepileptic effect.

Physical and chemical characteristics

Lamotrigine (3,5-diamino-6-[2,3-dichorophenyl]-1,2,4-triazine; molecular weight 256.1) is a triazine compound unrelated chemically to any other antiepileptic. It is a weak base, pK_a 5.7, and is poorly soluble in water or ethanol.

Mode of action

In its short life, a whole range of mechanisms of action has been postulated for lamotrigine, only later to be discounted. It seems now that the antiepileptic action is

Lamotrigine: pharmacokinetics – average adult values

Oral bioavailability	<100%
Time to peak levels	1–3 h (1–6 h in children)
Volume of distribution	0.90–1.31 L/kg
Biotransformation	Hepatic glucuronidation without phase 1 reaction
Elimination half-life	12–60 h (varies considerably with co-medication; monotherapy, 29 h; polytherapy with a combination of valproate and enzyme inducers: approximately 25 h; polytherapy with valproate without enzyme inducers: 60 h; polytherapy with enzyme inducers without valproate approx 13 h)
Plasma clearance	0.044–0.084 L/kg per h (varies considerably on co-medication)
Protein binding	55%
Active metabolite	None
Metabolism by hepatic enzymes	Only phase 2 glucuronidation via UGT1A4 (80%)
Inhibition or induction of hepatic enzymes	Iinducer of UGT1A4
Drug interactions	Common

largely due to its effect in blocking voltage-dependent sodium channel conductance, an action similar to that of carbamazepine or phenytoin. Indeed, the drug binds to the same amino acid residues as phenytoin, although it has different binding kinetics. Whether or not the drug has any more direct neurotransmitter action is uncertain, although antiglutamate and antiaspartate actions have been suggested, and also an action on kynurenic acid which may modulate the glycine-binding site on the N-methyl-D-aspartate (NMDA) receptor. Lamotrigine also modulates voltage-dependent calcium conductance at N-type calcium channels and potassium conductance. In experimental seizure models lamotrigine has a rather similar profile of action to that of phenytoin.

Pharmacokinetics
Absorption and distribution
Lamotrigine is well absorbed orally with a bioavailability approaching 100%. Peak concentrations occur within 1–3 h after dosing in adults (1–6 h in children), and a linear relationship exists between dose and concentration in the normal clinical dosing ranges. There is a second smaller lamotrigine peak after oral administration attributed to intestinal reabsorption of the drug sequestered in the stomach. Absorption is not affected by food. Lamotrigine is 55% bound to plasma proteins and has a volume of distribution of between 0.9 and 1.3 L/kg in adults and 1.5 L/kg in children. Brain concentrations are

1.5–2.5 times plasma concentrations. Lamotrigine is 55% bound to plasma proteins.

Metabolism and elimination
The drug undergoes extensive metabolism in the liver, largely to the inert glucuronide conjugate, most of which is renally excreted, and its metabolism results in complex pharmacokinetics. In chronic therapy, less than 10% of the drug is excreted unchanged in the urine. Metabolism is via the uridine diphosphate glucuronosyl transferase (UDPGT) enzymes, without prior involvement of the CYP family of enzymes.

Plasma clearance shows marked intraindividual variation and is affected strongly by age and co-medication. In monotherapy, plasma clearance values are higher in children (0.038 L/kg per h) than in adults (0.044–0.084 L/kg per h). Elimination half-lives are broadly similar in children and in adults (32 h in children vs 23–37 h in adults). Younger children have higher clearance values than older children, and older children and adults higher levels than elderly people.

These differences may be due to a relative reduction in liver size and hepatic blood flow in adolescents compared with young children, and diminished glucuronidation at older ages. A comparison of single 150 mg oral doses in healthy young and elderly volunteers revealed a 37% lower clearance in elderly people and a 27% higher maximum plasma concentration (C_{max}) and 55% higher values of plasma AUC. Some but not all investigators have shown autoinduction.

The plasma clearance of lamotrigine can greatly increase towards the end of pregnancy, and as a result doses of lamotrigine may need to be doubled during pregnancy to maintain constant serum levels. This change is reversed in the few days after delivery and so dose adjustments made in pregnancy should be rapidly reversed (see p. 142). Lamotrigine is excreted in considerable amounts in breast milk, which in combination with slow infantile elimination can result in similar plasma concentrations in the infant and mother – a potential hazard in breast-feeding.

Clearance is not significantly affected by renal impairment. Haemodialysis removes about 20% of lamotrigine in a 4-h session.

Gilbert syndrome, a common disorder of conjugation characterized by altered UDPGT activity, results in decreased clearance and prolongation (by approximately 35%) of the half-life.

Hepatic disease can have a marked effect on lamotrigine clearance. Mild-to-moderate disease reduces clearance by about 15% and severe disease by about 40%.

Drug interactions

The hepatic glucuronidation of lamotrigine is not via cytochrome P450 enzymes, and thus lamotrigine does not induce CYP activity and hence has little effect on the metabolism of other drugs, such as the enzyme-inducing antiepileptic drugs, the contraceptive pill or warfarin.

Unfortunately, the concomitant administration of other antiepileptic drugs does have a profound effect on the metabolism of lamotrigine. Enzyme inducers reduce the half-life from a mean of 29 h to 15 h in adults, and this effect is even greater in children (half-life of lamotrigine was reduced to 7–14 h in some clinical trials). Sodium valproate lengthens the half-life, by mechanisms that are unclear, four to ten times, to 60 h or more. In children, the half-life falls to <10 h in those co-medicated with enzyme-inducing antiepileptics and is between 15 and 27 h when valproate is given with inducers, and 44 and 94 h with valproate alone.

As a result of these major interactions, lamotrigine dosage needs to be modified according to concomitant therapy and, conversely, when the dose of co-medication is altered, lamotrigine levels will also change. In young children, pronounced peak–trough fluctuations may occur in co-medication with enzyme-inducing drugs, and more frequent dosing intervals may be required.

Drugs that are not hepatic enzyme inducers or inhibitors (e.g. ethosuximide, gabapentin, levetiracetam, pregabalin, tiagabine, vigabatrin and zonisamide) have no significant effect on lamotrigine pharmacokinetics. No clear differences have been observed in combination with felbamate, and co-medication with topiramate results in either slightly decreased or unchanged plasma concentrations.

The clearance of lamotrigine can be affected by non-antiepileptic enzyme-inducing drugs. A common example is the fall in half-life of lamotrigine by up to 50% when the oral contraceptive is added as co-medication, and this can require dosage change. This effect is not seen when valproate is taken in co-medication. Hormone replacement therapy in older women has a similar effect.

Adverse effects

In monotherapy, side effects of lamotrigine are generally slight and the drug has a reputation of being well tolerated. Certainly, in clinical trials, it has been slightly better tolerated than carbamazepine at the onset of therapy, although in chronic therapy there is little to choose between them. In polytherapy, the impact of side effects is much increased.

Central nervous system effects

The most common side effects of lamotrigine – noted in both adjunctive therapy and monotherapy – are headache, asthenia, rash, nausea, sleepiness and dizziness (Tables 8.10 and 8.11). Sedation can occur but is usually not prominent and the lack of sedation is an advantage of this drug over others. Other side effects are ataxia, and blurred and double vision. There have been reports of behavioural change, aggression, irritability, agitation, confusion, chorea, hallucinations and psychoses, but these side effects are uncommon.

In isolated individual cases, however, severe reactions do occur. Diplopia and unsteadiness seem particularly common when the drug is used in combination with carbamazepine, but whether this is a pharmacodynamic or a pharmacokinetic interaction is not known. Certainly, lowering either the carbamazepine or the lamotrigine dose in this situation will usually reverse the visual disturbance.

Lamotrigine causes few adverse psychomotor and cognitive effects. Motor function, as measured by body sway, adaptive tracking, smooth pursuit or saccadic eye movements, is unaffected by lamotrigine 100–300 mg. Similarly, no effect has been seen on psychomotor speed, sustained attention, verbal memory, language and mood measures in healthy volunteers.

Table 8.10 Adverse effects in newly diagnosed patients on monotherapy – pooled data from comparative trials of lamotrigine, carbamazepine and phenytoin.

Adverse effects	Lamotrigine ($n = 536$)	Carbamazepine ($n = 338$)	Phenytoin ($n = 95$)
Median–modal dose (mg/day)	100–200	600	300
Headache (%)	18	17	19
Asthenia (%)	15	20	29
Rash (%)	11	14	9
Nausea (%)	10	7	4
Sleepiness (%)	8	17	29
Dizziness (%)	9	13	12

Table 8.11 Adverse events reported by 10% of more of patients receiving lamotrigine in a double-blind study of lamotrigine tolerability.

Adverse events	Lamotrigine ($n = 334$)	Placebo ($n = 112$)
Dizziness (%)	50[a]	18
Headache (%)	37	36
Diplopia (%)	33[a]	11
Ataxia (%)	24[a]	5
Blurred vision (%)	23[a]	9
Nausea (%)	22	15
Rhinitis (%)	17	19
Somnolence (%)	14[a]	7
Pharyngitis (%)	13	12
Incoordination (%)	12	6
Flu-like symptoms (%)	11	9
Cough (%)	10	8
Rash (%)	10	5
Dyspepsia (%)	10	5
Vomiting (%)	10	9

[a]Significant difference compared with placebo.

Table 8.12 The rates of rash due to lamotrigine in children and adults in relation to co-medication with other antiepileptic drugs.

AED therapy	Total no. of patients	All rash (%)	DC rash (%)[a]	Hosp/ SJSrash (%)[b]
Paediatric (younger than 16 years)				
LTG + EIAED	394	9.6	4.1	0.8
LTG + VPA only	145	20.0	9.0	1.4
LTG + VPA + NEIAED	145	21.4	10.3	1.4
LTG alone	192	13.5	3.1	1.6
Adult (older than 16 years)				
LTG + EIAED	2240	6.7	2.0	0.1
LTG + VPA only	205	19.5	12.2	2.0
LTG + VPA + NEIAED	10	20.0	10.0	0
LTG alone	420	14.5	6.0	0

EIAED, enzyme-inducing antiepileptic drugs; NEIAED, non-enzyme-inducing antiepileptic drugs; LTG, lamotrigine; VPA, valproic acid.
[a]rash leading to discontinuation of treatment;
[b]rash leading to hospitalization or Stevens–Johnson syndrome (SJS).

Hypersensitivity

Idiosyncratic hypersensitivity has been a major concern, particularly in children, and predominantly affects the skin (Table 8.12). Many antiepileptic drugs cause allergic skin rash, but the incidence of rash and its severity separate lamotrigine from other antiepileptic drugs in this regard. The lamotrigine-associated skin rash is typically maculopapular or erythematous, associated with pruritus, and usually appears within the first 4 weeks of initiating treatment. Occasionally, the rash may be more severe (erythema multiforme) or progress to desquamation with involvement of the mucous membrane (Stevens–Johnson syndrome) and to toxic epidermal necrolysis.

The frequency of skin rash is higher in children than in adults, and early reports suggested that as many as 1 in 50 to 1 in 100 children developed a potentially life-threatening rash. This high frequency was probably due to the effects of valproate co-medication on lamotrigine levels, and the frequency of rash is greatly reduced with slow escalation of lamotrigine doses or its use in low doses or as monotherapy.

Rash resulting in hospitalization occurs in 8 per 1000 children started on lamotrigine. The rate of serious skin rash in adults is 0.8–1.3 per 1000.

Cross-reactivity is a nuisance, and the rate of rash is much higher in those who have already exhibited rash on phenytoin or other arene oxide antiepileptic drugs.

Hypersensitivity can be accompanied by a systemic illness with fever, malaise, arthralgia, lymphadenopathy and eosinophilia. Sporadic cases of multiorgan failure associated with disseminated intravascular coagulation have also been reported as part of a hypersensitivity reaction, sometimes associated with acute renal failure. Isolated cases of pseudolymphoma, agranulocytosis and hepatotoxicity have also been recorded.

Other adverse effects

Other side effects reported with lamotrigine include diarrhoea, abdominal pain, dyspepsia, rhinitis, tremor, infection, fever, bronchitis and flu-like symptoms. The drug can increase the requirement for therapy in diabetes insipidus and precipitate a flare-up of ulcerative colitis. A paradoxical increase in seizures occasionally occurs.

Lamotrigine has been shown to have less effect on female sex hormones and insulin than valproate in females, and less effect on testosterone levels and sexual functioning than carbamazepine in males. There is one report of an increased desmopressin requirement in children treated for diabetes insipidus. It has been suggested that the rate of sudden unexpected death in epilepsy (SUDEP) is slightly increased in those medicated on lamotrigine. Evidence is weak and conflicting. Several case reports of severe and unequivocal ECG QRS prolongation have been published, and this may increase the risk of cardiac arrhythmia.

Lamotrigine is associated with a slight increase in the risk of major malformations due to a teratogenic effect. In the manufacturer's pregnancy register, there were 23 live-born infants with major defects out 1145 pregnancies. A further three pregnancies were terminated because of major defects and one fetal death with major birth defects. A higher frequency of major malformations occurs in combination with valproate. In one large registry, lamotrigine effects were greater at higher doses.

Overdose

Cases of overdose up to 15 g have been reported, and can be fatal. Ingestion of up to 4500 mg is not associated with respiratory depression, although stupor, seizures, ataxia, and other cerebral and metabolic disturbances occur. Supportive therapy can be supplemented by gastric lavage and the use of activated charcoal, midazolam and fluid loads.

Antiepileptic effect
Partial-onset seizures

There have been 10 placebo-controlled trials exploring the use of lamotrigine as add-on therapy in refractory epilepsy. Nine of the ten showed lamotrigine to be significantly better than placebo, with a total decrease in seizures on lamotrigine of between 17 and 59%. Most trials showed a reduction in seizures of approximately 25–30%, and a 20–30% responder rate. In the largest of the trials, lamotrigine at a dose of 500 mg/day proved more effective than lamotrigine 300 mg/day or placebo as add-on therapy, reducing the total frequency of seizures by 36% and producing a reduction in seizure frequency of more than 50% in 34% of patients. Lamotrigine has also been studied in a large double-blind trial in 199 children, and a reduction in partial seizures of more than 50%, compared with the baseline frequency, was seen in 42% of lamotrigine-treated and 16% of placebo-treated children.

A meta-analysis of adjunctive therapy with lamotrigine in refractory partial epilepsy has been carried out in which lamotrigine was compared with other recently introduced antiepileptic drugs in chronic epilepsy. In general terms, these analyses suggest that lamotrigine is somewhat less effective than most other new antiepileptics, although equal in efficacy to gabapentin.

Generalized seizures

There is also now good evidence that lamotrigine is effective in generalized tonic–clonic, typical and atypical absence seizures. This is a significant advantage over other conventional antiepileptic drugs, and is, in this author's opinion, the drug's main merit. Lamotrigine can have a marked effect on seizures in the Lennox–Gastaut syndrome, and in one pivotal randomized controlled, double-blind study, for example, in a total of 169 patients, the median frequency of all major seizures decreased in the lamotrigine group from 16.4 to 9.9 vs 13.5 to 14.2 compared with placebo. Seizure reduction of >50% was seen significantly more often in the lamotrigine-treated patients (33% vs 16%).

The influence of lamotrigine on myoclonus is, however, variable. Some cases are improved, but in others the myoclonus is aggravated and lamotrigine can even precipitate myoclonic status epilepticus. Aggravation of severe myoclonic epilepsy in infancy (Dravet syndrome) and the progressive myclonic epilepsies (PMEs) is particularly common with lamotrigine. In myoclonus in the idiopathic generalized epilepsies, lamotrigine is not as effective as valproate, but it is a useful second-line therapy.

Lamotrigine has also been shown to be effective in neonatal seizures and infantile spasms, although it is not currently considered a drug of first choice in either clinical situation.

Newly diagnosed epilepsy

In monotherapy in newly diagnosed partial and generalized tonic–clonic seizures, lamotrigine has been shown to be as effective as carbamazepine or phenytoin. At least five RCTs compare lamotrigine and carbamazepine (three in elderly people) and show equal efficacy but slightly better tolerability of lamotrigine in the initial phase of therapy. Comparisons of lamotrigine with phenytoin and gabapentin have shown no differences in efficacy or tolerability in newly diagnosed patients, e.g. in one study of adults with newly diagnosed epilepsy randomized to lamotrigine 100–300 mg/day or carbamazepine 300–1400 mg/day for 48 weeks, the percentages of patients who remained free from seizures over the final 24 weeks of treatment were similar, in terms of overall seizures (39 vs 38%), partial seizures (35 vs 37%) and idiopathic generalized seizures (both 47%). In a study of 150 elderly patients, lamotrigine was shown to be as effective as carbamazepine and better tolerated.

Lamotrigine has been compared with valproate in two studies of newly diagnosed patients. In one study of mixed generalized and partial epilepsy, seizure freedom rates of 47% were found for both drugs, but valproate caused more side effects and weight gain. In the other study of generalized epilepsies, no overall differences were found although valproate was more effective in juvenile myoclonic epilepsy.

In the SANAD study (arm A – roughly equivalent to partial epilepsy), lamotrigine was shown to be significantly better than carbamazepine, gabapentin and topiramate for time to treatment failure, and carbamazepine had a non-significant advantage over lamotrigine, topiramate and oxcarbazepine for time to 12-month remission. In arm B (roughly equivalent to generalized epilepsy) lamotrigine was inferior to valproate in time to 12-month remission. Both drugs were better tolerated than topiramate in this study.

Lamotrigine has a useful action in newly diagnosed absence epilepsy. In one placebo-controlled trial, 30 of 42 patients (71%) aged 2–16 years became free from seizures at a median dose of 5 mg/kg per day, and 60% of 15 patients remained free from seizures with lamotrigine treatment compared with 21% of the 14 patients receiving placebo. Occasionally, absence seizures are exacerbated and there is a single case report of recurrent absence status epilepticus precipitated by lamotrigine therapy.

Clinical use in epilepsy

Lamotrigine is available in tablets containing 25, 50, 100 and 200 mg. Formulations of 5, 25 and 100 mg tablets are also available. There is no parenteral preparation.

The drug is usually prescribed on a twice-daily basis, although a single daily dose can be used if it is taken with valproate alone. The drug is currently licensed as first- and second-line treatment for primary generalized epilepsy or partial and secondarily generalized seizures, in polytherapy or as monotherapy. It is generally well tolerated but the risk of rash remains a clinical problem in children. If a rash develops, the drug should be stopped immediately, and it seems sensible to avoid using the drug in patients with severe hepatic impairment.

There is a general clinical consensus that the effectiveness of lamotrigine in chronic partial epilepsy is only moderate, comparable to that of gabapentin, but less effective than other first-line drugs. Its lack of sedative side effects is, however, a positive feature. In newly diagnosed epilepsy, it has comparable efficacy to other drugs and slightly better initial tolerability than its major comparators. It has a wide spectrum of activity, and is particularly useful in generalized epilepsies, e.g. the Lennox–Gastaut syndrome, and in patients with learning disability. However, it can exacerbate myoclonus. It has some use in the idiopathic generalized epilepsies, although it is not as effective as valproate against myoclonus in this condition.

Dosing regimens depend on age and co-medication (Tables 8.13–8.15).

Although plasma levels can be measured, and a therapeutic range has been postulated, there is only a loose relationship between serum concentration and clinical effectiveness (or indeed with side effects). The routine measurement of blood levels is therefore unnecessary. However, because of the complex effects of co-medication, monitoring of plasma levels when concomitant medication is changed can be helpful. This applies to the addition of both antiepileptic and non-antiepileptic drugs including the oral contraceptive. In later pregnancy, lamotrigine levels can fall precipitously (often to half the preconception levels), and plasma levels should be frequently measured; a rapid escalation of dose is sometimes required to maintain consistent levels.

Table 8.13 Lamotrigine dose regimens in monotherapy.

Patients aged >12 years
- Weeks 1 and 2: 25 mg every other day
- Weeks 3 and 4: 50 mg every day
- To achieve maintenance, doses may be increased by 50–100 mg/day every 1–2 weeks
- Usual maintenance dose, 200 mg/day

Patients aged 2–12 years
- Weeks 1 and 2: 0.3 mg/kg per day in one or two divided doses
- Weeks 3 and 4: 0.6 mg/kg per day in one or two divided doses
- Usual maintenance dose: 1–10 mg/kg per day in one or two divided doses (maximum 15 mg/kg per day)
- To achieve the usual maintenance dose, subsequent doses should be increased every 1–2 weeks (calculate 0.6 mg/kg per day)

Table 8.15 Lamotrigine dose regimens when co-medicated with enzyme-inducing antiepileptic drugs.

Patients aged >12 years
- Weeks 1 and 2: 50 mg/day in two divided doses
- Weeks 3 and 4: 100 mg/day in two divided doses
- Usual maintenance dose: 200–400 mg/day in two divided doses
- To achieve maintenance, doses may be increased by 100 mg/day every 1–2 weeks (maximum dose is 700 mg/day)

Patients aged 2–12 years
- Weeks 1 and 2: 0.6 mg/kg per day in two divided doses
- Weeks 3 and 4: 1.2 mg/kg per day in two divided doses
- Usual maintenance dose: 5–15 mg/kg per day in two divided doses (maximum 400 mg/day)
- To achieve the usual maintenance dose, subsequent doses should be increased every 1–2 weeks (calculate 1.2 mg/kg per day)

Table 8.14 Lamotrigine (LTG) dose regimens, when co-medicated with valproate.

Patients aged >12 years
- Weeks 1 and 2: 25 mg every other day
- Weeks 3 and 4: 25 mg every day
- To achieve maintenance, doses may be increased by 25–50 mg/day every 1–2 weeks
- Usual maintenance dose, when adding LTG to valproate alone, ranges from 100 mg/day to 200 mg/day

Patients aged 2–12 years
- Weeks 1 and 2: 0.15 mg/kg per day in one or two divided doses
- Weeks 3 and 4: 0.3 mg/kg per day in one or two divided doses
- Usual maintenance dose: 1–5 mg/kg per day in one or two divided doses (maximum 200 mg/day)
- To achieve the usual maintenance dose, subsequent doses should be increased every 1–2 weeks (calculate 0.3 mg/kg per day)

Levetiracetam

Levetiracetam (ucb L059) was first investigated in the early 1980s as a drug with cognitive enhancing and anxiolytic effects. More than 2000 patients were included in these early studies, the majority receiving doses ranging from 250 mg/day to 1000 mg/day, but the findings were disappointing. Pivotal clinical studies were then initiated in epilepsy, with excellent results, and clinical trials of the drug as adjunctive therapy in the treatment of partial-onset seizures began in 1991. The drug was licensed in 1999 in the USA and in 2000 in Europe. It is a powerful antiepileptic compound which has gained an important place in clinical practice. It is available in an oral and an intravenous formulation.

Physical and chemical characteristics

Levetiracetam bears a close structural similarity to piracetam, and is one of a large family of pyrrolidine drugs. Early studies in other indications used the racemic mixture, etiracetam. Levetiracetam is the S-enantiomer of etiracetam (the R-enantiomer, ucb L060, is inactive). It is a white powder (molecular weight 170.21) and is freely soluble in water, soluble in ethanol and chloroform.

Mode of action

Levetiracetam binds selectively and with high affinity to SV2A, a synaptic vesicle protein that is involved in synaptic vesicle exocytosis and presynaptic neurotransmitter release. This is a novel binding site, not shared by other conventional antiepileptic drugs, and exactly how binding confers antiepileptic action is unclear. It has an anti-kindling action and carries neuroprotective potential.

Levetiracetam has no action against the maximal electroshock and pentylenetetrazol seizure models, unlike

Proprietary name: Keppra[a]

Primary indications

Adjunctive therapy in partial-onset seizures in adults and children aged >1 month, and in myoclonic and tonic–clonic seizures in juvenile myoclonic epilepsy, age ≥12 years. Monotherapy in partial seizures with or without secondarily generalized seizures in patients aged ≥16 years

Commonly used as first-line drug

Yes

Usual preparations

Tablets: 250, 500, 750, 1000 mg; extended-release tablets 500, 750 mg. Oral solution: 100 mg/mL. Intravenous formulation 500 mg/5mL.

Usual dosage – adults

Initial: 125–250 mg/day; increased by increments of 250–500 mg/day every 2 weeks Maintenance: 750–4000 mg/day

Usual dosage – children

Initial: 10–20 mg/kg per day, increased by increments of 10–20 mg/kg per day every 2 weeks Maintenance 20–60 mg/kg per day

Dosing intervals

Twice a day

Is dose commonly affected by co-medication?

Occasionally

Is dose affected by renal/hepatic disease?

Renal disease

Does it affect dose of other drugs?

No

Does it affect the contraceptive pill?

No

Serum level monitoring

Not useful

Common/important adverse events

Somnolence, asthenia, infection, dizziness, headache, irritability, aggression, behavioural and mood changes, emotional lability, depersonalization, psychosis, nervousness, seizure exacerbation, rhinitis, cough, vomiting

Risk of hypersensitivity

Slight

Major mechanism of action

Action via binding to SV2A synaptic vesicle protein

Main advantages

Effective in partial and generalized seizures and generally well tolerated; mode of action not shared by other drugs

Main disadvantages

Mood and behavioural changes

Comment

Well-tolerated and powerful antiepileptic drug with a broad spectrum of activity

[a]Name of proprietary brand available in the UK.

Levetiracetam: pharmacokinetics – average adult values

Oral bioavailability	<100%
Time to peak levels	0.5–2 h
Volume of distribution	0.5–0.8 L/kg
Biotransformation	Hydrolysis in many body tissues. In monotherapy, 66% excreted unchanged
Elimination half-life	6–8 h
Plasma clearance	0.036 L/kg per h (varies with co-medication; faster in children)
Protein binding	None
Active metabolite	None
Metabolism by hepatic enzymes	No
Inhibition or induction of hepatic enzymes	No
Drug interactions	Minor only

many conventional antiepileptics, but does provide protection in a broad range of other models, especially those of chronic epilepsy.

Pharmacokinetics

Absorption
Levetiracetam is rapidly absorbed after oral administration. The peak concentration is reached at about 0.5–2 h after ingestion and oral bioavailability approaches 100%. The speed of absorption – but not its extent – is slowed by food. There is no protein binding. An extended-release formulation has been produced with a mean time to peak levels of 3 h.

Distribution
The drug is widely distributed, with a volume of distribution of approximately 0.5–0.7 L/kg. Despite its water solubility, it freely crosses the blood–brain barrier and it also crosses the placenta, and fetal and maternal plasma levels are similar. It is less than 10% bound to plasma proteins.

Metabolism and elimination
In monotherapy, levetiracetam is largely (66%) excreted unchanged. Most of the remainder (34%) is metabolized to a carboxylic acidic metabolite (ucb L057) by hydrolysis of the acetamide group. Metabolism occurs in various body tissues, including red blood cells, and does not involve the enzymes of the cytochrome P450 system. The half-life of levetiracetam in young healthy people ranges between 7 and 8 h and does not vary either with dose within the usual dose ranges, or with the frequency of dosing. The principal metabolite (ucb L057) is inactive. There is no autoinduction and the kinetics of the drug are linear in clinical dose ranges.

Age has an effect on metabolism and elimination. Levetiracetam clearance, normalized for weight, is 20–45% greater in infants and children than in adults. Higher doses are therefore sometimes required in younger patients.

Levetiracetam and its metabolites are excreted renally, with cumulative urinary excretion of unchanged levetiracetam and ucb L057 of 66% and 24%, respectively, after 48 h. In people with normal renal function, the renal clearance of levetiracetam is about 0.6 mL/min per kg. However, elimination is proportional to renal clearance, and the half-life increases in renal impairment. In a comparison of healthy controls and patients with severe renal impairment, the half-life of levetiracetam was 7.6 h in controls and 24.1 h in those with renal disease. Both the drug and its principal metabolite are removed from the plasma during haemodialysis. Dose reductions are needed in renal impairment, as shown in Table 8.16.

In severe hepatic impairment, the half-life and the exposure to both levetiracetam and ucb L057 are increased, but this is probably the result of coexistent renal disease, and hepatic impairment itself does not seem to affect the kinetics of the drug. The half-life in children (6–12 years of age) is about 6 h, the clearance 1.43 mL/min per kg and the C_{max} about 30% lower than in adults. In elderly people the half-life increases to 10–11 h, possibly due largely to a decrease in renal function. Serum level monitoring is possible, but wide ranges of serum levels are observed with marked individual variation and little correlation with clinical effect. Clearance of levetiracetam rises in the later stages of pregnancy, and dose changes may be required. This rise is probably due to increased renal blood flow.

Table 8.16 Levetiracetam dosing in patients with renal impairment.

Renal function	Creatinine clearance (mL/min per $1.73\,m^2$)	Dose administered twice daily (mg)
Normal	>80	500–1500
Mild	50–80	500–1000
Moderate	30–50	250–750
Severe	<30	250–500

Table 8.17 Frequency of adverse events – pooled results of the clinical trials of adjunctive therapy of levetiracetam in adults.

	Levetiracetam ($n = 769$)	Placebo ($n = 439$)
Asthenia (%)	15	9
Headache (%)	14	13
Infection (%)	13	8
Pain (%)	7	6
Depression (%)	4	2
Dizziness (%)	9	4
Somnolence (%)	15	8
Nausea (%)	4	4
Insomnia (%)	3	3
Nervousness (%)	4	2
Pharyngitis (%)	6	4
Rhinitis (%)	4	3

Drug interactions

Drug interactions do occur with levetiracetam, contrary to initial reports. The concomitant use of enzyme-inducing antiepileptic drugs increases the clearance of levetiracetam by between 20 and 37% in three studies. Dose changes are generally claimed not to be required, but it seems likely that some patients will need increased doses of levetiracetam in polytherapy. Quite how this interaction is mediated is not clear because the drug has no effect on CYP enzyme action. No effect of levetiracetam on the pharmacokinetics of other drugs has been shown.

Adverse effects

Levetiracetam is generally well tolerated, and has a good safety profile. The most commonly reported side effects in the adult population are somnolence, asthenia, a tendency to infection and dizziness (Table 8.17). In a pooled analysis, the most common side effect was somnolence, reported by 15% of patients with epilepsy treated with levetiracetam compared with 8.0% with placebo but the effect was not clearly dose related. In one study somnolence was seen in 20.4% of patients on levetiracetam 1000 mg and 18.8% on 3000 mg, compared with 13.7% of patients on placebo. The second most common side effect in clinical trials was asthenia, with an overall incidence of 15% compared with 9% with placebo, and again it was not clearly dose related. Other adverse effects are listed in Table 8.17. The incidence of side effects is greatest during titration, and slow titration improves tolerability significantly. Infections, including those of the upper respiratory tract (rhinitis and pharyngitis) and the urinary tract, were increased in some of the controlled trials, but the clinical relevance of this finding is still unclear.

Since licensing, by far the most troublesome side effects of levetiracetam, not appreciated in the clinical trials, are its effects on behaviour, and notably its propensity to cause agitation, hostility and anxiety. These effects can be marked, and levetiracetam should be used with extreme caution in patients with pre-existing anxiety or behavioural abnormalities. For the same reason, its use in those with learning disability should be carefully monitored, because behavioural effects can be particularly marked. Levetiracetam therapy can also occasionally precipitate acute psychosis, and this may persist in some cases in spite of drug withdrawal.

Other neurological side effects have included apathy, emotional lability, depersonalization and depression, and a small number of patients have psychotic symptoms and suicidal behaviour.

A marked increase in the frequency of seizures is noted in some patients in routine practice, and there is a suggestion that a paradoxical increase in seizures can occur at high doses, especially in those with generalized abnormalities on the EEG. If seizure exacerbation occurs, often lowering the dose will improve seizure control – and this is a not infrequently observed pattern in clinical practice. In the clinical trials, about 14% of patients experienced an increase in seizures.

A similar adverse event profile is seen in children, with behavioural disturbances being the most prominent problem, and these occur especially in those with a history of pre-existing behavioural disorder.

Hypersensitivity and skin rash are very uncommon, and there are no reports of serious idiosyncratic adverse effects. One severe side effect recently reported is enterocolitis, and this should be suspected in patients developing persistent diarrhoea.

Side effects in children
As a result of the experience in routine practice in adults, the paediatric trials of levetiracetam have looked carefully at behavioural aspects. The most common adverse events in studies in children are similar to those in adults, notably: somnolence, vomiting, anorexia, rhinitis, hostility, increased cough, pharyngitis and nervousness. Psychiatric and behavioural side effects occurring in more than 5% of patients in the clinical trials were: hostility (11.9% levetiracetam, 6.2% placebo), nervousness (9.9% levetiracetam, 2.1% placebo), personality disorder (7.9% levetiracetam, 7.2% placebo), emotional lability (5.9% levetiracetam, 4.1% placebo) and agitation (5.9% levetiracetam, 1.0% placebo). The incidence of psychiatric/behavioural events in children with partial-onset seizures treated with levetiracetam has been found to be 38.6% compared with 18.6% in adults. Various rating scales have been applied in other studies, and therapy with levetiracetam does not appear to adversely affect social skills, school and total competence scores, or other behavioural rating scores.

Side effects of intravenous formulation
The intravenous formulation is very well tolerated. Two studies have been performed to assess its safety profile; levetiracetam 2000–4000 mg i.v. over 15 min (or faster – 1500–3500 in 5 min) resulted in the following symptoms: dizziness 52.8%, somnolence 33.3%, fatigue 11.1%, headache 8.3%. After the 4-day twice-daily intravenous administration, clinical examination and laboratory parameters remained normal, there were no changes in cardiovascular parameters or in blood pressure, no respiratory depression, no clinically relevant changes in the ECG and no symptoms at the injection site.

Tolerance
Tolerance has been observed in an animal model, but has not been seen in the long-term extension arms of the clinical trials, nor does it appear to be much of an issue

in routine clinical practice. However, there is one interesting report of a patient with multiple seizures daily who became initially seizure free with levetiracetam therapy, but the effect was lost after a few weeks of treatment. Subsequently, she regained seizure control when levetiracetam was dosed only once a week, and this positive effect was maintained over years.

Teratogenicity
Levetiracetam is classified by the FDA as a category C drug. It is known to cause fetal anomalies and skeletal changes in rats exposed to the drug *in utero*. 45 pregnancies were recorded during clinical trials, of which 22 were either terminated or ended in spontaneous abortion or ectopic pregnancy. Of the 23 pregnancies ending in live births, there was one case with syndactyly, one with tetralogy of Fallot, one with heart block and one with dysplasia of the hip. All the malformations occurred after exposure to polytherapy that included levetiracetam. The remaining 19 live births had a normal outcome. In the UK pregnancy register, 117 infants exposed to levetiracetam were reported, of whom 3 (2.7%) had major malformations, but again all were exposed to polytherapy. In the registry there are relatively few monotherapy exposures, and no malformations have yet been recorded. This is promising, but it is currently too early to make any definitive statement about the teratogenic potential of the drug. Another recent conference presentation reported over 250 pregnancies (including polytherapy exposures) with a malformation rate of 3.1%.

Overdose
Overdose of levetiracteam is probably safe although no case series have been reported. In animal studies, doses of up to 5000 mg/kg per day produced only mild and transient signs. Haemodialysis would be expected to be effective therapy.

Antiepileptic effect
Adjunctive therapy in partial-onset seizures
In the clinical development programme of levetiracetam, four placebo-controlled studies of 1023 people were carried out in refractory partial epilepsy. Three had a similar parallel group randomized to placebo-controlled design and 904 patients were studied; it was on the basis of these that the drug was licensed. Efficacy was measured over a 12- to 14-week evaluation period at a daily dose of between 1 and 3 g of levetiracetam or placebo. The

three studies showed a statistically significant reduction in the weekly frequency of seizures compared with a baseline of 18–33% on 1 g, 27% on 2 g and 37–40% on 3 g (compared with a placebo rate of 6–7%). In all three studies the trend towards a larger improvement was seen in the highest dosage group. The responder rate, defined as the proportion of patients who had a reduction in frequency of partial seizures of at least 50%, was 23–33% on 1 g, 29–32% on 2 g and 40–42% on 3 g (compared with placebo rates of 10–17%). In a pooled analysis, seizure freedom during the stable dose period were 0.8%, 4.7%, 6.3% and 8.2% for placebo and levetiracetam 1000 mg/day, 2000 mg/day and 3000 mg/day, respectively

The proportion of patients entering the long-term extension studies and the retention rates in these studies was high (>90% and >70%, respectively), indicating the favourable effects of the drug without loss of efficacy.

A dose–response relationship is demonstrated only in some studies of levetiracetam, and in routine clinical practice many patients respond to lower doses than were used in the clinical trials. In most patients, raising the dose to levels above 4000 mg/day will have no additional beneficial effect.

In children, an RCT demonstrated a 50% reduction in partial seizure frequency per week in 44.6% of children on levetiracetam, compared with 19.6% on placebo ($P = 0.0002$). Seven (6.9%) children became seizure free during the entire 14-week double-blind treatment period, compared with one (1.0%) placebo-treated patient. In a multicentre, double-blind, randomized, placebo-controlled, parallel-group study, using video-EEG, the responder rate was significantly greater for levetiracetam (43.1%) than for placebo (19.6%; $P = 0.013$), with similar findings in all categories (1 month to <1 year, 1 year to <2 years and 2 years to <4 years).

Monotherapy in partial-onset seizures

A monotherapy study in patients with newly diagnosed epilepsy compared levetiracetam with controlled-release carbamazepine at optimized dosages: 73.0% (56.6%) of patients randomized to levetiracetam and 72.8% (58.5%) of those randomized to carbamazepine were seizure free for 6 months (1 year). Of all patients achieving 6-month (1-year) seizure freedom, 80.1% (86.0%) in the levetiracetam group and 85.4% (89.3%) in the carbamazepine group did so at the lowest dose level (levetiracetam 1000 mg/day, carbamazepine 400 mg/day). This was a useful study, showing that levetiracetam and controlled-release carbamazepine were of equivalent efficacy, often

at low doses, in newly diagnosed epilepsy using optimal dosing in a setting that was close to clinical practice.

Photosensitivity

Levetiracetam also has a marked effect on the photoparoxysmal response in patients with photosensitive epilepsy, and a single 750 or 1000 mg dose will diminish or abolish the photosensitivity in over 50% of photosensitive patients studied. The duration of suppression of photosensitivity greatly exceeds the plasma half-life of the drug in all patients, and an effect was noted for more than 24 h in a third of patients.

Generalized seizures

A large number of open studies have been carried out in other types of epilepsy showing undoubted efficacy, particularly in generalized seizure disorders, and a similar experience is noted in routine clinical practice.

In idiopathic generalized epilepsy (IGE), striking effects occur, especially in absence, myoclonus and tonic–clonic seizures. Initial clinical experience, confirmed subsequently, showed that the drug can be particularly effective in treating the myoclonic seizures in juvenile myoclonic epilepsy (JME) and the absence seizures in childhood (CAE). On the basis of this experience, an RCT was carried out in patients with refractory myoclonic seizures in IGE. Responder rates of 58.3% in the levetiracetam group were found compared with 23.3% in the placebo group ($P < 0.001$) and seizure freedom rates from myoclonic seizures were 25.0% on levetiracetam compared with 0% on placebo ($P = 0.004$). A second RCT studied tonic–clonic seizures in IGE and found a responder rate of 72.2% for the levetiracetam group and 45.2% for the placebo group ($P < 0.001$). During the 20-week study, seizure freedom rates were 34% for tonic–clonic seizures (vs 11% on placebo) and 24% for all seizures (vs 8% on placebo).

Open studies have provided confirmatory evidence of the efficacy in the various subgroups of IGE, including CAE, JME and eyelid myoclonia with absences. Striking effects are also reported in the progressive myoclonic epilepsies and in children with severe myoclonic epilepsy of infancy. The drug is also useful in cases of postanoxic myoclonus and in the Lennox–Gastaut syndrome, but studies in these areas are to date rather limited.

Clinical use in epilepsy

Levetiracetam is a highly effective antiepileptic drug, with a good safety and tolerability profile. It has a novel mode of action and the drug is effective in cases resistant to other antiepileptics. The pharmacokinetics of the drug are generally felicitous, and for all these reasons it has rapidly become a popular first-line therapy.

It is useful in a wide range of seizure types, both partial onset and generalized, and with good efficacy in myoclonus and absence seizures. It is effective as monotherapy and adjunctive therapy. Many patients in routine practice are well controlled on single drug therapy, often at low doses and at much lower doses than used in the clinical trials. The effects of the drug seem to be maintained during long-term follow-up. It is generally well tolerated and easy to use. For all these reasons, levetiracetam seems likely eventually to become a first-line drug in both partial and generalized epilepsies, rivalling carbamazepine and valproate in this role.

Somnolence is not an uncommon side effect but by far the most troublesome side effect is the tendency of the drug to cause behaviour change, particularly hostility, aggression, anxiety and agitation. It is these effects in routine practice that cause most difficulty. On rare occasions, these effects can be severe and patients should be warned about them. The behavioural effects seem only likely to occur in those who are already predisposed to anxiety or aggressive behaviour, and also in those with learning disability or impairment. Levetiracetam should be used only with caution in these groups of patients, and the effects carefully monitored.

Serum level monitoring seems not to be of any great clinical utility.

Levetiracetam is available in 250, 500 and 1000 mg tablets. In the clinical trials antiepileptic effect was noted at 2–4 g/day, but many patients respond to lower doses, and it is the author's current practice to aim initially for lower doses (750 mg/day) in many patients. The starting dose in routine practice can be 125–250 mg/day in adults, and the dose increased fortnightly by 250-mg steps in a twice-daily regimen. Doses above 4000 mg usually seem not to increase efficacy, and there is indeed a tendency for seizures to be exacerbated at higher doses.

Children metabolize levetiracetam faster, and therefore might be expected to require higher doses per unit of body weight than adults. Clinical trials in children aged 6–12 years used mean doses of 40 mg/kg per day, but initial doses used in children are typically 10–20 mg/kg per day. In patients with severe renal impairment and in elderly people, clearance is lowered and the dose should be reduced (see Table 8.16).

Oxcarbazepine

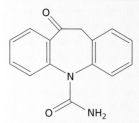

Proprietary name: Trileptal[a]

Primary indications
Monotherapy and adjunctive therapy in partial-onset seizures and generalized tonic-clonic seizures. Adults and children ≥6 years

Commonly used as first-line drug
Yes

Usual preparations
Tablets: 150, 300, 600 mg; oral suspension: 300 mg/5 mL

Usual dosage – adults
Initial: 300 mg/day; increased by increments of 300 mg/day every 2 weeks
Maintenance: 900–2400 mg/day

Usual dosage – children
Initial: 4–5 mg/kg per day, increased by 5 mg/kg per day increments weekly or 2 weekly as required
Maintenance: 20–45 mg/kg per day (maximum 60 mg/kg per day)

Dosing intervals
Twice a day

Is dose commonly affected by co-medication?
Yes

Is dose affected by renal/hepatic disease?
Severe renal disease

Does it affect dose of other drugs?
Yes (but less than carbamazepine)

Does it affect the contraceptive pill?
Yes

Serum level monitoring
Useful (measures of MHD derivative)

Target range
50–140 μmoL; 3–35 mg/L (MHD derivative)

Common/important adverse events
Somnolence, headache, dizziness, diplopia, ataxia, rash, hyponatraemia, weight gain, alopecia, nausea, gastrointestinal disturbance

Risk of hypersensitivity
Yes – but less than carbamazepine

Major mechanism of action
Inhibition of sodium channel conductance. Also effects on potassium conductance, N-type calcium channels, NMDA receptors

Main advantages
Similar to carbamazepine, but adverse event profile is different and fewer drug interactions

Main disadvantages
Higher incidence of hyponatraemia than with carbamazepine, side effects can be marked at higher doses

Comment
Powerful antiepileptic for use in partial-onset epilepsy. Clinical indications and effects similar to those of carbamazepine

[a]Name of proprietary brand available in the UK.
MHD, monohydroxylated derivative (metabolite) (10,11-dihydro-10-hydroxy-5*H*-dibenz[*b,f*]azepine-5-carboxamide); NDMA, *N*-methyl-D-aspartate.

Oxcarbazepine: pharmacokinetics – average adult values (and figures given where indicated for active metabolite MHD)

Oral bioavailability	<100%
Time to peak levels	4–6 h (MHD)
Volume of distribution	0.7–0.8 L/kg (MHD)
Biotransformation	Hepatic reduction to MHD, then conjugation
Elimination half-life	8–10 h (MHD)
Plasma clearance	0.04–0.05 L/h per kg (MHD) (varies with co-medication)
Protein binding	38% (MHD)
Active metabolite	MHD
Metabolism by hepatic enzymes	Aldo-ketoreductase enzymes (not via CYP) and then glucuronidation
Inhibition or induction of hepatic enzymes	Inhibits CYP2C19, induces CYP3A (less than carbamazepine), UGT1A4
Drug interactions	Some drug interactions

MHD, monohydroxylated derivative (metabolite) (10,11-dihydro-10-hydroxy-5*H*-dibenz[*b,f*]azepine-5-carboxamide).

Oxcarbazepine is the 10-keto analogue of carbamazepine. Although it was synthesized in 1963, clinical trials did not begin until 1977 and its clinical development was initially slow and irregular, reflecting, perhaps, a lack of clarity by the manufacturers about its role vis-à-vis carbamazepine. It was introduced into clinical practice early in Denmark and was widely accepted, but, by the time more general licensing was considered, a second set of modern clinical trials was required for regulatory purposes. These were completed in the 1990s and the drug was introduced into EU countries in 1999 and into the USA in 2000. The drug underwent trials in monotherapy initially, which is unusual for an antiepileptic drug, and is available for single and combination drug therapy. Oxcarbazepine is metabolized first by reduction, and thus avoids the oxidative step that carbamazepine undergoes, an important difference because the oxidative metabolite of carbamazepine (CBZ epoxide) is responsible for some of its side effects. Although oxcarbazepine has a different range of side effects and drug interactions compared with carbamazepine, its antiepileptic effects are very similar.

Physical and chemical characteristics
Oxcarbazepine (10,11-dihydro-10-oxo-5*H*-dibenz[*b,f*]azepine-5-carboxamide; molecular weight 252.3) is chemically speaking very similar to carbamazepine. It is a neutral lipophilic compound, and similar to carbamazepine it is very insoluble in water. Its monohydroxylated derivative (MHD) is more soluble. An aqueous solution of MHD, which may allow parenteral administration, is under development, but at present only an oral preparation is available. It is not clear whether oxcarbazepine is as unstable in humid conditions as carbamazepine.

Mode of action
The pharmacological action of oxcarbazepine is exerted almost exclusively through its 10-monohydroxy metabolite MHD (10,11-dihydro-10-hydroxy-5*H*-dibenz[*b,f*]azepine-5-carboxamide). The primary mechanism of action is very similar to that of carbamazepine: blockade of voltage-sensitive sodium channels resulting in stabilization of hyperexcited neural membranes, inhibition of repetitive neuronal firing and inhibition of the spread of discharges. Unlike carbamazepine, MHD also increases potassium conductance and modulates high-voltage N- and P-type calcium channel activity. Similar to carbamazepine, it has actions on NMDA receptors, but it has no action on serotonin, GABA or acetylcholine (ACh) receptors.

Pharmacokinetics
Absorption and distribution
Oxcarbazepine is absorbed almost completely after oral ingestion, and this is an advantage over carbamazepine. Absorption is not affected by food. Oxcarbazepine is rapidly reduced to the biologically active 10-monohydroxy metabolite MHD, and its pharmacological action is due to this metabolite (Figure 8.4). MHD reaches peak levels 4–6 h after oxcarbazepine ingestion and it is widely distributed to the brain and other lipid tissues. The volume of distribution of oxcarbazepine is 0.3–0.8 L/kg, and of MHD 0.7–0.8 L/kg. MHD is 38% bound to plasma proteins. Fetal and maternal plasma concentrations of oxcarbazepine and MHD are similar, and the plasma:breast milk ratio of both compounds is approximately 0.5.

Biotransformation and excretion
Oxcarbazepine is rapidly and extensively metabolized in the liver, and less than 1% of the drug is excreted unchanged in the urine. The main metabolic pathway is via the cytosolic aldo-ketoreductase enzymes in the liver to monohydroxycarbazepine (MHD 96%). Aldo-ketoreductases are practically non-inducible enzymes. A small fraction of oxcarbazepine (4%) is oxidized to an inactive dihydroxy derivative (DHD). MHD is partly glucuronidated by microsomal transferases to the UDPGTs. MHD is responsible for the antiepileptic action of the drug. The half-life of conversion is 1–2.5 h and the elimination half-life is 8–10 h.

In contrast to carbamazepine, there is no autoinduction. This metabolic pathway avoids the oxidation step (to the epoxide) of carbamazepine, which is mediated via CYP3A4 and CYP2C8, and it is these steps that render the metabolism of carbamazepine so prone to enzyme induction and drug interaction.

The clearance of the drug in children aged >8 years is similar to that of adults, but in younger children it is 30–40% higher. In elderly people clearance may be reduced, but usually in proportion to changes in renal function. Serum MHD levels have been reported to drop by a third or more during pregnancy, and to return to baseline values shortly after delivery.

The disposition of oxcarbazepine or MHD is not greatly influenced by hepatic disease or by mild renal disease. However, in patients with creatinine clearance <30 mL/min, doses should be reduced by 50% or more. MHD levels can be measured, and levels of 20–200 μmol/L are associated with an antiepileptic effect. The place of monitoring in routine practice has not been established.

Drug interactions

Oxcarbazepine has the advantage of not inhibiting or inducing hepatic microsomal enzymes to anything like the same extent as carbamazepine, but some interactions do occur.

Of the CYP enzymes, CYP2C19, CYP3A4 and CYP3A5 can be inhibited by both oxcarbazepine and its MHD. The inhibition of CYP2C19 can result in elevation of phenytoin, carbamazepine epoxide and phenobarbital levels. Lamotrigine levels can fall on co-medication by up to a third in some patients. Co-medication with the same three drugs reduces MHD concentrations by 30–40%. Valproate has a slight effect and can lower MHD levels by between 0 and 18%.

As is the case with carbamazepine, oral contraceptive levels may be lower on co-medication with oxcarbazepine (via CYP3A family enzymes) and this may render low oestrogen contraceptives ineffective. No interactions have been noted with warfarin, cimetidine, viloxazine or erythromycin.

Adverse effects

The side-effect profile of oxcarbazepine is generally similar in nature to that of carbamazepine (at least in so far as side effects on initiation of therapy are concerned). Although oxcarbazepine is probably generally better tolerated than standard formulations of carbamazepine, the tolerability of oxcarbazepine has not been extensively compared with slow-release carbamazepine. This would be of interest, because carbamazepine tolerability is itself significantly improved by the use of the slow-release formulation. The discontinuation rates due to side effects in the monotherapy studies were significantly lower for oxcarbazepine than carbamazepine (14% vs 26%) or phenytoin, but were similar to those of valproate. In add-on studies in adults, the reported discontinuation rates due to side effects were 12%, 36% and 67% on oxcarbazepine 600, 1200 and 2400 mg/day, respectively, compared with 9% on placebo. It is common clinical experience that oxcarbazepine is not well tolerated at high doses, possibly because of peaking of the parent drug concentrations.

Neurological and gastrointestinal side effects

The most common are effects on the CNS (Table 8.18) and include headache, dizziness, somnolence, fatigue, double vision and ataxia, and the side-effect profile in this regard is very similar to that of carbamazepine. Nausea and vomiting can also be prominent, especially in children. Other side effects include weight increase, tremor, vertigo, alopecia, nervousness, oculogyric crises

Table 8.18 The five most common CNS side-effects on oxcarbazepine (OXC) therapy. Comparison of initial monotherapy with adjunctive therapy studies.

Side-effect	Initial monotherapy trials		Adjunctive trials[a]	
	OXC (n = 440)	Placebo (n = 66)	OXC (n = 705)	Placebo (n = 302)
Headache	37	12	26	21
Somnolnce	22	6	26	12
Dizziness	20	4	30	11
Ataxia	2	0	17	5
Diplopia	0.5	0	24	3

[a]Combined data from randomized placebo-controlled studies of oxcarbazepine add-on therapy in refractory partial epilepsy in adults and children.

and gastrointestinal disturbance. Two formal controlled studies have shown no impairment of cognitive function after 4–12 months of therapy with oxcarbazepine.

Hyponatraemia

Oxcarbazepine, similar to carbamazepine, results in hyponatraemia, probably as a result of an alteration in the regulation of antidiuretic hormone or increased renal tubular sensitivity. The effect is, however, more common and more severe with oxcarbazepine and is a particular problem in elderly patients. In one study comparing sodium levels in patients switched from carbamazepine to oxcarbazepine, a mean drop in sodium levels of 9 mmoL/L was observed. Between 25 and 50% of patients on chronic therapy have serum sodium levels <135 mmoL/L, but this is usually asymptomatic. If the serum sodium level falls to <125 mmoL/L (as is reported in <5% of patients) careful monitoring is advised, and dose reductions should be made if symptoms of hyponatraemia are present. It also seems sensible to advise dose reduction or drug withdrawal if the level falls to <120 mmoL/L even in the absence of symptoms.

Hypersensitivity

The risk of serious life-threatening idiosyncratic side effects is low, and lower than that of carbamazepine. However, skin rash is relatively common (about 3–10% of all patients) and was the main reason for discontinuation of the drug in the comparative monotherapy studies (10% vs 16% on carbamazepine in one study). Although the rate of occurrence of rash is somewhat lower with carbamazepine, there is significant cross-reactivity, with oxcarbazepine-induced rash occurring in 25–30% of those experiencing rash on carbamazepine. A few cases of Stevens–Johnson syndrome and toxic epidermal necrolysis have been reported.

Teratogenicity

In animal studies, oxcarbazepine was associated with an increased incidence of craniofacial, skeletal and cardio-vascular malformations, decreased fetal body weights and increased rates of fetal death. In a retrospective database review, six congenital malformations occurred among 248 infants born to women who had received oxcarbazepine monotherapy during pregnancy (a rate of 2.4%), suggesting that it is relatively safe in comparison with other antiepileptic drugs, but data are not sufficient to be certain about its safety. It is licensed by the FDA as a pregnancy category C compound.

Overdose

Six cases are reported with a maximum dose of 24 g and all recovered. Potential risks include cardiac arrhythmia, respiratory depression, anticholinergic effects and gastro-intestinal effects. By analogy with experience with carba-mazepine, in addition to supportive therapy, gastric lavage, activated charcoal and dialysis are likely to be helpful.

Antiepileptic effect

Oxcarbazepine has been subjected to a large number of randomized double-blind trials, including eight in mono-therapy. Comparisons have been made with placebo and between high and low doses of oxcarbazepine. All these studies demonstrated effectiveness. Comparative RCTs have also been conducted in which the drug has been compared with carbamazepine, phenytoin, valproate and levetiracetam. This trial programme is generally more extensive than other drugs, and a consistent picture of efficacy has been established.

Monotherapy studies preceded add-on studies, uniquely in modern antiepileptic drug development programmes, largely because safety had been established in older open studies. There are, in fact, more monotherapy data on this drug than on any other new antiepileptic.

In newly diagnosed epilepsy, oxcarbazepine mono-therapy has been shown to have similar efficacy to val-proate, carbamazepine and phenytoin, in studies including almost 1000 patients. Overall, about 50–60% of newly diagnosed patients become free of seizures on initiation of oxcarbazepine therapy.

In refractory patients, two outpatient 'conversion to monotherapy' studies have been carried out. The primary end-points were 'exit' if there was a twofold increase in partial seizure frequency over baseline. The rates on low dose (300 mg/day) were 89–93% compared with 41–59% on high-dose (2400 mg/day) oxcarbazepine therapy. Monotherapy vs placebo studies have also been carried out in patients undergoing presurgical monitoring. To the author's mind, however, it is doubtful whether these studies, with their highly artificial designs, provide many data of clinical utility.

Two large, randomized, double-blind, add-on studies have been carried out in refractory adult patients with partial seizures, and the superiority of oxcarbazepine over placebo was demonstrated in both. The median reduction in the frequency of partial seizures was between 26% at 600 mg/day and 50% at 2400 mg/day. Twenty-two per cent of patients on 2400 mg/day were free of seizures. This is an impressive result for adjunctive therapy in refractory patients, but may be high partly because the duration of treatment with 2400 mg was relatively short for patients who dropped out early as a result of adverse effects.

In a randomized, double-blind, placebo-controlled study in children, 41% of patients treated with oxcar-bazepine had a reduction in the frequency of seizures of at least 50%, and a 34.8% reduction in the median frequency of seizures. Recent trials in children have shown excellent results with higher doses than previously used (up to 60 mg/kg per day), extending the dose range and potential of oxcarbazepine in paediatric practice.

Three controlled studies have compared the efficacy of oxcarbazepine with carbamazepine, and no overall dif-ferences were found. However, it is known that some patients converting from carbamazepine to oxcarbaze-pine show an improvement, so overall figures may hide individual differences. In newly diagnosed patients, the efficacy of oxcarbazepine has been shown to be the same as that of phenytoin, carbamazepine or valproate. In the SANAD study, no differences in efficacy were found when oxcarbazepine was compared with carbamazepine, lamotrigine, gabapentin and topiramate.

Clinical use in epilepsy

The indications for oxcarbazepine are similar to those for carbamazepine. Its efficacy is similar to that of other first-line drugs, including carbamazepine, and it is reasonably well tolerated. It has fewer enzyme-inducing effects than some other antiepileptic drugs, including carbamaze-pine, and thus fewer interactions. If the drug is being substituted for carbamazepine, care is needed, because the removal of the carbamazepine enzyme-inducing effects could alter levels of the concomitant medication.

Oxcarbazepine, however, interacts with the contraceptive pill, and low-dose oestrogen contraceptives should not be used. There are few human data concerning pregnancy. Oxcarbazepine is currently classed as a category C teratogen.

The most common chronic effect is hyponatraemia, but this is usually mild and of no clinical significance. The hyponatraemia is due in part at least to a marked antidiuretic effect, and the consumption of large volumes of fluid (including large quantities of beer) should be discouraged.

Oxcarbazepine is available only as an oral preparation. It can be introduced more quickly than carbamazepine. In adults a starting dose of 600 mg/day can be increased 2 weekly by 300 mg increments to a usual maintenance dose of 900–2400 mg/day, in two or three daily doses, although infrequently doses up to 3000 mg/day are used.

It has been claimed that carbamazepine can be abruptly substituted with oxcarbazepine (in a dosing ratio of 200:300), although there is widespread anecdotal evidence that a rapid switch carries a real risk of severe seizure exacerbations, and should not be routinely carried out. It has also been suggested that oxcarbazepine and carbamazepine can be combined to obtain high combined doses without the side effects that would be expected at equivalent doses in monotherapy, but again in routine practice this seems not to be the case, and high-dose combinations of the two drugs are frequently poorly tolerated.

In children the usual initial dosage is 4–5 mg/kg per day, given in divided doses, and increasing in steps of 5 mg/kg. The usual maintenance dose for a child is 30 (range 20–45) mg/kg per day and the maximum dose for a child is 60 mg/kg per day. In severe renal disease (creatinine clearance <30 mL/min) oxcarbazepine should be started at half the usual dose, and the dose incremented at a slower than usual rate until the desired clinical response is attained.

In routine practice, serum level monitoring of MHD has some role, but experience is not as favourable as for carbamazepine. Serum sodium should be measured as a baseline, after 1–2 months of establishing therapy in all patients and then at regular intervals depending on clinical circumstances.

Phenobarbital

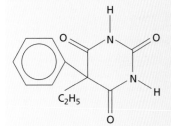

Proprietary name: Luminal[a]

Primary indications
Monotherapy and adjunctive therapy in partial or generalized seizures (including absence and myoclonus) in adults and children. Also status epilepticus, the Lennox–Gastaut syndrome, other childhood epilepsy syndromes, febrile convulsions, neonatal seizures

Commonly used as first-line drug
Yes – in some countries

Usual preparations
Tablets: 15, 30, 50, 60, 100 mg; elixir: 15 mg/5mL; injection: 200 mg/mL

Usual dosage – adults
Initial: 30 mg/day; increased by increments of 15–30 mg every 2 weeks
Maintenance: 30–120 mg/day (maximum 180 mg/day)

Usual dosage – children
Neonates: 3–4 mg/day; initially 1–2 mg/day
Children 1month–12 years: initially 1–1.5 mg/kg per day, increased by 2 mg/kg per day as required
Usual maintenance dose 3–8 mg/kg per day
Children ≥12 years 30–180 mg/day; initially 15 mg/day

Dosing intervals
Once a day

Is dose commonly affected by co-medication?
Yes

Is dose affected by renal/hepatic disease?
Severe hepatic and renal disease

Does it affect dose of other drugs?
Yes

Does it affect the contraceptive pill?
Yes

Serum level monitoring
Very useful

Target range
50–130 μmol/L

Common/important adverse events
Sedation, ataxia, dizziness, insomnia, hyperkinesis (children), dysarthria, mood changes (especially depression), behaviour change, aggressiveness, cognitive dysfunction, impotence, reduced libido, folate deficiency and megaloblastic anaemia, vitamin K and vitamin D deficiency, osteomalacia, Dupuytren contracture, frozen shoulder, shoulder–hand syndrome, connective tissue abnormalities, rash. Risk of dependency. Potential for abuse

Risk of hypersensitivity
Slight

Major mechanism of action
$GABA_A$-receptor agonist. Also depresses glutamate excitability, and affects sodium, potassium and calcium conductance

Main advantages
Highly effective and low-cost antiepileptic drug

Main disadvantages
CNS side effects, especially in children; a controlled drug in many countries

Comment
Highly effective well-tried antiepileptic. Often reserved for second-choice therapy because of potential for side effects

---

ᵃName of proprietary brand in the UK.

Phenobarbital: pharmacokinetics – average adult values

Oral bioavailability	80–100%
Time to peak levels	0.5–4 h
Volume of distribution	0.36–0.73 L/kg
Biotransformation	Hepatic oxidation, glucosidation and hydroxylation, then conjugation
Elimination half-life	75–120 h
Plasma clearance	0.006–0.009 L/kg per h
Protein binding	45–60%
Active metabolite	None
Metabolism by hepatic enzymes	CYP2C9, CYP2C19, CYP2E1, UGT1A4
Inhibition or induction of hepatic enzymes	Induces CYP2B6, CYP2C9, CYP2C19, CYO3A4, UGT1A4
Drug interactions	Common

Phenobarbital is a remarkable drug. It was introduced into practice in 1912, and is still, in volume terms, the most commonly prescribed antiepileptic drug in the world. It is highly effective, and its introduction opened a new chapter in the history of epilepsy treatment. Its efficacy has not generally been bettered by any subsequent drug, it is well tolerated by many people and it is by far the cheapest of the antiepileptic drugs commonly available. As a result of its efficacy and low cost, it is recommended by the World Health Organization as first line for partial and tonic–clonic seizures in developing countries in all age groups.

Physical and chemical characteristics

Phenobarbital (5-ethyl-5-phenylbarbituric acid; molecular weight 232.23) is a substituted barbituric acid with a crystalline structure. It is a free acid, soluble in non-polar solvents but relatively insoluble in water (the sodium salt is readily soluble, but can be unstable in solution). The pK_a of phenobarbital is 7.2, similar to the physiological pH of plasma. Changes in pH, common in active epilepsy, can result in substantial shifts of phenobarbital between compartments.

Mode of action

Phenobarbital seems to act in a relatively non-selective manner, both limiting the spread of epileptic activity and elevating the seizure threshold. It binds strongly to the $GABA_A$ receptor, and its major action is at this receptor, postsynaptically, where it increases the duration of channel opening without affecting the frequency of opening; it differs from the benzodiazepine drugs, which bind to adjacent sites, and has more effect on frequency than duration. This difference is due to the different binding to individual $GABA_A$-receptor subunits by the barbiturates and benzodiazepines. At higher concentrations, it directly reduces sodium and potassium conductance. It also reduces presynaptic calcium influx and depresses glutamate excitability.

Pharmacokinetics

Absorption

Phenobarbital can be administered by intramuscular, intravenous or oral routes. It has a bioavailability of 80–100% in adults after oral or intramuscular administration. Peak plasma concentrations occur 0.5–4 h after oral administration, but can be significantly delayed in patients with poor circulation or reduced gastrointestinal motility. After intramuscular administration, peak serum concentrations usually occur within 4 h (range 2–8 h),

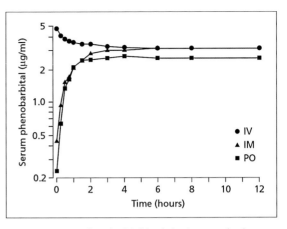

Figure 8.5 Mean phenobarbital levels in six normal volunteers after single IV or IM injections of 130 mg or a single oral dose of 100 mg. This demonstrates the complete absorption of the drug after IM and oral ingestion and their comparable rates of absorption.

and peak plasma concentrations are similar to those after oral administration (Figure 8.5). Absorption is affected by the type of preparation administered (e.g. free acid or salt, crystal size), gastric blood flow, gastric emptying time, gastric acidity, and slowed by the presence of food and neutralizing agents. Absorption occurs mostly in the small intestine because of its larger surface area and longer intraluminal dwell time, and disease at this site can markedly reduce absorption. In newborn and young infants, bioavailability is reduced and oral absorption is incomplete compared with that after intramuscular injection.

Distribution

Phenobarbital is distributed rapidly throughout body tissues. Acidosis enhances transfer from plasma to tissue. In adults, the relative volume of distribution ranges from 0.36 L/kg to 0.73 L/kg after intramuscular administration and from 0.42 L/kg to 0.73 L/kg after oral dosing. The volume of distribution is larger in newborns, where it ranges from 0.39 L/kg to 2.25 L/kg after intravenous or intramuscular injection. The distribution of phenobarbital is very sensitive to variations in the plasma pH and acidosis results in an increase in the transfer of phenobarbital from plasma into tissue. This is of potential importance in the treatment of, for example, status epilepticus. After intravenous administration, phenobarbital relatively slowly enters brain tissue (12–60 min) but in status epilepticus, because of focal acidosis and increased blood flow, the transfer of phenobarbital into the brain is much faster. Phenobarbital is 40–60% bound to plasma protein. Binding in newborns is lower (35–45%). The concentration of phenobarbital in CSF in adults is about 50% of that in plasma, and correlates well with the unbound phenobarbital plasma concentrations. The brain:plasma concentration ratios in human epileptic brain specimens vary widely, ranging from 0.35 to 1.13. Phenobarbital rapidly crosses the placenta, so that maternally derived plasma phenobarbital concentrations in neonates are similar to those in the mother. Phenobarbital is also secreted in breast milk, in which its concentrations are about 40% of those in plasma.

Metabolism and elimination

Phenobarbital has a median half-life of 75–120 h, the longest among any of the commonly used antiepileptic drugs. This is age dependent. Premature and full-term newborns have the longest phenobarbital half-lives (ranging from 59 h to 400 h), infants (aged 6 weeks to 12 months) the shortest, and the half-life diminishes from an average of 115 h to 67 h between birth and the first month of life. By the time the child is 6 months old, however, the half-life is between 21–75 h. The elimination of phenobarbital is reduced when the urine has acidified, and by age, genetic factors, nutritional status and drug interactions.

Phenobarbital is subject to extensive biotransformation in the liver. The major metabolite of phenobarbital is p-hydroxyphenobarbital, and approximately 8–34% of the daily dose is converted to this metabolite, which is then largely excreted as the glucuronide conjugate. N-Glucosidation is another important metabolic pathway, inactive at birth and becoming effective only after about 2 weeks of life. Hydroxylation is catalysed primarily by the isoenzyme CYP2C9, with minor contributions from CYP2C19 and CYP2E1. N-Glucosidation is a more recently identified metabolic pathway. This pathway becomes effective only after 2 weeks of life, and may be the cause of the long phenobarbital half-life in newborns. Other metabolites include an epoxide, a dihydrodiol catechol and methylcatechol derivatives, but these are of less clinical significance.

The amount of drug excreted unchanged is very variable between individuals, with mean values of 20–25% of the total dose (range 7–55%). Although phenobarbital is a powerful inducer of hepatic microsomal enzymes, it does not exhibit autoinduction in humans. The total renal clearance of phenobarbital ranges from 0.006 L/kg per h to 0.009 L/kg per h in adults, and is considerably less than the glomerular filtration rate, indicating extensive resorption. Acidification of the urine increases resorption, and a combination of sodium bicarbonate administration to alkalinize the urine and forced diuresis can increase clearance by up to fivefold. There is no enterohepatic recirculation and faecal excretion of phenobarbital is of little consequence. Elimination is linear at normal dose rate ranges. Oral administration of activated charcoal can assist elimination, by increasing intestinal absorption.

Drug interactions
Effect of phenobarbital on other drugs
Phenobarbital is a potent inducer of hepatic enzyme activity and increases the metabolism of other drugs including a number of analgesics and antipyretics (antipyrine, amidopyrine, meperidine, methadone, paracetamol), antiasthma agents (theophylline), antibiotics (chloramphenicol, doxycycline, griseofulvin), anticoagulants (bis-hydroxycoumarin, warfarin), antiulcer agents (cimetidine), immunosuppressants (ciclosporin), psychotropic drugs (chlorpromazine, haloperidol, desipramine, nortriptyline, benzodiazepines), oral steroid contraceptives and antiepileptic agents.

Among the antiepileptic drugs, phenobarbital particularly induces the metabolism of valproate. It has also been suggested that induction of valproate metabolism by phenobarbital may contribute to valproate hepatotoxicity, by stimulating the production of several valproate metabolites. Phenobarbital may cause a decline in plasma carbamazepine levels in some patients, but the effect is often negligible. The effect on phenytoin is complex, involving induction and competitive inhibition, and is difficult to predict in any individual. The conversion of carbamazepine, diazepam and clobazam to active metabolites is also accelerated by phenobarbital.

Effects of other drugs on the pharmacokinetics of phenobarbital
Phenobarbital is involved in a number of pharmacokinetic drug interactions, the magnitude of which varies greatly from person to person depending on genetic factors and concomitant medication.

Phenytoin, valproate and felbamate inhibit phenobarbital metabolism leading to elevation of phenobarbital levels. The interaction with valproate is clinically the most significant and is complex. Severe somnolence or even stupor can be induced by this combination, a side effect not entirely explained by high serum levels. The increase in serum phenobarbital concentrations appears to be greater in children (112.5%) than in adults (50.9%). The primary mechanism of this interaction is a decrease in the biotransformation of phenobarbital to *p*-hydroxyphenobarbital by inhibition of CYP2C9 and/or CYP2C19. The use of vigabatrin in combination with phenobarbital has sometimes been associated with a small but significant decrease in serum phenobarbital concentration. The mechanism of this interaction is unknown.

Among the non-epileptic drugs, rifampicin is a powerful enzyme inducer and may lower phenobarbital levels, and drugs such as dextropropoxyphene inhibit metabolism and increase levels.

Adverse effects
Neurological side effects

The most important side effects are alterations of behaviour, sedation and cognitive impairment. Sedation and cognitive impairment occur in adults and children. Impairments include motor slowness, memory disturbance, loss of concentration and mental slowness. To what extent these problems are common is uncertain, but it is a clinical impression that in adults at low doses these deficiencies are usually of minor importance. The frequency of sedation was no greater on phenobarbital than on phenytoin or carbamazepine in the large Veterans' Administration (VA) cooperative study. Changes in cognitive function have been measured by various standardized neuropsychological tests. A slight decrease in verbal and performance IQ scores has been observed in children treated with phenobarbital compared with normal controls or patients receiving valproate or carbamazepine. Memory and concentration scores, visuomotor performance and spatial memory, and short-term memory can also be significantly impaired, especially in children.

In contrast to the sedative effects in adults, phenobarbital can cause behavioural changes, primarily hyperactivity, irritability and aggressiveness in children, and also in elderly people and those with organic brain damage. In one study 42% of children developed these paradoxical behavioural changes after febrile seizures. The disturbances were not correlated with plasma phenobarbital concentrations, and improved in all children when phenobarbital was discontinued. In another study comparing phenobarbital with other first-line agents in newly diagnosed epileptic children, phenobarbital was associated with the highest chance of withdrawal because of behavioural problems. Problems with memory or compromised work and school performance can develop even in the absence of sedation or hyperkinetic activity. As a result of these behavioural disturbances, great caution should be exercised in using phenobarbital in children, especially those with learning disabilities or organic brain syndromes.

Alteration of affect, particularly depression, also occurs. A complex picture including depression, apathy, impotence, dysthymia, decreased libido and sluggishness is sometimes observed in adults. In the VA cooperative study, decreased libido and/or potency was found to be more common in patients treated with phenobarbital than in those taking phenytoin or carbamazepine. During chronic therapy other side effects include nystagmus and ataxia, and more rarely peripheral neuropathy and dyskinesia. Elderly patients with organic cerebral disease may also become confused and irritable rather than sedated.

Dysarthria, ataxia, dizziness, blurring of vision and nystagmus may appear if serum levels exceed 40 mg/L. Dyskinesia and peripheral neuropathy are very rare effects induced by phenobarbital. Exacerbation, or the new appearance, of absence seizures has been reported with phenobarbital.

Drug dependency and withdrawal symptoms

Phenobarbital use can be associated with physical dependence, and withdrawal symptoms after abrupt discontinuation. A withdrawal syndrome may also be observed in neonates born to mothers who received phenobarbital during pregnancy. This includes hyperexcitability, tremor, irritability and gastrointestinal upset, and can last for days or even weeks. Seizure exacerbation, novel convulsive seizures and even status epilepticus can occur during withdrawal. For all these reasons, when being withdrawn, phenobarbital should be tapered very gradually.

Effects on blood, bone and connective tissue

Phenobarbital commonly lowers the serum folate level but frank megaloblastic anaemia is rare. A severe coagulation defect has been reported in neonates born to mothers with epilepsy taking phenobarbital due to drug-induced vitamin K deficiency, and supplementation of vitamin K at birth will prevent this complication. Phenobarbital can affect calcium and vitamin D metabolism, by inducing hydroxylation of vitamin D, but only occasionally resulting in overt rickets or osteomalacia. The extent to which phenobarbital induces osteoporosis is unclear, but it is likely to be clinically relevant only in postmenopausal women or in infirm individuals. Regular measurements of bone density, and calcium and vitamin D supplements, are nevertheless advisable in high-risk populations.

The drug has marked effects on connective tissue, resulting in an increased tendency to fibrosis, with increased rates of Dupuytren contractures with palmar nodules, frozen shoulder, plantar fibromatosis, Peyronie disease, heel and knuckle pads, and generalized joint pain. The incidence of these disorders ranges from 5% to 38%, depending on the population studied, e.g. in one study a shoulder–hand syndrome was observed in 28% of 126 neurosurgical patients treated with barbiturates but in none of 108 control patients receiving carbamazepine or phenytoin.

Hypersensitivity and immunological reactions

Mild skin reactions, usually maculopapular, morbilliform or scarlatiniform rashes, occur in 1–3% of all patients receiving phenobarbital.

Serious skin reactions, such as exfoliative dermatitis, erythema multiforme, Stevens–Johnson syndrome or toxic epidermal necrolysis, are extremely rare. A barbiturate hypersensitivity syndrome, characterized by rash, eosinophilia and fever, is also rare. An immunologically mediated hepatitis has been reported. Systemic lupus erythematosus and acute intermittent porphyria may be unmasked or precipitated by phenobarbital.

Teratogenicity

In spite of its use for over 90 years, the extent of the teratogenic potential of phenobarbital is quite unclear. Although a barbiturate fetal syndrome has been identified, there are few reports of major malformations; 6.5% of 77 children exposed to phenobarbital were born with major malformations, including cardiac defects (coarctation of the aorta with abnormal valves, tetralogy of Fallot, pulmonary atresia) and cleft lip and palate, in an American registry – a greater risk than with any antiepileptic other than valproate. Other registries have shown much lower risks, however, and data are inadequate to make definitive recommendations.

Overdose

Levels of phenobarbital >350 μmol/L are potentially fatal, and many deaths from overdose are reported. Characteristic cerebral and EEG changes are seen as levels increase (Figure 8.6). Drug-naïve patients are much more sensitive to the effects, and coma occurs in most cases with levels >300 μmol/L. Coma, respiratory depression and hypothermia are leading symptoms. Supportive treatment is, however, usually successful, and additional effective measures include forced diuresis, the alkalinization of urine, and the use of activated charcoal and ion-exchange resins.

Antiepileptic effect

Phenobarbital has been extensively used in a wide variety of epileptic seizure types for many years. As a result of its venerable age, the drug has not been subjected to the usual panoply of prelicensing controlled trials, and indeed there are very few controlled data to document the extent of its self-evident effectiveness.

In the VA cooperative double-blind study, the efficacy and tolerability of four drugs (phenobarbital, primidone, carbamazepine and phenytoin) were assessed in 622 adults with previously untreated or under-treated partial and secondarily generalized tonic–clonic seizures. Similar rates of overall seizure control were obtained with each drug (36%, 35%, 47% and 38%, respectively). Carbamazepine, however, provided better total control of partial seizures (43%) than phenobarbital (16%) or primidone (15%). Interestingly, phenobarbital was associated with the lowest incidence of motor, gastrointestinal or idiosyncratic side effects.

In another large, long-term, prospective randomized, pragmatic trial the comparative efficacy and toxicity of phenobarbital, phenytoin, carbamazepine and valproate were assessed in both adults and children newly diagnosed with epilepsy. In 243 adults, the overall control of seizures on all 4 drugs was similar, with 27% of patients being free from seizures throughout the follow-up, and 75% entering 1 year of remission by 3 years of follow-up. Similar results were reported in 167 children (aged 3–16 years) who entered the study. Twenty per cent remained free from seizures and 73% achieved 1-year remission by 3 years of follow-up. Again there was no difference in efficacy between the drugs for either measure of efficacy at 1, 2 or 3 years of follow-up in adults; in children, only 10 continued the study because there was a high incidence of behavioural side effects and the phenobarbital arm was discontinued prematurely.

Both these studies show that phenobarbital is useful in the treatment of generalized tonic–clonic seizure and partial seizures. Similarly, in drug-resistant patients, there are small trials showing equivalent efficacy of phenobarbital with other established drugs. There are, however, no large randomized controlled studies in refractory epilepsy.

Idiopathic generalized epilepsy

Phenobarbital has also been shown to be effective in the treatment of seizures (generalized tonic–clonic, myoclonic) in the syndrome of IGE, and is a useful alternative if valproate is ineffective or not well tolerated. The effects of phenobarbital on absence seizures seem

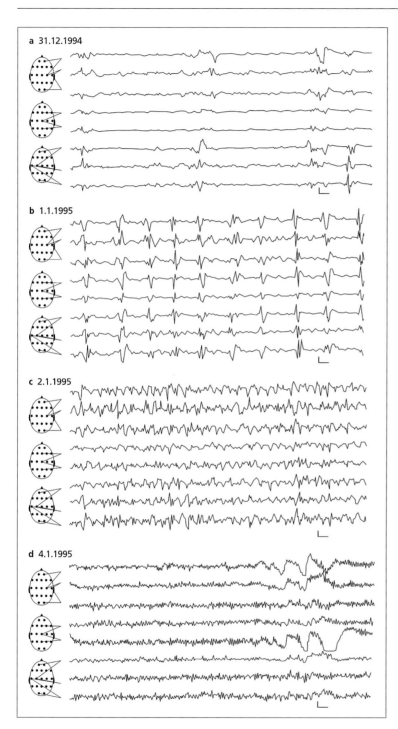

a 31.12.1994

b 1.1.1995

c 2.1.1995

d 4.1.1995

Figure 8.6 PB overdose in a 47-year-old woman with a 34-year history of focal motor and secondarily generalized seizures, on chronic treatment with PB 100 mg daily. There was no apparent aetiology for epilepsy. The patient was found comatose in her bed; on admission to the hospital, the patient was in deep coma and required assisted ventilation; the EEG showed a burst-suppression pattern (a). The plasma levels of PB were 82 µg/ml. On the subsequent day, there was some improvement of the EEG, with shortening of the 'inter-bursts' flattenings (b). The corresponding plasma levels were 60 µg/ml. Progressive improvement of the EEG continued (c), with a normal tracing on the fifth day (d) after overdose. When awake, the patient admitted to have taken 'many' pills to attempt suicide.

rather variable, and indeed absence seizures can be exacerbated.

Neonatal seizures

Phenobarbital is traditionally considered the drug of choice for the treatment of neonatal seizures. This reflects long familiarity and experience rather than any superiority over other drugs (there is none) in this very heterogeneous condition.

In three open trials, an intravenous loading dose of 15–20 mg/kg resulted in seizure control in 32–36% of cases. High-dose phenobarbital therapy in newborns at term with severe perinatal asphyxia has also been shown to improve neurological outcome. In a randomized prospective study, phenobarbital at a dose of 40 mg/kg i.v. resulted in a 27% reduction in the incidence of seizures and a significant improvement in neurological outcomes at 3 years of age.

Status epilepticus

Phenobarbital is a drug of choice in the established stage of convulsive status epilepticus (see pp. 299–300). The usual adult dose is 10 mg/kg at a rate of 50–75 mg/min, and in children and neonates the dose is 15–20 mg/kg at a rate of 100 mg/min. These doses may be followed by a maintenance daily dose of 1–4 mg/kg (adults) or 3–4 mg/kg (children and neonates). It is as effective as a combination of diazepam and phenytoin and more effective than phenytoin alone.

The best evidence for the efficacy of phenobarbital in generalized convulsive status epilepticus stems from a double-blind, multicentre trial which compared four intravenous regimens: diazepam (0.15 mg/kg) followed by phenytoin (18 mg/kg), lorazepam (0.1 mg/kg), phenobarbital (15 mg/kg) and phenytoin (18 mg/kg). The study included 518 patients with either overt generalized convulsive status epilepticus or subtle status epilepticus. In the group with overt generalized convulsive status epilepticus (386 patients), lorazepam was successful in 64.9% of cases, phenobarbital in 58.2%, diazepam plus phenytoin in 55.8% and phenytoin in 43.6%. The major side effects of phenobarbital in this indication are respiratory depression and hypotension, and the full panoply of intensive care monitoring and life support is needed.

Febrile convulsions

Phenobarbital has also been extensively used as an anticonvulsant for the prophylaxis of febrile seizures. However, the potential adverse effects associated with continuous anticonvulsant treatment are now thought to outweigh the relatively minor risks associated with simple febrile seizures. Thus, long-term prophylaxis is now hardly used, and reserved only for children with preexisting neurological abnormalities, or those who are at risk of repeated prolonged seizures. If long-term prophylaxis is required, one study compared 59 patients with 72 untreated children, and found a recurrence rate of 13% in the phenobarbital group compared with 20% in the control group. Where phenobarbital levels were between 16 and 30 mg/L, the recurrence rate was 4%. In a metaanalysis of the efficacy of various medications in the prevention of recurrent febrile seizures, the risk of recurrence was significantly lower in children receiving continuous phenobarbital therapy than in those receiving placebo.

Cerebral malaria in children

In cerebral malaria, phenobarbital has been the traditional treatment of choice, but a recent study showed that, although the frequency of seizures was significantly lower in a phenobarbital group than in a placebo group (11% vs 27%), the mortality rate was doubled (18% vs 8% deaths). The drug is therefore not recommended in this indication.

Clinical use in epilepsy

There is no large pharmaceutical company promoting or marketing phenobarbital, and as a result its value is underestimated. It has a strikingly low cost and ease of use, which renders phenobarbital an important antiepileptic drug, especially in the developing world. It can be given once a day, and has a low risk of idiosyncratic reactions and probably also of teratogenicity. Its efficacy is not in question, but its general use as a first-line drug is limited by its potential to cause sedation and mental slowness in adults and the risk of paradoxical reactions in children. To what extent the sedative potential of small doses of phenobarbital is actually greater or less than that of other antiepileptics has not really been very clearly established, and studies in developing countries suggest that this is seldom a major issue, especially at low doses. Individuals can experience severe sedation, but many patients take the drug without any noticeable side effects.

Nevertheless, in the western world, its use is now largely confined to second-line therapy in adult patients with focal or generalized seizures intractable to other more modern first-line alternatives. Other indications are in refractory IGE, first-line therapy for neonatal seizures, and as second-line therapy for severe secondarily generalized seizure disorders. The drug is valuable in status epilepticus. In children, because of the sometimes severe disturbance of behaviour that is not uncommonly the result of phenobarbital therapy, the drug is less useful.

Phenobarbital is available in a large number of formulations and preparations. Tablet sizes include 30, 50, 60 and 100 mg sizes, and elixirs (15 mg/5 mL) and injections (200 mg in 1 mL) or propylene glycol and water (90%/10%) are also in common use. In adults the starting dose is 30–60 mg, given at night. The dose can be increased in 15 or 30 mg increments for a maintenance dose of between 60 and 180 mg/day, the most common dose for adults being between 60 and 120 mg/day. Too rapid an initiation of therapy can produce drowsiness, which may persist for several weeks, and it is usually better to introduce the drug slowly.

Many patients are well controlled on low serum levels and low doses. Indeed, it seems likely that low-dose phenobarbital therapy is as effective as any other first-line therapy, with few side effects, at least in adults, and the low cost of the drug (US$2–5 per year) confers remarkable value. There is a need for randomized head-to-head comparisons against the newer drugs, but none has been carried out. In adults, the side effects develop mainly at the higher doses, which are anyway largely redundant in contemporary practice. In children the usual starting dose is 3 mg/kg per day, with maintenance doses in the range 3–6 mg/kg per day. Twice-daily dosing may be necessary in younger children because of the shorter half-life. The drug is widely used in neonatal seizures, where rapid seizure control is needed, and intravenous administration is used. Loading doses of 15–20 mg/kg, intravenously followed by maintenance doses of 3–4 mg/kg per day, are usually used. Side effects (particularly behavioural changes and hyperkinetic behaviour) are more severe in children than in adults, and these effects need to be particularly monitored. In elderly people, paroxysmal agitation and irritability can also occur, as they can in patients with learning difficulty or cerebral damage. The use of the drug in these patients should, therefore, be circumspect.

Serum level measurement of phenobarbital has been widely used, and for most patients concentrations of 40–170 µmol/L are associated with optimal seizure control. Some patients will, however, experience good seizure control above or below this limit and, although side effects are usually not too troublesome when levels are maintained in this range, there is a relatively inconsistent relationship between side effect and level. This is possibly because of the tendency for tolerance to phenobarbital to develop over time.

Phenytoin

Proprietary name: Epanutin[a]

Primary indications
Monotherapy and adjunctive therapy in partial-onset seizures and generalized tonic–clonic seizures. Also status epilepticus. Adults and children

Commonly used as first-line drug
Yes – in some countries

Usual preparations
Capsules: 25, 30, 50, 100, 200 mg; chewtabs: 50 mg; liquid suspension: 30 mg/5 mL, 125 mg/50 mL; injection: 250 mg/5 mL

Usual dosage – adults
Initial: 200 mg at night; increased by 25–100 mg/day increments every 2 weeks.
Maintenance: 200–450 mg/day
(higher doses can be used; guided by serum level monitoring)

Usual dosage – children
Child: 1 month to <12 years: initially 1.5–2.5 mg/kg per day, usual maximum 7.5 mg/kg per day
12–18 years 75–150 mg/day; initially 75 mg/day. Usual maximum 300 mg/day
(higher doses can be used; guided by serum level monitoring)

Dosing intervals
Once or twice a day

Is dose commonly affected by co-medication?
Yes

Is dose affected by renal/hepatic disease?
Severe hepatic disease

Does it affect dose of other drugs?
Yes

Does it affect the contraceptive pill?
Yes

Serum level monitoring
Very useful

Target range
40–80 µmol/L (10–20 mg/L)

Common/important adverse events
Ataxia, dizziness, lethargy, sedation, headaches, dyskinesia, acute encephalopathy (phenytoin intoxication), hypersensitivity, rash, fever, blood dyscrasia, gingival hyperplasia, folate deficiency, megaloblastic anaemia, vitamin K deficiency, decreased immunoglobulins, mood changes, depression, coarsened facies, hirsutism, peripheral neuropathy, osteomalacia and osteoporosis, hypocalcaemia, hormonal dysfunction, loss of libido, hepatitis, coagulation defects

Risk of hypersensitivity
Yes – marked risk

Major mechanism of action
Inhibition of sodium channel conductance

Main advantages
Highly effective and low-cost antiepileptic drug

Main disadvantages
CNS and systemic side effects; non-linear elimination kinetics; drug interaction profile

Comment
Powerful antiepileptic drug. Use reserved increasingly for second-choice therapy because of side effects and pharmacokinetic properties

aName of proprietary brand available in the UK.

Phenytoin: pharmacokinetics – average adult values

Oral bioavailability	95%
Time to peak levels	4–12 h
Volume of distribution	0.5–0.8 L/kg
Biotransformation	Hepatic oxidation, glucosidation, hydroxylation, and then glucuronidation
Elimination half-life	7–42 h (varies with plasma level and co-medication)
Plasma clearance	0.003–0.02 L/kg per h (varies with plasma level and co-medication)
Protein binding	80–95%
Active metabolite	None
Metabolism by hepatic enzymes	CYP2C9, CYP2C19, CYP3A4, UGT1A4
Inhibition or induction of hepatic enzymes	Induces CYP2B6, CYP2C9, CYP2C19, CYP3A4, UGT1A4
Drug interactions	Common

Phenytoin was introduced into clinical practice in 1938 – as Lennox put it 'a year of jubilee' for people with epilepsy. Since then phenytoin has been a major first-line antiepileptic drug in the treatment of partial and secondarily generalized seizures. When it was introduced, only potassium bromide and phenobarbital showed equal effectiveness, but phenytoin was found to cause less sedation. Although phenobarbital continues to be used, the introduction of phenytoin meant that bromides were finally, after nearly 100 years of prescription, redundant. Now many alternative drugs are available, and the use of phenytoin has diminished. Nevertheless, it has both low cost and strong antiepileptic effects, and is still considered a drug of first choice in some parts of the world. It has had a huge effect on the treatment of epilepsy over the last 50 years, and has been a paradigm for epilepsy clinical and experimental therapeutics and drug development. Phenytoin has also been used as second-line treatment in trigeminal neuralgia, neuropathic pain, certain cardiac arrhythmias, as a prophylactic in occasional varieties of migraine, and in paroxysmal choreoathetosis and myotonia.

Physical and chemical characteristics

Phenytoin (5,5′-diphenylhydantoin) is usually available as the free acid (molecular weight 252.3) or, more commonly, as the sodium salt (molecular weight 274.3). It is a white crystalline solid, a weak acid with a pK_a of 8.3–9.2, and is relatively insoluble in water. A parenteral formulation is available with a pH of about 12. The storage of phenytoin capsules under conditions of high temperature and humidity may reduce the oral bioavailability of the drug.

Mode of action

Phenytoin exerts its antiepileptic effect largely by binding to, and thus prolonging the inactivation of, voltage-dependent sodium ion channels in neuronal cell membranes (a mechanism discovered in 1983, more than 40 years after its introduction and worldwide use). This effect is greater when the cell membrane is depolarized than when it is hyperpolarized. Phenytoin binds to the same site on the outer surface of the cell membrane sodium ion channel as carbamazepine and lamotrigine; however, the drugs have different binding affinities. Phenytoin at high concentration may also inhibit axonal and nerve terminal calcium ion channels, an action that stabilizes axonal cell membranes and diminishes neurotransmitter release at axon terminals in response to action potentials. The drug has no effect on the function of the T-type calcium ion channels in the thalamus. At high concentrations, phenytoin inhibits Ca^{2+} calmodulin-mediated protein phosphorylation. The drug also binds to the peripheral type of benzodiazepine receptor in brain membranes, but it is not clear whether this action leads to any antiepileptic effect. Phenytoin also has mild dopamine antagonist effects.

Pharmacokinetics
Absorption and distribution

Phenytoin is usually given to patients as the sodium salt, a crystalline preparation that is absorbed rather slowly from the gastrointestinal tract. Absorption through the stomach is relatively poor because phenytoin is very insoluble at the pH of gastrointestinal juice. The high pH of the small intestine, however, enhances phenytoin solubility and absorption. The presence of food alters phenytoin absorption, as do diseases of the small bowel. In an average healthy person, the oral bioavailability is about 95%, and the time to peak levels after oral administration is 4–12 h. Any factor that interferes with the dissolution of phenytoin in the gastrointestinal tract will retard or prevent absorption. There is a wide intra- and interindividual variability in absorption, and occasional patients have very unusual patterns for no obvious reason. Pregnancy reduces absorption, occasionally to extreme levels. Neonates absorb the drug poorly and erratically. The difference in formulation of some generic preparations of phenytoin can result in altered absorption, and so it is usually recommended that the same formulation of phenytoin be dispensed – this is particularly important in patients where metabolism is close to saturation levels. Phenytoin can also be given intravenously (see p. 312). Intramuscular phenytoin must not be given, because the drug precipitates in muscle resulting in a profound delay in absorption and sometimes in muscle necrosis. The bioavailability of rectal phenytoin is also low, around $24 \pm 3\%$.

Phenytoin is distributed throughout total body water with relatively little selective regional concentration. The apparent volume of distribution is about 0.5–0.8 L/kg. The drug achieves a slightly higher concentration in the brain than in plasma, and is at higher concentration in white than in grey matter. Phenytoin is probably transported, partially at least, out of the brain by P-glycoprotein activity. Phenytoin is 70–95% bound to plasma proteins. The concentration of free phenytoin is higher in neonates than adults, in elderly people, in later pregnancy, in the presence of hypoalbuminaemia as occurs in malnutrition, liver disease, nephrotic or uraemic states, and with high levels of glycated albumin as in people with diabetes. The CSF levels of phenytoin are equal to the free plasma fraction, as are the salivary and tear levels. Bioavailability is not significantly altered during pregnancy, and the phenytoin breast milk:plasma ratio is about 0.2, so breast-feeding is safe. A number of acidic drugs, e.g. salicylates and valproate, and certain endogenous substances (fatty acids, bilirubin) displace phenytoin from its plasma protein-binding sites, but these effects are rarely of importance clinically.

Metabolism and excretion

Phenytoin is extensively metabolized by the hepatic cytochrome P450 mixed oxidase system, and at normal doses 90% of the metabolism is by the isoenzyme CYP2C9 activity. The first step involves zero-order kinetics, accounting for the non-linear dose to serum level relationship (see below). The p-hydroxylation step is mainly followed by glucuronidation, although there is a range of other minor metabolites. None of the phenytoin metabolites has anticonvulsant activity, and all are excreted via the kidney. The major metabolite of phenytoin found in urine, p-hydroxyphenytoin (HPPH), accounts for the elimination of some 60–80% of usual doses of the drug. This particular oxidative metabolite is probably formed via a short-lived arene oxide intermediate in a reaction catalysed by the cytochrome P450 isoenzymes CYP2C9 and CYP2C19. The glucuronide conjugate S-isomer of p-hydroxyphenytoin is the predominant one in human urine, accounting for 75–95% of the total phenytoin metabolite present. None of these metabolites has any known biological activity. There is some evidence that the postulated arene oxide intermediate and also epoxide products can interact with tissue proteins, and that the reaction products formed in this way are responsible for some unwanted effects of the drug. About 1 in 500 of the Japanese population is a slow hydroxylator of phenytoin, and hereditary poor metabolizers of the drug have more rarely been encountered in other populations. Variations in the *CYP2C9* gene appear to be responsible for the slow metabolism (Figure 8.7). Minor degrees of autoinduction occur in phenytoin metabolism.

As the first step in the enzymatic degradation of phenytoin is rate limited, the dose to serum level ratio is not linear. As the dose is increased, plasma levels initially rise linearly until the point of enzymatic saturation is reached, and then in a much steeper fashion. There is marked interindividual variability (Figure 8.8). The clearance and half-life of phenytoin therefore both vary considerably within populations, and also depend on the plasma level.

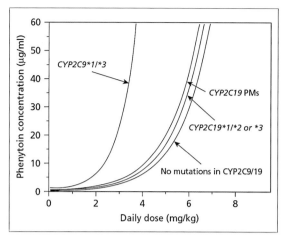

Figure 8.7 Estimated phenytoin dose–concentration relationships in groups of patients with differing CYP2C9 and CYP2C19 genotypes–showing the importance of CYP genotype in determining rates of phenytoin metabolism.

At higher plasma concentrations, the half-life is much longer and the clearance much reduced owing to saturation of the enzyme systems. The time to steady state will also vary non-linearly with dose (but linearly with plasma level) and as many as 28 days may need to elapse before steady state is reached after certain dose changes. The Michaelis–Menten constant of phenytoin is around 6 mg/L (24 µmol/L), lower than the usual plasma concentration in clinical practice.

Neonates eliminate phenytoin more slowly and young children more rapidly than adults. In elderly people, metabolism is less rapid than in younger adults. Phenytoin doses need to be reduced in severe hepatic failure. In renal failure phenytoin levels fall, although those of its major metabolite rise. Haemodialysis has little effect on phenytoin plasma concentrations. In pregnancy, phenytoin metabolism is increased, the elimination half-life of phenytoin shortens and total plasma levels fall, especially in the last trimester, although free levels may be maintained, and doses only occasionally need to be increased to maintain therapeutic effects. Pre-pregnancy values are regained within a few weeks of childbirth.

Drug interactions

Phenytoin is probably the antiepileptic drug with the most problematic drug interaction profile (Table 8.19). This is partly because of the saturable kinetics of phenytoin itself, which results in different interaction behaviour at different doses/serum levels. Phenytoin also

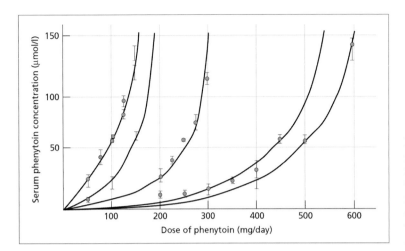

Figure 8.8 Relationship between serum phenytoin concentration and daily dose in five patients. Each point represents the mean (±SD) of three to eight measurements of serum phenytoin concentration at steady state. The curves were fitted by computer using the Michaelis–Menten equation.

is a strong enzyme inducer, prone to induction and inhibition, and is highly protein bound. In addition, some drugs interfere with phenytoin absorption.

The effect of other antiepileptic drugs on phenytoin levels
Carbamazepine and phenobarbital
There is a complex pattern of interactions between phenytoin and these two drugs. Phenytoin levels can be raised or lowered by carbamazepine or phenobarbital co-medication, as both induce and compete for hepatic enzyme metabolism. The overall effect on phenytoin levels is highly variable.

Valproate
Valproate displaces phenytoin from its protein-binding sites and also inhibits its metabolism. There is a transient rise in free levels, but within weeks, owing to redistribution, the free levels return to their previous values, although total levels may be somewhat lower (and dosage should not be increased). Near saturation levels, however, the combination of protein-binding displacement and metabolic inhibition can result in marked rises in phenytoin levels and toxicity. Care therefore needs to be taken, particularly when high phenytoin doses are used or when pre-interaction serum levels are near the top of the therapeutic range.

Vigabatrin
Vigabatrin leads to an approximately 25% fall in phenytoin levels in most patients when introduced as co-medication. The mechanism of this interaction is not known.

Other antiepileptics
Felbamate, oxcarbazepine and stiripentol act as competitive inhibitors of CYP2C9 and CYP2C19 and thus often elevate phenytoin levels. Sultiame co-medication markedly increases plasma phenytoin levels.

The effect of non-antiepileptic drugs on phenytoin levels
Phenytoin levels are affected by a wide range of other drugs (Table 8.20). These are all more marked when phenytoin is close to the top of its therapeutic level. Amiodarone increases serum phenytoin concentrations by as much as 100–200% and its signs of toxicity are similar to those of phenytoin. Antacids and protein hydrolysates and theophylline can reduce the bioavailability of phenytoin, although the effect is variable, reflecting the complex effects on phenytoin dissolution, chelation and gastrointestinal motility. Dosing should be separated by at least 2 h. Some nutritional formulas can reduce phenytoin absorption by up to 75%; Isocal and Osmolite are the main culprits, while Ensure apparently does not have a marked effect. Other drugs that, in co-medication, can reduce phenytoin concentrations include: aciclovir, aspirin, cisplatin, dexamethazone, doxycycline, diazoxide, methotrexate, nitrofurantoin and vinblastine.

Drugs that inhibit CYP2C9 and CYP2C19 will elevate phenytoin concentrations, by impairing oxidation to *p*-hydroxyphenytoin. Such drugs include: sulfaphenazole, phenylbutazole, fluconazole, azapropazone, co-trimoxazole, dextropropoxyphene, disulfiram, fluvoxamine, fluoxetine, ketoconazole, losartan, metronidazole, miconazole, paroxetine, proguanyl, propranolol, sertraline,

Table 8.19 Pharmacokinetic interactions between phenytoin (PHT) and other antiepileptic drugs.

	Effect of phenytoin on the drug	Effect of the drug on phenytoin
Carbamazepine (CBZ)	↑CBZ epoxide and ↓ CBZ concentration	Variable ↓↑
Ethosuximide (ESM)	↓ ESM concentration	No effect
Felbamate (FLM)	↓ FLM concentrations	↑ PHT concentrations
Lamotrigine (LTG)	↓ LTG concentration	No effect
Oxcarbazepine (OXC)	↓ OXC concentrations	↑ PHT concentrations
Phenobarbital (PB)	Variable ↓↑ in PB concentration	Variable ↓↑ in PHT concentration
Primidone (PRM)	↓ PRM concentration	Variable ↓↑ PHT concentrations
Tiagabine (TGB)	↓ TGB concentrations	No effect
Topiramate (TPM)	↓ TPM concentration	No effect
Valproate (VPA)	↓ VPA concentration	↑ PHT concentration at high levels
Vigabatrin (VGB)	No effect	↓ PHT concentrations
Zonisamide (ZNS)	↓ ZNS concentration	No effect

Gabapentin, levetiracetam and pregabalin have no interactions with phenytoin.

trimethoprim, omeprazole, cimetidine, imipramine and diazepam. Cimetidine is a potent inhibitor of phenytoin metabolism and can rapidly cause phenytoin toxicity if phenytoin metabolism is close to saturation. Isoniazid markedly inhibits phenytoin metabolism, and symptoms of phenytoin intoxication are common within days of the introduction of isoniazid as co-medication. The effects are greatest in those individuals who are slow acetylators of isoniazid, and who therefore have higher isoniazid levels. Azapropazone, diazoxide, phenylbutazone, salicylate, sulfafurazone, sulfamethoxypyrine and tolbutamide displace phenytoin from its protein-binding sites (in the same way as valproate) and will affect phenytoin dosage only when levels are close to saturation.

The effect of phenytoin on levels of other drugs
Phenytoin is a potent enzyme-inducing agent. Co-medication with phenytoin results in falling concentrations of carbamazepine, clobazam, clonazepam, ethosuximide, felbamate, lamotrigine, midazolam, primidone, tiagabine, topiramate, valproate and zonisamide. The effect of phenytoin on phenobarbital concentrations is variable, and levels may rise or fall.

The most clinically common interactions with non-antiepileptic drugs include the inhibition of warfarin metabolism, and clotting times need to be monitored frequently if phenytoin dosage changes are made. Corticosteroid metabolism (including dexamethazone) is induced, and doses may need to be twice normal to obtain the desired therapeutic effects. The levels, and thus effectiveness, of busulfan and possibly other anti-mitotic agents can also be significantly affected by phenytoin co-medication. Theophylline levels can be lowered by as much as 35–75% by phenytoin co-medication. Furosemide clearance can be increased by as much as 50% and ciclosporin clearance is increased by 75%. Serum folate levels are reduced in about 50% of patients receiving phenytoin. Praziquantel levels are reduced by a mean of 75% by phenytoin co-medication; this compares with a 10% reduction by carbamazepine, which may therefore be the drug of first choice in treating active cysticercosis. Enhanced metabolism of the combined oral contraceptives renders low-oestrogen contraceptives potentially inactive. Other drugs affected include: atorvastatin, chloramphenicol, dicoumarol, digoxin, disopyramide, doxycycline, haloperidol, methadone, mexiletine, isoniazid, nortriptyline, pethidine, phenazone, quinidine, simvastatin and the tricyclic antidepressants.

Adverse effects
Phenytoin is one of the oldest drugs in the pharmacopoeia (although outflanked in this regard by phenobarbital, which is even longer in the tooth) and the most studied. There is therefore a large body of information about adverse effects. It is salutary to contemplate how long some, even common, side effects took to be recognized. Many patients taking phenytoin, however, have no or only minimal side effects even after decades of therapy

Table 8.20 Metabolic interactions involving phenytoin. The level of evidence for these interactions varies across substances, and not all potential interactions occur consistently in all subjects.

Interacting substances causing raised phenytoin concentrations
Allopurinol, amiodarone[a], amphotericin, azapropazone[a], brivaracetam, bupropion, carbamazepine[b], chloramphenicol, chlordiazepoxide, chlorpromazine, cimetidine[b], clinafloxacin, clobazam, clofibrate, co-trimoxazole[a], dexamethasone, dextropropoxyphene[a], diazepam[b], dicoumarol, diltiazem, disulfiram, erythromycin, ethanol (acute intake), ethosuximide, famotidine, felbamate[b], fluconazole[a], flucytosine, 5-fluorouracil, fluvoxamine[a,b], fluoxetine[b], halothane, 10-hydroxyoxcarbazepine, imipramine[b], isoniazid[a], itraconazole, ketoconazole[b], losartan[a], methsuximide, methoin[b], methylphenidate, methylphenobarbital[b], metronidazole[a], miconidazole[a], nafimidone, nifedipine, nor-diazepam[b], omeprazole[b], paroxetine[a], phenylacetylurea, pheneturide, phenylbutazone[a], phenyramidol, pindolol, prochlorperazine, progabide, proguanyl[b], propoxyphene, propranolol[b], ranitidine, remacemide, sertraline[a], stiripentol[a], sulphaphenazole[a], sulthiame, tacrolimus, thioridazine, ticlopidine[a,b], tolbutamide[a], topiramate[b], torsemide[a], trazodone, trimethoprim[a], troxidone, valproic acid, verapamil, viloxazine, voriconazole, [S]-warfarin[a]

Interacting substances causing lowered phenytoin concentrations
Aciclovir, aspirin, bleomycin, carbamazepine[d], carmustine, ciprofloxacin, cisplatin, dexamethasone, diazepam, diazoxide, dichloralphenazone, doxycycline, evening primrose oil, ethanol (chronic intake), folate, methotrexate, nelfinavir, nitrofurantoin, oxacillin, phenobarbital, pyridoxine, reserpine, rifampicin[c,d], salicylates, theophylline, tolbutamide, vigabatrin, vinblastine

Phenytoin causing raised concentrations of other substances
Chloramphenicol, phenobarbital, tirilazad, warfarin

Phenytoin causing lowered concentrations of other substances
Albendazole, antipyrine, atorvastatin, bromphenac, campothecin, carisbamate, carbamazepine, chloramphenicol, cisactracurium, clobazam, clonazepam, clozapine, ciclosporin, cyclophosphamide, dexamethasone, dicoumarol, digoxin, disopyramide, doxycycline, efavirenz, ethosuximide, felbamate, felodipine, flunarizine, haloperidol, 10-hydroxycarbazepine, irinotecan, itraconazole, lamotrigine, lidocaine, losartan, methadone, methotrexate, metyrapone, mexiletine, midazolam, mirtazepine, misonidazole, nimodipine, nisoldipine, nortriptyline, oral contraceptives, oxazepam, paracetamol, pethidine, phenobarbital, prednisolone, primidone, praziquantel, quetiapine, quinidine, retigabine, all-*trans*- and ±-*cis*-retinoic acid, simvastatin, sirolimus, tacrolimus, taxanes, teniposide, theophylline, thiotepa, tirilazad, topiramate, topotecan, tricyclic antidepressants, valproic acid, vecuronium, vinca alkaloids, voriconazole, warfarin, zonisamide

[a]known substrate and/or inhibitor of CYP2C9;
[b]known inhibitor and/or substrate of CYP2C19;
[c]known inducer of CYP2C9;
[d]known inducer of CYP2C19.

– an important point to emphasize when discussing the pros and cons of therapy.

Phenytoin intoxication and encephalopathy
Acute dose-related effects of phenytoin are usually seen at serum levels >80 μmol/L, although there is individual variation, and some patients have no side effects at much higher levels. These effects, known as 'phenytoin intoxication', include ataxia, dysarthria, motor slowing, lethargy and sedative mental changes. A reversible encephalopathy can occur at high doses (levels usually >160 μmol/L) with mental changes, confusion progressing to stupor or even coma (at levels >200 μmol/L), and a paradoxical exacerbation of seizures.

Chronic neurological side effects
The most common neurological side effects are the acute dose-related side effects listed above, and these reverse when the blood levels of phenytoin are lowered. Phenytoin also has more chronic side effects that occur at normal levels, usually after years of chronic therapy; common side effects include lethargy, nausea

and dizziness. A phenytoin-induced permanent cerebellar syndrome has been postulated, although its existence has been disputed, and it is most likely to be produced by phenytoin overdose. A similar partial loss of colour vision has been reported. Occasionally asterixis, headache, dystonia, orofacial dyskinesia and ophthalmoplegia have occurred. Phenytoin can also induce a peripheral neuropathy, and two patterns are described: a reversible demyelinating neuropathy associated with phenytoin intoxication, and a mild usually asymptomatic sensorimotor neuropathy on chronic therapy. Phenytoin has been reported clinically to cause chronic motor slowing or mental dulling, although rigorous studies have failed to detect any clear-cut effects.

Hypersensitivity and immunologically related side effects

Phenytoin hypersensitivity is idiosyncratic and immunologically mediated (Table 8.21). Skin rash occurs in about 5% of patients started on phenytoin, and is most common in the first 4 weeks of treatment. The rash is usually minor and recedes when the drug is discontinued. It is occasionally associated with fever, leucopenia and lymphadenopathy, and very occasionally evolves into the anticonvulsant hypersensitivity reaction, exfoliative

Table 8.21 Signs and symptoms in 38 cases of phenytoin hypersensitivity reaction.

Sign or symptom	Percentage of patients
Rash	
Morbilliform or licheniform	66
Erythema multiforme	18
Stevens–Johnson syndrome	13
Total	74
Fever	13
Abnormal liver function tests	29
Lymphoid hyperplasia	24
Eosinophilia	21
Blood dyscrasias	
Leucopenia	16
Thrombocytopenia	5
Anaemia	16
Increased atypical lymphocytes	3
Total	31
Serum sickness	5
Albuminuria	5
Renal failure	3

dermatitis, toxic epidermal necrolysis or Stevens–Johnson syndrome. The incidence of phenytoin-related rashes is higher in postoperative patients or those receiving radiotherapy. Serious agranulocytosis, thrombocytopenia and red cell aplasia have been recorded but are fortunately rare. Patients who experience rash on phenytoin have a much higher incidence of rash also on carbamazepine or lamotrigine.

Phenytoin can suppress both humoral and cellular mechanisms. However, there is no clear evidence that patients taking phenytoin are more prone to infection, and the immunological effects are largely subclinical. Very rarely, pulmonary fibrosis has occurred in patients taking phenytoin and may be due to an immune complex disorder. Lymph-node enlargement is not uncommon on phenytoin therapy, and this has led to a controversy about the relationship of phenytoin therapy and malignant lymphoma. Most cases take the form of 'pseudo-lymphomas', which resolve when phenytoin therapy is withdrawn, but a small number of persisting lymphomas have also been recorded in patients on phenytoin therapy. In addition an illness similar to systemic lupus erythematosus has been reported but the immunological markers of drug-induced cases differ from those of the idiopathic form. Phenytoin exacerbates myasthenia gravis, and has been recorded to precipitate the condition. Acute hepatitis and hepatic necrosis have been rarely caused by phenytoin, usually in the context of an acute hypersensitivity reaction. A 'serum sickness'-like syndrome of rash, fever, arthralgia and atypical lymphocytes has also been recorded, as have cases of autoimmune nephritis and thyroiditis.

Connective tissue effects

Gum hypertrophy occurs in up to 10–40% of adult patients on phenytoin and there is possibly a higher incidence in children. In the past, before the widespread availability of plasma level monitoring, gum hypertrophy was often severe, but the effects nowadays are usually mild. The reduction in frequency is due to the introduction of serum level monitoring, and thus the avoidance of high phenytoin levels, and also an emphasis on better dental hygiene. Gum hypertrophy usually develops within 3 months of starting phenytoin therapy and will regress within 6 months of discontinuing the drug, and can be reduced by good dental hygiene and periodic gingivectomy. The cause of the gingivitis is uncertain, but it has been suggested that, as phenytoin is metabolized in gum tissue to *p*-hydroxyphenytoin, the resulting arene-oxide metabolic intermediate forms adducts with various tissue proteins in the gums, leading to gum overgrowth. An alternative hypothesis is that gum hypertrophy is due to increased serum concentrations of basic fibroblast growth factor, which is elevated by phenytoin. Facial changes including coarsening, enlargement of the lips and nose, hirsuitism and acne, and pigmentation can result from chronic phenytoin therapy. The overgrowth of body hair can be marked and of cosmetic importance, especially in dark-haired females. These effects too have become much less prominent since the introduction of drug level monitoring.

Haematological effects

Mild leucopenia is very common in patients taking phenytoin, and does not require attention unless the neutrophil count falls to <1200/mm^3. Macrocytosis occurs in up to a third of patients on chronic therapy, a subnormal folate level in at least half the patients and low CSF folate levels in up to 45%. Despite this, less than 1% develop a frank megaloblastic anaemia. The mechanism of the folate deficiency is uncertain, but may reflect impaired absorption. Folate supplementation is not usually required unless the patient develops a megaloblastic anaemia, or in pregnancy. In up to 10% of patients, low serum vitamin B_{12} levels are also noted. Evidence that the folate deficiency results in depression or mental side effects is weak.

Neonatal blood coagulation defects due to a relative deficiency of vitamin K-catalysed clotting factors can occur in neonates exposed to phenytoin during pregnancy, carrying the risk of neonatal haemorrhage. This is prevented by prophylactic vitamin K administration immediately after birth.

Endocrine and biochemical effects

Phenytoin affects a range of endocrine values, but these changes are, in most cases, of no clinical significance. The drug impairs the absorption of vitamin D and calcium, and increases the hepatic metabolism of vitamin D. Biochemical abnormalities include an elevated plasma alkaline phosphatase and reduced plasma calcium and plasma 2-hydroxycholecalciferol. This can result in loss of bone density, and occasionally in frank osteomalacia, especially in institutionalized patients and in Asian immigrants to northern climates – reflecting the contribution of dietary factors and sunlight exposure. There may also be secondary hyperparathyroidism. The osteomalacia may lead to repeated fractures, and sometimes presents with a painful proximal myopathy. Asymptomatic biochemical changes require no specific treatment, but long-

term therapy with vitamin B can be given. Osteomalacia or rickets reverses with appropriate therapy.

To what extent phenytoin causes osteoporosis is not clear, but, in view of the potential risk, it is recommended that all patients aged >60 years, and also symptomatic patients of any age, on chronic phenytoin therapy should have regular dual X-ray absorptiometry (DEXA) bone density scans to monitor osteopenia and osteoporosis.

Phenytoin can displace thyroxin from its plasma globulin binding. This may result in a decrease in total thyroxine levels, but triiodothyronine (T_3) and thyroid-stimulating hormone (TSH) levels are usually normal and the patients are clinically euthyroid. The acute administration of phenytoin can increase adrenocorticotrophic hormone (ACTH) and cortisol levels but this reverses on chronic administration. Phenytoin can affect the result of the dexamethasone suppression test. Free testosterone levels are lowered by chronic phenytoin therapy, and follicle-stimulating hormone (FSH), luteinizing hormone (LH) and prolactin levels are raised. Phenytoin treatment in experimental models does not affect fertility, but there is a higher incidence of hyposexuality and sperm abnormalities recorded in patients taking phenytoin.

Other biochemical effects, which are usually asymptomatic, include: raised serum or plasma levels of high-density lipoprotein (HDL)-cholesterol, ceruloplasmin, copper, prolactin and sex hormone-binding globulin. It has also been associated with reduced concentrations of fibrinogen, vitamin K, vitamin E, oestrogens, progesterone, free testosterone, pyridoxal phosphate, tryptophan and thiamine. The reduction of sex hormones may affect sexual drive and libido. Phenytoin can also very rarely induce deficiency of IgA, IgG, IgE, IgM, and thus immunological insufficiency. In neonates, the induced deficiency of vitamin k can induce deficiencies of vitamin-K-catalysed clotting factors and the risk of bleeding.

Phenytoin intake can precipitate attacks of porphyria in those who have the disorder, and it can diminish insulin secretion from the pancreas, resulting in a tendency to hyperglycaemia.

Cardiovascular effects

Intravenous phenytoin, especially if the rate of administration exceeds 50 mg/min in adults or 1–3 mg/min per kg in children, or if the dose exceeds the recommended levels, causes hypotension, cardiovascular collapse, atrial and ventricular conduction depression, and ventricular fibrillation.

Teratogenicity

Phenytoin is an FDA category D teratogen (i.e. a drug in which studies have shown a fetal risk in humans). Fetal abnormalities due to phenytoin were first recorded in 1970, but much still remains to be discovered about the extent of the risk and its mechanisms. The individual role of phenytoin has been difficult to interpret, partly because of the tendency to treat the teratogenicity of antiepileptic drugs as a class effect, and also because of the large number of women in the earlier studies who were on multiple drug therapy. Although these initial reports attributed to phenytoin a marked teratogenic potential, more recent studies have not shown this. In an analysis of five prospective European studies of malformation rates after fetal exposure to antiepileptic drugs during pregnancy, the malformation rate for phenytoin monotherapy was 6%, and the relative risk for phenytoin being associated with malformations, compared with the background risk, was 2.2 (95% CI 0.7–6.7). In that study, phenytoin in monotherapy seemed safer than other established major antiepileptic drugs. It seems therefore that, in monotherapy and particularly at low doses, the teratogenic risk is not high and may be less than that of alternative drugs.

A range of different malformations has been reported. The most severe include facial clefts, diaphragmatic hernias, hip dysplasias and congenital heart abnormalities. That these can be due to phenytoin therapy seems well established, and animal experimentation has confirmed this. Phenytoin is less likely to cause serious spinal malformations than carbamazepine or valproate.

A 'fetal hydantoin syndrome' has been described (first in 1975), comprising characteristic facies with wide-spaced eyes, deformities of the fingernails, slender and shortened terminal phalanges, mild learning disability, and poor infantile growth and development. Many of these minor abnormalities become unrecognizable within the first few years of life. Partial rather than full syndromes are more commonly encountered, and the extent to which there are really teratogenic effects or simply variations in healthy development, unrelated to phenytoin exposure, is unclear. The mechanism of teratogenicity may relate to the production of reactive metabolic intermediates, notably arene oxide derivatives, which form adducts with fetal tissue proteins. Free radical intermediates produced by the activity of tissue peroxidases may also play a part. The arene oxide adducts would be more likely to be present at higher concentrations if the activity of the enzyme epoxide hydrolase (which catalyses the further metabolism of arene oxides and epoxides) is deficient, and there is evidence that low levels of the enzyme epoxide hydrolase in amniocytes and fetal fibroblasts are associated with the fetal hydantoin syndrome.

Antiepileptic effect

Phenytoin was introduced for the treatment of partial and tonic–clonic seizures on the basis of a small number of open uncontrolled investigations. In the first study in the late 1930s, phenytoin was added for 2–11 months to 142 patients with active seizures on phenobarbital and bromides. Bromides were withdrawn but the phenobarbital was continued, and 'complete relief' was obtained in 58% of the 118 patients with frequent 'grand-mal' seizures, and there was a 'marked decrease' in seizures in another 32%. The corresponding figures for the 74 patients with 'petit mal' (probably some cases would now be classified as having complex partial seizures) were 35% and 49%, respectively, and for the 6 with 'psychomotor seizures' 67% and 33%. It is salutary also to note that the drug was in wide global use within a year or two of the first patient taking the drug in the first clinical trial, a speed of market penetration that would be the envy of the modern pharmaceutical industry.

Similar excellent findings were reproduced in many other open studies. In the past decade, blinded controlled comparisons of new drugs with phenytoin, phenobarbital and carbamazepine have been carried out (notably the VA study and studies from King's College Hospital in London). None of these demonstrated any significant differences in antiepileptic effect between phenytoin and either phenobarbital or carbamazepine in the control of either partial or generalized tonic–clonic seizures. In a series of similar studies of partial and generalized tonic–clonic seizures, phenytoin has also been compared in a controlled fashion with valproate, carbamazepine, clobazam and lamotrigine, without significant differences in efficacy or withdrawal rates due to toxicity. In one study only, of newly diagnosed patients, was phenytoin found to control tonic–clonic seizures better than carbamazepine (but not valproate). There is, therefore, consensus that phenytoin is as effective as any other first-line drug in partial and tonic–clonic seizures (especially when secondarily generalized). Dispute exists about its relative tolerability.

The effectiveness of phenytoin in partial and secondarily generalized seizures is clearly dependent on serum level. In any individual, better control is consistently obtained at higher serum levels. The concept of a therapeutic range was established on the basis of experience with phenytoin, and applies more to phenytoin than to any other antiepileptic drug. The upper limit of the target range is 80 μmol/L, although there are patients who respond better to higher levels without serious side effects. Equally, there are large numbers of patients with low serum levels that are quite adequate for seizure control. At least 70% of patients (78% in one study) with newly diagnosed epilepsy (partial or tonic–clonic seizures) will be controlled by phenytoin monotherapy A recent study showed that functional polymorphisms in the *CYP2C9* gene and an intronic polymorphism in the *SCNIA* gene were related to the dosage of phenytoin (and, in the latter case, carbamazepine) needed in clinical practice, although this study has not been replicated and the validity of its results are now doubted.

There is also general agreement that phenytoin is ineffective for treating myoclonic seizures (irrespective of the age of onset or epilepsy syndrome), typical absence seizures (petit mal), atonic seizures or atypical absence seizures of the Lennox–Gastaut syndrome. In some of these seizure types phenytoin can cause an exacerbation of seizures, although this is unusual. The drug can worsen myoclonus in patients with progressive myoclonic epilepsy. The drug has also proved ineffective in treating two reasonably common varieties of situation-related human epilepsy, namely febrile convulsions of infancy and the eclamptic seizures of pregnancy, where there is a controlled study showing phenytoin to be less effective than magnesium sulphate in eclampsia.

Intravenous phenytoin has been used successfully in treating neonatal seizures and status epilepticus.

Clinical use in epilepsy

Phenytoin is still one of the most commonly used antiepileptics in the world, e.g. in North America until recently phenytoin accounted for almost 50% of all new prescriptions and 45% of the total antiepileptic drug market, eclipsing carbamazepine and valproate. In the UK and Scandinavia, phenytoin is used less commonly than carbamazepine or valproate, but in other countries it remains a drug of first choice. As the efficacy of the major antiepileptic drugs in partial and secondarily generalized epilepsy has not been shown to differ, the rational choice of a drug will depend on other factors such as cost, ease of use and the side-effect profile. Phenytoin is extremely cheap. However, its use requires serum level monitoring, and the list of side effects is

long. In most patients on chronic therapy with non-toxic blood levels, no serious side effects are experienced, and evidence of any general difference in tolerability between phenytoin and other old (or new) drugs is weak.

In the author's practice, phenytoin is a drug of second choice in partial and secondarily generalized seizures, and also in primary generalized tonic–clonic seizures. The difficult pharmacokinetics of the drug, rather than its side-effect profile, weigh against its first-line use. As a result of the non-linear kinetics of phenytoin, blood level monitoring is essential. The therapeutic range of plasma phenytoin concentrations is usually considered to be 40–80 μmol/L (10–20 mg/100 mL). However, many patients achieve total control of seizures at lower levels, and others require higher levels (100–120 μmol/L). It is often claimed that lower levels are required to control tonic–clonic seizures than partial seizures. Drug interactions are common, complex and troublesome, and where possible phenytoin should be used as monotherapy. Once a satisfactory phenytoin dosage regimen has been achieved in a particular patient, it will rarely be necessary to alter that regimen over many years.

Phenytoin is also often recommended after head trauma or neurosurgical procedures, although the frequency of rash and immunologically mediated side effects seems greater in these acute situations than in routine therapy. Phenytoin is, after phenobarbital, a drug of choice in neonatal seizures when administered parenterally. The drug also has a major role in the treatment of status epilepticus.

Phenytoin is available in tablets and capsules of 25, 50, 100 and 200 mg sizes. It is also available as a solution for intravenous injection and as a suspension and chewable tablet. In most patients it is given on a once, or more commonly twice, daily basis. A typical starting dose in an adult is 200 mg/day and this can be increased up to 450 mg as initial maintenance therapy, although the dose will depend to some extent on the serum level and some patients require higher doses. Serum concentrations usually take about a week to reach steady state after a change in dose, but occasionally steady state may not be reached for up to 4 weeks. In children the usual starting dose is 5 mg/kg per day and the drug given twice a day. Phenytoin can also be loaded intravenously or orally in emergency situations, the oral loading dose being 15 mg/kg in three doses at 1-hourly intervals. A serum level in the low therapeutic range is usually achieved 12 h after such a loading dose.

Pregabalin

Proprietary name: Lyrica[a]

Primary indications
Adjunctive therapy in partial-onset seizures. Adults only

Commonly used as first-line drug
No

Usual preparations
Capsules: 25, 50, 75, 150, 300 mg

Usual dosage – adults
Initial: 50 mg/day; increased by increments of 50 mg/day
Maintenance: 150–400 mg/day (maximum 600 mg/day)

Dosing intervals
2 or 3 times/day

Is dose commonly affected by co-medication?
No

Is dose affected by renal/hepatic disease?
Dose reductions needed in renal disease

Does it affect dose of other drugs?
No

Does it affect the contraceptive pill?
No

Serum level monitoring
Not useful

Common/important adverse events
Weight gain, somnolence, dizziness, ataxia, asthenia, tremor, blurred vision, double vision, amnesia, depression, insomnia, nervousness, anxiety, cognitive effects and confusion

Risk of hypersensitivity
No

Major mechanism of action
Action on α_2–δ subunit of the voltage-gated calcium channel. Also reduces release of glutamate and other excitatory neurotransmitters

Main advantages
Effective and well tolerated

Main disadvantages
Limited routine clinical experience to date

Comment
Recently licensed drug for adjunctive therapy in partial-onset epilepsy in adults

[a]Name of proprietary brand available in the UK.

Pregabalin: pharmacokinetics – average adult values	
Oral bioavailability	>90%
Time to peak levels	1 h
Volume of distribution	0.56 L/kg
Biotransformation	None
Elimination half-life	5–7 h
Plasma clearance	0.042–0.06 L/kg per h
Protein binding	None
Active metabolite	None
Metabolism by hepatic enzymes	No
Inhibition or induction of hepatic enzymes	No
Drug interactions	None

Pregabalin was discovered in 1989 by the medicinal chemist Professor Richard Silverman working at Northwestern University in the USA. The drug was licensed to Pfizer and its effects in epilepsy, anxiety and pain were studied. Pregabalin was approved for use in the EU in 2004 for epilepsy, in the USA for epilepsy, diabetic neuropathy pain and postherpetic neuralgia in 2005, and then in 2007 for fibromyalgia. Its effects in neuropathic pain have been exceptionally profitable and, within 2 years of its launch in late 2005 in the USA, it had brought in US$1.2 billion in sales, and the sales of the drug for epilepsy are, similar to that of its sister drug gabapentin, dwarfed by those for pain.

Physical and chemical properties

Pregabalin (S-(+)-3-isobutyl-γ-aminobutyric acid) is a structural analogue of GABA (molecular weight 159.23). It is a white stable solid, freely soluble in water and organic solvents, with pK_a values of 4.2 and 10.6. Although pregabalin has structural similarities to gabapentin, the potency in animal models of epilepsy, pain and anxiety is significantly greater.

Mode of action

Pregabalin binds in a very potent fashion to the α_2–δ protein subunit of the voltage-gated calcium channel, binding much more strongly, for example, than gabapentin. Its binding reduces calcium influx in response to depolarization possibly by influencing trafficking of the calcium channels to the membrane), and this in turn reduces nerve terminal release of neurotransmitters including glutamate. This is likely to be responsible for the antiepileptic effect, although it is possible that it has

other additional mechanisms of action. It has strong analgesic and anxiolytic actions, probably due to the same binding properties. The S-isomer binds 10 times more strongly than the R-isomer, and only the S-isomer has antiepileptic action. In spite of its close structural similarity to GABA, pregabalin is inactive at $GABA_A$ and $GABA_B$ receptors and it is not converted metabolically into GABA or a GABA-receptor antagonist, nor does it, like gabapentin, alter GABA uptake or degradation. It has no effect on GABA in the retina or optic nerve, in contrast to vigabatrin. In animal experimentation, pregabalin has a similar profile to gabapentin in all animal models tested, but pregabalin was consistently three- to sixfold more potent on a milligram per kilogram dose basis. It is effective in a wide range of animal models of epilepsy.

Absorption and distribution

Pregabalin is rapidly absorbed with a bioavailability of over 90%, and peak levels are reached within 1 h. The serum level concentration rises linearly with dose and there is little intraindividual variation. Steady state is reached within 24–48 h after repeated administration. It is transported into the brain by the system L active transport system.

Metabolism and elimination

Pregabalin is not metabolized to any extent in humans. Pregabalin has linear pharmacokinetics in the normal dosing ranges. Its plasma half-life is approximately 6 h, independent of dose and repeated administration. Food has no clinically significant effect on absorption, in contrast to tiagabine, for example. Plasma pregabalin concentration–time profiles are similar after two- or three-times-daily dosing. It does not bind to plasma proteins.

Approximately 98% of the drug can be recovered unchanged in the urine. The amount excreted is independent of dose and is not significantly different whether given as single or repeated administrations, but it is affected by severe renal disease. A 50% reduction in dose is recommended in those with a creatinine clearance of 30–60 mL/min and daily doses should be reduced by 50% for each additional 50% reduction in clearance.

There are no data on the disposition of the drug in pregnancy. No differences in pharmacokinetic parameters have been noted in different ethnic groups or by gender and, although only limited data are available, the pharmacokinetics seem to be unchanged in elderly people (matched for renal function).

Drug interactions

Pregabalin has no effect or action on the cytochrome P450 system in humans at therapeutic doses, nor is it protein bound. There have been no reports of drug interactions and, on the basis of its pharmacology, none would be expected. There is no interaction with the combined contraceptive pill.

Adverse effects

The major side effects in routine practice are drowsiness, sedation and weight gain.

Weight gain was reported as an adverse event, reported overall by 24% of patients in the clinical trials and long-term follow-up studies. In the latter, the mean weight gain was approximately 5 kg, with 44% of patients experiencing a 7% or greater weight increase. Similarly, in a 6-month study which had as primary outcome the assessment of weight gain in patients treated with less than 300–450 mg/day pregabalin, the median body weight gain was 4.0 kg, and 41% of patients who completed the study had a body weight increase of more than 5 kg.

In the epilepsy clinical trials adverse events resulted in discontinuation of pregabalin in between 10 and 14% of patients at 300 mg/day and in 19–26% of patients at 600 mg/day, with no difference between two- and three-times-daily regimens. Common adverse events were dizziness, somnolence, ataxia and asthenia, and these appear to be dose related. Other side effects include increased appetite, blurred vision, diplopia, dry mouth, constipation, peripheral oedema and weight gain. Most adverse events were transient and mild to moderate in intensity.

Overall, pregabalin seems reasonably well tolerated, and 83% of pregabalin-treated patients in the clinical trials enrolled in the open-label extension phases: 0.3% of all patients on pregabalin developed myoclonus vs 1.5% for all epilepsy controlled trials. Only 0.37% of patients discontinued due to myoclonus. No life-threatening adverse events have been recorded. In the four fixed dose clinical trials of pregabalin versus placebo, the most common side effects were (range 50–600 mg/day): dizziness (9–34%), somnolence (10–26%), ataxia (3–20%), fatigue (6–18%), headache (7–10%) and weight gain (1–17%). In longer-term studies, the most frequently reported adverse events were dizziness, somnolence, ataxia, difficulties with concentration, tremor, amnesia, depression, insomnia, nervousness, anxiety and confusion. Other recorded adverse events headache, asthenia, and diplopia.

There is not enough information available on the effect of pregabalin on pregnancy to make any recommendations, and although pregabalin is not teratogenic in mice or rabbits, teratogenicity has been observed in rats at high doses.

Antiepileptic effect

The definitive efficacy data are largely from three multi-centre, double-blind, placebo-controlled, parallel-group, randomized trials of pregabalin as add-on therapy in patients with refractory partial epilepsy (Table 8.22).

The first trial enrolled 453 patients in the USA and Canada, and reported percentage reductions in the frequency of seizures between baseline and treatment

Table 8.22 Mean seizure reductions on placebo and pregabalin in three clinical trials as adjunctive therapy in refractory partial epilepsy (expressed as RRatio).

	Placebo	Pregabalin dose			
		50 mg	150 mg	300 mg	600 mg
Simple and complex partial seizures	1.2	−5.1	−10.6/−28.3[a,c]	−28.3[c]	−29.1/−32.5[c]
Secondarily generalized seizures	−3.7	18.5	1.5/6.8	−24.7	−30.6/−35.3[a,b]
All partial-onset seizures	−0.8	−6.2	−20.5/−11.6[b,c]	−27.8[c]	−32.5/−34.0[c]

The table shows the RRatio, which was the primary end-point of the study (RRatio is the mean response rate – transformed symmetrical change in seizure frequency). The two values in the 150 and 600 mg dose columns refer to different trials.
[a]Significant difference compared with placebo, $P \leq 0.05$;
[b]significant difference compared with placebo, $P \leq 0.001$;
[c]significant difference compared with placebo, $P \leq 0.0001$.

periods were 7%, 12%, 34%, 44% and 54% for the placebo and pregabalin 50, 150, 300 and 600 mg/day without titration, respectively. Seizure reduction for all partial seizures was statistically significantly greater in the pregabalin 150, 300 and 600 mg/day groups compared with the placebo group. Responder rates were 14%, 15%, 31%, 40% and 51% across all treatment groups, respectively, and the rate was significantly greater than for placebo in the pregabalin 150, 300 and 600 mg-treated groups. Seizure-free rates for the intention-to-treat (ITT) population were 8%, 5%, 6%, 11% and 17%, respectively.

The second study enrolled 287 patients in Europe and South Africa and studied placebo and pregabalin at two doses (150 and 600 mg/day). Seizure reduction for all partial seizures was found to be statistically significantly greater in both the pregabalin groups. Responder rates were 6%, 14% and 40% for placebo and pregabalin 150 mg and 600 mg/day respectively. Seizure-free rates were 1%, 7% and 12%, respectively for the ITT population.

The third study enrolled 312 patients at 43 centres in the USA and Canada, and compared twice- and three-times-daily dosing at 600 mg with placebo. There was a percentage reduction in the frequency of seizures between baseline and treatment periods of 1%, 48% and 36% for the placebo, pregabalin 600 mg/day three-times-daily and pregabalin 600 mg/day twice-daily groups, respectively. The percentage reduction in seizure rate for the pregabalin two- and three-times-daily groups were similar and not statistically significantly different. Responder rates were 9%, 49% and 43%, respectively; the responder rates for the pregabalin two- and three-times-daily groups were similar. Seizure-free rates were 3%, 14% and 3%, respectively for the intent-to-treat population.

The mean reduction in seizures in all three studies combined is shown in Table 8.22, which uses the RRatio (defined as the difference between treatment and placebo rates divided by the sum of the two rates) to compare treatment with placebo rates. This ratio was accepted as a primary end-point of the study, and is a transformed ratio that allows statistical comparisons to be made. As the figures in Table 8.22 show, there were highly significant reductions in the frequencies of seizures at doses between 150 and 600 mg/day for partial seizures and at 600 mg/day for secondarily generalized seizures. It was notable too that significant reductions in seizure frequency were recorded from day 2 onward of the titration phase (with a dosage of 150 mg/day). Between 3 and 17% of patients were seizure free in the last 28 days of treatment (compared with 0.0–1.0% on placebo).

The long-term studies of pregabalin have included 1480 patients with an overall exposure to pregabalin of 3150 patient-years. In these, 77% of patients had received at least 6 months of pregabalin treatment, 59% at least 1 year of treatment, 35% at least 2 years and approximately 20% at least 5 years. In patients who took treatment for at least 6 months or 1 year, 9.2% (103/1119) were seizure free for the last 6 months, and 8.1% (71/877) for the last 12 months, respectively. In the long-term follow-up, responder rates among patients still treated with pregabalin ranged between 41 and 66%. Although these results are likely to be influenced to a great extent by the self-selected nature of the cohort, they do suggest that pregabalin has persisting effectiveness over long time periods in a significant number of cases.

Clinical use in epilepsy

Pregabalin is licensed in Europe, the USA and 40 additional countries as adjunctive therapy in partial-onset epilepsy in adults, and its place in routine therapy has yet to be fully ascertained. The results from the clinical trials are encouraging, and the lack of interactions and its excellent pharmacokinetic properties make pregabalin an easy drug to use. Pregabalin has a reasonable side-effect profile, and the frequency of adverse effects may be reduced by slow titration. The main side effects are weight gain, which can be marked, drowsiness and sedation. No life-threatening or serious idiosyncratic effects have been recorded. In addition to its effects in epilepsy, pregabalin shows a marked analgesic effect, especially against neuropathic pain, and the drug is now widely licensed for this indication. The usual starting dose in routine clinical practice is 150 mg/day given in two or three divided doses, and dose escalation up to 600 mg/day will depend on individual tolerability and response to the drug. The drug should not be used in pregnancy because there is insufficient information on its safety.

Primidone

Primidone was introduced into clinical practice in 1952. Although it has strong advocates, most clinicians feel that it functions simply as a prodrug of phenobarbital, with little clinical advantage (and significant disadvantages) compared with the parent drug. In most countries it is not, similar to phenobarbital, a drug of abuse and therefore it is not subject to special controls – a practical (and rather illogical) benefit enjoyed by the drug.

Proprietary name: Mysoline[a]

Primary indications

Monotherapy and adjunctive therapy in partial-onset seizures and generalized tonic–clonic seizures. Adults and children

Commonly used as first-line drug

No

Usual preparations

Tablet: 250 mg

Usual dosage – adults

Initial: 62.5–125 mg/day; increased by increments of 125–250 mg/day every 2 weeks
Maintenance 250–1000 mg/day (maximum 1500 mg/day)

Usual dosage – children

Initial 1–2 mg/kg per day
Maintenance 10–20 mg/kg per day

Dosing intervals

1–2 times/day

Is dose commonly affected by co-medication?

Yes (as for phenobarbital)

Is dose affected by renal/hepatic disease?

Severe hepatic and renal disease

Does it affect the contraceptive pill?

Yes

Serum level monitoring

Very useful (measures of derived phenobarbital)

Target range

25–50 μmol/L (and derived phenobarbital 50–130 μmol/L)

Common/important adverse events

As for phenobarbital. Also dizziness and nausea on initiation of therapy

Risk of hypersensitivity

Slight

Major mechanism of action

As for phenobarbital – $GABA_A$-receptor agonist. Also depresses glutamate excitability, and affects sodium, potassium and calcium conductance

Main advantages

Not a controlled drug; less risk of abuse than phenobarbital

Main disadvantages

Adverse event profile, as for phenobarbital

Comment

A prodrug of phenobarbital with probably some minor additional efficacy

[a]Name of proprietary brand available in the UK.

Primidone: pharmacokinetics – average adult values

Oral bioavailability	<100%
Time to peak levels	0.27–3.2 h
Volume of distribution	0.64–0.72 L/kg
Biotransformation	Hepatic metabolism to phenobarbital, and then biotransformation as for phenobarbital
Elimination half-life	3.3–22.4 h (varies with co-medication)
Plasma clearance	0.035–0.052 L/kg per h (varies with co-medication)
Protein binding	25%
Active metabolite	Phenobarbital
Metabolism by hepatic enzymes	CYP2C9, CYP2C19 and then glucuronidation
Inhibition or induction of hepatic enzymes	Induces CYP2B6, CYP2C, CYP3A (derived phenobarbital)
Drug interactions	Common

Physical and chemical characteristics and mode of action

Primidone (5-ethyldihydro-5-phenyl-4,6-(1*H*,5*H*)-pyrimidine-dione; molecular weight 218.25) is a deoxybarbiturate that differs from phenobarbital by the absence of a carbonyl group in position 2 of the pyrimidine ring (Figure 8.9). It is a crystalline powder with very low solubility in water. The main action of primidone is due to the derived phenobarbital, and whether either primidone itself or a second active metabolite, phenylethylmalonamide, adds anything to its antiepileptic properties is controversial.

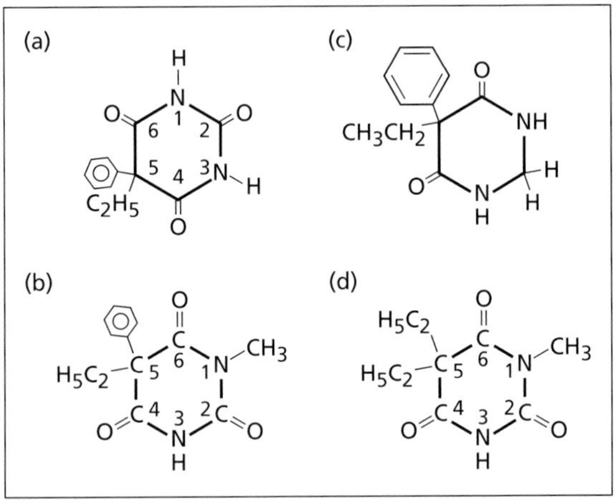

Pharmacokinetics
Absorption and distribution
Primidone is well absorbed orally, with a bioavailability approaching 100%, although there does seem to be quite significant intraindividual variation (and possibly differences in different formulations). Time to peak plasma concentrations of primidone is between 2.7 and 3.2 h in adults and 4 and 6 h in children. The drug is 25% bound to proteins and concentrations in fluids, including CSF, saliva and breast milk, approach those in plasma. The distribution of the drug through tissues is similar to that of phenobarbital.

Metabolism, elimination and drug interactions
About 90% of primidone is excreted unchanged in the urine. Of the remaining 10%, most is rapidly metabolized into phenobarbital, which is its primary metabolite, and phenylethylmalonamide (PEMA). After a first dose of primidone, PEMA was detected in blood within a few hours, whereas phenobarbital was often not measurable

Figure 8.9 Structural formulae of (a) phenobarbital, (b) methylphenobarbital, (c) primidone and (d) metharbital.

during the first 24 h. The elimination half-life of primidone is very variable (range 3–22.4 h) and of the derived phenobarbital 40–60 h. In adults co-medicated with enzyme-inducing antiepileptic drugs, half-life values are generally in the range 3.3–11 h; the ability of newborns to metabolize primidone to phenobarbital is limited, and in neonates the half-life of primidone is 23 h on average, with a range of 8–30 h.

As primidone is metabolized by the cytochrome oxidase system, there is a potential for drug interactions, not only between primidone and other drugs but also between primidone and the derived phenobarbital. Phenytoin and carbamazepine markedly increase the rate of conversion of primidone to phenobarbital, and primidone lowers carbamazepine levels. Morning trough levels of primidone are reduced by about 50% compared with monotherapy levels, and phenobarbital levels were raised by a factor of 1.6 in patients co-medicated with phenytoin and/or carbamazepine. Thus, with phenytoin or carbamazepine co-medication, the average primidone dose required to achieve a given phenobarbital concentration is 1.6 times lower than with primidone monotherapy. In addition, the morning trough serum concentration ratio of phenobarbital to primidone is more than three times higher in co-medicated patients, and toxicity may be caused if phenytoin or carbamazepine is added to pre-existing primidone therapy.

There is a complex interaction with valproate, which usually elevates the ratio of phenobarbital to primidone. The ratio primidone:phenobarbital in the plasma also seems variable, depending on co-medication, age, duration of therapy, and factors such as pregnancy and disease. Valproate can have variable and unpredictable effects on the rate of conversion of primidone to phenobarbital. In contrast to other antiepileptic drugs, clonazepam seems to increase primidone levels and this drug combination often causes marked drowsiness.

Serum level monitoring

There is a poor correlation between the oral dose of primidone and the plasma levels of primidone itself and its metabolite phenobarbital. Although a therapeutic range of about 3–12 mg/L has been suggested for primidone, monitoring primidone levels has very limited clinical value, and monitoring the levels of metabolically derived phenobarbital is of far more use in guiding therapy.

Overdose

Primidone overdose causes CNS depression and hypotonia in overdose. These seem to correlate better with plasma and CSF primidone levels than with phenobarbital or PEMA levels. The management of primidone overdose follows the same procedures as for phenobarbital overdose.

Adverse effects

The side effects are largely those of phenobarbital (see pp. 214–215). The drug is, however, often considered to be less well tolerated, and this is because of intense dizziness, nausea and sedation which occur commonly at the onset of therapy (sometimes after only one tablet). These reactions are probably due to the initially high concentration of the parent drug. These side effects disappear over a week or so, but it is always advisable to start primidone at a low dose.

Antiepileptic effects

There is an unresolved debate as to the extent to which primidone itself (or its other metabolite phenylethylmalonamide) exerts a significant antiepileptic action over and above that of its derived phenobarbital. A number of studies appear to demonstrate independent action, but, although this evidence is reasonably strong, it is not conclusive. Perhaps the best clinical study is the VA cooperative study, in which primidone, phenobarbital, carbamazepine and phenytoin were compared. The efficacy of primidone and phenobarbital was similar but primidone showed fewer behavioural side effects than either phenobarbital or phenytoin. There is also an interesting report of a patient in whom primidone generic formulations were substituted on two occasions for the proprietary formulation (Mysoline), with loss of seizure control on both occasions. The phenobarbital level was virtually unaltered but the primidone level was reduced by 53%. These and other studies suggest that primidone does have independent actions, but these are probably relatively slight.

Clinical use in epilepsy

Primidone is available as 250 mg tablets, which have similar efficacy to 60 mg phenobarbital. Measurement of the derived phenobarbital (and not primidone) levels is usually carried out if plasma concentration monitoring is required. An average starting dose for an adult would be 62.5–125 mg at night, with increments every 2–4 weeks to an average maintenance dose of 250–1000 mg/day in one or two divided doses. A low starting dose is essential to avoid the risk of intense side effects on drug initiation. In routine therapy, the efficacy of primidone can be assumed to be close to that of phenobarbital. However, it is doubtful whether there is any advantage in prescribing primidone rather than phenobarbital, other than in exceptional circumstances.

Rufinamide

Rufinamide is a newly licensed antiepileptic drug developed initially by Ciba-Geigy in the 1980s (and known as CGP-33101 and then RUF-331) and acquired by Eisai in 2004 (and henceforth known as E2080). It was licensed for use in Europe in 2009, under the orphan drug mechanism for adjunctive use only in the Lennox–Gastaut syndrome.

Proprietary name: Inovelon[a]

Primary indications
Adjunctive therapy in the Lennox–Gastaut syndrome, ≥4 years of age

Commonly used as first-line drug
No

Usual preparations
Tablets: 100 mg, 200 mg, 400 mg

Usual dosage – adults
Initial: 400 mg at night; increased by increments of 400 mg/day every 2 weeks
Usual maintenance dose:
30–50 kg – 1200–1800 mg/day
51–70 kg – 1200–2400 mg/day
71 kg or more – 2400–3200 mg/day

Usual dosage – children
Initial: <30 kg: 200 mg; increased by 200 mg/day increments weekly
Maximum:
<30 kg not receiving valproate: 1000 mg/day
<30 kg receiving valproate medication, 600 mg/day

Dosing intervals
Twice a day

Is dose commonly affected by co-medication?
Yes

Is dose affected by renal/hepatic disease?
No effects in renal disease. Insufficient data in hepatic disease

Does it affect dose of other drugs?
Slight effect

Does it affect the contraceptive pill?
Yes

Serum level monitoring
Utility not established

Common/important adverse events
Headache, dizziness, somnolence, fatigue, nausea, diplopia, blurred vision, ataxia

Risk of hypersensitivity
None to date

Mechanism of action
Inhibition of sodium channel conductance

Main advantages
Efficacy in the Lennox–Gastaut syndrome

Main disadvantages
Limited clinical experience

Comment
New antiepileptic drug, licensed in 2009

[a]Name of proprietary brand available in the UK.

Rufinamide: pharmacokinetics – average adult values

Oral bioavailability	<85% with food, but affected by dosage; lower without food
Time to peak levels	4–6 h
Volume of distribution	0.8 L/kg
Biotransformation	Hydrolysis
Elimination half-life	8–12 h (in monotherapy); varies with co-medication, dose and age
Plasma clearance	0.09 L/kg per h (in monotherapy; varies with co-medication, dose and age)
Protein binding	30%
Active metabolite	None
Metabolism by hepatic enzymes	Metabolized by the carboxylesterase enzymes, not via CYP enzymes
Inhibition or induction of hepatic enzymes	Induces CYP3A4
Drug interactions	Common

Physical and chemical characteristics

Rufinamide, 1-(2,6-difluorophenyl)methyl-1H-1,2,3-triazole-4-carboxamide, is a slightly soluble compound with a molecular weight of 238.20.

Mode of action

Rufinamide's main antiepileptic action is the modulation of sodium channel function, largely by increasing the duration of the inactive state of the channel. It has no known effect on the glutamate or GABA receptor.

Pharmacokinetics

Absorption

Rufinamide is only slowly absorbed, and absorption is limited by its slow dissolution. As a result of this, the bioavailability of the drug is dose dependent, and the fraction absorbed decreases with increasing doses. This results in a non-linear relationship between steady-state plasma concentration and dosage. One study found that the steady-state plasma rufinamide concentration:dose ratio at a dose of 3600 mg twice daily was approximately half that recorded at a dose of 400 mg twice daily. Bioavailability is also reduced by about 30–40% higher after a high-fat meal compared with a fasting state. It is recommended that rufinamide always be taken during meals.

Distribution

The plasma protein binding of rufinamide is 26–34%. The volume of distribution is about 0.8 L/kg at a dose of 3200 mg/day, and rufinamide is concentrated in erythrocytes and plasma. In experimental animals, the concentrations in breast milk were similar to those of plasma.

Biotransformation and elimination

Rufinamide is extensively metabolized, with only 4% recovered unchanged. The main metabolite is a carboxylic acid derivative, and the main metabolic pathway is hydrolysis by carboxylesterases, which are non-CYP hepatic enzymes. Carboxylesterase activity is induced by the same drugs that induce CYP enzymes and this explains the increase in rufinamide clearance by such drugs as phenytoin and carbamazepine. The elimination half-life is 8–12 h, but falls by 30% in patients on concomitant enzyme-inducing antiepileptic drug therapy. Body size affects clearance values. Rufinamide clearance is about 30% higher in young children than in adults. There are no major differences in elderly people or those with renal impairment. The effect of hepatic disease is not known.

Drug interactions

Enzyme-inducing drugs such as carbamazepine, phenytoin and phenobarbital reduce rufinamide serum levels, in one study by an average of 19–26%. Valproate increases serum concentration by 12–70% with the highest increases recorded in children, requiring dosing adjustments. Serum rufinamide levels are not affected by lamotrigine or topiramate.

Rufinamide does not affect activity of CYP isoenzymes, and has only a slight effect on the levels of co-medicated antiepileptic drugs. In one study, there was a mean increase of 8–13% in the levels of phenobarbital and of 7–21% in the levels of phenytoin, a decrease in levels of 7–13% of lamotrigine and carbamazepine, and no effect on the levels of topiramate or valproate. Rufinamide increases the metabolism of the contraceptive steroids, and probably reduces the effectiveness of the contraceptive pill.

Side effects

In the clinical trials in adults, headache, dizziness, fatigue, nausea and somnolence were the most commonly reported adverse events. These were mild and the rate of discontinuation due to side effects was 10% on rufinamide and 6% on placebo. The adverse events are dose related. In trials in the Lennox–Gastaut syndrome (largely in children), the most common side effects, compared with placebo, were headache (22.9% vs 8.9%), dizziness (15.5% vs 9.4%), fatigue (13.6% vs 9%), somnolence (11.8% vs 9.1%) and nausea (11.4% vs 7.6%). The drug was discontinued in 8.1% compared with 4.3% on placebo. No idiosyncratic reactions were recorded. Cognitive testing has been studied and did not reveal any differences before and after rufinamide therapy.

Antiepileptic effect

Rufinamide has a rather complex history of antiepileptic drug trials. A total of nine double-blind efficacy studies have been conducted and one large-scale study of adjunctive therapy in partial epilepsy is under way. Monotherapy studies were undertaken in partial epilepsy and were found to be largely negative. Two of three adjunctive studies in partial epilepsy in adults showed significant effects, but not the third, and a multicentre study of partial epilepsy in children was also negative. A study in primarily generalized tonic–clonic seizures was also negative. It has been suggested that the somewhat mixed results were due to failure to account for the effects of food on rufinamide absorption or the effects of co-medication, and further studies are ongoing.

In a multicentre, double-blind, parallel-group study of adjunctive therapy in the Lennox–Gastaut syndrome, 74 patients on rufinamide were compared with 64 on placebo. There was a statistical difference in all three of the primary efficacy variables on rufinamide: a 32.7% median reduction in total seizure frequency compared with 11.7% on placebo ($P = 0.015$); a 42.5% median reduction in tonic–atonic seizure frequency compared with a 1.4% median increase on placebo ($P = 0.0001$); and a reduction in seizure severity in 53.4% of patients compared with 30.6% on placebo ($P = 0.0041$). Some 124 patients entered an open extension phase for up to 36 months and the median reduction in total seizures after 12 was over 43%, and over 58% in tonic–atonic seizures. Post-marketing experience of rufinamide is, at the time of writing, extremely limited.

Clinical use of rufinamide

Rufinamide has shown efficacy in the trial in the Lennox–Gastaut syndrome, and was approved for this indication in Europe under the orphan drug designation. Its studies in partial and primarily generalized epilepsy have been to date negative and it is not approved for these indications at present. The recommended dosing schedules for rufinamide are complex. The drug should be given in two divided daily doses, and taken during meals.

In children weighing <30 kg and not receiving valproate, treatment should be initiated at a daily dose of 200 mg, increased by 200 mg/day increments weekly to a maximum dose of 1000 mg/day. In children weighing <30 kg also receiving valproate medication, a lower maximum dose of 600 mg/day is recommended.

In adults and children aged ≥4 years and weighing ≥30 kg, treatment should be initiated at a daily dose of 400 mg and increased by 400 mg/day increments, to a maximum recommended dose as follows: 30–50 kg – 1800 mg/day; 51–70 kg – 2400 mg/day; ≥71 kg – 3200 mg/day.

Doses of up to 4000 mg/day (in patients in the 30–50 kg range) or 4800 mg/day (in patients >50 kg) have been studied in a limited number of patients. There is limited information on the use of rufinamide in elderly people, but the pharmacokinetic parameters suggest that dosage adjustment is not required. No dose adjustment is needed in those with renal impairment, but the use in patients with hepatic impairment has not been studied and caution should be applied.

It is too early to predict the place in therapy of rufinamide, but its effect, particularly on the multiple seizure types of the Lennox–Gastaut syndrome, is promising.

Tiagabine

Tiagabine was introduced into clinical practice in 1998, first in the UK. It is the last of the 'GABA-wave' drugs to be introduced. It has been the subject of a well-conducted programme of clinical trials, but post-licensing experience is rather disappointing and the drug is now relatively little used.

Chemical and physical characteristics

Tiagabine (molecular weight 412.0) is a derivative of the GABA-uptake inhibitor nipecotic acid ((−)-(R)-1-[4,4-bis(3-methyl–2-thienyl)-3-butenyl]-3-nipecotic acid hydrochloride), rendering the parent compound

Proprietary name: Gabitril[a]

Primary indications
Adjunctive therapy in partial and secondarily generalized seizures in patients aged ≥12 years

Commonly used as first-line drug
No

Usual preparations
Tablets: 2, 4, 12, 16 mg (USA); 5, 10, 15 mg (Europe)

Usual dosage – adults
Initial: 15 mg/day; increased by increments of 4–5 mg/day every 2 weeks. Maintenance: 30–45 mg/day

Dosing intervals
2–3 times/day

Is dose commonly affected by co-medication?
Yes

Is dose affected by renal/hepatic disease?
Hepatic disease (of any severity)

Does it affect dose of other drugs?
No

Does it affect the contraceptive pill
No

Serum level monitoring
Utility not established

Common/important adverse events
Dizziness, tiredness, nervousness, tremor, diarrhoea, nausea, headache, confusion, psychosis, flu-like symptoms, ataxia, depression, word-finding difficulties, encephalopathy, non-convulsive status epilepticus

Risk of hypersensitivity
No

Major mechanism of action
Inhibition of postsynaptic GABA reuptake

Main advantages
Effectiveness.

Main disadvantages
Poorly tolerated; three-times-a-day administration

Comment
Drug of second choice in partial-onset epilepsy in adults, not widely used

[a]Name of proprietary brand available in the UK.

Tiagabine: pharmacokinetics – average adult values

Oral bioavailability	<100%
Time to peak levels	1–2 h
Volume of distribution	1.0 L/kg
Biotransformation	Hepatic oxidation then conjugation
Elimination half-life	5–9 h (in monotherapy)
Plasma clearance	0.109 L/kg per h (varies with co-medication)
Protein binding	96%
Active metabolite	None
Metabolism by hepatic enzymes	CYP3A4 and then glucuronidation
Inhibition or induction of hepatic enzymes	No
Drug interactions	Common

lipid soluble by the attachment of a lipophilic side chain. Tiagabine is thus able freely to cross the blood–brain barrier, unlike the parent compound. It is also freely water soluble.

Mode of action

Tiagabine greatly increases cerebral GABA concentrations, via inhibition of GABA transporter-1 (GAT-1), which is one of at least four specific GABA-transporting compounds that carry GABA from the synaptic space into neurons and glial cells. Measurements in human and experimental models have confirmed that extracellular GABA concentrations are indeed raised after administration of tiagabine. The action of tiagabine on GAT-1 is reversible (unlike the action of vigabatrin on GABA-T), and its affinity is greater for glial than for neuronal uptake. Although its primary effect is similar to that of vigabatrin, the range of pharmacological changes differs, and tiagabine does not result in the widespread increase in brain GABA levels that accompanies vigabatrin therapy, nor does it increase retinal GABA levels. Its effect seems remarkably specific, and studies have shown little or no effect at other receptor systems, including the glutamate, benzodiazepine, 5HT (serotonin), dopamine 1 and 2, adenosine, serotonin, glycine, adrenergic and muscarinic receptors. Tiagabine also appears not to affect the sodium or calcium channels. It has antiepileptic effects in a wide range of animal models, and an experimental profile that differs from that of vigabatrin.

Pharmacokinetics
Absorption and distribution

The oral bioavailability of the drug approaches 100% and absorption is almost complete at all ages. Drug concentrations are linear over the range of usual clinical dosages, and peak concentrations occur about 30–90 min after intake. A second peak of the plasma concentration of tiagabine is seen 12 h after ingestion, and is presumably due to enterohepatic recycling. Food slows down absorption by two or three times; however, the total amount absorbed is unchanged by food. The peak concentration (C_{max}) is also reduced by food and, in view of the rapid absorption and short half-life, taking the drug with food avoids excessive peak blood levels and greatly improves tolerability. It is therefore recommended that the drug always be taken with food, preferably at the end of a meal. The volume of distribution is about 1 L/kg, and the drug is extensively bound (96%) to human plasma proteins, but does not displace other antiepileptics from their protein-binding sites.

Metabolism and excretion

Tiagabine is extensively metabolized in the liver. This is a relative disadvantage of the drug, although one shared by many other antiepileptics. In vitro studies suggest that the main enzymatic degradation is by the isoenzyme CYP3A of the cytochrome P450 family. At least five major metabolites are found both in plasma and in urine and there are additional metabolites in faeces. None of these known metabolites has any antiepileptic action. After oral ingestion of a single dose, less than 3% of the drug appears in the urine unchanged.

The plasma half-life of tiagabine is about 5–9 h in healthy volunteers, and 2–3 h in patients with epilepsy co-medicated with enzyme-inducing drugs. The shorter half-life in patients is presumably due largely to the hepatic-inducing effects of other antiepileptics. The plasma clearance of tiagabine has been found to be 0.12 L/kg/h in patients without concomitant therapy and is faster in those receiving adjunctive therapy with enzyme-inducing antiepileptic drugs. Clearance is about 30% lower in elderly people. The kinetics in young children seem to be more variable and are less well studied, but generally speaking the clearance of tiagabine is greater in children.

Co-medication with enzyme-inducing drugs greatly increases metabolism in children as in adults, and the tiagabine half-life can fall to 2–3 h. The elimination of the drug is reduced in patients with mild-to-moderate liver impairment. In a study of four individuals with mild hepatic impairment, three with moderate impairment and six matched normal controls, tiagabine half-life was found to be 16, 12 and 7 h, respectively, and similar affects were found on C_{max} and AUC. The patients with hepatic impairment also have more neurological side effects, and the drug should be used only with caution in those with hepatic disease. The pharmacokinetics of tiagabine are unaffected in patients with renal impairment or in those with renal failure requiring haemodialysis.

Drug interactions

Tiagabine does not itself induce or inhibit hepatic metabolic enzymatic activity, and therefore should not alter the concentration of other adjunctive antiepileptic drugs, and this has been confirmed in formal interaction studies with carbamazepine, phenytoin, theophylline, warfarin, digoxin, cimetidine, alcohol and triazolam. Tiagabine does not alter plasma concentrations of the contraceptive pill.

However, the metabolism of tiagabine itself is markedly changed by co-administration of hepatic-inducing drugs such as carbamazepine, phenytoin and primidone. In one large population kinetic analysis, the clearance of tiagabine was increased by two-thirds, and the AUC and C_{max} are similarly reduced in patients taking concomitant enzyme-inducing antiepileptic drugs. Higher tiagabine doses are therefore necessary for those receiving concomitant enzyme-inducing antiepileptic drug therapy. Valproate, cimetidine and erythromycin have been found not to affect tiagabine plasma concentrations.

Adverse effects
Neurological and other side effects

In the randomized placebo-controlled trials, 91% of the 675 patients taking tiagabine reported at least one side effect compared with 79% of those taking placebo. The most common adverse events are listed in Table 8.23. Other side effects – which included somnolence, headaches, abnormal thinking, abdominal pain, pharyngitis, ataxia, confusion, psychosis and skin rash – occurred at a similar frequency in treated and placebo groups. Most of these side effects were categorized as mild or moderate in severity, and 15% of patients on tiagabine withdrew from therapy because of side effects.

In the clinical trials, these CNS-related adverse events occurred at greater frequency in patients on tiagabine than in those on placebo only in the titration period. There is now also the recognition that the dizziness, lightheadedness and unsteadiness occurring within 1–2 h of taking a tiagabine dose are due to peaking of the drug

Table 8.23 Adverse effects of tiagabine in the randomized placebo-controlled studies as add-on therapy in refractory partial epilepsy in adults (%).

	Tiagabine, ($n = 675$)	Placebo, ($n = 276$)
Dizziness	30	13
Tiredness	24	12
Nervousness	12	3
Tremor	9	3
Diarrhoea	7	2
Depressed mood	5	1

This table lists the adverse events that occurred significantly more frequently on tiagabine than placebo, from combined data from the placebo-controlled randomized clinical trials.

concentration. This has led to the practice of titrating tiagabine slowly, and taking the drug after food, which has greatly improved tolerability. On an empty stomach, many patients find the drug impossible to take.

As a result of its action on GABA-ergic mechanisms, the question has been raised of whether tiagabine, similar to vigabatrin, can result in visual field abnormalities. To date, however, there is no evidence of an increased risk of concentric visual field defects, in spite of careful testing. Both prospective and cross-sectional studies have been carried out, without a single tiagabine-treated patient showing abnormalities.

Again, on the basis of the experience with vigabatrin, the potential of tiagabine to cause psychosis, depression or severe behavioural disturbance has been carefully studied. In the three main clinical trials the incidence of psychosis was 0.8% in the tiagabine-treated patients and 0.4% in the placebo-treated patients, which was a nonsignificant difference. However, depression occurred more often on tiagabine than on placebo (5% vs 2%). As a result of this, tiagabine should be carefully monitored in patients with a history of behavioural problems or depression.

No adverse effect on cognitive abilities has been demonstrated in extensive neuropsychological studies of tiagabine add-on therapy and monotherapy. Indeed, there is evidence that monotherapy with tiagabine results in modest improvements in cognitive abilities and adjustment and also causes less fatigue when compared with standard antiepileptic drugs.

Non-convulsive status epilepticus and encephalopathy

Several cases of non-convulsive status epilepticus have been reported, usually in patients with spike–wave epilepsy. The extent of this risk is unclear, and at least some of the reported cases were probably not cases of status epilepticus but rather drug-induced encephalopathy.

However, in view of this clear risk, tiagabine should not be used routinely in patients with generalized epilepsy, especially those with a history of absence or myoclonic seizures, spike-and-wave discharges on EEG or non-convulsive status epilepticus.

Idiosyncratic side effects and changes in laboratory parameters

No idiosyncratic reactions have as yet been linked to the use of tiagabine. There are no systematic abnormalities in haematological values or common biochemical parameters, and routine monitoring of laboratory values is not required. The relationship of adverse events has correlated more strongly with dose than with the plasma concentration of tiagabine, and there is therefore no need to check plasma concentrations routinely.

Teratogenicity

There is no definitive information on the teratogenic risk of tiagabine in humans and the drug cannot therefore be recommended for treatment during pregnancy. Effects were seen in the offspring of rats exposed to maternally toxic doses of tiagabine, but not in animals receiving non-toxic doses.

Overdose

Forty-seven cases are reported and all survived. One patient took 400 mg and developed convulsive status epilepticus. In addition to respiratory and cerebral depression, other symptoms included agitation and myoclonus. Treatment with simple supportive measures is effective.

Antiepileptic effect

Partial-onset seizures

Tiagabine has been the subject of a series of clinical trials designed to demonstrate efficacy, including five double-blind, placebo-controlled studies of the drug as adjunctive therapy, three trials (one open and two double-blinded) in monotherapy and six long-term open studies.

The randomized, double-bind, placebo-controlled studies in refractory partial epilepsy in adults form the core of the definitive efficacy studies. Pooling the results, 661 of the 951 enrolled patients were entered into a double-blind phase, and 23% of patients showed a reduction of more than 50%, versus 9% of patients on placebo. The overall frequency of seizures was also reduced, by 25% on tiagabine versus 0.1% on placebo. Tiagabine was effective at doses of 32 and 56 mg/day. A meta-analysis across all three trials for 50% responders showed an odds ratio of 3.03 (95% CI 2.01–4.58) in favour of tiagabine, with no significant differences in efficacy among tiagabine, gabapentin, lamotrigine, topiramate, vigabatrin and zonisamide.

The summary odds ratios for each dose indicated increasing efficacy with increasing dose, with no suggestion that the effect of the drug had reached a plateau at the doses examined in these studies. A 16 mg dose has a fairly small effect of 2.40 (95% CI 0.65–8.87), and this was substantially increased with doses of 30 or 32 mg with an odds ratio of 3.17 (95% CI 2.03–4.96).

Randomized studies have also been performed to compare two- and three-times-daily dosing, and greater numbers of patients completed the study in the three-times-daily group, suggesting that this regimen is better tolerated. The proportion of responders is similar whatever regimen is chosen. Studies of combination therapy with carbamazepine and phenytoin have been carried out. These did not show that any particular drug combination was more efficacious, although tiagabine combinations were better tolerated than the combination of phenytoin and carbamazepine. In the long-term extension studies (i.e. of responders in the short-term clinical trials), a total of 772 patients were treated with tiagabine (at <80 mg/day), with a reduction in the frequency of seizures of at least 50% in about 30–40% of patients treated for between 3 and 6 months. For partial seizures this effect was maintained during 12 months, but not for secondarily generalized seizures.

In open studies in 2248 patients, of whom more than half were treated with tiagabine for more than 1 year, 30–40% of the patients obtained considerable treatment effect, which was maintained after 12 months of treatment. Daily doses in the long-term studies were between 24 and 60 mg in most patients and mean and median doses were 45 mg/day for most studies. However, up to 15% of patients received a dose of between 80 and 120 mg/day after their first year of treatment.

Monotherapy

Tiagabine has also been studied in three monotherapy studies. In chronic partial epilepsy, withdrawal-to-monotherapy studies have been conducted comparing

6 mg/day tiagabine with 36 mg/day after gradual withdrawal of other antiepileptic drugs over 29 weeks. Thirty-three per cent of the patients on the low dose completed the study compared with 47% taking the higher dose, and in both groups the median complex partial seizure rates decreased significantly during treatment compared with baseline. However, a higher proportion of patients in the 36 mg/day group experienced a reduction in complex partial seizures of at least 50% compared with the 6 mg/day group (31 vs 18%). A second double-blind, randomized trial has compared a slow and fast switch to tiagabine monotherapy from another monotherapy: 34 (85%) of the 40 patients were successfully switched to tiagabine monotherapy, finding a retention rate for 12 weeks on tiagabine monotherapy of 63% (25/40) and 48% for 48 weeks (19/40). A third study compared monotherapy with carbamazepine in newly diagnosed partial epilepsy and found carbamazepine to be more effective, with 41% (77 out of 144) in the tiagabine group and 53% (77 of 144) in the carbamazepine group seizure free or having only one seizure ($P < 0.05$, although it has been argued that the dose of tiagabine compared with carbamazepine in this trial was too low, and greater efficacy would have been likely at higher doses).

Children

Tiagabine has also been studied as adjunctive therapy in children in several studies. Effectiveness is reported in partial seizures, to a similar extent as in adults, and tiagabine was also shown to be effective in atypical absence, tonic and atonic seizures (the seizure types of the Lennox–Gastaut syndrome). In an American RCT, in several hundred children, the median seizure reduction was 16% in the placebo group and 25% in the tiagabine group. The tiagabine 50% responder rate was 31% compared with 19% in the placebo group ($P = 0.021$). In the open-label extension study, of 140 evaluable patients, 10 were seizure free with tiagabine add-on therapy and 13 achieved seizure freedom with tiagabine monotherapy (for periods ranging from 9 weeks to 109 weeks). The dose range in this study was from 4 mg/day to 66 mg/day, and the average dose was 23.5 mg/day.

Clinical use in epilepsy

Tiagabine is available for use as add-on therapy in refractory patients with partial or secondarily generalized seizures, in adults and in children aged >12 years. It has been claimed, on the basis of anecdotal experience, that the drug has a particular place in patients with lesional epilepsy (e.g. tumoral epilepsy), and in patients who are prone to agitation or anxiety. In this author's practice, however, these impressions do not seem to be borne out.

It is a reasonably effective drug, but its use is complicated by the need to titrate slowly, the potential for drug interactions, the frequent need for three-times-daily dosing and the side effects. In adults tiagabine should be initiated at a dose of 4–5 mg/day and incremented by weekly increments of 4–5 mg until a maintenance dose is reached. This titration rate is slower than that used in the labelling or in the clinical trials, but minimizes CNS-related side effects. Initial doses can be given twice a day, but a change to three-times-daily dosing is recommended with doses >30–32 mg/day. Tiagabine should always be taken with food, and preferably at the end of meals, to avoid rapid rises in plasma concentrations, and taking it with food will greatly improve tolerability. Individual dosing four times daily may also be helpful, at least with higher doses.

The recommended initial target maintenance dose is between 30 and 32 mg/day in patients co-medicated with enzyme-inducing drugs, and 15–16 mg/day for those who are not. The usual maximum recommended dose is 50–56 mg/day in patients taking enzyme-inducing drugs, and 30–32 mg/day for those not taking enzyme-inducing drugs. However, high daily doses of at least 70–80 mg have been used in occasional patients and seem to be well tolerated. At an anecdotal level, there is a general view that the higher doses of tiagabine particularly can be strikingly effective, and certainly there are series of patients reported, by different authorities, who had been resistant to all previous antiepileptic therapies and who gained total seizure control with tiagabine. Patients taking a combination of inducing and non-inducing drugs (e.g. carbamazepine and valproate) should be considered to be enzyme induced. Routine tiagabine withdrawal should be carried out at rates of no greater than 5 mg/week.

Although dose-related side effects are common, the frequency of idiosyncratic drug-related reactions, including cutaneous reactions, is very low, and an advantage of tiagabine over other conventional drugs is its favourable cognitive profile. It does not have the major side effects encountered with vigabatrin, namely psychosis and depression, or the induction of visual-field defects. However, if there is a history of depression, treatment with tiagabine should be initiated at a low initial dose under close supervision because there may be an increased risk of recurrence.

In view of the risk of inducing an encephalopathic state (with stupor and confusion) or non-convulsive status epilepticus, tiagabine should not be used in patients with generalized epilepsy, especially those with a history of absence or myoclonic seizures, with a history of spike-and-wave discharges or non-convulsive status epilepti-cus. Tiagabine is contraindicated in severe hepatic impairment. Dosage recommendations in children are not yet available. The drug should not be used in pregnant or lactating women.

Topiramate

Proprietary name: Topamax[a]

Primary indications
Adjunctive therapy for partial-onset seizures and for the Lennox–Gastaut syndrome, ≥2 years of age. Monotherapy for partial-onset and generalized seizures, ≥6 years of age

Commonly used as first-line drug
Yes

Usual preparations
Tablets: 25, 50, 100, 200 mg; sprinkle: 15, 25, 50 mg

Usual dosage – adults
Initial: 25–50 mg/day; increased by 25–50 mg/day increments every 2 weeks. Maintenance: 75–300 mg/day (maximum 600 mg/day)

Usual dosage – children
Initial: 0.5–1 mg/kg per day
Maintenance: 5–9 mg/kg per day

Dosing intervals
Twice a day

Is dose commonly affected by co-medication
Yes

Is dose affected by renal/hepatic disease
Renal disease

Does it affect dose of other drugs?
Uncommonly, and usually slight effect only

Does it affect the contraceptive pill?
Yes

Serum level monitoring
Potentially useful

Target range
10–60 µmoL/L

Common/important adverse events
Dizziness, ataxia, headache, paraesthesia, tremor, somnolence, cognitive dysfunction, confusion, agitation, amnesia, depression, emotional lability, nausea, diarrhoea, diplopia, weight loss

Risk of hypersensitivity
No

Major mechanism of action
Inhibition of sodium channel conductance, potentiation of GABA-mediated inhibition at the $GABA_A$ receptor, reduction of AMPA receptor activity, inhibition of high-voltage calcium channels, carbonic anhydrase activity

Main advantages
Powerful antiepileptic action; weight loss a common side-effect

Main disadvantages
Potential for CNS and other side effects

Comment
Drug of first choice in partial epilepsy, with additional action in generalized epilepsies

[a]Name of proprietary brand available in the UK.
AMPA, aminohydroxymethylisozole propionic acid.

Topiramate: pharmacokinetics–average adult values

Oral bioavailability	<100%
Time to peak levels	2–4 h
Volume of distribution	0.6–1.0 L/kg
Biotransformation	In monotherapy, most of the drug is excreted without metabolism. In polytherapy with enzyme-inducing drugs, a proportion of topiramate undergoes hydoxylation or hydrolysis and then conjugation
Elimination half-life	19–25 h (varies with co-medication)
Plasma clearance	0.022–0.036 L/kg per h; higher in children than in adults
Protein binding	13–17%
Active metabolite	None
Metabolism by hepatic enzymes	In monotherapy only minor metabolism
Inhibition or induction of hepatic enzymes	Induces CYP3A4, inhibits CYP2C19
Drug interactions	Some drug interactions

Topiramate was initially developed as an antidiabetic drug. It was found to have striking antiepileptic action in animal models on routine screening, and then underwent a series of controlled trials in North America and Europe. It was licensed, first in the UK, in 1994 and subsequently in the USA and Europe and many countries worldwide. Its strong antiepileptic action has differentiated topiramate from some other newer antiepileptics, and it has gained a reputation as a powerful antiepileptic drug, effective in some patients in whom all other medications have failed.

Physical and chemical properties
Topiramate (2,3:4,5-*bis*-O-(1-methylethylidene)-α-D-fructo-pyranose sulphamate; molecular weight 339.36) is a sulphamate-substituted monosaccharide, derived from D-fructose, a naturally occurring sugar. It is mildly acidic, pK_a of 8.61, moderately soluble in water and its solubility is increased in alkaline solutions. It is freely soluble in ethanol and other organic solvents.

Mode of action
Topiramate appears to have multiple actions that potentially contribute to its antiepileptic potential. The relative contribution of each mechanism is not known, and probably varies in different individuals and types of epilepsy. The drug exerts an inhibitory effect on sodium conductance in neuronal membranes. This action is similar to that of phenytoin and carbamazepine although its action is not as rapid or as complete as that of phenytoin or lamotrigine. It also enhances $GABA_A$-receptor activity and, as do phenobarbital and the benzodiazepine drugs, increases GABA-mediated chloride influx into neurons. However, topiramate does not bind at the benzodiazepine-binding site, and the exact mechanism of action at the GABA site is not known. Topiramate also inhibits glutamate receptors, particularly of the aminohydroxymethylisozole propionic acid (AMPA) subtype, but has no action on NMDA-receptor activity. It is unique among the antiepileptic drugs in this regard. It also reduces L-type high-voltage-activated calcium

channel activity. Finally, topiramate is a weak inhibitor of carbonic anhydrase, 10–100 times less potent than acetazolamide in this regard. Topiramate exerts a powerful antiepileptic action in a wide range of experimental models of epilepsy. There is also a body of experimental work suggesting a promising potential for neuroprotection, but no human studies have yet been carried out to explore this.

Pharmacokinetics
Absorption and distribution
Topiramate is rapidly absorbed after oral dosing with a bioavailability approaching 100%. The time to peak blood levels is usually between 2 and 4 h. Food delays absorption by several hours, but does not affect its extent and the drug need not be given at any fixed time in relation to food. Topiramate is widely distributed in tissues, including the brain. The volume of distribution is between 0.6 and 1.0 L/kg, although this falls at higher doses. Approximately 13–17% of topiramate is bound to plasma protein. Plasma concentrations increase linearly with dose within the normal dosing range.

The mean milk:maternal plasma concentration ratio was 0.86 (range 0.67–1.1) 2–3 weeks after delivery, and this ratio was similar at 1 and 3 months postpartum. Low levels of topiramate were found in the blood of the breast-fed infants.

Metabolism and elimination
Topiramate is metabolized in the liver by the cytochrome P450 microsomal enzymes. At least eight metabolites have been identified, formed by hydroxylation, hydrolysis or cleavage of the sulphamate group. None of the metabolites has antiepileptic action. The plasma elimination half-life of topiramate is between 19 and 25 h, and is independent of dose over the normal clinical range. In monotherapy metabolism is slight, plasma concentrations show little intraindividual variability and most of the drug (85%) is excreted unchanged in the urine. In polytherapy, however, metabolism is much more extensive, presumably due to enzyme induction. The elimination of topiramate and its metabolites is via renal mechanisms.

In children, topiramate clearance is higher than in adults. In older children, clearance values are about 50% higher than in adults. In children between the ages of 4 and 7 years, renal clearance is 40% higher than in children aged over 8 years. In infants, topiramate clearance is further increased, and the dose requirement in infants (milligrams per kilogram per day) necessary to maintain

a similar plasma concentration is twice that of adults. No change in clearance or elimination half-life of topiramate has been seen among elderly adults with healthy renal function. Topiramate clearance is reduced by 42% in patients with moderate renal impairment and 54% in patients with severe renal impairment, and topiramate doses should be reduced in such patients. However, topiramate is cleared rapidly by haemodialysis, and supplemental dosing may be required during haemodialysis. Severe hepatic disease results in about a 30% decrease in clearance and about a 30% increase in plasma concentrations.

Drug interactions
Topiramate is a mild inhibitor of the P450 isoenzyme CYP2C19 at very high doses, but in most patients in practice topiramate does not affect the steady-state concentrations of other antiepileptic drugs. However, where phenytoin metabolism is close to saturation, the inhibitory action of topiramate may cause phenytoin levels to increase. It has been shown to have no effect on carbamazepine or CBZ epoxide levels and no consistent significant effect on valproate concentrations. In children, co-medication has been shown to result in a slight decrease in lamotrigine levels. Topiramate also slightly increases the clearance of warfarin and the oestrogen component of the oral contraceptive, the latter only at high doses.

Enzyme-inducing antiepileptic drugs such as phenytoin, phenobarbital and carbamazepine decrease topiramate serum concentrations by approximately 50% and, as a result of this interaction, topiramate dosage in combination therapy with these drugs needs to be increased. Valproate administration has no effect on topiramate concentrations. A similar effect is noted in children, and studies have shown a reduction in average half-life from 15.4 to 7.5 h in the presence of enzyme-inducing drugs. In infants, treatment with enzyme inducers has been shown to reduce the half-life of topiramate to 6.4 h.

Adverse effects
Topiramate side effects have been extensively studied in the controlled trials, and also during the extensive open experience of the drug. The adverse effects noted as adjunctive therapy in the regulatory RCTs of topiramate in adults are shown in Table 8.24. These included doses that are much higher than used in routine clinical practice (where doses in excess of 400 mg are rare). In the early trials, 14% of those randomized to topiramate withdrew prematurely because of adverse events, but this rate

Table 8.24 Side effects in adults: percentage of adults with side effects at different doses – a pooled analysis from the add-on clinical trials of topiramate.

Side effect	Percentage of patients receiving the daily topiramate dose[a]					
	Placebo	200 mg/kg	400 mg/kg	600 mg/kg	800 mg/kg	1000 mg/kg
Dizziness	13	36	22	32	32	40
Fatigue	6	13	18	32	49	32
Diplopia	12	7	19	8	18	30
Somnolence	10	27	27	17	20	28
Confusion	5	9	1	18	15	28
Abnormal thinking	2	20	12	29	28	26
Ataxia	8	20	22	17	16	21
Anorexia	3	4	4	8	9	21
Impaired concentration	1	11	9	12	15	21
Headache	26	29	25	30	25	7

[a]Events occurring at frequency of 20% or more in any treatment group. Dose assigned to in the clinical trials.

is less in subsequent studies, which have used lower doses and slower rates of titration. Adverse events seen in trials in children are shown in Table 8.25 and, as in adults, these effects were more prevalent in polytherapy than monotherapy, and with a more rapid titration of the dose.

Neurological side effects

The most prominent side effects noted in clinical practice are somnolence, impairment of concentration, mental slowing and cognitive effects, with a particular effect on word finding and language. Cognitive testing has shown significant effects, particularly on word fluency, list learning and verbal IQ. These are very much dose related and their frequency increases markedly at higher doses and with fast titration.

Other side effects are not uncommon and include dizziness, ataxia, fatigue, paresthesias in the extremities, ataxia, disturbance of memory, depression and agitation.

These adverse events are prominent in about 15% of patients, and topiramate is badly tolerated by a higher proportion of patients than other less effective medication. However, tolerance to many of the side effects does develop within a few weeks if the drug is continued, and it is worth emphasizing this point in clinical practice.

Furthermore, the adverse events can be greatly reduced by slow titration of the drug, and the high frequency of

Table 8.25 Side effects in children: percentage of children with side effects – a pooled analysis from the add-on and monotherapy trials of topiramate.

Adverse event	Placebo (in add-on studies)	Topiramate (in add-on studies)[a]	Topiramate (in monotherapy studies)[b]
Somnolence	16	26	10
Anorexia	15	24	13
Fatigue	5	16	19
Nervousness	7	14	4
Concentration/ attentional difficulty	2	10	8
Aggressiveness	4	9	4
Weight loss	1	9	5
Memory difficulties	0	5	5

Events with a 5% or more difference in frequency vs placebo.
[a]Pooled analysis, dose of 6 mg/kg per day.
[b]Pooled analysis of all doses, 25–500 mg/day of topiramate.

side effects noted in the clinical trials largely occurred as the dose was being rapidly titrated upwards, often to high doses. The importance of slow titration was emphasized in a randomized, parallel, double-blind study evaluating two rates of titration, in which incremental steps of 100/200 mg/day resulted in twice the withdrawal rate of 50 mg/day increments.

Topiramate can affect cognition and in particular word-finding and verbal fluency. The rate of titration is important. In healthy young adults, the cognitive profile at baseline was compared, after rapid titration, with that at 2 and 4 weeks of treatment with topiramate 5.7 mg/kg per day, lamotrigine 7.1 mg/kg or gabapentin 35 mg/kg. The verbal fluency rate of the topiramate group dropped an average of 50% per individual compared with a negligible change for the other two groups, and a threefold error occurred for the visual attention task. At the 2- and 4-week test periods only those receiving topiramate continued to display adverse cognitive effects from drug administration. In a second study, the cognitive effects of topiramate were compared with those of valproate with slow titration to a dose of 200–400 mg/day for topiramate (weekly increments of 25 mg) and 1800 mg/day for valproate. Of ten baseline to end-point comparisons, only one test (measuring short-term verbal memory) showed a statistically significant worsening for topiramate and improvement for valproate. None of the tests of mood or subjective complaints showed significant differences between the treatments.

Weight loss

Topiramate also causes weight loss in many patients. This effect is dose related and greatest in those who are overweight. In the early clinical trials, mean decreases were 1.1 kg at 200 mg/day and 5.9 kg at doses >800 mg/day, and the mean loss in patients >60 kg was 8%, compared with 3% in those <60 kg. The weight loss can be marked, sometimes >10 kg, and patients need to be warned about this to prevent misinterpretation. The effect is probably due to a suppressive effect on appetite, although this has not been unequivocally shown. To some patients, weight loss is welcome, and counters the tendency of other antiepileptic drugs (notably valproate, gabapentin, pregabalin and vigabatrin) to promote weight gain.

Other side effects

Topiramate causes a variety of side effects due to its inhibitory effect on carbonic anhydrase. The most important is the risk of renal calculi which are reported to occur in one patient per 1000 per year (symptomatic calculi),

and topiramate should be used cautiously in those with a history of renal calculi or a family history. Patients should be encouraged to drink plenty of fluids because of this risk. Parasthesias are also common, but usually of minor importance. A decrease in serum bicarbonate may occur, particularly in children, and a mild metabolic acidosis is relatively common but usually asymptomatic. However, very low serum bicarbonate levels can occur, especially in infants and in those predisposed, for example, by a ketogenic diet. Clinical and biochemical monitoring is essential in these patients and discontinuation of treatment with topiramate if symptomatic. Chronic metabolic acidosis can also cause osteomalacia and/or osteoporosis, reduced growth in children and renal calculi. So children with persisting metabolic acidosis, in whom drug withdrawal is not decided upon, may require oral bicarbonate treatment. Hypohidrosis can occur and result in hyperpyrexia, especially in children; mothers should be cautioned about this.

There are no reports of significant cardiotoxicity or gastrointestinal toxicity. Ocular side effects include blurring of vision, diplopia, and occasionally acute angle-closure glaucoma, acute myopia and ciliochoroidal detachment. Other rare idiosyncratic reactions include ciliochoroidal effusion, anterior displacement of the lens and then secondary acute angle-closure glaucoma. These resolve with discontinuation of therapy.

Allergic rash is extremely rare. One case of fulminant hepatic failure has been reported, and also hyperammonaemia, especially when topiramate is given with valproate. Those with inborn errors of metabolism or reduced hepatic mitochondrial activity are probably at higher risk of liver dysfunction with topiramate and/or valproate. There have been no reports of haematological toxicity with topiramate.

Side effects in children

Adverse effects reported in children are generally similar to those in adults. The CNS effects and anorexia/weight loss are the most common. Somnolence, anorexia, fatigue, dizziness, psychomotor slowing, speech difficulties and concentration difficulties were the most frequent effects in the clinical trials. Hypohidrosis and hyperthermia are much more common in children than in adults. Children taking topiramate should be monitored for increased body temperature during hot weather and/or vigorous exercise. Weight loss can also occur in children as in adults, but the possible long-term implications of weight loss in children are uncertain, and further studies are required.

There are no definitive data on the teratogenic effects of topiramate in humans, although teratogenicity has been reported in isolated cases and was also found in the animal screening. The drug is therefore not recommended for use in pregnancy.

Antiepileptic effect
Partial-onset seizures
Topiramate has been intensively studied in various types of epilepsy and in various syndromes over the past 10 years. The initial studies were, as with all antiepileptic drugs, in adults with refractory partial epilepsy.

The Cochrane collaboration analysis reviewed 10 randomized, placebo-controlled, double-blind trials with 1312 randomized participants. Topiramate was found to be highly effective, with a relative risk of 2.85 (95% CI 2.27–3.59) for a 50% or greater reduction in seizure frequency compared with the placebo. A meta-analysis of the five regulatory trials has been carried out (Table 8.26). A reduction in the frequency of seizures of at least 50% (treatment responders) was seen in 35–50% of participants, and this was a greater effect on topiramate than on any of the other drugs in the analysis. In the number-needed-to treat analysis, significantly smaller numbers of patients were required to find a responder to topiramate treatment than to gabapentin or lamotrigine. The first pivotal studies included patients randomized to high doses (600–1000 mg/day), and it was quickly realized that the gains in efficacy were outweighed by poor tolerability at these high levels. Thus, subsequent double-blind, placebo-controlled studies were carried out at 300 and 200 mg/day. In these studies, 48% and 45% of patients showed a reduction in seizures of at least 50% compared with 13% and 24% of placebo-treated patients. In these low-dose studies, only 8% of topiramate-treated patients and 2% of patients receiving placebo discontinued the trial as a result of adverse events. Most of these patients were receiving other enzyme-inducing antiepileptics and, even in these cases, 100–200 mg/day appears to be an appropriate target dosage.

Table 8.26 The results of five double blind, placebo-controlled clinical trials of topiramate in adults with partial epilepsy.

Placebo topiramate (mg/day)	No. of subjects	Median percent reduction in monthly seizure rate	Percentage of patients with 50% decrease in seizures	Percentage of patients with 75–100% decrease in seizures
Placebo	24	1	8	4
Topiramate 400	23	41[a]	35[b]	22
Placebo	30	−12[f]	10	3
Topiramate 600	30	46[c]	47[d]	23
Placebo	28	−18[f]	0	0
Topiramate 800	28	36[d]	43[d]	36
Placebo	45	13	18	9
Topiramate 200	45	30[d]	27	9
Topiramate 400	45	48[e]	47[b]	22
Topiramate 600	46	45[d]	46[b]	22
Placebo	47	1	9	0
Topiramate 600	48	41[d]	44[d]	23
Topiramate 800	48	41[d]	40[d]	13
Topiramate 1000	47	38[d]	38[d]	13

[a] $P = 0.065$.
[b] $P \le 0.05$.
[c] $P \le 0.005$.
[d] $P \le 0.001$.
[e] $P \le 0.01$.
[f] negative number indicates an increase in seizure rate.

Data from open studies have confirmed the effectiveness of topiramate in partial seizures, and one pragmatic study of 901 adults, for example, showed a median reduction in seizures of 73%, with 68% of patients achieving a 50% or more reduction. In a retrospective review, the 1-year retention rates in the open extension phases of clinical trials were 52% for topiramate compared with 46% for lamotrigine and 23% for gabapentin. At 5 years, retention rates were 28% (topiramate), 12% (lamotrigine) and 2% (gabapentin). Perceived lack of efficacy resulted in treatment withdrawal in 19% of topiramate-treated patients compared with 39% of those receiving lamotrigine and 34% of those treated with gabapentin.

Partial-onset seizures in children

In children with partial-onset seizures, similar results have been obtained in formal regulatory studies. In the pivotal randomized, double-blind, controlled trial in children with partial-onset seizures, the addition of topiramate reduced the median seizure frequency by 33% (compared with 11% in the placebo group, $P = 0.03$). No child discontinued topiramate treatment because of adverse events in the trial period. Five per cent of children receiving topiramate were free from seizures during the 16-week study and none in the placebo-treated group. No children discontinued topiramate treatment because of adverse events. In an open-label extension study of the RCT (for a mean of 2.5 years), 14% of children became seizure free for at least 6 months and seizure frequency over the last 3 months of therapy was reduced in 57% of children. Six per cent of children discontinued treatment because of adverse events and 13% because of inadequate seizure control.

Monotherapy

Topiramate has been extensively evaluated also as monotherapy. In a pivotal regulatory study, a dose of 400 mg/day was compared with 50 mg/day in an RCT in newly diagnosed partial (with or without secondary generalization) or primarily generalized tonic–clonic seizures. A greater proportion of patients were seizure free at 6 and 12 months on 400 mg/day ($P < 0.01$). In an open trial of topiramate monotherapy in 692 patients with partial or generalized epilepsy who were treatment naive or had failed with prior treatment using one antiepileptic drug, 76% of patients were reported to have had a >50% reduction in seizure frequency, with 44% of patients rendered seizure free. In these monotherapy studies, 40–82% of those with partial seizures and 62–85% of those with generalized seizures were free of seizures. In a compara-

tive RCT of 613 patients with newly diagnosed epilepsy, the time to trial exit, the time to the first seizure and the proportion of seizure-free patients were found to be similar for topiramate (110–200 mg/day), carbamazepine (600 mg/day) and valproate (1250 mg/day). The 6-month seizure-free rates with 100 and 200 mg/day were 49% and 44%, compared with 44% on carbamazepine and valproate. The discontinuation rates owing to adverse events for 100 mg/day topiramate, 200 mg/day topiramate, carbamazepine, and valproate were 19%, 28%, 25% and 23%, respectively. In an open flexible-dose studies of monotherapy in recently diagnosed epilepsy, topiramate therapy was shown to be highly effective at low doses. At doses of 100–125 mg/day, 80% of patients exhibited a >50% reduction in seizures and, at months 7 and 13 of therapy, 44% and 35% respectively of patients had remained seizure free. In the generalized seizure arm of the SANAD study (see p. 89) topiramate performed less well than valproate or lamotrigine in time to treatment failure (defined as 'time to cessation of treatment because of adverse events, inadequate seizure control or the addition of another antiepileptic drug'), but was more effective than lamotrigine (but not valproate) in the time taken to achieve a 1-year period of remission from seizures. In the partial seizure arm, topiramate was less effective than carbamazepine or lamotrigine for time to treatment failure (largely owing to adverse events).

Primarily generalized seizures

There have also been two double-blind, placebo-controlled, add-on trials of topiramate in primarily generalized tonic–clonic seizures. There was a statistically significant reduction of seizures in one study but not the other. When data from both studies were pooled, the median percentage reduction was 57% in topiramate-treated patients and 27% in the placebo group. Fifty-five per cent of topiramate-treated patients had a reduction of seizures of at least 50% compared with 28% in the placebo group. The effects were similar in children and adults. Adverse events led to discontinuation of therapy in 10% of the topiramate-treated patients and 8% in the placebo group. These good results are confirmed at an anecdotal level in routine clinical practice. Topiramate has also been shown to reduce myoclonus and absence seizures (petit mal) in patients with JME and IGE.

Lennox–Gastaut syndrome

In adult patients and children with the Lennox–Gastaut syndrome, the pivotal study compared the addition of topiramate with placebo. Topiramate was started at

1 mg/kg per day and increased at weekly intervals to 3 mg/ kg per day and then 6 mg/kg per day. Stabilized dosages were maintained for an additional 8 weeks. There was a significantly greater reduction in all major seizure types including drop attacks with topiramate. On topiramate, the median percentage of reduction in drop attacks was 15% compared with a 5% increase in patients receiving placebo ($P = 0.04$). The median percentage reduction in major motor seizures (drop attacks and tonic–clonic seizures combined) was 26% with topiramate treatment compared with a 5% increase with placebo ($P = 0.02$). The proportion of patients achieving at least 50% reduction in drop attacks was higher in the topiramate group than in placebo-treated patients (28% versus 14%, $P = 0.07$), with 33% of topiramate-treated patients and 8% of placebo-treated patients achieving at least 50% reduction in major motor seizures ($P = 0.002$).

In the open-label extension, the effect of topiramate was sustained. Drop attacks were reduced by at least 50% in 55% of patients receiving topiramate. Even though the mean number of drop attacks before topiramate was introduced was 90 per day, 15% of patients had no drop attacks for at least 6 months. Substantial reductions were also observed in atypical absence, myoclonic and tonic–clonic seizures. During follow-up for up to 3.4 years, only 12% of patients discontinued treatment as a result of inadequate seizure control and 10% discontinued due to adverse events.

Other epilepsy studies

Open studies have also shown effectiveness in various other epilepsy syndromes and situations. These include the following.

West syndrome

A number of studies have shown efficacy in West syndrome. In one study of 11 patients, infantile spasms were reduced in 9 patients (82%), and 5 patients (45%) became spasm free.

Severe myoclonic epilepsy of infancy

In an open study of 18 patients with severe myoclonic epilepsy of infancy (SMEI), after a mean period of 10 months of treatment, 72% of the patients had achieved a reduction in seizure rate of at least 50% and 16.6% were seizure free.

Childhood absence epilepsy

Topiramate can have a variable effect in absence seizures and there are a number of anecdotal case reports and small series reporting some patients to be rendered seizure free and others to be worsened by the drug.

Angelman syndrome

In one study of five children, after a mean 8.8 months on topiramate two were seizure free.

Status epilepticus

Pilot work suggests that topiramate is highly effective in controlling tonic–clonic status epilepticus.

Learning difficulty

There is a general view that topiramate is especially effective in the epilepsy associated with learning disability. In one open study, in 64 patients with refractory epilepsy and learning disability, 70% achieved at least 50% seizure reduction with topiramate adjunctive therapy, and 16 patients (25%) became seizure free, including 10 who were receiving topiramate doses of 200 mg/day. However, it must be recognized that responses can be variable and some patients become worse and some develop acute and severe side effects.

Elderly patients

A recent 24-week study compared topiramate 50 mg/day and 200 mg/day as add-on or monotherapy in 77 elderly patients (mean age 68 years). Seizure control was similar with the two dosages when the drug could be used as a monotherapy, but 200 mg/day was more effective in patients requiring adjunctive therapy. A total of 14 patients (7 in each group) discontinued topiramate use as a result of adverse events. This study shows the efficacy of low-dose topiramate in elderly people in particular.

Clinical use in epilepsy

Topiramate is a powerful antiepileptic drug. It has been extensively studied in regulatory and also post-licensing studies – more so than most other new-generation antiepileptic drugs. It is clearly effective in a broad spectrum of epilepsies and epilepsy syndromes, but has a particular place in the treatment of resistant focal seizures, and those with severe symptomatic generalized epilepsies. It is useful in children, adults and elderly people, and in those with learning disability.

The drug is available as 50, 100 and 200 mg tablets, and as a sprinkle and syrup. There are currently no parenteral preparations.

The early clinical trials were carried out at higher doses than are currently recommended and, although these studies showed marked efficacy, the rate of neurological and cognitive side effects was also high. The drug gained a reputation for being strikingly effective, but also poorly tolerated. However, subsequent experience has shown that lower doses are also effective and confer much better tolerability. In routine practice, the rate of side effects is thus lower than initially feared. The risk of side effects can also be greatly reduced by starting the drug at a very low dose and titrating upwards slowly. The most common side effects are effects on cognitive function (notably effects on language and word finding), paraesthesias and weight loss. These are reversible when doses are reduced.

In adults on adjunctive therapy, the author's own practice is to initiate therapy at 25–50 mg/day and increase this 2 weekly to 50 mg, 100 mg and then increase in 50 mg increments to an initial maintenance dose of between 100 and 200 mg/day (and higher dose ranges in patients co-medicated with enzyme-inducing antiepileptic drugs).

The drug is given in two divided doses. The usual maximum maintenance dose is 600 mg/day, but very occasionally up to 1000 mg/day has been given without side effects.

Much lower doses are needed in newly diagnosed patients, and in monotherapy, and it is the author's practice to aim for maintenance doses of 75–150 mg/day initially in adults, building the dose up slowly in 25 mg increments every 2–3 weeks. On this regimen, good efficacy is usually obtained with very few side effects.

In children on adjunctive therapy, the usual recommended dose is 0.5–1 mg/kg per day for the first week, with weekly increments of 0.5–1 mg/kg per day until an initial maintenance dose of 4–6 mg/kg per day is reached. Higher doses, up to 20–30 mg/kg per day, have been used and are sometimes necessary, especially in those co-medicated with enzyme-inducing drugs.

Blood levels can be measured, but are not routinely useful.

Valproate

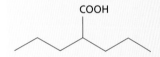

Proprietary names: Epilim, Episenta, Orlept[a]

Primary indications
Monotherapy and adjunctive therapy in partial-onset and generalized seizures, including myoclonus and absence, and for the seizures associated with the Lennox–Gastaut syndrome. Idiopathic generalized epilepsy, febrile convulsions, other childhood epilepsy syndromes. Adults and children

Commonly used as first-line drug
Yes

Usual preparations
Enteric-coated tablets: 200, 500 mg; crushable tablets: 100 mg; capsules: 150, 300, 500 mg; syrup: 200 mg/5 mL; solution or syrup: 250 mg/5 mL; sustained-release microspheres, sachets: 100, 250, 500, 750, 1000 mg; divalproex tablets delayed release: 125, 300, 500 mg; divalproex sprinkle 125 mg; divalproex tablets extended release: 250, 500 mg; intravenous solution 100 mg/mL

Usual dosage – adults
Initial: 200–500 mg/day; increasing by 200–500 mg increments every 2 weeks
Maintenance: 500–2000 mg/day (maximum 3000 mg/day)

Usual dosage – children
Neonates: initial and maintenance: 20 mg/kg
Children 1 month to 12 years: initial: 10–15 mg/kg; maintenance 25–30 mg/kg (up to 60 mg/kg in infantile spasms)

Dosing intervals
2–3 times/day

Is dose commonly affected by co-medication?
Yes

Is dose affected by renal/hepatic disease?
Avoid in hepatic disease

Does it affect dose of other drugs?
Yes

Does it affect the contraceptive pill?
No

Serum level monitoring
Useful

Target range
300–700 µmol/L (50–100 mg/L)

Common/important adverse events
Nausea, vomiting, hyperammonaemia and other metabolic effects, endocrine effects, severe hepatic toxicity, pancreatitis, drowsiness, cognitive disturbance, aggressiveness, tremor, weakness, encephalopathy, thrombocytopenia, neutropenia, aplastic anemia, hair thinning and hair loss, weight gain, polycystic ovarian syndrome

Risk of hypersensitivity
Yes

Major mechanism of action
Effects on GABA and glutaminergic activity, calcium (T) conductance and potassium conductance

Main advantages
A wide spectrum of activity; drug of choice in most patients with idiopathic generalized epilepsy; mood stabilizing effects

Main disadvantages
Weight gain, CNS and other side effects; risk of severe hepatic disturbance in children; teratogenicity

Comment
Drugs of first choice in a wide spectrum of epilepsies.

aNames of proprietary brands available in the UK.

Valproate: pharmacokinetics – average adult values

Oral bioavailability	<100%
Time to peak levels	0.5–2 h (sodium valproate; but longer in different preparations and affected by food)
Volume of distribution	0.13–0.30 L/kg
Biotransformation	Hepatic oxidation, epoxidation, reduction and glucuronidation (and some metabolism by non-cytochrome enzymes)
Elimination half-life	13–16 h (varies with co-medication)
Plasma clearance	0.010–0.115 L/kg per h (varies with co-medication)
Protein binding	70–95%
Active metabolite	None (but see text)
Metabolism by hepatic enzymes	CYP2C9, CYP2C19, CYP2B6, UGT1A4
Inhibition or induction of hepatic enzymes	Inhibits CYP2C9, UGT1A4 (and a very weak inhibitor of CYP2C19 and CYP3A4)
Drug interactions	Common

Valproate was first synthesized in 1882 as an organic solvent. Its antiepileptic properties were recognized in the 1960s, entirely by accident, while being used as a solvent for the screening of new antiepileptic compounds. It was licensed in Europe in the early 1960s, where it became very widely used, and then in the USA in 1978. It has been marketed as a magnesium or calcium salt, an acid and also as sodium hydrogen divalproate (divalproex sodium; Depakote). Sodium valproate is the usual form in the UK and sodium hydrogen divalproate in Europe. Valpromide (dipropylacetamide), a prodrug of valproate, is also marketed, as is a delayed-release formulation of sodium valproate. The term 'valproate' is usually adopted to refer to all these forms and, although properties vary to some extent, none of these formulations has been shown to confer any real superiority over the others.

Valproate is widely available, is one of the most commonly prescribed antiepileptic drugs throughout the world and is the drug of first choice for many types of epilepsy.

Physical and chemical properties

Valproic acid is a simple molecule (molecular weight 144.21), a branched-chain carboxylic acid, similar in clinical structure to endogenous fatty acids. It is slightly soluble in water and very soluble in organic solvents. Its pK_a is 4.8. The sodium salt is extremely soluble in water, whereas the calcium and magnesium salts are insoluble. Sodium hydrogen divalproate (divalproex sodium) is a stable combination compound of equal parts of valproic acid and sodium valproate.

Mode of action

Despite its venerable age, and its wide usage, the mechanism of action of valproate is not entirely clear. Valproate has a number of actions at the $GABA_A$ receptor, e.g. increasing synaptosomal GABA concentrations through the activation of the GABA-synthesizing enzyme glutamic acid decarboxylase, and also inhibiting GABA catabolism through inhibition of GABA transaminase and succinic semialdehyde dehydrogenase. However, valproate also inhibits excitatory neurotransmission mediated by aspartic acid, glutamic acid and γ-hydroxybutyric acid. Valproate reduces conductance at the voltage-dependent sodium channel. In hippocampal slices, it reduces the threshold for calcium and potassium conductance. The relative importance of these mechanisms in human epilepsy is unclear. In animal models valproate is highly effective against a range of seizures.

Pharmacokinetics

The pharmacokinetics of valproate are complex.

Absorption and distribution

Sodium valproate is rapidly absorbed with a bioavailability approaching 100%. The peak plasma concentration after oral administration is usually reached within 30 min to 2 h. Other formulations have slightly different absorption properties, and administration with food slightly delays the absorption of most forms, but not their extent. Sodium valproate is available in an enteric-coated formulation, which results in peak plasma concentrations within 3–8 h (and as metabolism is rapid, levels may actually fall in the few hours after ingestion – so trough levels may be experienced in late morning or early afternoon) and this is the commonly used form in the UK. Rectal administration also results in about 80% and the extended-release formulations in between 80 and 95% of absorption.

Valproate has a restricted distribution, probably mainly in the vascular compartment and extracellular fluid, and has a relatively low apparent volume of distribution of 0.13–0.19 L/kg (adults) and 0.20–0.30 L/kg (children). High concentrations are, however, found in the liver, intestinal tract, gallbladder, kidney and urinary bladder. Valproate also enters the CSF compartment and brain rapidly, via an active transport mechanism that is saturatable, rendering absorption at high doses much less efficient. Peak concentrations can be achieved in the brain within minutes. The CSF concentration is lower than the free plasma concentration, with mean total CSF:plasma ratio of about 0.15. Valproate is removed from the brain by a probenecid-sensitive monoamine transport system. This has implications for its use in acute seizures or status epilepticus.

Valproate is 70–95% bound to plasma proteins, with complicated kinetics. The free faction is concentration dependent and at higher plasma concentrations (>700 μmol/L) protein binding decreases markedly, e.g. the average unbound fraction of valproic acid in adults is reported to be 7% at 50 mg/L, 15% at 100 mg/L and 30% at 150 mg/L. Thus, with a threefold increase in total serum valproic acid concentration from 50 mg/L to 150 mg/L, the unbound concentration would increase more than 10 times, from 3.5 mg/L to 45 mg/L. Protein binding is reduced in renal and hepatic disease and during pregnancy, and other drugs may displace valproate from its protein-binding sites (e.g. aspirin, phenylbutazone). The other antiepileptics do not influence binding, however.

Metabolism and elimination

Valproate is rapidly eliminated from the body by hepatic metabolism. Uniquely among antiepileptics, the enzymes involved are mainly not those of the cytochrome P450 system. There are a variety of pathways, the main one being β-oxidation followed by glucuronidation. At least 30 metabolites have been identified, some of which may be responsible for adverse side effects (notably the 4-ene metabolite related to hepatic toxicity and teratogenicity). Two metabolites have antiepileptic activity, but are present in the serum only in very low concentrations. One of these is the 2-ene-valproic acid, and this accumulates in the brain, where it is cleared more slowly than valproic acid itself, and might be an explanation for the dissociation between the time courses of valproic acid concentrations in plasma and the onset of antiepileptic activity. The levels of the 4-ene metabolite are influenced by the cytochrome P450 enzymes and this might be an explanation for the greater hepatic toxicity of valproate in polytherapy.

Less than 4% of the drug is excreted unchanged. The elimination half-life is between 12 and 15 h in young adults and between 14 and 17 h in elderly people. The half-life is shorted to approximately 9 h in those co-medicated with antiepileptic drugs. In children, the mean half-life is 11.6 h in monotherapy and 7.0 h in polytherapy. In neonates the drug is slowly metabolized and the half-life is 20–40 h.

The clearance of valproate and its metabolites follows linear kinetics at most dosage ranges, although at higher plasma concentrations reduced protein binding results in increased clearance.

As a result of the relatively short half-life of the drug, there are marked diurnal variations in plasma levels (100% differences between peak and trough levels) on twice-daily dosing. Also there is marked intraindividual variation.

Valproate is relatively contraindicated in hepatic disease, because of concern about its toxicity, but in cirrhosis there is slowed clearance of the unbound drug. Its pharmacokinetic properties are not altered by renal impairment. The protein binding of valproate decreases during pregnancy and the total concentration is also reduced as a result of an increased volume of distribution. The free drug fraction concentration is relatively stable but may increase in the late stages of pregnancy. Concentrations of valproate in breast milk range from 1% to 10% of those in maternal plasma, and breast-fed infants have serum concentrations between 4 and 12% of the maternal concentration.

Drug interactions

Valproate is involved in a number of interactions with other antiepileptic drugs, the mechanisms of which are often obscure. It can inhibit the metabolism of other drugs, and there are also interactions at the protein-binding level; these vary at different doses and in different individuals. Thus, the clinical consequences are often difficult to predict. Although most interactions do not pose much of a clinical problem in most patients, they can occasionally be very marked. Its own metabolism is greatly affected by co-medication with enzyme-inducing antiepileptic drugs that can greatly influence valproate clearance. The common interactions with other antiepileptic drugs are shown in Table 8.27.

Table 8.27 Pharmacokinetic interactions between valproate (VPA) and other antiepileptic drugs.

Drug	Effect of VPA on the drug	Effect of the drug on VPA
Benzodiazepines	↑ Benzodiazepine concentration	No significant effect[a]
Carbamazepine (CBZ)	↑ CBZ-epoxide (25–100%)	↓ VPA (30–40%)
Ethosuximide (ESM)	↑ ESM concentration (50%)	No effect
Felbamate (FLM)	↑ FLM concentration	↑ VPA concentration
Lamotrigine (LTG)	↑ LTG concentration (up to 164%)	No effect
Phenytoin (PHT)	↑ PHT unbound fraction	↓ VPA (30–40%)
Phenobarbital (PB)	↑ PB concentration (30–40%)	↓ VPA (30–40%)
Primidone (PRM)	↑ PB concentration (30–40%)	↓ VPA (30–40%)
Vigabatrin (VGB)	No effect	No effect
Zonisamide	↓ ZNS (15%)	No effect

Gabapentin, levetiracetam, oxcarbazepine, tiagabine and zonisamide have no interactions with VPA;
[a]clobazam co-medication can result in an increase in VPA levels.

Phenytoin, phenobarbital and carbamazepine can induce the hepatic metabolism of valproate, and levels can be reduced by co-medication by as much as 50%. In children these interactions can be particularly marked – and, in one study in children, the withdrawal of co-medication with enzyme-inducing antiepileptic drugs resulted in rises in valproate levels of 122% after withdrawal of phenytoin, 67% after withdrawal of phenobarbital and 50% after withdrawal of carbamazepine. The addition of lamotrigine may decrease valproate levels by about 25%, and felbamate, stiripentol and clobazam elevate valproate serum levels.

Valproate is a potent inhibitor of both oxidation and glucuronidation, and via this mechanism elevates phenobarbital levels by 57–81%, and also levels of diazepam and lorazepam, phenytoin, rufinamide, felbmate, ethosuximide, carbamazepine and particularly carbamazepine 10,11-epoxide. Valproate can lengthen the half-life of lamotrigine by two to three times and cause a profound elevation of lamotrigine levels.

The effect on phenytoin action is complex. Valproic acid displaces phenytoin from plasma proteins and can inhibit phenytoin metabolism. Thus, total phenytoin levels can be unchanged but the unbound phenytoin concentration can be significantly increased. In all patients, in co-medication with valproate, total phenytoin serum levels of phenytoin can be misleading and underestimate the concentrations of the unbound, pharmacologically active drug.

Valproate also interacts with non-antiepileptic drugs. Co-medication with the carbapenem group of antibiotics, particularly meropenem, results in dramatic falls in valproate levels (and in serious seizure exacerbations), although the mechanisms underlying this interaction are unclear. Valproic acid levels may also be lowered by rifampicin, the anti-HIV agent ritonavir and the oestrogen-containing contraceptive steroids.

Fluoxetine, isoniazid and salicylate increase valproate levels. Doxorubicin and cisplatin have been shown to impair the absorption of valproate. Naproxen, phenylbutazone and salicylate displace valproate from its albumin-binding sites and occasionally result in significant toxicity.

The metabolism of some drugs is inhibited by valproate, notably of nimodipine, levels of which can be almost doubled. Other drugs affected include tricyclic antidepressants and zidovudine.

In contrast to enzyme-inducing antiepileptic drugs, valproate acid does not affect the serum levels or efficacy of oral contraceptives.

Adverse effects

As valproate was introduced before the wide use of large controlled and blinded studies, the frequency of side effects has not been fully established. However, clinical experience has led to the view that the drug is in general as well tolerated as carbamazepine, phenytoin or the newer antiepileptic drugs. There are, however, a number of side effects not shared by other drugs.

Neurological side effects

There are distinctive neurological side effects. Tremor is a particularly common effect and occurs in about 10% of patients on valproate. It is dose related but usually mild. Sedative side effects, typical of many antiepileptic drugs, also occur with valproate, and severely so in about 2% of patients, and are sometimes associated with other neurological symptoms such as confusion and irritability. Parkinsonism and asterixis are other uncommon but unusual side effects of valproate therapy, usually developing on long-term treatment and reversible on drug withdrawal. Their mechanism is unclear.

Encephalopathy

Rarely, severe sedation amounting to stupor or even coma has been reported (valproate encephalopathy). Encephalopathy usually occurs in the first weeks of treatment but may appear months after the initiation of therapy. It is also said to commonly occur within a few days of adding another antiepileptic drug to valproate therapy (or valproate to another antiepileptic drug). In some cases, serum concentrations and serum ammonia levels are within healthy limits. The encephalopathy worsens if treated with benzodiazepines, and an improvement with flumazenil (a benzodiazepine receptor antagonist) has been reported. Occult carbamyl phosphate synthetase-1 deficiency may be responsible for some cases at least. Co-medication with phenobarbital also seems to induce severe sedation or even stupor, and this seems to be a pharmacodynamic reaction. The EEG usually shows high-voltage slow activity and the stupor or coma rapidly reverses when valproate is withdrawn. The encephalopathy should be differentiated from the encephalopathy associated with valproate-induced hyperammonaemia (see below).

Gastrointestinal side effects and weight gain

The common dose-related side effects include nausea, vomiting and gastrointestinal effects, common on initiation of therapy, and are avoided by the administration of enteric-coated formulations.

Weight gain is a frequent side effect (seen in 30% of all patients), often troublesome and occasionally profound, especially in women. It is less of a problem in children. This is dose related and a problem mainly only at higher doses. A recent study showed a mean gain of 5.8 kg after 8 months of treatment at a mean dose of 1800 mg/day. The cause of weight gain is not completely known, but is likely to be due to insulin resistance and an increase in appetite due to impaired β-oxidation of fatty acids with hyperinsulinaemia. It has also been shown that patients who developed obesity on valproic acid had increased leptin levels and decreased ghrelin and adiponectin levels.

Metabolic and endocrine effects

Valproate has various metabolic effects resulting from interference in mitochondrially based intermediate metabolism. The common results are hypocarnitinaemia, hyperglycinaemia and hyperammonaemia. These metabolic effects are a problem in those predisposed by genetically determined enzymatic defects or where enzymatic pathways are already stressed by illness or co-medication.

Ammonia levels are often slightly raised on valproate therapy. Hyperammonaemia is usually asymptomatic and routine monitoring of ammonia is not warranted. If the levels exceed 60 μmol/L, symptoms of drowsiness and encephalopathy may occur. Occasionally hyperammonaemia is severe, and stupor, coma or even death can result. Hyperammonaemia should be suspected whenever drowsiness occurs on valproate therapy. Severe rises in ammonia levels occur in predisposed individuals, and particularly in patients with urea cycle disorders. Valproate should not be used in patients with such conditions or in those with hepatic disease. The most common predisposing enzymatic defect is partial deficiency (heterozygosity) of ornithine transcarbamylase (OTC), which may be asymptomatic until valproate is prescribed or until valproate and metabolic stress combine to precipitate acute hyperammonaemia. The resulting hyperammonaemic encephalopathy can be severe and is occasionally fatal.

Endocrine effects

Valproate also has endocrine effects. The importance of these is uncertain, and data are somewhat conflicting. Polycystic ovarian syndrome (PCOS) – a syndrome with polycystic ovaries, hyperandrogenism, obesity, hirsutism, anovulatory cycles and menstrual disorders – occurs more frequently in women with epilepsy than in the general population (prevalence rate of 13–25% vs 4–6%, respectively). It has been particularly, but not exclusively, associated with valproate therapy. Polycystic ovaries are a common finding in young women and do not necessarily imply PCOS. Assessment is further complicated by the confounding effects of weight gain and other medications. However, the presence of a menstrual disorder, hirsutism or weight gain should trigger a thorough evaluation, and favours discontinuation of valproate. The mechanism of this valproate effect is not fully understood, but probably involves valproate-induced insulin resistance and alterations in hormone concentrations.

Other effects: on hair, pancreatic function, viral replication in HIV

Another unusual side effect of valproate is its propensity to cause hair changes – sometimes hair loss, change in colour or more usually curling of hair. Some degree of hair loss occurs in up to 12% of patients. The mechanism is unclear, but it may be due to the formation of abnormal metabolites. The hair curling can sometimes be profound, and striking changes of appearance (not always unwelcome) may result. It is said that the hair changes reverse if therapy is continued, but in the author's experience this is certainly not true in all cases.

Treatment with valproate may increase serum amylase concentration in up to 24% of asymptomatic patients. This requires no particular action, provided that other hepatic and pancreatic enzymes (lipase, trypsin) are within healthy limits. However, valproate can also induce acute pancreatitis. This is a rare but serious complication, due possibly to a drug-induced reduction in free radical-scavenging enzyme activity. Pancreatitis usually presents with progressive epigastric pain, nausea and vomiting, three-quarters of reported patients are aged <20 years and a third are <10 years. A quarter occurred during valproate monotherapy, half within 3 months of initiating therapy and two-thirds within 12 months of the initiation of treatment. The pancreatitis appears not to be related to dose or serum concentration. In most cases the illness is relatively mild, although occasional fatalities have been reported. It is not appropriate to rechallenge patients after pancreatitis because there is a high risk of relapse.

Valproate appears to increase the viral burden in patients infected with HIV by potentiating viral replication. The clinical consequences of this effect for HIV-positive patients are unknown. Recently, a 14% reduction in bone mineral density during long-term treatment with valproate was reported in both men and women.

Hypersensitivity, haematological and hepatic side effects

Acute allergic rashes have only rarely been reported, as have severe bone marrow depression and neutropenia. Minor haematological changes are common and of no significance. The most troublesome haematological effects of valproate are those on clotting; these include thrombocytopenia, inhibition of platelet aggregation, reduction of factor VII complex and fibrinogen depletion. Thrombocytopenia is the most frequent haematological side effect and is dose dependent. This can, with other valproic acid-induced disturbances of haemostasis, such as impaired platelet function, fibrinogen depletion and coagulation factor deficiencies, cause bruising or bleeding. Usually mild, these are of little clinical significance except during surgical intervention, and it is sometimes advised that valproate is withdrawn before intracranial surgery (including epilepsy surgery). It is also sometimes recommended that valproate be withdrawn 1 month before elective surgery where blood loss is common, although the actual risks of valproate in this situation are not known. Valproate also occasionally causes neutropenia and bone marrow suppression.

The serious idiosyncratic side effect that has caused most concern is acute hepatic failure. This has been most frequently observed in children under the age of 2 years on polytherapy and with neurological handicaps. The risk of fatal hepatotoxicity on polytherapy was initially estimated to be: 1 in 600 of those aged <3 years, 1 in 8000 in range 3–10 years, 1 in 10 000 in range 11–20 years, 1 in 31 000 between 21 and 40 years and 1 in 107 000 aged >40 years. On monotherapy, the risk is much lower: from 1 in 16 000 at age 10 years to 1 in 230 000 at age 21–40 years. However, some of these initial cases are now recognized as being multifactorial, with valproate precipitating an already existing diathesis and, with more careful prescribing to avoid high-risk cases, the rate of valproate-induced hepatic failure is considerably lower (0.2 cases per 10 000).

The risk factors for hepatotoxicity seem to be: young age (<3 years), use in polytherapy, presence of psychomotor retardation and the presence of certain underlying metabolic disorders (organic acidaemias, mitochondrial disorders, Alpers disease).

Hepatotoxicity usually appears during the first 3 months of therapy. The pathology is microvesicular steatosis with necrosis, and may be caused by an unsaturated 4-ene metabolite of the drug (2-n-propyl-4-pentenoic acid) that is a potent inducer of microvesicular steatosis. Hepatic failure has occasionally occurred in older children and adults, but no fatalities associated with valproate monotherapy have occurred in patients over the age of 10 years.

However, routine measurement of ammonia and other metabolites has not been useful in predicting hepatic disease, nor have routine measurements of bilirubin or liver function tests. The most important step in the diagnosis of hepatic failure is the early recognition of the clinical symptoms (e.g. nausea, vomiting, anorexia, lethargy, jaundice, oedema and at times loss of seizure control). In addition to the usual general and supportive measures, it has been suggested that an infusion of intravenous L-carnitine, 100 mg/kg per day, up to a maximum of 2 g/day, should be given.

Oral L-carnitine has also been advocated by some authorities in those on valproate with: symptomatic hyperammonaemia, risk factors for hepatotoxicity, infants and young children, those on the ketogenic diet who have hypocarnitinaemia, those on dialysis and premature infants who are receiving total parenteral nutrition.

Hepatic hypersensitivity should be differentiated from dose-related elevations of liver enzymes, which are present in up to 44% of valproate-treated patients. These elevations are usually not associated with clinical symptoms and resolve with drug reduction or withdrawal.

Teratogenicity

There are three aspects to consider:

Major malformations

Overall risks of major malformations in the offspring of women treated with valproate monotherapy are between 4 and 9%. This includes a 1–2% increased risk of spina bifida and other congenital anomalies such as cardiovascular malformations and craniofacial defects. The rate of major malformation is thus somewhat worse than that on carbamazepine or lamotrigine (risks of 2–4%). Many of these abnormalities can be detected prenatally, however, and termination of pregnancy reduces the risk in live offspring to almost baseline rates.

Fetal valproate syndrome

Valproate can cause a 'fetal valproate syndrome'. This comprises minor changes in facial appearance and skeletal effects such as a high forehead, long digits, long philtrum and small flat nose. To what extent these are simply healthy population variations, or if 'unhealthy' are related to genetic influences or are drug related, is unknown, as is the frequency of these effects.

Learning disability

There is a possibility that maternal valproate therapy can result in learning disability and behavioural problems in the offspring, often manifest only in the school years. Evidence on these points is rather weak, and is based on retrospective series with potential for bias and with data that exhibit internal inconsistencies (see p. 141). Nevertheless, these effects might be common, and the possibility (even if unproven) will preclude the use of valproate during pregnancy unless there are pressing reasons.

If valproate is to be given during pregnancy, the dose should be reduced (to <1000 mg/day), and monotherapy used, wherever possible. The daily dose should be divided into three or more administrations per day to avoid high peak plasma levels of valproate and its metabolites (as these may be a mechanism for teratogenic effects) and the controlled-release formulation should be used. It is also possible that administration of folic acid during pregnancy will reduce the risk of spina bifida, and, although not formally studied in valproate-treated women, folic acid supplements (5 mg/day) should be given from the onset of pregnancy.

Counselling on all these points is essential in all fertile women contemplating pregnancy; not to do so is now negligent practice.

Overdose

Overdose causes: coma, convulsions and respiratory depression; cardiac conduction defects, hypotension; and gastrointestinal and multiple metabolic effects. Profound coma occurs at doses >200 mg/kg. Death is rare but has been reported. Supportive treatment should be supplemented by gastric lavage and the use of activated charcoal. Haemodialysis and haemoperfusion may be helpful. Naloxone has been reported to reverse coma, and L-carnitine infusions may prevent hepatic damage.

Antiepileptic effect

Valproate has been the subject of many open and uncontrolled studies, in many types of epilepsy, since its introduction in the 1960s. The standards of monitoring and documentation do not match modern regulatory studies, yet these investigations showed indubitable effectiveness.

Partial-onset seizures

Existing evidence suggests that the drug has approximately similar efficacy to other main-line therapies,

although most clinicians use carbamazepine as a first choice, a decision based, mainly, on a large and influential study that compared valproate and carbamazepine in 480 previously untreated adults with partial-onset epilepsy. In this study, both drugs were similarly effective in controlling secondarily generalized seizures, but a greater percentage of patients with partial seizures remained free from seizures on carbamazepine. However, other controlled studies have not found differences between valproate and other drugs. In randomized, double-blind monotherapy studies in newly diagnosed patients, for example, similar efficacy was found when comparing valproate and oxcarbazepine (seizure-free rates of 54% and 57%, respectively, over 1 year in 249 adults) and valproate and lamotrigine (26% on valproate and 29% on lamotrigine free from seizures at 8 months).

A meta-analysis of a number of trials comparing valproate and carbamazepine concluded that carbamazepine was more effective than valproate in reducing time to first seizure and time to 12 months of remission.

The absolute effect of valproate can be estimated from two randomized controlled studies that compared valproate and placebo in uncontrolled partial epilepsy, in one of which a 38% responder rate (at a dose of 1200 mg/day) was found (and in both valproate was significantly more efficacious than placebo), a rate that compares favourably with that of many more modern drugs. Also, a controlled comparison of the effect of low-dose and high-dose valproate (defined by plasma concentrations of 25–50 and 80–150 µg/mL) found 30% and 70% median reductions of complex partial seizures and tonic–clonic seizures, respectively, in the high-dose group, compared with 19% and 22% in the low-dose (active control) group.

In children, several large prospective open-label studies have compared valproate with carbamazepine and phenytoin in newly diagnosed patients on monotherapy, finding no differences in efficacy between the drugs (and comparisons with phenobarbital showed that valproate was better tolerated).

Generalized tonic–clonic seizures

Valproate is a drug of first choice for the treatment of tonic–clonic seizures in IGE and also a drug of first choice, with carbamazepine, in secondarily generalized seizures. In one study of monotherapy in 36 patients with primarily generalized tonic–clonic seizures, of whom 24 had been treated previously with other antiepileptic drugs, seizures were fully controlled in 33. In another study, tonic–clonic seizures were fully controlled by the addition of valproate in 14 of 42 patients with previously intractable seizures. In a comparison with phenytoin in 61 previously untreated patients with generalized tonic–clonic, clonic or tonic seizures, seizure control was achieved in 73% on valproate and 47% on phenytoin. In another study of previously untreated patients, a 2-year remission was achieved in 27 (73%) of 37 patients with valproate and in 22 (56%) of 39 patients with phenytoin. In two studies of generalized tonic–clonic seizures in IGE, complete seizure control was achieved in 79% of 114 patients.

Typical absence seizures

In typical absence seizures, valproate was found to control all seizures in over 90% of patients in a variety of open-label studies, with control most likely if the seizures did not coexist with other seizure types. Two double-blind RCT studies have compared valproate with ethosuximide in children with absence epilepsy in a cross-over design. Both drugs had similar effects on absence seizures, but valproate was more effective in controlling convulsive seizures.

Myoclonic seizures

Valproate is the drug of choice for myoclonic seizures, regardless of aetiology or syndrome. Effectiveness varies in different syndromes, being high in JME, lower in the Lennox–Gastaut syndrome and lowest in the progressive myoclonic epilepsies.

The most common form of myoclonic epilepsy is JME. In open studies in this condition, around 85% of patients were rendered free from seizures. In one open study of 142 young patients with generalized epilepsy, 50% of whom were having daily seizures before therapy, valproate completely controlled the epilepsy in 63% of all cases overall, and a further 18% showed improvement >50%. Of the 69 patients with 3 Hz spike-wave discharges, 81% became free from seizures, as did 77% of those with myoclonic jerks.

Idiopathic generalized epilepsy

Valproate is often considered the drug of first choice for IGE and all its subgroups. It is effective in the three seizure types in this syndrome (myoclonic, generalized absence and generalized tonic–clonic seizures).

Lennox–Gastaut and West syndromes

The effectiveness of valproate in the Lennox–Gastaut syndrome has been shown in numerous open studies, and one small controlled investigation. In another study of 100 children, most of whom had the Lennox–Gastaut syndrome, seizure control was achieved on valproate in 12 of 27 children with 'absences and other seizures' and in 9 of 39 children with atonic seizures. The drug in another study was said to control seizures in about 10% of cases and reduce attacks by 50% or more in a third. This seems optimistic and experience suggests more modest outcomes.

In West syndrome, high-dose valproate is sometimes used if steroids and vigabatrin are ineffective or contraindicated, but not now usually as first-line therapy. One series reported a 90% rate of seizure control, but other studies report far less good results. The dose used varies between 20 and 60 mg/kg per day.

Other syndromes

Valproate is also a drug of first choice in the progressive myoclonic epilepsies, although it seldom fully controls the myoclonus in these cases. Valproate also controlled the seizures in 8 of 32 patients with myoclonic–astatic epilepsy, and 8 of 32 were improved by more than 50%. Valproate is as effective in controlling photosensitivity and abolishes it in more than half the patients. In patients with photosensitive seizures, total seizure control is attained in 84%. It has been used in neonatal seizures and to prevent febrile seizures, although other drugs are preferable in children aged <2 years in view of the potential hepatotoxic effects. Benign myoclonic epilepsy of infancy also responds very well to valproate. In postanoxic intention myoclonus, valproate is one of the more successful drugs, but this condition is often refractory to treatment. The use of valproate in status epilepticus is discussed on pp. 299–300, 302, 304–306, 313.

Clinical use in epilepsy

Valproate is still one of the most commonly used antiepileptics throughout the world. It is a drug of first choice in all seizure types (absence, myoclonus, tonic–clonic) in IGE (including JME). It is strikingly more effective than lamotrigine and topiramate in this indication, and more useful than the benzodiazepines or barbiturates. Whether levetiracetam can compete with its effectiveness is not yet clear, but seems unlikely. It is a drug of first choice in the Lennox–Gastaut syndrome, where it controls atypical absence and atonic seizures better than most other first-line drugs. It is also a drug of first choice in the syndromes of myoclonic epilepsy and the progressive myoclonic epilepsies, and for epilepsies with photosensitivity and/or generalized spike–wave electrographically.

In partial and secondarily generalized epilepsy, carbamazepine is usually tried before valproate, although there is no real evidence that valproate is less effective in new or mild cases.

Valproate is presented in different formulations in different countries, and this can be very confusing. It exists as the sodium, calcium and magnesium salts, as the acid, as sodium hydrogen divalproate or as valpromide. Enteric-coated, immediate and slow-release formulations also exist, as well as syrup, sprinkle, intravenous forms and a rectal suppository. There are no convincing therapeutic differences between any of these forms, although the enteric-coated form reduces gastrointestinal side effects, and rates of absorption differ in different formulations. The pharmacokinetics of individual patients vary much more than any difference in formulation, and there is little logic in having so many different manufactured products. In the UK the most popular form of sodium valproate is as 200 and 500 mg enteric-coated tablets.

The usual starting dose for an adult is 200 mg at night increasing in 2-weekly steps by 200 or 500 mg increments to a usual maintenance dose of between 600 and 1500 mg. Doses as high as 3000 mg/day are occasionally given. Twice-daily dosing is usual.

Valproate has complex interactions, and general rules are difficult to make. However, generally, patients on co-medication require higher doses than those on monotherapy. In children, the usual starting dose is 20 mg/kg per day and the maintenance dose is 40 mg/kg per day, and on combination therapy doses may need to be higher.

Although a target serum level range has been suggested by clinical studies, the levels fluctuate widely during a 24-hour period even on three-times-daily doses, although the antiepileptic effectiveness is not influenced by these fluctuations. The controlled-release formulation lessens this fluctuation, but does not improve seizure control.

Serum level estimations can be made, but there is a poor relationship between level and effect. Moreover, the marked diurnal swings in blood levels on two- or three-times-daily dosing often render measurements rather meaningless. There is little point in rigid adherence to the so-called therapeutic range (300–700 µmoL/L).

Side effects remain a problem, and it is because of these that enthusiasm for valproate has waned in recent years. Weight gain is common and often problematic. Other side effects, such as the neurotoxic effects and effects on hair growth, are also common, but often are only slight and usually not a reason for drug withdrawal.

In female patients, the suggestion that valproate increases the frequency of polycystic ovaries, causes menstrual irregularities and reduces fertility is enough for many to avoid its use. Scientific evidence on these points is, however, generally slight, and has tended to come from potentially unreliable sources. Valproate teratogenicity is a major concern and is a further reason for avoiding valproate in female patients where pregnancy is an issue. Its use in young children, especially those <2 years, carries a small but definite risk of hepatic failure and, where other drugs are available, these tend to be used now. It is contraindicated in the presence of hepatic or pancreatic disease.

Vigabatrin

Proprietary name: Sabril[a]

Primary indications
West syndrome. Also, partial-onset seizures where other therapy has been ineffective and the risk vs benefit ratio is appropriate. Adults and children.

Commonly used as first-line drug
No

Usual preparations
Tablets: 500 mg; powder sachet: 500 mg

Usual dosage – adults
Initial 500; increasing in 500 mg/day increments every 2 weeks
Maintenance: 1000–3000 mg/day (maximum 4000 mg/day)

Usual dosage – children
Body weight 10–15 kg: 40 mg/kg per day or 500–1000 mg/day; initially 125 mg/day
Body weight 15–30 kg: 1000–1500 mg/day; initially 250 mg/day
Body weight >30 kg: 1500–3000 mg/day; initially 500 mg/day

Dosing intervals
Twice a day

Is dose commonly affected by co-medication?
No

Is dose affected by renal/hepatic disease?
Renal disease

Does it affect dose of other drugs?
Sometimes, but usually slight in extent

Does it affect the contraceptive pill
No

Serum level monitoring
Not useful

Common/important adverse events
Mood change, depression, psychosis, aggression, confusion, weight gain, insomnia, changes in muscle tone in children, tremor and diplopia. Irreversible visual field constriction

Risk of hypersensitivity
No

Major mechanism of action
Inhibition of GABA transaminase activity

Main advantages
Highly effective antiepileptic drug. Excellent effect in West syndrome

Main disadvantages
Adverse effect on visual fields and potential for cognitive and behavioral side effects

Comment
Prescribing now restricted to last-resort use in partial epilepsy. Drug of choice in infantile spasm, especially when due to tuberous sclerosis

ᵃName of proprietary brand available in the UK.

Vigabatrin: pharmacokinetics – average adult values

Oral bioavailability	<100%
Time to peak levels	0.5–2 h
Volume of distribution	0.8 L/kg (for racemate)
Biotransformation	None
Elimination half-life	4–7 h
Plasma clearance	0.102–0.114 L/kg per h
Protein binding	None
Active metabolite	None
Metabolism by hepatic enzymes	No
Inhibition or induction of hepatic enzymes	No
Drug interactions	None

Recognition in the 1970s that γ-aminobutyric acid was an important inhibitory neurotransmitter in the CNS raised the possibility that boosting GABA action might suppress seizures. This led the worldwide pharmaceutical industry to turn their attention to GABA analogues. The first developed and the most successful was vigabatrin. This was synthesized in 1974 and then underwent trials in epilepsy, was licensed in the UK in 1989, and subsequently in 65 other European countries and worldwide, but not in the USA. It was the first of a long series of novel antiepileptic drugs introduced in the last 20 years. It was marketed as the prime example of a 'designer drug' engineered to produce a specific and rational mechanism of action, presaging a new chapter in epilepsy therapy, and was heavily marketed as such. It had gained an important role in the treatment of epilepsy and then, in 1997, the first case of visual failure was reported. This resulted in a dramatic decline in the use of the drug, and within a few years vigabatrin become almost completely eclipsed, saved only by the discovery of its value in infantile spasms.

Physical and chemical characteristics

Vigabatrin (γ-vinyl-γ-aminobutyric acid; 4-amino-hex-5-enoic acid; molecular weight 129.16) is a close structural analogue of GABA. The drug is a racemic mixture, but only the S-(+)-enantiomer is biologically active. It is a crystalline substance, highly soluble in water but only slightly soluble in ethanol.

Mode of action

Vigabatrin is a close structural analogue of GABA and acts on GABA transaminase, the enzyme that metabolizes GABA in the synaptic cleft. Vigabatrin binds irreversibly to the enzyme, and binding results in non-competitive inhibition of the enzyme.

Pharmacokinetics

Vigabatrin has simple pharmacokinetics, which poses few problems in the clinical arena. As the drug acts by irreversibly inhibiting the cerebral enzyme GABA transaminase, its effect is dependent on the rate of production of new enzyme rather than on any pharmacokinetic parameters, and the measurement of blood vigabatrin levels has no clinical utility. The biological half-life of the drug, i.e. the time taken for the enzyme concentrations to recover to half their previous level, is several days, even after a single dose. The plasma half-life is only 4–7 h.

Absorption and distribution

Absorption is rapid after oral ingestion, with a peak concentration at about 2 h. The oral bioavailability is at least 60–70%. Food has little effect on the rate or extent of absorption. There is no appreciable protein binding in plasma, and the volume of distribution of the drug is 0.8 L/kg. The drug is distributed widely. The CSF concentration of vigabatrin is about 10% that of the plasma. In neonates and young children, bioavailability and C_{max} of the active S-(+)-enantiomer are somewhat lower than in adults. Only a small amount of the drug crosses the placenta. The ratio of drug levels in breast milk compared with plasma is <0.5.

Metabolism and excretion

Vigabatrin is only minimally metabolized by humans (<5%), and is eliminated primarily by renal excretion.

Vigabatrin does not induce the activity of hepatic enzymes. The elimination half-life in people with healthy renal function is between 4 and 7 h, and is not dose dependent. The plasma clearance is 0.102–0.114 L/kg per h. Elimination is slower in elderly people. A steady state is attained after stable dosing regimens within 2 days. Sixty per cent of the drug is removed by haemodialysis and so extra dosage is needed in these circumstances. In neonates, C_{max} and AUC values of the active S-enantiomer of vigabatrin were significantly lower than in adults or older children.

Drug interactions

Vigabatrin has virtually no pharmacokinetic or pharmacodynamic interactions with any other antiepileptic drug, except phenytoin. The addition of vigabatrin can result in a fall on plasma concentration of phenytoin by a mean of 25%, usually within a few weeks of polytherapy. The mechanism of this effect is uncertain, but presumably it is due to impairment of phenytoin absorption because phenytoin protein binding, metabolism and excretion are unchanged. Serum levels of phenobarbital can also be slightly reduced. Vigabatrin has no effect on the metabolism of the oral contraceptive, or any known effects on other non-antiepileptic drugs.

Adverse effects

The adverse effects of vigabatrin have proved severe, and the once highly feted vigabatrin has become a vagabond on the periphery of epilepsy therapy because of these.

Intramyelinic oedema

One facet of the preclinical animal toxicology caused great concern and this was the finding, in rats and dogs, of widespread vigabatrin-induced intramyelinic vacuolization throughout the brain on pathological examination. This could also be demonstrated in vivo by magnetic resonance spectroscopy (MRS). Primate studies, human surgical and postmortem pathology, human MRS and human evoked potential studies, however, failed to demonstrate any similar changes, and on the basis of these generally reassuring data the drug was licensed. However, many expressed unease about this, and vigilance was recommended particularly over prolonged treatment periods. Recently, there have been reports of transient MRI hyperintensities on T2- and diffusion-weighted images in the basal ganglia and brain stem in infants and children treated with vigabatrin, and it is considered likely that these represent intramyelinic oedema. Most of

Table 8.28 Adverse effects due to vigabatrin (% of patients affected); pooled data from 2692 patients from the clinical trials of vigabatrin.

Adverse event	Frequency
Drowsiness	18.6
Fatigue	15.1
Headache	12.7
Dizziness	10.3
Weight gain	7.9
Agitation	6.9
Abnormal vision	5.3
Diplopia	5.1
Tremor	5.1
Depression	5.1

these MRI abnormalities resolve, even in those who remained on vigabatrin therapy.

Neurological side effects

Minor neurological side effects were noted in about 40% of all patients taking vigabatrin in the clinical trials, and the most common are fatigue, drowsiness, dizziness, agitation, amnesia, ataxia, confusion and mood change (Table 8.28).

More troublesome is the occasional tendency of vigabatrin to cause severe neuropsychiatric adverse events, notably depression, agitation or confusion, and in a few cases psychosis, with paranoid features and visual hallucinations. In a review of 717 patients in the RCTs, vigabatrin was associated with a significantly higher incidence, when compared with placebo, of depression (12.1% vs 3.5%) and psychosis (2.5% vs 0.3%). These psychotic reactions often occurred when seizure control had been improved, and some cases at least have been attributed to the process of forced normalization (a rather dubious concept – see p. 113) rather than to a direct toxic effect of the drug. The vigabatrin-induced depression can be severe, and is occasionally a threat to life. Disturbances of mood were (before the discovery of the visual field deficits) the most common reason for discontinuation of vigabatrin therapy in clinical trials.

The effect of vigabatrin on cognition has been formally studied, in a double-blind, placebo-controlled manner, and a dose-dependent decrease in performance was detected in only one of eight tests (digit cancellation).

Weight gain

An increase in body weight of more than 10% is seen in about 10–15% of adults taking long-term vigabatrin therapy and is a troublesome side effect. Weight gain seems particularly to develop in the first 6 months of therapy, but the mechanism is unknown.

Peripheral visual field loss

In 1997 – 8 years after the licensing of the drug and 15 years after its introduction into clinical trials – three cases of constriction of the peripheral visual fields were reported. In the following year, other cases were noted, and it has now become clear that between 30% and 40% of people treated with vigabatrin therapy develop this side effect. The longer the treatment with vigabatrin, and the higher the cumulative dose, the higher the prevalence.

The prevalence in children is less easy to determine, partly because field testing is more difficult, but is probably lower. In a study from Finland, visual field constriction was observed in 19% of children. Of course, as vigabatrin is now used to treat infantile spasms, concern has been raised about the risks of field deficits in infants in whom detailed field testing is not possible. Preliminary data from prospective long-term follow-up studies of those infants exposed to vigabatrin have shown a lower frequency of visual field and it seems possible, but not certain, that very young children are least susceptible to this adverse effect of vigabatrin.

Typically, the visual field loss is asymptomatic, although a number of patients (perhaps 10% of all those taking vigabatrin) notice deterioration in peripheral vision and occasionally this deterioration is severe. Visual fields show the pattern of bilateral nasal then concentric constriction (tunnel vision), with central vision preserved (Figure 8.10). The changes seem to be irreversible, even if vigabatrin therapy is withdrawn and, if chronic therapy with vigabatrin is to be contemplated, baseline field testing should be carried out and repeated initially 6 monthly and then annually. The patients should be fully counselled about this risk.

Field testing to confrontation in the clinic is usually normal, and the visual field disturbances are picked up often only by careful testing by experienced personnel using techniques such as Goldman perimetry and the computerized Humphries testing battery.

The mechanism of this effect is likely to be due to GABA inhibition in the retina, which is a structure rich in $GABA_C$ receptors, and GABA levels in the retina have been shown to be considerably raised on treatment with vigabatrin.

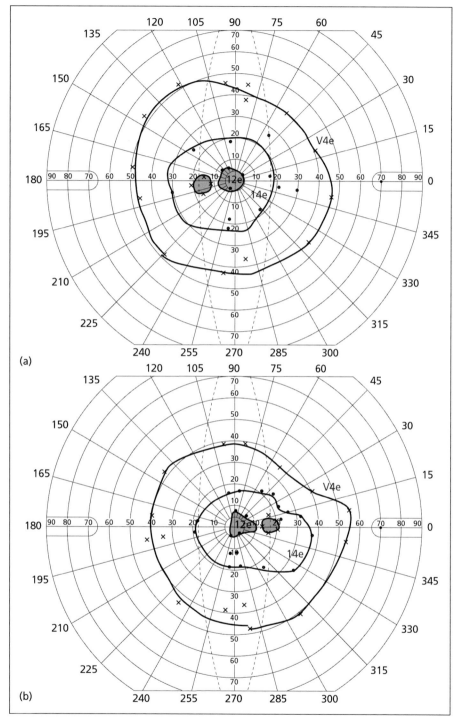

Figure 8.10 Perimetry showing severe bilateral visual field constriction caused by vigabatrin therapy.

Hypersensitivity and other effects

Acute idiosyncratic immunological adverse events (e.g. rash, hepatic disturbance, marrow dysplasia) are extremely rare, and vigabatrin has proved a safe drug in this regard. One case of fatal hepatotoxicity has been reported, but was probably due to an undetected metabolic disorder rather than vigabatrin.

One unusual effect of vigabatrin is to increase levels of α-aminoadipic acid in plasma and urine, and this can mimic α-aminoadipic aciduria, causing diagnostic confusion. Similar confusion can be caused by abnormal urinary amino acid measurements due to inhibition of β-alanine metabolism.

Antiepileptic effect
Partial-onset seizures

Adults with refractory partial epilepsy were the first target group in clinical trials in the clinical evaluation of vigabatrin. The pivotal European studies were of 479 such patients, in an add-on parallel group design. These demonstrated a 50% or greater response rate in 40–50% of adult patients with refractory partial seizures. Up to 10% of patients in these clinical trials became free from seizures. Essentially similar figures were then shown in similar studies from the USA, with 40–50% response rates at doses of 2–4 g/day. These are evidence of very good efficacy, and of the newer drugs only topiramate showed better response rates. In paediatric studies, too, vigabatrin had a good effect against complex partial seizures, with seizure-free rates of between 10 and 40% in some studies.

Monotherapy was also been extensively studied, but the results of vigabatrin were less good than as adjunctive therapy in refractory partial epilepsy. In a large randomized, double-blind, parallel-group comparison with carbamazepine in newly diagnosed epilepsy, 53% of 229 patients on 2 g vigabatrin daily and 57% of 230 patients on 600 mg carbamazepine daily achieved 6-month remission. However, significantly more patients on vigabatrin withdrew due to lack of efficacy than with carbamazepine, and time to first seizure after the first 6 weeks from randomization also showed carbamazepine to be more effective. Longer-term efficacy has been investigated in a number of open long-term retention studies with between 39% and 72% of patients remaining on vigabatrin for more than 3 years.

Generalized seizures

Vigabatrin has little efficacy either in primarily generalized tonic–clonic seizures or against absence seizures or myoclonus; indeed these seizure types are frequently worsened by vigabatrin. In placebo-controlled trials in refractory epilepsy, 20% of children and 5% of adults showed an increase in seizures. Absence status can be precipitated by vigabatrin therapy. Patients with Angelman syndrome may be particularly prone to seizure exacerbation on vigabatrin. Similarly, secondarily generalized seizures are notably less well controlled than partial seizures, and less well controlled than with other first-line antiepileptic drugs, even where the two seizure types coexist. Experience suggests that vigabatrin has little utility in patients with the Lennox–Gastaut syndrome, although studies have shown conflicting results. Case reports described favourable effects of vigabatrin in neonatal seizures due to Ohtahara syndrome and in the Landau–Kleffner syndrome.

Infantile spasms

Infantile spasms are currently the only major indication for vigabatrin therapy. ACTH or corticosteroids had been, for decades, the gold standard treatment for infantile spasms, but, in 1990, vigabatrin was also found to be effective, and now these drugs are universally recommended as alternative first-line therapies. An RCT in 40 children with newly diagnosed infantile spasms compared vigabatrin and placebo. At the end of a 5-day double-blind phase, seven (35%) vigabatrin-treated children were spasm free and five (25%) had a resolution of hypsarrhythmia, compared with two (10%) and one (5%) respectively in the placebo group. A comparison has also been made with ACTH. In a cross-over study, there was complete control of spasms in 48% of infants in the vigabatrin group and 74% in the ACTH group. The response to vigabatrin occurred within 14 days, and follow-up data for up to 44 months identified only one case of relapse of spasms. In the ACTH group, six patients relapsed 40–45 days after termination of ACTH. A multicentre study randomly assigned 142 infants to low-dose (18–36 mg/kg per day) or high-dose (100–150 mg/kg per day) vigabatrin treatment in which 8 of 75 (10.6%) patients in the low-dose group and 24 of 67 (35.8%) in the high-dose group responded. The UK Infantile Spasms Study (UKISS) was a multicentre RCT that compared the efficacy of vigabatrin with that of prednisolone or tetracosactide. Of 52 infants randomized to vigabatrin (100–150 mg/kg per day), 28 (54%) were spasm free within 2 weeks, compared with 70% (21 of 30) of infants who received prednisolone. Adverse events were reported in 54% of the infants on vigabatrin (mainly drowsiness and gastrointestinal symptoms) and in 55% of the infants on hormonal therapy (mainly high blood pressure, irritability and gastrointestinal symptoms). There have been numerous other reports of the use of vigabatrin in newly diagnosed or drug-refractory infantile spasms, with fairly consistent findings. All show that the response to vigabatrin occurs relatively rapidly and complete disappearance of spasms and hypsarrhythmia can be expected in over 50% of infants.

Vigabatrin has been shown to be particularly effective in the treatment of infantile spasms due to tuberous sclerosis complex. In a prospective randomized trial performed comparing vigabatrin and hydrocortisone, 100% of those randomized to vigabatrin (150 mg/kg per day) became seizure free compared with fewer than 50% of those on hydrocortisone and, when crossed over to vigabatrin, all became seizure free. It has been postulated that epileptogenesis in tuberous sclerosis complex may be caused by an imbalance of decreased inhibition secondary to molecular changes in GABA receptors in giant cells and dysplastic neurons, but the exact mechanisms underlying the preferential response of these patients to vigabatrin are still unknown.

Clinical use in epilepsy

In the first few years after licensing, vigabatrin gained a significant place in the therapy of partial epilepsy in adults and children, especially as adjunctive therapy. This has completely changed, however, with the finding of irreversible drug-induced visual field deficits. In adults, vigabatrin is now used only as add-on therapy for patients with refractory partial epilepsy who were placed on vigabatrin before the risk of visual field effects was recognized, who do not have any field deficits and in whom vigabatrin had proved superior to all other therapy. In such cases, the balance of risk and benefit is in favour of the maintenance of vigabatrin therapy; this is a very small number of cases. Very few patients indeed are now started anew on vigabatrin.

The usual starting dose for an adult is 250–500 mg once or twice a day, increasing by 250–500 mg incremental steps every 1–2 weeks. The average maintenance dose is between 1 and 2 g/day, although 25% of patients have better control on 3 g than on 2 g. The maximum dose is 4 g. In children, 40 mg/kg per day is the usual starting dose, with maintenance doses of 80–100 mg/kg per day. Lower doses should be used in patients with renal impairment, especially when the creatinine clearance is <60 mL/min. When the drug is being withdrawn it is recommended that this be done slowly, with 250 or 500 mg decrements every 2–4 weeks. The drug has significant side effects in addition to visual field defects. These include the risk of psychosis or depression and there remains constant anxiety about the possibility of drug-induced intramyelinic oedema (an anxiety fuelled by the recent reports of MRI changes in children on vigabatrin).

It is likely that the drug would have disappeared altogether were it not for its emergence as a drug of first choice for infantile spasm, and one particularly useful where the spasms are due to tuberous sclerosis. This is a niche indication, and in infants the positive effects can be dramatic. The role of vigabatrin vis-à-vis steroid therapy is outlined in more detail on pp. 93–94.

Zonisamide

CH$_2$SO$_2$NH$_2$

Proprietary name: Zonegran[a]

Primary indications
Adjunctive therapy in partial-onset seizures in adults ≥18 years (in Europe and the USA). Monotherapy and adjunctive therapy in children and adults for a broad range of epilepsy (in Japan and Asia)

Commonly used as first-line drug
No

Usual preparations
Capsules: 25, 50, 100 mg; tablets: 100 mg (Japan, Korea); powder: 20% (Japan, Korea)

Usual dosage – adults
Initial: 50 mg/day; increase by increments of 50 mg/day every 2 weeks
Maintenance 200–400 mg/day (maximum 600 mg/day)

Usual dosage – children
Initial: 2–4 mg/kg per day
Maintenance: 4–8 mg/kg per day

Dosing intervals
Once or twice a day

Is dose commonly affected by co-medication?
Yes

Is dose affected by renal/hepatic disease?
Avoid in severe renal disease

Does it affect dose of other drugs?
No

Does it affect the contraceptive pill?
No

Serum level monitoring
Potentially useful

Target range
30–140 µmol/L; 10–40 mg/L

Common/important adverse events
Somnolence, ataxia, dizziness, fatigue, nausea, vomiting, irritability, anorexia, impaired concentration, mental slowing, itching, diplopia, insomnia, abdominal pain, depression, skin rashes, hypersensitivity. Significant risk of renal calculi, metabolic acidosis, weight loss and oligohidrosis. Risk of heat stroke

Risk of hypersensitivity
Yes

Major mechanism of action
Inhibition of sodium channel conductance, T-type calcium currents, glutaminergic transmission, carbonic anhydrase; enhancement of GABA-ergic action

Main advantages
Shown to be effective in broad spectrum of epilepsies; also a particular place in the Lennox–Gastaut syndrome, infantile spasm and progressive myoclonic epilepsies

Main disadvantages
Side-effect profile

Comment
Drug of second choice in wide spectrum of epilepsies

[a]Name of proprietary brand available in the UK.

Zonisamide: pharmacokinetics – average adult values

Oral bioavailability	<100%
Time to peak levels	2.4–4.6 h
Volume of distribution	1.1–1.7 L/kg
Biotransformation	Hepatic reduction, *N*-acetylation and then glucuronidation
Elimination half-life	49–69 h (varies with co-medication)
Plasma clearance	0.0089–0.001 L/kg per h (varies with co-medication)
Protein binding	40–50%
Active metabolite	None
Metabolism by hepatic enzymes	CYP3A4, acetylation and glucuronidation
Inhibition or induction of hepatic enzymes	No
Drug interactions	Common

Zonisamide is a sulphonamide derivative chemically distinct from any of the previously established antiepileptic drugs. Its antiepileptic action was discovered by chance in 1974, and it was approved for use in Japan in 1989 and in the USA in 2003, and licensed in Europe in 2005. It was subjected to intensive study in Japan in the 1980s and then a further three pivotal clinical studies were carried out in the USA and Europe. Its current regulatory licence is for monotherapy and adjunctive therapy in a wide spectrum of epilepsies in Japan, but as adjunctive therapy in refractory partial epilepsy in adults only in the USA, the UK and Europe.

Chemical and physical properties

Zonisamide (1,2-benzisoxazole-3-methanesulphonamide; molecular weight 212) is a white crystalline powder, slightly soluble in acidic and neutral aqueous solutions, with a pK_a of 10.2. Solubility markedly increases as pH increases.

Mode of action

Zonisamide has a number of different properties that contribute to its antiepileptic effect. It reduces conductance at the voltage-gated sodium channel by affecting the kinetics of sodium-channel inactivation, an action similar to that of phenytoin but with different kinetics. It also affects T-type calcium currents, increasing the proportion of channels in the inactivated state. It binds to the benzodiazepine $GABA_A$ receptor, where it has valproate-like actions. It also has effects on excitatory glutaminergic transmission and acetylcholine metabolism, and it inhibits dopamine turnover and carbonic anhydrase activity, but the relevance of these actions to its anticonvulsant action is unclear. It is effective in a wide variety of animal models of epilepsy. In addition to its antiepileptic action, it has marked neuroprotective properties in some experimental models, by its ability to scavenge free radicals and its antioxidant properties.

Pharmacokinetics
Absorption and distribution

Zonisamide is rapidly and completely absorbed, and peak concentrations are achieved usually within 2.4–4.6 h. Bioavailability is close to 100% and not affected by food. The mean volume of distribution is between 1.1 and 1.7 L/kg. The drug is widely distributed in the body, involving active transport systems, and is particularly highly concentrated in erythrocytes. Concentrations in the cerebral cortex are higher than in the midbrain. Protein binding is 30–60%. There is a linear dose to serum level relationship at doses up to 800 mg, but the C_{max} and AUC increase disproportionately at higher doses, perhaps owing to saturation of the binding to red blood cells. It is not known to what extent the drug is excreted in breast milk.

Metabolism and excretion

Zonisamide is metabolized largely by acetylation and cleavage of the isoxazole ring, by the CYP3A species of the cytochrome P450 system, followed by conjugation with glucuronic acid. N-Acetylation also occurs. The plasma half-life is between 49 and 69 h in monotherapy, but lower in co-medication with enzyme-inducing drugs. The drug exhibits first-order kinetics at normal doses. In monotherapy, therefore, steady state is reached within 7 days and diurnal variations in the levels are small, with peak–trough differences of only 14–27% at steady-state concentrations. The metabolites are not active and are excreted in the urine. In chronic therapy about 35% of the drug is excreted unchanged. Zonisamide does not induce its own metabolism. Plasma clearance is low, in various studies between 0.0089 and 0.001 L/kg per h in patients who are not receiving enzyme-inducing co-medication. It increases to about 0.015 L/kg per h in co-medicated patients. In renal disease clearance is markedly reduced (35% reduction in those with a creatinine clearance of <20 mL/min).

Drug interactions

Zonisamide does have drug interactions that might be expected to alter dosing requirements in some situations. As a result of enzyme induction, adjunctive administration of enzyme-inducing antiepileptic drugs reduced the half-life of zonisamide, in one study, from 52–66 h to <27 h with phenytoin, 38 h with carbamazepine and 38 h with phenobarbital. The effect of valproate is inconsistent, but one study showed a reduction of half-life to 46 h. Lamotrigine usually has no effect on the metabolism of zonisamide. Other drugs inducing the CYP3A4 system such as rifampicin will also be expected to induce zonisamide metabolism.

Conversely, as zonisamide is not a strong enzyme inducer or inhibitor, co-medication with zonisamide generally has no effect on concentrations of phenytoin, carbamazepine or valproate. There is no autoinduction. Zonisamide has no effect on the contraceptive pill. Zonisamide is a weak inhibitor of P-glycoprotein and so may change the brain levels of substrates (such drugs as digoxin or quinidine), but there is no definite evidence that this is relevant to other antiepileptic drugs.

Adverse effects
Neurological and other side effects

In the pooled data of three double-blind, placebo-controlled studies in the USA and Europe, the incidence of adverse drug reactions was 78.1%, compared with 61.3% on placebo. Side effects that occurred at an incidence >5% in the placebo-controlled studies are listed in Table 8.29; 11.5% of the treated patients and 6.5% of the placebo group discontinued treatment because of side effects, mainly sedation and effects on behaviour and cognition. Speech and language problems were also recorded, especially after 6–10 weeks of therapy and at doses >300 mg/day, similar to the effect of topiramate. In the placebo-controlled studies, 2.2% of patients were hospitalized for depression and 2.2% were hospitalized for psychosis. Other neurological and psychiatric side effects include fatigue, lability of affect, anxiety, insomnia, tremor and bradyphrenia.

Weight loss is a common side effect, often welcomed by patients. Abdominal pain, constipation, diarrhoea and nausea are relatively common side effects. Pancreatitis has been reported.

Table 8.29 Adverse effects of zonisamide (%) in double-blind placebo controlled studies; pooled data: effects occurring in more than 5% of patients.

Adverse effect	Placebo (n = 230)	Zonisamide (n = 269)
Somnolence	12.2	19.3
Ataxia	5.7	16.7
Anorexia	6.1	15.6
Dizziness	10.9	15.6
Fatigue	10.4	14.1
Nausea and/or vomiting	11.7	11.5
Irritability	5.2	11.5
Diplopia	4.3	8.9
Headache	8.3	8.6
Decreased concentration	0.9	8.2
Insomnia	3.5	7.8
Abdominal pain/discomfort	1.7	7.4
Depression	3.0	7.4
Forgetfulness	2.2	7.1
Rhinitis	6.1	6.7
Confusion	1.3	5.6
Anxiety	2.6	5.6
All effects	*61.3*	*78.1*

Renal stones, metabolic acidosis and oligohidrosis

One striking difference that has been noted between the Japanese studies and the US and European studies is the occurrence of renal stones. In pre-approval studies in Japan, only two patients (0.2%) developed urinary stones, compared with a rate of 2.6% in the early studies in the USA and Europe. In another US study, the occurrence of renal stones was assessed by means of renal ultrasonography, repeated annually during the study, in 501 patients treated with zonisamide and 85 patients with placebo. Calculi were demonstrated in 2 of 85 patients (2.4%) during placebo treatment, and in 17 of 501 patients (3.4%) treated with zonisamide. In the subsequent controlled trials in the USA and Europe and the open-label extensions, symptomatic calculi were reported in 9 of 626 (1.4%) patients, and overall in Europe and the USA in 15 of 1296 (1.2%) of patients taking the drug for up to 8.7 years.

The risk of symptomatic renal stones, during the developmental studies of zonisamide, was 28.7 per 1000 patient-years of exposure in the first 6 months, 62.6 per 1000 patient-years of exposure between 6 and 12 months, and 24.3 per 1000 patient-years of exposure after 12 months.

Zonisamide had a mild effect on renal function in some clinical studies. A mean 8% elevation of serum creatinine occurred in some studies during the first 4 weeks of therapy, and this returned to baseline values on discontinuation of the drug. It is advised that zonisamide not be used in patients with severe renal failure (glomerular filtration rate <30 mL/min).

Hyperchloraemic metabolic acidosis (decreased serum bicarbonate without chronic respiratory alkalosis) can be caused by zonisamide, due to inhibition of carbonic anhydrase. Bicarbonate levels are often slightly reduced (average decrease of approximately 3.5 mmol/L at daily doses of 300 mg in adults) and rarely more severely decreased. Conditions or therapies that predispose to acidosis (such as renal disease, severe respiratory disorders, diarrhoea, surgery, ketogenic diet and certain drugs) can exacerbate this metabolic effect and cause symptoms.

Oligohydrosis (impairment of sweating) is another unusual side effect of zonisamide. This was identified in 17–25% of cases in two studies in children, but less than 1% in post-marketing surveillance. Zonisamide can be shown to suppress the sweating response to acetylcholine loading in humans. This adverse effect is a particular problem in infants and young children and may predispose to heat stroke. As a result of this, zonisamide should not be used with other carbonic anhydrase inhibitors or anticholinergic drugs.

Hypersensitivity

Zonisamide is a benzisoxazole derivative, which contains a sulphonamide group, and the hypersensitivity associated with such a chemical structure also occurs in zonisamide. Of patients in the controlled trials 2.2% withdrew from the drug because of the occurrence of rash, and across all trials the rate of rash is 12 events per 1000 patient-years of treatment. Eighty-five per cent of the rashes occurred within 16 weeks of the initiation of therapy in the US studies.

Two cases of aplastic anaemia and one case of agranulocytosis were reported during the first 11 years post-marketing of zonisamide in Japan. Forty-nine cases of the Stevens–Johnson syndrome and toxic epidermal necrolysis were reported in the same period (with seven deaths) – a rate of 46 cases per million patient-years of exposure. All patients were taking other drugs. No cases have been reported in the European or US development programmes.

Teratogenicity

Zonisamide has demonstrated teratogenic potential in animal studies. Of 25 known human pregnancies in which zonisamide was taken in combination with other antiepileptics, one infant had anencephaly (with co-medication with phenytoin) and one an atrial septal defect (with co-medication with valproate and phenobarbital). It is classified as a category C teratogen by the FDA.

Overdose

One patient is reported who took 7400 mg zonisamide. It is thought that her peak levels may have reached 200 μg/mL. She developed coma and respiratory depression. She was treated with supportive measures, fluids and gastric lavage, and recovered.

Antiepileptic effect
Partial-onset epilepsy

In the four definitive placebo-controlled studies in the USA and Europe, zonisamide (400, 200 or 100 mg/day) was used in 845 patients with refractory partial or generalized epileptic seizures. In three studies, responder rates (i.e. those showing a reduction in seizures of at least 50%) were 41.8% at 400 mg/day, 29.0% at 200 mg/day and 28.0% at 100 mg/day (compared with 22.2%, 15.0% and 12.0% on placebo). The median reduction in seizures was 40.5% at 400 mg/day, 27.2% at 200 mg/day and 29.5% at

100 mg/day (compared with 9.0%, −3.2% and −1.1% on placebo). In one of the trials, dose effects could be studied; in this trial the median reduction in seizures: at 100 mg/day was 24.7% (8.3% on placebo); at 200 mg/day 20.4% (4.0% on placebo); and at 400 mg/day 40.5% (9% on placebo). All (bar one) of these findings showed significant improvements compared with placebo (at $P < 0.05$).

A randomized comparison of zonisamide and carbamazepine in 123 patients with refractory partial epilepsy showed mean reductions in seizures of 68.4% on zonisamide compared with 46.6% on carbamazepine (69.7 and 70.2% for tonic–clonic seizures), and responder rates were 81.8% and 70.7%, respectively. These were not significant differences. Zonisamide (mean daily dose of 7.3 mg/kg per day) was compared with valproate (mean daily dose 27.6 mg/kg per day) in 34 children with refractory generalized seizures, with overall improvement rates of 50.0% on zonisamide and 43.8% on valproate.

The responder rates from the pooled data of 1008 adults and children who had been enrolled in the controlled studies and non-comparative multicentre studies are shown in Table 8.30. Among the partial seizures, responder rates were similar in temporal lobe epilepsy (54%; $n = 428$) and those with extratemporal lobe

Table 8.30 Clinical efficacy of zonisamide in 1008 patients from the clinical trials of the drug.

Seizure type	No. of patients	Responder rate (%)
Partial		
Simple partial	63	57
Simple partial followed by complex partial	82	50
Complex partial	362	50
Partial-onset generalized tonic–clonic	168	60
Generalized		
Generalized tonic–clonic	46	59
Generalized tonic	74	26
Atypical absences	9	67
Typical absences	4	50
Atonic	10	50
Myoclonic	7	43
Clonic	1	100
Combination	129	41

epilepsy (51%; $n = 224$). Sixty-six per cent (of 41 patients) with idiopathic epilepsy responded, as did 32% of 132 patients with the Lennox–Gastaut syndrome and 22% of 9 patients with the West syndrome. Controlled studies in these conditions would be valuable but have not been thus far reported.

Progressive myoclonic epilepsy

Zonisamide seems to have a specific effect in patients with progressive myoclonic epilepsy (PME), at least on the basis of evidence from open studies and case series. Dramatic improvements in all seizure types (tonic–clonic and myoclonic) were first reported in 1988 and have been repeatedly confirmed. In one study 10 of 30 patients with PME had a sustained 50% reduction in seizure frequency. The improvement occurs in patients with both Unverricht–Lundborg disease and Lafora body disease, and in mitochondrial disease.

Clinical use in epilepsy

Zonisamide is a chemically distinctive drug with striking effectiveness in a broad range of seizure types and epilepsies, and notably also in epilepsy syndromes that are otherwise often resistant to therapy. The effects are maintained and there is no evidence of tachyphylaxis. It may have a particular role in the PMEs, and also has intriguing possibilities as a neuroprotective agent. As a result of its long usage in Japan, there are now over 2 million patient-years of experience and its side-effect profile is well understood. The CNS side effects can be prominent but can be lessened by starting at a low dose and incrementing the dose slowly at a rate of 50 mg every 2 weeks in adults.

Other side effects are less common, but can be troublesome and include renal stones, metabolic acidosis and oligohidrosis, and a risk of hypersensitivity. It is licensed currently in the USA, the UK and Europe only for adjunctive therapy in adults with partial epilepsy (± secondary generalization), but has much wider indications in Asia.

The initial recommended dose is 25 mg twice daily in adults and 2–4 mg/kg per day in children. The dose can be increased at 50 mg increments every 2 weeks. Usual maintenance doses are 200–400 mg/day in adults (maximum dose 600 mg/day) and 4–8 mg/kg per day in children (maximum dose 12 mg/kg per day). The drug can be given once or twice a day. The half-life is long in monotherapy, but considerably reduced in adjunctive therapy. Serum level monitoring is not usually needed, but it has been suggested that the usual range of therapeutic levels is 30–140 µmoL/L.

As a result of the risk of hypersensitivity, patients should report to their physicians immediately if a skin rash, fever, sore throat or bruising occurs. Renal function should be monitored and the drug avoided in renal failure. It has some unusual side effects relating to its propensity to induce oligohidrosis and occasionally cause heat stroke or difficulty with temperature control on exercise, especially in children. As a result of the risk of acidosis and of renal stones, the drug should not used in co-medication with other carbonic anhydrase inhibitors (including acetazolamide or topiramate) or anticholinergic drugs.

Other drugs used in the treatment of epilepsy

In 1861, Sir Edward Sieveking closed the treatment chapter in his book on epilepsy with the famous words 'there is scarcely a substance in the world capable of passing through the gullet of man that has not at one time or other enjoyed the reputation of being an antiepileptic'. Things have changed, but still unsubstantiated claims are made about numerous medicinal and non-medicinal products, with varying degrees of hope or cynicism.

Among prescribed medicines there are a number with claims that are based on highly unsatisfactory open studies, often in small numbers of patients and for short periods of time. Some of these are listed in Table 8.31, and some are still occasionally encountered in clinical practice.

There are, however, other drugs for which utility is proven, and which are occasionally used in the treatment of epilepsy, and these are outlined here.

Table 8.31 Prescription drugs licensed for other indications that have also been reported to have been used as antiepileptics.

Allopurinol
Calcium channel blockers (diltiazem, nimodipine, nifedipine, verapamil)
Carbenoxolone
Furosemide (and other diuretics)
Mannitol
Propranolol and other beta-blockers
Quinidine
Vitamin E

Acetazolamide

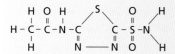

Proprietary name: Diamox[a]

Primary indications
All seizure types. Catamenial epilepsy

Commonly used as first-line drug
No

Usual preparations
Tablets: 250 mg

Usual dosage – adults
Initial: 250 mg/day
Maintenance: 250–750 mg/day

Usual dosage – children
Initial: 10 mg/kg per day
Maintenance: 30 mg/kg per day

Dosing intervals
Once or twice daily

Is dose commonly affected by co-medication?
No

Is dose affected by renal/hepatic disease?
Avoid in renal and hepatic disease

Does it affect dose of other drugs?
No

Does it affect the contraceptive pill?
No

Serum level monitoring
Not useful

Common/important adverse events
Acidosis, drowsiness, anorexia, irritability, nausea and vomiting, loss of appetite, weight loss, enuresis, headache, thirst, dizziness, hyperventilation, flushing, loss of libido, renal stones. Severe hypersensitivity affecting skin and blood

Risk of hypersensitivity
Yes – marked risk

Major mechanism of action
Carbonic anhydrase inhibition

Main advantages
Broad-spectrum action; can be used as intermittent therapy (e.g. in catamenial epilepsy)

Main disadvantages
Tolerance to the antiepileptic effects; hypersensitivity reactions; other side effects

Comment
Drug of second choice in refractory epilepsy. Also used in catamenial epilepsy

[a]Name of proprietary brand available in the UK.

Acetazolamide: pharmacokinetics (average adult values)	
Oral bioavailability	<90%
Time to peak levels	1–3 h
Volume of distribution	0.2 L/kg
Biotransformation	None
Elimination half-life	10–12 h
Plasma clearance	insufficient data
Protein binding	90–95%
Active metabolite	None
Metabolism by hepatic enzymes	No
Inhibition of induction of hepatic enzymes	No
Drug interactions	None

Acetazolamide, 2-acetylamido-1,3,4-thiadiazole-5 sulphonamide (molecular weight 222), is a sulphonamide derivative ($C_4H_6N_4O_3S_2$); it is a carbonic anhydrase inhibitor and this is probably the mechanism of its antiepileptic action. It has a clear effect in animal models of epilepsy, and its antiepileptic action was first reported in humans in the 1950s. The drug has had a place in therapy ever since.

Pharmacokinetics
Acetazolamide is a poorly soluble crystalline substance. It is a weak acid with a pK_a of 7.4. The drug is absorbed largely in the duodenum and upper jejunum. The oral bioavailablity is more than 90% in the dose range used in epilepsy. The peak plasma concentrations (10–18 µg/mL) are reached 1–3 h after oral ingestion of a single 250 mg dose. The volume of distribution of acetazolamide is 0.21 L/kg, and the drug is preferentially concentrated in erythrocytes (as is zonisamide) and other tissues where carbonic anhydrase concentrations are high. Acetazolamide is 90–95% bound to plasma proteins. About half the unbound drug exists in the plasma in the unionized form, and this diffuses into tissues where it binds strongly to carbonic anhydrase as an enzyme inhibitor complex. The plasma half-life of freely available acetazolamide is about 2 h, although by 24 h after ingestion most of the drug is in the form of an enzyme inhibitor complex, which has a half-life of 10–12 h. The concentration in brain is rather lower than in other tissues owing to an active transport system of the drug out of the brain.

The drug is not metabolized; 20% of the elimination is by glomerular filtration and 80% by renal tubular excretion. The whole of a single oral dose of acetazolamide is recovered in the urine in 24 h. Less than 0.7% of the dose per kilogram of body weight of the mother is transferred in breast milk, and breast-feeding is therefore likely to be harmless.

There are no significant drug interactions, except at the level of protein binding.

Side effects
Idiosyncratic reaction
Like any sulphonamide drug, acetazolamide can cause acute hypersensitivity, and this its most serious risk. The Stevens–Johnson syndrome, aplastic anaemia, agranulocytosis, acute thrombocytopenia and acute renal failure can occur. These are uncommon but patients should be warned about the risk. There is cross-sensitivity to other sulphonamide drugs, which should therefore be avoided.

Renal calculi
Renal calculi can be caused by acetazolamide, owing to renal tubular acidosis with resultant hypercalciuria and hypocitraturia. The frequency of stone formation has varied between studies from 0% to 43%. Citrate supplementation and hydration may be effective in reducing stone formation.

Other side effects
Mild side effects are common (recorded in 10–30% of most series). In one study, 11% of 277 patients reported the following side effects in descending order of frequency: drowsiness, anorexia, irritability, nausea, vomiting, enuresis, headache, thirst, dizziness and hyperventilation. Other effects that are commonly recorded include paraesthesias of the hands and feet, diarrhoea, loss of libido, diuresis and transient distortion of healthy taste sensations.

A metabolic acidosis, and hyperventilation, can be induced by acetazolamide, due to inhibition of carbonic anhydrase activity in the proximal renal tubules. In 44 of 92 (48%) patients treated with acetazolamide for chronic glaucoma, malaise, fatigue, weight loss, depression, anorexia and loss of libido were common and attributed to acidosis. Treatment with sodium bicarbonate 56–70 mmol/day orally may alleviate some of these effects.

Acute closed-angle glaucoma can occur.

Teratogenicity
There are no adequate studies in pregnancy and the risk of malformations has not been established. However, animal experimentation has demonstrated a teratogenic potential, and there are at least two human case reports of major malformations. The drug should be avoided in pregnancy.

Antiepileptic effect

Acetazolamide has a very broad spectrum of activity. It is effective in most forms of generalized seizures including tonic–clonic, generalized absence and myoclonic seizures, and also partial and secondarily generalized seizures. This efficacy has been confirmed in numerous open case series. In absence seizures, early studies have shown up to 90% control. In myoclonic seizures, similarly dramatic responses are recorded and in one study 20% of patients showed a 90–100% improvement. Similar excellent results in tonic–clonic seizures are recorded in some open studies showing 40–50% seizure-free rates. There is one double-blind, placebo-controlled study of 14 children with refractory post-traumatic seizures, and this showed initial therapy with acetazolamide to be superior to placebo, and comparable to phenytoin. Eight of the fourteen patients (57%) had a seizure reduction of at least 75%.

The drug will have an initial effect in most patients. However, there is an almost universal tendency for the effects of therapy to diminish over time (a phenomenon known as 'tolerance'), and this has been demonstrated in all seizure types. In one study, for example, the control of absence seizures fell from over 90% of cases initially to only 7% at 3 years of therapy. Similarly, about 30% of patients with complex partial seizures became seizure free within the first 3 months of therapy, but the proportion fell to about 10% at 1 and 2 years.

As a result of this tendency for tolerance, the drug is often given intermittently, notably in catamenial epilepsy. It is usually given at dosages of 250–750 mg/day for 5–7 days to women before the onset of the menstrual period and for its duration. There are a variety of case reports recommending its use in this way, although the author's own clinical experience is less positive, and most women with catamenial exacerbations of seizures seem to derive little benefit from the drug. Clobazam used in this way is probably more efficacious.

In one retrospective study, the drug was given as adjunctive therapy continuously in 55% and intermittently in 45% of individuals. A 59% decrease in the frequency of seizures was reported by 40% (both of focal and generalized seizures), and there was no difference in effectiveness between continuous and intermittent regimens. Loss of efficacy was reported by 15% of patients over 6–24 months.

Clinical use in epilepsy

Acetazolamide is an interesting broad-spectrum antiepileptic drug. It has a place in modern therapy, and is probably generally under-employed. Indeed, it can have a spectacular effect, and is worth a trial in any patient with severe epilepsy in whom other more conventional therapies have failed. It is usually given as adjunctive therapy, and has the advantage of not interacting with other antiepileptic drugs. The recommended dose in children is between 10 and 30 mg/kg, and in adults 250 and 500 mg/day, given twice daily. The usually quoted plasma levels are 10–14 μg/mL, but serum level monitoring is generally not worthwhile. The antiepileptic effect is immediate, and so it can be quickly evaluated.

The major drawback of the drug is the frequent development of tolerance, which can occur weeks or months after initiating therapy, and this limits its usefulness. Once tolerance has developed the drug should be withdrawn. Its restitution after a period of 'drug holiday' sometimes restores its effect, and cyclical regimens may also reduce the development of tolerance. Acetazolamide is often used as adjunctive therapy in catamenial epilepsy for this reason.

The drug is generally simple and easy to use and well tolerated. However, because of the risk of acute and severe hypersensitivity (a risk shared with all sulphonamide drugs), a blood count should be obtained before initiating treatment. Patients should be warned of the possibility of hypersensitivity, and acetazolamide should not be used if there is a history of allergy to any sulphonamide, or topiramate or zonisamide. The drug should be avoided in renal failure, and also in hepatic failure, because alkalinization of the urine diverts ammonia of renal origin from urine into the systemic circulation, causing hepatic encephalopathy. It increases potassium loss and should not be used in Addison disease or adrenal insufficiency. It should be used cautiously in combination with carbamazepine and oxcarbazepine because of its tendency to cause hyponatraemia, and should not be given with topiramate or zonisamide because of the risk of renal calculi.

Benzodiazepines

The benzodiazepines are first introduced into practice in 1960 (chlordiazepoxide) and since then over 4000 related compounds have been synthesized. Benzodiazepines have antiepileptic, anxiolytic, hypnotic and antispastic properties, and several have been widely adopted for use in epilepsy.

Diazepam, lorazepam and midazolam are commonly prescribed for the acute treatment of seizures (including febrile convulsions) and in status epilepticus, and the

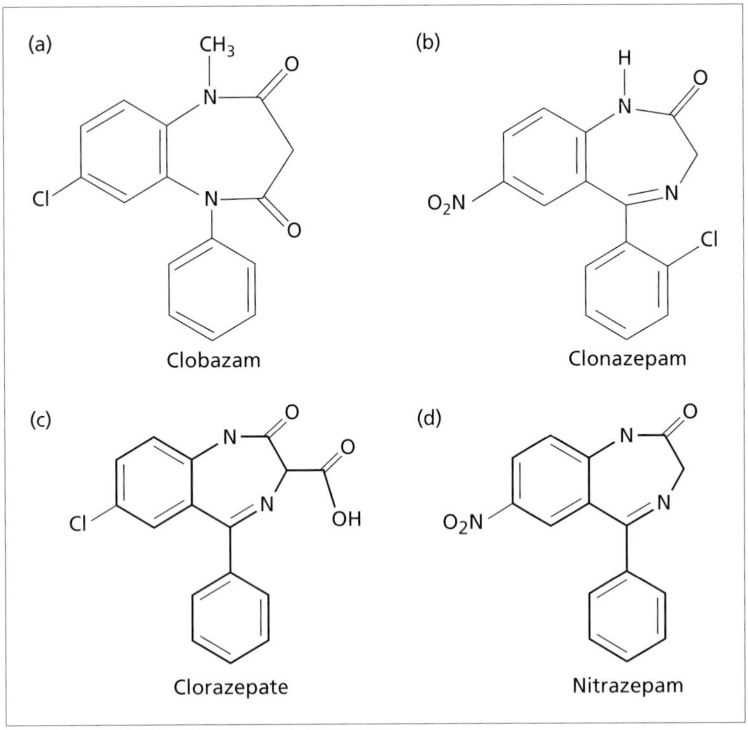

Figure 8.11 Structures of four benzodiazepine drugs used in epilepsy.

usage in these indications is outlined elsewhere (see chapter 9).

In chronic epilepsy, clobazam and clonazepam are the most commonly used benzodiazepines, and are described earlier in this chapter, but three other benzodiazepines – diazepam, clorazepate and nitrazepam – still have a minor role.

The benzodiazepines all bind to the GABA$_A$ receptors and exert their antiepileptic action by enhancing inhibitory neurotransmission. Differences between the drugs relate to their differential binding at the receptor and their pharmacokinetic properties. The similarities between the drugs are greater than the differences (Figure 8.11).

Diazepam

Diazepam was the first benzodiazepine to be used in epilepsy. It is highly lipophilic, allowing rapid entry into the brain, but this high lipid solubility also results in rapid subsequent redistribution into peripheral tissues. It is 90–99% bound to plasma proteins. The volume of distribution for the free component of diazepam (i.e. the active, unbound fraction) is 1.1 L/kg. The distribution half-life of 5–10 mg diazepam after intravenous injection is <20 min,

but the elimination half-life is between 18 and 100 h (mean 20–40 h). Enterohepatic circulation results in a second peak in blood levels 6–8 h after ingestion. Diazepam undergoes demethylation to *N*-desmethyldiazepam (DMD; nordiazepam), a metabolite with anticonvulsant activity and a long half-life (>40 h), and then slow hydroxylation to oxazepam, which is also active. Both metabolites are conjugated with glucuronic acid in the liver, with an elimination half-life of 24–48 h. Diazepam induces the cytochrome P450 enzyme CYP2B, and enhances the metabolism of phenobarbital and phenytoin. Valproate displaces diazepam bound to plasma proteins, leading to increased free diazepam levels. Concentrations in breast milk are low.

Drowsiness, fatigue, amnesia, mental slowing, depression, sleep disturbances and ataxia are common side effects in chronic therapy. Less common are dizziness, weakness, headache, agitation or restlessness, aggression, and mood and personality changes. Occasionally hallucinations and delirium occur. Hypersensitivity includes neutropenia or thrombocytopenia, nephritis, skin reactions and anaphylaxis.

There is significant potential for abuse and dependency, and this is a major drawback of therapy.

The teratogenicity of diazepam has not been clearly quantified, but is probably relatively slight. However, a 'fetal syndrome' and major malformations have been described.

Diazepam is mainly used intravenously or rectally in acute seizures (see pp. 287–288) but is sometimes given as a long-term antiepileptic, especially in the presence of anxiety. It is used largely as adjunctive therapy in severe partial and generalized epilepsy, and also in the Lennox–Gastaut syndrome. The dose is usually 5–10 mg/day, but long-term use is limited by the sedative side effects, the risk of dependency and the marked potential for tolerance.

Clorazepate

Clorazepate is a benzodiazepine used in adjunctive treatment of seizure disorders, anxiety and alcohol withdrawal. It is a prodrug that is rapidly converted to nordiazepam (DMD), the major active metabolite of diazepam. Ninety per cent of orally administered clorazepate is converted in the stomach to nordiazepam in <10 min, and so its effects are almost identical to those of diazepam. Clorazepate is around 100% bioavailable by the intramuscular route, and conversion to nordiazepam occurs more slowly in the blood.

Clorazepate and nordiazepam are 96–98% protein bound. The time to peak concentration is 0.7–2 h. The volume of distribution ranges from 0.9 L/kg to 2.2 L/kg, and is greater in elderly people and obese individuals. The elimination half-life of clorazepate is 2.3 h, but the half-life of nordiazepam is 40 h or longer (the longest half-lives are in elderly people and neonates). Nordiazepam is excreted predominantly by the kidneys (62–67%) with renal clearance of 0.15–0.27 mL/min per kg. Plasma nordiazepam levels of 0.5–1.9 µg/mL are said to be those producing optimal antiepileptic activity. There are minor drug interactions with other enzyme-inducing drugs, and also reportedly with herbal medicines including the Chinese herb dong quai. Pharmcodynamic interactions also occur with CNS depressant agents including phenobarbital and, where possible, co-medication with these should be avoided.

The side effects of clorazepate are identical to those of diazepam (see above). Hepatotoxicity and transient skin rashes have also been reported, and clorazepate has a teratogenic potential (and FDA category D status), although this has not been quantified and is probably slight. However, where possible, it should not be used in pregnancy.

Open and blinded studies of its antiepileptic effect have been performed, and one double-blind, add-on study found no difference in control of seizures between clorazepate and phenobarbital or phenytoin.

Its contemporary use is restricted to add-on therapy in refractory partial and generalized epilepsy. The drug is available as 3.75 mg, 7.5 mg and 15 mg tablets. The recommended initial dose of clorazepate for the adjunctive treatment of epilepsy is 7.5 mg two or three times a day (adults) with slow incremental increases in 3.75 or 7.5 mg steps, to a maximal daily dose of 90 mg in two- or three-times-a-day regimens.

Nitrazepam

Nitrazepam is a benzodiazepine derivative with a nitro group at the 7 position of the benzodiazepine ring. Oral bioavailability is about 78%. Peak concentrations are reached in 1.3–2.5 h. Nitrazepam is 85–88% protein bound. The volume of distribution is 2.4–2.9 L/kg, and is higher in elderly people. The plasma half-life is about 27 h, but the drug is rapidly taken up into the CSF and brain tissue, and the CSF elimination half-life is 68 h. Nitrazepam is metabolized in the liver by nitro reduction to the inactive aromatic amine (7-aminonitrazepam), followed by acetylation to 7-acetoamidonitrazepam. Excretion occurs in both urine (45–65%) and faeces (14–20%), with the remainder bound in tissues for prolonged periods.

Similar to most benzodiazepines, nitrazepam can produce sedation, disorientation, sleep disturbance, nightmares, confusion, drowsiness, aggression, hallucinations and ataxia. Hypotonia, weakness, hypersalivation, drooling, and impaired swallowing and aspiration seem to be particularly common with nitrazepam, particularly in young children. Confusion and pseudodementia can occur in elderly people. Withdrawal symptoms include delirium, mood and behavioural change, insomnia, involuntary movements, paraesthesia and confusion.

A risk of sudden death in young children due to nitrazepam therapy has been reported, probably because of pharyngeal hypotonia in children given nitrazepam doses >0.7 mg/kg. In a rather alarming retrospective analysis of 302 patients treated for periods ranging from 3 days to 10 years, 21 patients died, 14 of whom were taking nitrazepam at the time of death. In patients younger than 3.4 years, the death rate was 3.98 per 100 patient-years, compared with 0.26 deaths per 100 patient-years in patients not taking nitrazepam. Conversely, nitrazepam was found to have a slight protective effect (death rate of 0.50 vs 0.86) in children older than 3.4 years. Nitrazepam is in the FDA pregnancy category C (teratogenic effects demonstrated in animals but no studies in humans) and should be avoided where possible in pregnancy.

Nitrazepam has been used mainly in the West syndrome, febrile seizures, the Lennox–Gastaut syndrome and myoclonic epilepsy, and as adjunctive therapy for refractory epilepsy, particularly in children. Its main residual use is in refractory childhood epilepsy. One study showed a reduction in average daily seizure number from 17.7 to 7.2 in 36 infants and children (aged 3 months to 12 years) when nitrazepam was added to existing therapy. Myoclonic seizures particularly improved. In another study of 31 children with learning disability, aged between 2 months and 15 years, complete control of seizures was obtained in 7 patients and moderate control in 10. In the West syndrome, a study of 52 patients (aged 1–24 months) demonstrated similar efficacy when nitrazepam (0.2–0.4 mg/kg per day in two divided doses) and ACTH (40 IU intramuscularly daily) were compared. Both regimens resulted in a reduction in seizure frequency of 75–100% in 50–60% of patients.

The usual initial dose is 1–6 mg/day, and the maintenance dose is usually 0.25–10 mg/day in children. Optimal seizure control has been related to a mean plasma concentration of 114 ng/mL. Occasionally, very high maintenance doses have been used (up to 60 mg/day). There was also a common practice among paediatricians, up until the 1980s, of using very small doses (1.25–5.0 mg a day), sometimes on alternate days – a practice that seems to have no published evidential support. However, in view of the alarming suggestion of increased mortality rates, nitrazepam should be used with extreme caution, if at all, in children younger than 4 years.

Corticosteroids and ACTH

Since the 1950s ACTH and corticosteroids have been used to treat a variety of seizure types and epileptic syndromes. In 1958, the first report of the effect of steroids in the West syndrome was made, and since then it has a niche position in this condition and has remained a drug of first choice in this indication. Their role in the chronic treatment of other epilepsies is now vanishingly small, although high-dose steroids have maintained a place in the acute therapy of refractory status epilepticus. Although these compounds have a clear antiepileptic action, the mechanisms of the effects are quite unclear.

Pharmacokinetics

Prednisone is converted to prednisolone and this is the active metabolite. Prednisone has a bioavailability of about 70% (in terms of its conversion to prednisolone) and the derived prednisolone has peak levels within 1–2 h, a volume of distribution of 0.5–0.9 L/kg, 55–75% protein binding and a half-life of 1–3/4 h. It metabolized in the liver by oxidation and then conjunction. Naturally occurring and synthetic ACTH is used in some countries (the common synthetic ACTH preparations are Synacthen Depot and Cortrosyn-Z). ACTH has to be administered by intramuscular or subcutaneous routes, and is metabolized by enzymatic hydrolysis outside the liver and has a half-life of 15 min.

Adverse effects

Steroids (including ACTH) produce serious side effects that severely limit their usefulness, particularly as long-term therapy. Most children will develop cushingoid features and behavioural changes, especially irritability. Hypertension develops in 4–33% of children with infantile spasms, and infections – including pneumonia, septicaemia, urinary tract infections, gastroenteritis, ear infections, candidiasis and encephalitis – are more common. Hypokalaemia may sometimes occur in patients receiving higher doses and longer durations of hormonal therapy. Myocardial hypertrophy develops in 72–90%, but this reverses within months of discontinuation of ACTH therapy.

Clinical use in epilepsy

Steroids are used mainly for the treatment of the West syndrome (see p. 93 for details). Where formal comparisons have been made, ACTH and corticosteroids seem to be of equal efficacy, although many paediatricians still opt for ACTH. ACTH has also been reported to be effective in the occasional patient with intractable seizures. It also maintains a place in the therapy of refractory convulsive status epilepticus and epilepsia partialis continua.

Felbamate

Felbamate, a carbamate drug (2-phenyl-1,3-propanediol dicarbamate; molecular weight 238.43), was synthesized in 1954, investigated in the Antiepileptic Drug Development Program of the National Institutes of Health and licensed for use in the USA in 1993. It was rapidly adopted, but, within a year, reports of aplastic anaemia and liver failure emerged and the drug was withdrawn. However, because of its effectiveness,

Proprietary name: Felbatrol[a]

Primary indications
Refractory partial and secondarily generalized epilepsy and the Lennox–Gastaut syndrome as last resort therapy

Commonly used as first-line drug
No

Usual preparations
Tablets: 400, 600 mg; syrup: 600 mg/5 mL

Usual dosage – adults
Initial: 1200 mg/day
Maintenance: 1200–3600 mg/day

Usual dosage – children
Initial: 15 mg/kg per day
Maintenance: 45–80 mg/kg per day

Dosing intervals
2–3 times/day

Is the dose commonly affected by co-medication?
Yes

Is the dose affected by renal/hepatic disease?
Dose reductions needed in renal disease. Avoid in hepatic disease

Does it affect dose of other drugs?
Yes

Does it affect the contraceptive pill?
Yes

Serum level monitoring
Potentially useful

Target range
30–60 mg/L

Common/important adverse events
Severe hepatic disturbance and aplastic anaemia, insomnia, weight loss, gastrointestinal symptoms, fatigue, dizziness, lethargy, behavioural change, ataxia, visual disturbance, mood change, psychotic reaction, rash, neurological symptoms

Risk of hypersensitivity
Yes – marked risk

Major mechanism of action
Inhibition of NMDA receptor (glycine recognition site) and sodium-channel conductance

Main advantages
Powerful broad-spectrum action; well tolerated (aside from hypersensitivity)

Main disadvantages
Severe hypersensitivity reactions

Comment
Drug used only by specialists as last-resort therapy

[a]Name of proprietary brand available in the UK.

Felbamate: pharmacokinetics – average adult values	
Oral bioavailability	<100%
Time to peak levels	1–4 h
Volume of distribution	0.75 L/kg
Biotransformation	Hepatic hydroxylation and conjunction
Elimination half-life	11–25 h (varies with co-medication)
Plasma clearance	0.027–0.032 L/kg per h (varies with on co-medication)
Protein binding	20–25%
Active metabolite	None
Metabolism by hepatic enzymes	CYP3A4, CYP2E1, UDPGT
Inhibition of induction of hepatic enzymes	Induces CYP3A4, inhibits CYP2C19
Drug interactions	Common

it remains available, with special precautions for specialist use, in the USA, the UK and many other countries.

Mode of action

Felbamate blocks the NMDA receptor, and also modulates sodium channel conductance. It has no major effect on the $GABA_A$ receptor. It is active in a wide variety of seizure models and, in addition to its antiepileptic action, felbamate seems to possess neuroprotective action.

Absorption and distribution

Felbamate is rapidly and almost completely absorbed after oral administration, the time to peak plasma concentration being 1–4 h, and is unaffected by food. It is distributed rapidly and widely to many tissues, including the brain. The apparent volume of distribution is estimated at about 0.8 L/kg; 20–25% of the total concentration is protein bound.

Biotransformation and excretion

Felbamate is extensively metabolized in the liver via hydroxylation and conjugation. A number of potentially pharmacoactive and toxic metabolites may be formed, including 2-phenylpropenal, an α,β-unsaturated aldehyde (atropaldehyde). The latter compound is suspected to be largely responsible for hepatic failure and bone marrow suppression; 40–49% of the drug is excreted unchanged in the urine. The half-life of felbamate is approximately 20 h (range 13–23 h) in monotherapy and shortened to 13–14 h (range 11–20 h) in co-medication

with enzyme-inducing drugs. In renal failure lower doses are required. In children, clearance is faster and higher doses are needed. Patients with severe renal failure require lower doses.

Drug interactions

Felbamate is both an inhibitor of some drugs and an inducer of others. Phenytoin metabolism is inhibited by felbamate, and phenytoin dose decreases of about 20% were needed in the add-on felbamate study to maintain stable phenytoin concentrations. Carbamazepine concentrations are lowered by felbamate, and CBZ epoxide concentrations elevated by up to 30%. Valproate levels are increased by felbamate by 20–30%.

Felbamate metabolism is also affected by co-medication; the half-life of felbamate is shortened by about 30% on co-medication with phenytoin or carbamazepine and can be doubled on co-medication with valproate. There are few other formal studies, but felbamate is a strong inhibitor of the CYP2C19 enzymes.

Adverse effects
Neurological and other effects

In the clinical trials felbamate was found to be well tolerated, a fact that figured prominently in its advertisements, ironically in view of subsequent developments. The most common side effects of felbamate as monotherapy were anorexia, vomiting, insomnia, nausea and headache. One case of urolithiasis has been reported and one case of crystalluria and renal failure. Toxic epidermal necrolysis after initiation of felbamate has also been reported.

Marrow aplasia

Scattered case reports of marrow aplasia began to occur within 12 months of the launch of the drug. The incidence has subsequently been calculated to be approximately 127 per million patients (in a range lying between 27 and 209) compared with a general population risk of about 2 per million. In the cases studied, a prior history of antiepileptic drug allergy or toxicity, especially rash, was observed in 52%, a history of prior cytopenia in 42% and evidence of immune disease, especially lupus erythematosus, in 33%. If two of the above three factors were present, the patient's relative risk for aplastic anaemia quadrupled. Aplastic anaemia developed after 23–339 days (mean 173 days) and, although most cases occur within 1 year, a single case has been reported in a patient taking the drug for 8 years.

Hepatic failure

Hepatic failure was also recorded within a year of the drug being licensed, and in total 18 cases have been reported, with a clear relationship to felbamate therapy in 7. The overall risk has been estimated to be 1 per 18 500–25 000 drug exposures, using 7 cases as the numerator, or 1 case per 9000–12 000 if one assumes that all 18 cases were related to felbamate therapy. This compares to hepatic-related fatality estimates of one case in 10 000–49 000 in patients treated with valproate. Although the overall risk is similar to that of valproate, felbamate cases occurred largely in adults.

Antiepileptic effect

Various randomized controlled, blinded and open studies have been undertaken, in adults and in children, and in polytherapy and monotherapy. In all, felbamate was shown to be highly efficacious. It has demonstrated effectiveness in partial and secondarily generalized epilepsy, in primary generalized tonic–clonic and absence seizures, and in the various seizure types in the Lennox–Gastaut syndrome. In a double-blind study in the Lennox–Gastaut syndrome, a 34% decrease in the frequency of atonic seizures ($P = 0.01$) and a 19% decrease in the frequency of all seizures were observed.

Clinical use in epilepsy

After the catastrophe of a series of cases exhibiting hypersensitivity, 1 year after licensing, felbamate was close to being withdrawn. However, it is now recognized that the drug still has a place in therapy, in view of its outstanding efficacy. It should be used only by experienced specialists, and after full counselling. Its current use is solely confined to therapy in patients with severe epilepsy, unresponsive to other more conventional antiepileptics.

A full haematological evaluation is needed before initiation of felbamate therapy, and blood counts should be monitored frequently during therapy. Liver function tests are recommended every 4 weeks. Patients should be warned to report any symptom such as lethargy, nausea and vomiting, flu-like symptoms, easy bruising and unusual bleeding, and haematological and biochemical parameters should immediately be checked.

There is no definite 'therapeutic range', but concentrations between 40 and 100 µg/mL are commonly found in individuals who respond favourably.

Felbamate is available in 400 mg tablets (largely for children) and 600 mg tablets and a suspension (600 mg/5mL). In adults therapy should be initiated at 1200 mg/day in three divided doses, with increases to 2400 or 3600 mg/day in weekly or bi-weekly increments of 600 or 1200 mg steps, as tolerated, as outpatients. Some patients have tolerated doses as high as 7200 mg/day as monotherapy. In children, recommended starting doses have been 15 mg/kg per day with weekly incremental increases to 45–80 mg/kg per day. Combination therapy can be complex and monotherapy should be a goal, but where adjunctive therapy is used, blood levels may need to be monitored. Doses of felbamate and concomitant therapy may need modification in polytherapy.

Piracetam

Piracetam is a drug with an unusual clinical history. It was developed in 1967 by the research laboratory of UCB-Pharma in Belgium and deployed in clinical practice as a 'memory enhancing drug'. Its efficacy in this role has been highly contentious and the drug was not been licensed for this indication in either the USA or the UK, although it is widely used in other, particularly developing, countries (the manufacturers report over a million prescriptions). Recent controlled trials do show a small but definite effect in improving memory, but a Cochrane analysis considered that the evidence of effectiveness is inconclusive. In 1978 its antimyoclonic effect was first noted in a case of postanoxic myoclonus after cardiac arrest, where it was being given as a neuroprotective agent. In the last 10 years or so the remarkable effectiveness of this drug in cortical myoclonus of various aetiologies has been confirmed by controlled trials. It has

Proprietary name: Nootropil[a]

Primary indications
Myoclonus, especially in progressive myoclonic epilepsies. Adults and children.

Commonly used as first-line drug
No

Usual preparations
Tablets or capsules: 400, 800, 1200 mg; solution: 20%, 33%

Usual dosage – adults
Initial: 2.4 g/day
Maintenance: up to 32 g/day

Dosing intervals
2–3 times/day

Is dose commonly affected by co-medication
No

Is dose affected by renal/hepatic disease?
Severe renal disease

Does it affect dose of other drugs?
No

Does it affect the contraceptive pill?
No

Serum level monitoring
Not useful

Common/important adverse events
Dizziness, insomnia, nausea, gastrointestinal discomfort, hyperkinesis, weight gain, tremulousness, agitation, drowsiness, rash

Risk of hypersensitivity
No

Major mechanism of action
Probably via binding to the SV2A protein. Other properties include enhancement of oxidative glycolysis, anticholinergic effects, rheological effects

Main advantages
Highly effective in some resistant cases; very few side effects and well tolerated

Main disadvantages
Not effective in many cases

Comment
Drug of second choice in refractory myoclonus

[a]Name of proprietary brand available in the UK.

Piracetam: pharmacokinetics (average adult values)

Oral bioavailability	<100%
Time to peak levels	30–40 min
Volume of distribution	0.6 L/kg
Biotransformation	None
Elimination half-life	5–6 h
Plasma clearance	86 mL/min (renal clearance in healthy young individuals)
Protein binding	None
Active metabolite	None
Metabolism by hepatic enzymes	No
Inhibition of induction of hepatic enzymes	No
Drug interactions	None

received a licence in the UK and elsewhere for its use in this indication. Interestingly, levetiracetam, which is the ethyl ester of the laevo-isomer of piracetam, has a much more marked and broad-spectrum antiepileptic action as well as an antimyoclonic effect.

Physical and chemical properties and mode of action

Piracetam, 2-oxo-1-pyrrolidine acetamide, is a crystalline powder, closely related in structure to levetiracetam (Figure 8.12). It binds to the SV2A receptor although weakly (Figure 8.13), and this may be its main mechanism of action. However, it also has effects on brain vasculature, affects the rheology of membranes and mitochondrial function, enhances oxidative glycolysis and has anticholinergic effects, but whether these are related to its antimyoclonic effects is unknown. Piracetam appears to have no effect on brain GABA-ergic function, nor to affect cerebral serotonin or dopamine levels.

Pharmacokinetics

The drug has an oral bioavailability of 100%. The time to peak levels is usually between 30 and 40 min. Absorption of the drug is not affected by food. Piracetam is not bound to plasma proteins. The volume of distribution is 0.5–0.75 L/kg. The drug does not undergo metabolism and is completely excreted by the kidneys, with an elimination half-life of 5–6 h and almost complete elimination from the body after 30 h. There are no drug interactions. The elimination from CSF occurs with a half-life of about 7 h. It readily crosses the placenta and into breast milk.

Adverse effects

The drug is very well tolerated and there is a low incidence of reported side effects. Those that do occur (at a frequency of <10%) include dizziness, insomnia, nausea, gastrointestinal discomfort, hyperkinesis, weight gain, tremulousness and agitation. Rash occurs at a frequency of <1% and there have been no serious idiosyncratic reactions. In a placebo-controlled, double-blind, cross-over study, the only adverse effects were a sore throat and headache in one patient and single seizures in two, and these side effects may well not have been treatment related. At the very high doses used in the treatment of myoclonus, most patients report a few side effects, although there are no formal studies of side effects at these very high doses. There is no information regarding its safety in pregnancy.

Use in myoclonus

Piracetam is useful in cortical myoclonus of various types and causes. The drug has been shown to be effective in postanoxic action myoclonus, some cases of PME, myoclonus due to carbon monoxide poisoning, some cases of primarily generalized epilepsy with myoclonus, post-electrocution myoclonus, myoclonus in Huntington disease and in other symptomatic metabolic disorders (e.g. sialidosis). Initial case reports and then case series were followed by a well-conducted, double-blind, placebo-controlled study in 21 patients with severe myoclonus. A medium 22% improvement was noted on piracetam on global rating scales of disability, and some patients became free from seizures. The results were impressive in this severe condition, and on this basis the drug was licensed for myoclonus in the UK and elsewhere. Longer-term follow-up of some of the patients in these trials has confirmed the effect of piracetam, and in at least one of the cases (treated by the author), the effect was profound and maintained without evidence of tolerance. This 21-year-old patient was under the author's care with myoclonus and occasional generalized epileptic seizures of unknown aetiology, and was bedbound and dependent before piracetam therapy. There was an immediate response to piracetam, and immediate relapse on the three occasions that the drug had been withdrawn. After 12 years of piracetam monotherapy (at a daily dose of 21 g) she is still almost entirely free of myoclonus, has completed a university education, produced two healthy babies and lives a normal life. A more recent double-blind cross-over study in Finland compared placebo and three dosage regimens of piracetam (each for 2 weeks) in

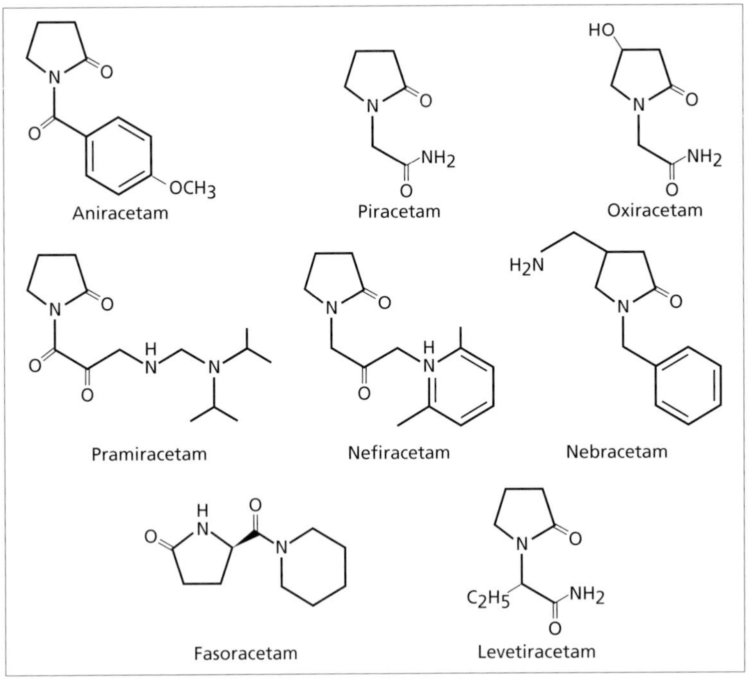

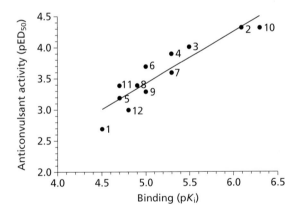

Figure 8.12 Structure of piracetam and seven other pyrrolidone drugs which are either licensed or in clinical development.

Figure 8.13 Piracetam has weak binding to the SV2A binding site compared with levetiracetam. Here is shown a comparison between the affinity of (S)homologues of levetiracetam at the [³H]levetiracetam binding site with the anticonvulsant activity of these compounds in the audiogenic mouse test. $r^2 = 0.84$, $P < 0.0001$, $n = 12$. 1, piracetam; 2, levetiracetam.

improvement in functional disability was also found with daily doses of 9.6 g and 16.8 g. The dose–effect relation was linear and significant. There are now numerous reported cases of complete 'cure' of severe myoclonus by the drug, often in cases where all other therapy had failed, and indeed it may be the only drug that improves myoclonus in some patients.

Cortical myoclonus may produce profound disabilities. The jerks are often exacerbated by actions and patients may be bedbound and immobile, unable to move without severe jerking disrupting all motor activity. In some cases (but not all), piracetam can have a remarkable effect in suppressing the myoclonus and reversing completely even severe disability. There does not seem to be a loss of the antimyoclonic effect over time. It has been said that the drug works best in combination, say with clonazepam, although there is no doubt that monotherapy with piracetam can be highly efficacious.

20 patients with Unverricht–Lundborg disease. A daily dose of 24 g piracetam produced significant and clinically relevant improvement in the primary outcome measures of motor impairment, functional disability, and in global assessments by both investigator and patient. Significant

Clinical use in epilepsy

Piracetam is indicated only in myoclonus, and is used usually as a second line for patients resistant to treatment with valproate or benzodiazepine drugs. Its effectiveness in some patients, even with severe and disabling myoclonus, combined with its almost complete lack of side effects, gives the drug a special place in the therapy of myoclonus. The extent to which this place will be superseded by the use of levetiracetam remains to be seen.

It is available as 800 and 1200 mg tablets and as a solution. The initial dose is 4.8–8 g/day and this may be rapidly increased (in 1600 mg incremental steps weekly) to 18–24 g/day. Some patients require up to 32 g/day. The drug can be given in two or three divided doses, and is usually given in combination with other antimyoclonic drugs. The major drawback at these higher doses is the number of tablets taken (sometimes 30 or 40 a day) and their bulk. Serum level monitoring is not available. Dosage reductions in patients with moderate or severe renal disease are recommended and the drug is contraindicated in patients with creatinine clearances <20 mL/min. There is no published experience of the drug in children. Withdrawal needs to be gradual (2-weekly decrements of 800 or 1600 mg), and abrupt cessation has been associated with a severe exacerbation of seizures.

Stiripentol

Stiripentol is a drug that has been under development for over 30 years, but which was in 2008 licensed under the orphan drug designation by the European Medicines Agency for a very small indication – the treatment of treatment of refractory generalized tonic–clonic seizures in the syndrome of severe myoclonic epilepsy in infancy (SMEI, Dravet syndrome), used with valproate and clobazam. This is the first antiepileptic drug licensed for children in this scheme.

Physical and chemical properties and mode of action
Stiripentol (4,4-dimethyl-1-[(3,4-methylenedioxy)phenyl]-1-penten-3-ol) is an insoluble racemate mixture, with a molecular weight of 234. The antiepileptic activity of stiripentol was discovered in the 1970s, but, although it has been shown to act as an agonist at the $GABA_A$ receptor, it is not clear if this is the mechanism of action.

Pharmacokinetics
It is rapidly absorbed, with peak serum levels reached at 0.5–2 h. The drug should be taken with food because it degrades rapidly in an acidic environment, such as in the stomach in a fasting state, but should not be taken with milk, dairy products, carbonated drinks, fruit juices, or food and drinks that contain caffeine. It is 99% bound to plasma proteins. It has, similar to phenytoin, non-linear kinetics and a half-life in the range 4.5–13 h, but this increases with increasing dose. It is extensively metabolized in the liver and is subject to enzyme induction. It is a potent inhibitor of CYP1A2, CYP2C9, CYP2C19, CYP2D6 and CYP3A4 and this inhibition is also subject to enzyme induction. There are therefore many drug interactions. The clearance of stiripentol is increased by 300% by carbamazepine, phenobarbital and phenytoin. Conversely it inhibits the metabolism of phenytoin, phenobarbital and carbamazepine, requiring their doses to be reduced by 25–50% on co-medication. Stiripentol also greatly increases the serum concentrations of other drugs including the active metabolite of clobazam, N-desmethylclobazam.

Adverse effects
Stiripentol seems to be relatively well tolerated. The common side effects are usually mild and include drowsiness, hyperactivity and aggressiveness. Other effects include ataxia, tremor, hypotonia, dystonia, behaviour disorder, insomnia, nausea, anorexia, weight loss, vomiting, neutropenia and thrombocytopenia.

Antiepileptic effect
Stiripentol originally underwent trials in refractory complex partial epilepsy, with promise in open studies, but no effect demonstrated in the regulatory RCTs in adult patients. In 1995, its development for this indication was discontinued. However, in an open paediatric study, in 2006, its effect on SMEI was noted, and an RCT in 41 children was carried out which demonstrated a more than 50% reduction of seizure frequency in 71% of children after stiripentol (50 mg/kg per day) when added to valproate and clobazam. Nine of these 41 children became free of clonic or tonic–clonic seizures. It was not known then, and is still knot known, whether the dramatic effects of the drugs are due to its inherent antiepileptic action or because of its interaction with clobazam.

Current place in therapy
The studies in adult partial epilepsy were disappointing. In contrast, its effects on SMEI were dramatic and unparalleled. On the basis of this, stiripentol was granted orphan drug status and was licensed for use in Europe in 2008. The recommended mean dose in children is

50 mg/kg per day, in two to three divided doses, and administered during a meal. Treatment is usually started with a lower dose, and is gradually increased to the recommended dose over 3 days. It is still not clear whether it is equally effective when not combined with valproate and clobazam, and its interactions with other drugs make it a difficult drug to use. How it will fare in routine practice is not yet clear.

9

The Emergency Treatment of Epilepsy

How to deal with a seizure

General measures

Short-lived tonic–clonic seizures do not require emergency drug treatment. The patient should be made as comfortable as possible, preferably lying down (or eased to the floor if seated), the head should be protected (by a cushion if possible) and tight clothing or neckwear released. During the attack measures should be taken to avoid injury, e.g. from hot radiators, hot water, stairs, road traffic. No attempt should be made to open the mouth or force anything solid between the teeth, as this can break teeth (a soft flexible mouth guard is available for sale and can be safely used). After the convulsive movements have subsided, roll the person into the recovery position, and check that the airway is not obstructed and that there are no injuries. Ensure that there is no apnoea and that the pulse is maintained. The patient should be attended until full consciousness has returned and there is no confusion. When fully recovered, the patient should be comforted and reassured. An ambulance or emergency treatment is required only if:

- injury has occurred
- convulsive movements continue for longer than 10 min, or longer than is customary for the individual patient
- the patient does not recover consciousness rapidly
- seizures rapidly recur
- the cardiorespiratory system is impaired.

Non-convulsive seizures are less dramatic but can still be disturbing to onlookers and embarrassing to the victim. Again, drug treatment is not indicated in short attacks. If consciousness is not lost, the patient should be treated sympathetically and with the minimum of fuss. If consciousness is impaired or, in the presence of confusion, it is necessary to prevent injury or danger (e.g. from wandering about), but at the same time minimizing restraint as attempts at restraint will often increase confusion and cause agitation or occasionally violence. Again the patient should be attended until the confusion has passed.

If a person with epilepsy is likely to have a seizure in any particular situation (e.g. at school or at work) it is usually best to inform those who might be present (e.g. fellow students, workmates, supervisors), and to provide simple advice about first-aid measures. This lessens the impact of a sudden epileptic seizure, which can be particularly frightening and disturbing if unexpected.

Emergency antiepileptic drug therapy

This is needed in convulsive attacks if the convulsions:
- persist for more than 10 minutes
- recur rapidly or last longer than is customary for the individual patient.

It is usual to give a fast-acting benzodiazepine. The traditional choice is diazepam, administered either intravenously or rectally. Intravenous diazepam is given in its undiluted form at a rate not exceeding 2–5 mg/min, using the Diazemuls® formulation. As a result of the high lipid solubility of diazepam, injections given at a faster rate carry the risk of high first-pass concentrations causing respiratory arrest or cardiovascular collapse. Rectal administration is either as the intravenous preparation infused from a syringe via a plastic catheter or as the ready-made proprietary rectal tube preparation (Stesolid®), which is convenient and easy. Diazepam suppositories should not be used, as absorption is too slow. The adult bolus intravenous or rectal dose is 10–20 mg, and in children the equivalent bolus dose is 0.2–0.3 mg/kg.

Intravenous lorazepam is an alternative with some advantages over intravenous diazepam. It is longer lasting and, as it is less lipid soluble, the intravenous injection can be given faster without the need to limit the rate of injection. The potentially dangerous first-pass effects possible with diazepam are not a risk with lorazepam. The dose is 4 mg in adults or 0.1 mg/kg in children.

Handbook of Epilepsy Treatment, 3rd Edition. By Simon Shorvon. Published 2010 by Blackwell Publishing Ltd.

Midazolam has the advantage that it can be given by buccal or intranasal instillation or intramuscular injection. The usually favoured method of administration now is a buccal instillation. The adult dose used is 10 mg drawn up into a syringe and instilled via a catheter into the mouth or between the cheeks and gums (a proprietary preparation, with a charged syringe and catheter is Epistatus®). A published randomized trial has shown that buccal midazolam has equal efficacy and as rapid an action as rectal diazepam, and is more convenient, potentially faster to administer, far more socially acceptable and less stigmatizing.

Precautions needed with parenteral benzodiazepines

Although benzodiazepines are the drugs of first choice for emergency therapy, they do carry a risk of respiratory depression, hypotension and cardiorespiratory collapse. In a well-controlled study in anaesthetic practice, for example, diazepam 10 mg was given intravenously to 15 patients and resulted in a drop in blood pressure of 10 mmHg or more in 8 patients, a mean 28% decrease in ventilation and a 23% decrease in tidal volume. The effects on cardiorespiratory function are as great (or even greater) with midazolam or lorazepam. In the occasional patient, the cardiorespiratory effects can be extremely severe, and for this reason it is essential that no patient given parenteral benzodiazepine should be left unattended until confusion has cleared and the patient is fully alert. After parenteral benzodiazepine administration (buccally, intranasally, rectally, intramuscularly or intravenously), pulse, respiration, blood pressure and (where possible) oxygen saturation should be frequently monitored, until the patient has recovered full consciousness. Resuscitation is occasionally needed, and deaths have occurred owing to lax post-administration care.

Serial seizures

Serial seizures are defined as seizures recurring at frequent short intervals, with full recovery between attacks, and in the latter sense differ from status epilepticus. The premonitory stage of status, however, often takes the form of serial seizures, and drug therapy is advisable even if the individual seizures are short. The emergency antiepileptic drug treatment is as outlined above for acute seizures.

Seizures occurring in clusters

In some patients clusters of seizures regularly occur, often at certain times (e.g. around menstruation in females). In a cluster, seizures typically recur over periods of hours or days. Acute therapy after the first seizure can be given in an attempt to prevent subsequent attacks. Clobazam (10–20 mg) is a common choice. An oral dose of clobazam will take effect within 1 h and last for 12–24 h. Clobazam has the advantage that it causes much less sedation than either diazepam or lorazepam.

A cluster of seizures is sometimes the result of the withdrawal or dose reduction of an antiepileptic drug. The reintroduction of the drug will usually terminate the seizure cluster.

Intermittent prophylactic treatment

In a minority of patients, the timing of seizure occurrence is predictable, e.g. in relation to menstruation (catamenial epilepsy). Occasionally, in such patients, intermittent therapy with either clobazam (10–20 mg/day) or acetazolamide (250–500 mg/day) can be given for a few days to cover the risky period. Such an approach is usually, however, unsuccessful, and seizures seem simply to be delayed rather than prevented.

In other seizures disorders, a single dose of clobazam (10 mg) can be taken in situations where seizures would be particularly hazardous (e.g. on the day or travel or examinations) or in susceptible individual at times when seizures are particularly likely to occur (e.g. after sleep deprivation, alcohol, labour or delivery). The use of occasional intermittent clobazam in these settings, as a 'booster' to conventional therapy, can be highly effective and is an underused resource in my experience.

Status epilepticus

Classification of status epilepticus

Status epilepticus is defined as a condition in which epileptic activity persists for 30 min or more. The seizures can take the form of prolonged seizures or repetitive attacks without recovery in between. There is a variety of types with clinical features that are dependent on age, seizure type, syndrome and aetiology. A simplified classification of the types of status epilepticus is shown in Table 9.1.

Pharmacokinetics and pharmacodynamics in status epilepticus

The pharmacokinetic properties of antiepileptic drugs in status epilepticus are noteworthy for a number of reasons:
• Rapid action is needed.
• The pharmacokinetics of a drug administered parenterally in large doses can differ greatly from those of the drug chronically administered orally.

Table 9.1 Classification of status epilepticus (SE)

1 SE in the neonatal and infantile epilepsy syndromes:
  – West syndrome
  – Ohtahara syndrome
  – Severe myoclonic encephalopathies of infancy (including SMEI)
  – SE in other forms of neonatal or infantile epilepsy
2 SE confined to childhood:
  – SE in early onset benign childhood occipital epilepsy (Panayiotopoulos syndrome)
  – SE in other forms of childhood epileptic encephalopathies, syndromes and aetiologies, e.g. ring chromosome X, Angelman syndrome, myoclonic–astatic epilepsy, other childhood myoclonic encephalopathies
  – ESES (electrical status epilepticus in slow-wave sleep)
  – Landau–Kleffner syndrome
3 SE occurring in childhood and adult life:
  With epileptic encephalopathy:
  – Non-convulsive SE in the Lennox–Gastaut syndrome and similar syndromes: (1) atypical absence status epilepticus and (2) tonic status epilepticus
  – Other forms of non-convulsive SE in patients with learning disability or disrupted cerebral development (cryptogenic or symptomatic)
  Without epileptic encephalopathy:
  – Tonic–clonic SE
  – Typical absence SE
  – Myoclonic SE
  – Myoclonic SE in coma (NCSE in diffuse cerebral injury).
  – Complex partial SE: (1) limbic and (2) non-limbic
  – Non-convulsive SE occurring in the postictal phase of tonic–clonic seizures
  – Subtle SE (myoclonic SE occurring at the late stage of tonic–clonic SE
  – Aura continua
4 NCSE confined to late adult life:
  – New absence status epilepticus of late onset
5 Boundary syndromes:[a]
  – Cases of epileptic encephalopathy
  – Cases of acute brain injury, often with irregular myoclonus (myoclonic SE in coma)
  – Drug-induced or metabolic confusional states with epileptiform EEG changes
  – Cases of epileptic behavioural disturbance or psychosis

[a]Boundary syndromes are defined as cases in which it is not clear to what extent the continuous epileptiform electrographic abnormalities contribute to the clinical impairment.

• Drug distribution can be affected by seizures.
• Drug effectiveness can lessen the longer the seizures continue (the phenomenon of acute tolerance).

Rapid action and parenteral pharmacokinetics
Fast drug absorption is essential in the treatment of status epilepticus, and thus almost all drugs need to be administered intravenously. Midazolam is the only drug that is absorbed fast enough by the intramuscular, intranasal or buccal routes, and buccal midazolam has become a favoured out-of-hospital therapy. Diazepam and other drugs can be given rectally in out-of-hospital situations, but in hospital the intravenous route is favoured. The onset of action of these therapies is usually within 5–10 min.

In order to act rapidly, the drugs need to cross the blood–brain barrier readily, and thus the drugs that are effective in status epilepticus usually have a high lipid solubility. The intravenous infusion of lipid-soluble drugs carries, however, the particular problem of drug accumulation, especially if the elimination half-life is long and the volume of distribution large. During parenteral administration, the drug first enters the central compartment (blood and the extracellular spaces of highly perfused organs) and then is rapidly redistributed to peripheral compartments such as fat and muscle, which act as 'sumps'. Thus, large doses are needed, because this redistribution leads to rapid falls in plasma levels. The initial drug half-life depends on redistribution and elimination, the former being much more important. The half-life of redistribution – the distribution half-life – is usually very short. As these 'sumps' become saturated, redistribution begins to fail, and the half-life of the drug then depends on elimination via hepatic and renal mechanisms (as in chronic therapy). The elimination half-life is much longer than the distribution half-life. Thus, the dose–serum level relationship changes as the duration of therapy lengthens, sometimes dangerously. This is a problem with drugs given by repeated bolus injections or by continuous infusions. The high doses needed initially (because of redistribution) become dangerously high as time passes and, unless this is recognized, continued administration may lead to sudden and persistent rises in blood level (as redistribution ceases), which can result in respiratory or cardiovascular collapse. The phenomenon occurs of 'sudden collapse at the end of a needle' and many iatrogenic deaths have occurred because of the failure to recognize this problem. This phenomenon occurs with the benzodiazepine drugs, barbiturates and clomethiazole in particular. Midazolam infusion, because of its rapid elimination, is much safer than diazepam in this regard.

Kinetics of drugs during seizures

Seizures (especially convulsive seizures) can affect both the peripheral and the central pharmacokinetics of drugs. During convulsive seizures there is a fall in the pH of the blood, resulting in a change in the degree of ionization (and thus lipid solubility) of drugs in plasma. This will affect the distribution half-lives, the ability to cross the blood–brain barrier and the protein binding. Blood pH decreases to a greater degree than brain pH, and this pH gradient facilitates the movement of a weakly acidic drug from blood to brain. This effect is prominent, for example, with phenobarbital. Other peripheral pharmacokinetic changes occur during status epilepticus, resulting from increased blood flow to muscle, and hepatic and renal compromise. The permeability of the blood–brain barrier increases during convulsive seizures, especially at the seizure foci where blood flow increases. As a result of these changes, cortical blood flow can largely determine the rate at which some drugs, notably phenobarbital, cross the blood–brain barrier. The

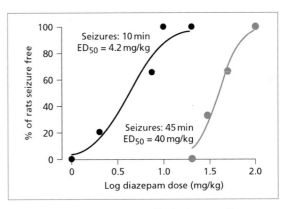

Figure 9.1 Diazepam was more effective in controlling seizures when given early (before 10 min) than when given later (45 min) in the lithium–pilocarpine rat model of status epilepticus.

concentration of these drugs at the seizure foci, where blood flow is greatest, enhances their effectiveness.

Drug responsiveness

As status epilepticus progresses it becomes more difficult to treat, largely because of brain receptor changes triggered by continued seizure activity. The most important change is of the rate of trafficking of receptors to and from the membrane surface, which changes within minutes of the development of a seizure. Many treatments effective in the initial stages thus become increasingly ineffective as the duration of the seizure lengthens. This reduction in potency is known as acute tolerance (Figure 9.1). This affects γ-aminobutyric acid (GABA)-ergic drugs and non-GABA-ergic drugs such as phenytoin, and the effect is so great that, for example, phenytoin is generally largely ineffective once status has been present for more than an hour or two.

Clinical features of tonic–clonic status epilepticus

Tonic–clonic status epilepticus is the classic form of status epilepticus, and its clinical form was first comprehensively described in the early nineteenth century. It is a common and important type of status epilepticus, not least because urgent therapy is required to prevent consequent permanent cerebral damage.

Tonic–clonic status epilepticus is defined as a condition in which prolonged or recurrent tonic–clonic seizures persist for 30 min or more. The annual incidence has been estimated to be approximately 18–28 cases per 100 000 people, with the highest rates in children, learning-disabled individuals and those with structural cerebral pathology, especially in the frontal lobes. About two-thirds of cases develop anew, without a prior history of epilepsy, and such cases are almost always due to acute cerebral disturbances; common causes are cerebral infection, trauma, cerebrovascular disease, cerebral tumour, acute toxic or metabolic disturbances, or childhood febrile illness. In patients with pre-existing epilepsy, tonic–clonic status can be precipitated by drug withdrawal, intercurrent illness, metabolic disturbance or the progression of the underlying disease, and is more common in symptomatic than in idiopathic epilepsy (Table 9.2). There is a range of other less common causes reported (Table 9.3). About 5% of all adult patients attending an epilepsy clinic will have at least one episode of status in the course of their epilepsy, and in children the proportion is higher (10–25%).

The mortality rate of tonic–clonic status is about 5–10%, most patients dying of the underlying condition rather than the status itself or its treatment. Permanent neurological and mental deterioration may result from status, particularly in young children. The risks of morbidity are greatly increased the longer the duration of the status episode.

Clinical evolution of tonic–clonic status epilepticus

At the onset of status, the attacks typically take the form of discrete tonic–clonic seizures. The motor activity then becomes continuous and the seizures become very prolonged. As neuronal function becomes progressively impaired, the jerking begins to fade and, if the status is allowed to progress, the motor activity may cease altogether or take the form of irregular myoclonus. This is the stage of subtle status epilepticus, by which time the

patient will be deeply unconscious and often in need of respiratory support. This stage develops in some patients within a few hours of the onset of status and indicates severe cerebral compromise. The EEG also shows progressive change, mirroring the changing motor signs. It initially shows discrete seizure activity, which becomes continuous or virtually continuous, and then this is interrupted by periods of EEG quiescence, and ultimately all that remains of cerebral activity are periodic lateralized epileptiform discharges (PLEDs or PEDs).

There is also often a premonitory stage of several hours before the onset of the status – particularly in patients with pre-existing epilepsy. During this phase, epileptic activity increases acutely in frequency or severity from its habitual level. This clinical deterioration is a warning of impending status and is often recognized as such by patients or carers in those who have had previous episodes of status. It is important to recognize this phase, because immediate urgent therapy can prevent the evolution into full-blown status.

Physiological changes in tonic–clonic status epilepticus

The physiological changes in status can be conceptualized (albeit as a simplification) as being divided into two phases, the transition from phase 1 to phase 2 occurring after about 30–60 min of continuous seizures (Table 9.4 and Figure 9.2).

Phase 1 (phase of compensation)

The initial consequence of a prolonged convulsion is a massive release of plasma catecholamines, with resulting increases in heart rate, blood pressure and plasma

Table 9.2 Common causes of tonic–clonic status epilepticus.

Underlying condition	Those without a prior history of epilepsy (%)	Those with a prior history of epilepsy (%)	All patients (%)
Cerebral trauma	12	17	1
Cerebral tumour	16	10	13
Cerebrovascular disease	20	19	20
Cerebral infection	15	6	11
Acute metabolic disturbance	12	5	9
Antiepileptic drug reduction or withdrawal or other acute event	25	44	33

Aetiology of tonic–clonic status epilepticus derived from 554 patients in 5 case series.

Table 9.3 Uncommon causes of status epilepticus.

Type	Examples
Immunological disorders	Paraneoplastic encephalitis; Hashimoto encephalopathy; anti-NMDA receptor encephalitis; anti-VGKC receptor encephalitis; Rasmussen encephalitis; cerebral lupus; thrombotic thrombocytopenic purpura; antibody-negative limbic encephalitis
Mitochondrial disorders	Alpers disease; occipital lobe epilepsy/MSCAE; MELAS; Leigh syndrome; MERRF
Uncommon infectious disorders	*Bartonella* sp./cat-scratch disease; *Coxiella burnetii* (Q fever); *Mycoplasma pneumoniae*; Creutzfeldt–Jakob disease; paracoccidioidomycosis; HIV and HIV-related infections; West Nile encephalitis; progressive multifocal leucoencephalopathy (JC virus); measles encephalitis; rubella encephalitis; St Louis encephalitis
Genetic and chromosomal disorders	Ring chromosome 20; Angelman syndrome; ring chromosome 17; porphyria; focal cortical dysplasias; hemimegalencephaly; polymicrogyria; heterotopias; schizencephaly; Sturge–Weber syndrome; tuberous sclerosis; Dravet syndrome; Lafora disease; DRPLA
Drug and toxin induced	Antiepileptic drugs (especially carbamazepine, gapapentin, pregabalin, tiagabine and vigabatrin); antimicrobials and antiviral drugs (especially cephalosporins, quinolones, isoniazid, antimalarials); antidepressants; antipsychotics; contrast media; chemotherapeutic agents; other drugs (especially theophylline, lithium and baclofen); toxins (especially aluminium-containing biomaterial, domoic acid, ecstasy, lead, star fruit and tetramine)
Others	Electroconvulsive therapy; neurosurgery (including temporal lobectomy); multiple sclerosis; hypertension-induced PRES; neuroleptic malignant syndrome; ulcerative colitis; coeliac disease

DRPLA, dentato-rubral-pallido-luysian atrophy; MELAS, mitochondrial encephalopathy, lactic acidosis and stroke-like episodes; MERRF, myoclonic encephalopathy with ragged red fibres; MSCAE, mitochondrial spinocerebellar ataxia and epilepsy; NMDA, *N*-methyl-D-aspartate; PRES, posterior reversible encephalopathy syndrome; VGKC, voltage-gated K$^+$ channel.

glucose. During this stage cardiac arrhythmias frequently occur and can be fatal. As the seizure continues, there is a steady rise in the core body temperature, and prolonged hyperthermia (above 40°C) can itself cause cerebral damage and carries a poor prognosis. Acidosis also commonly occurs, and in one series 25% of the patients had an arterial pH < 7.0. This acidosis is mainly the result of lactic acid production, but there is also a rise in carbon dioxide tension that can, in itself, result in life-threatening narcosis. The acidosis increases the risk of cardiac arrhythmias and hypotension, and in conjunction with the cardiovascular compromise may result in severe pulmonary oedema. The autonomic activity also results in sweating, bronchial secretion, salivation, and hypersecretion and vomiting.

However, within the brain, homoeostatic physiological mechanisms (autoregulation) are initially sufficient to compensate for these changes. There is a massive increase in cerebral blood flow, and the delivery of glucose to the active cerebral tissue is maintained. At this stage neuronal integrity is maintained, the blood–brain barrier is not impaired and there is little risk of cerebral damage.

Phase 2 (phase of decompensation)

The status epilepticus may then enter a second late phase in which cerebral protective measures progressively fail. The main systemic characteristics of this phase are a fall in systemic blood pressure and progressive hypoxia. Hypotension is due to seizure-related autonomic and cardiorespiratory changes and drug treatment, and in the later stages can be severe and intractable. At a critical stage cerebral autoregulation begins to fail and the control of blood flow then becomes dependent on systemic blood pressure. This is potentially hazardous, as falling blood pressure leads to a failure of cerebral perfusion. The high metabolic demands of the epileptic

Table 9.4 Physiological changes in tonic–clonic status epilepticus.

Phase I: compensation

During this phase, cerebral metabolism is greatly increased because of seizure activity, but physiological mechanisms are sufficient to meet the metabolic demands, and cerebral tissue is protected from hypoxia or metabolic damage. The major physiological changes are related to the greatly increased cerebral blood flow and metabolism, massive autonomic activity and cardio-vascular changes.

Cerebral changes	Systemic and metabolic changes	Autonomic and cardiovascular changes
Increased blood flow	Hyperglycaemia	Hypertension (initial)
Increased metabolism	Lactic acidosis	Increased cardiac output
Energy requirements matched by supply of oxygen and glucose (increased glucose and oxygen utilization)		Increased central venous pressure
		Massive catecholamine release
Increased lactate concentration		Tachycardia
Increased glucose concentration		Cardiac dysrhythmia
		Salivation
		Hyperpyrexia
		Vomiting
		Incontinence

Phase II: decompensation

During this phase, the greatly increased cerebral metabolic demands cannot be fully met, resulting in hypoxia and altered cerebral and systemic metabolic patterns. Autonomic changes persist and cardio-respiratory functions may progressively fail to maintain homoeostasis.

Cerebral changes	Systemic and metabolic changes	Autonomic and cardiovascular changes
Failure of cerebral autoregulation; thus cerebral blood flow becomes dependent on systemic blood pressure	Hypoglycaemia	Systemic hypoxia
	Hyponatraemia	Falling blood pressure
Hypoxia	Hypokalaemia/ hyperkalaemia	Falling cardiac output
Hypoglycaemia		Respiratory and cardiac impairment (pulmonary oedema, pulmonary embolism, respiratory collapse, cardiac failure, dysrhythmia)
Falling lactate concentrations	Metabolic and respiratory acidosis	
Falling energy state		
Rise in intracranial pressure and cerebral oedema	Hepatic and renal dysfunction	
	Consumptive coagulopathy, DIC, multi-organ failure	Hyperpyrexia
	Rhabdomyolysis, myoglobulinuria	
	Leucocytosis	

DIC, disseminated intravascular coagulopathy.
Note: the physiological changes listed above do not necessarily occur in all cases. The type and extent of the changes depend on aetiology, clinical circumstances and the methods of therapy employed.

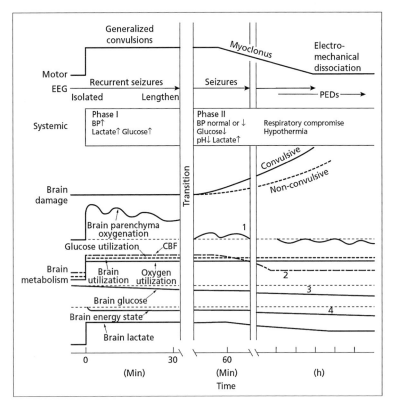

Figure 9.2 Temporal changes that occur as tonic–clonic status epilepticus progresses. Motor activity lessens, the EEG evolves and profound physiological changes occur, both systemically and cerebrally. In the first 30 min or so, physiological changes are largely compensatory, but as the seizures continue these compensatory mechanisms break down. The biphasic evolution is emphasized. PED, periodic epileptic discharge; 1, loss of reactivity of brain oxygen tension; 2, mismatch between the sustained increase in oxygen and glucose utilization and a fall in cerebral blood flow; 3, a depletion of cerebral glucose and glycogen concentrations; 4, a decline in cerebral energy state.

cerebral tissue cannot be met and this results in ischaemic, excitotoxic or metabolic damage. The hypotension can be greatly exacerbated by intravenous antiepileptic drug therapy, especially if infusion rates are too fast. Intracranial pressure can rise dramatically in late status, and the combined effects of systemic hypotension and intracranial hypertension cause cerebral oedema, particularly in children.

Physiological changes are not confined to brain metabolism (Table 9.5). Pulmonary hypertension and pulmonary oedema occur, and pulmonary artery pressures can exceed the osmotic pressure of blood, causing oedema and stretch injuries to lung capillaries. Cardiac output can fall owing to decreasing left ventricular contractility and stroke volume, and cardiac failure can ensue.

Profound hyperpyrexia is a common consequence. There are many metabolic and endocrine disturbances in status, the most common and most important being acidosis (including lactic acidosis), hypoglycaemia, hypo-/hyperkalaemia and hyponatraemia. Other potentially fatal metabolic complications include acute tubular necrosis, renal failure, hepatic failure and disseminated intravascular coagulation (DIC). Rhabdomyolysis, resulting from persistent convulsive movements, can precipitate renal failure if severe.

Risk of cerebral damage

The major reason for treating tonic–clonic status epilepticus as a medical emergency is because prolonged seizures carry the risk of causing permanent cerebral damage, a consequence amply demonstrated in animal and human studies. Status-induced brain damage has a number of mechanisms. Hypoxia, ischaemia or metabolic disturbances can certainly be a cause, but the predominant risk is of excitotoxic brain damage. This is damage due to the continuous electrographic activity itself, and the repeated depolarization of neurons that occurs during continuous seizures. The electrographic activity results in progressively increasing calcium influx into the affected neurons, and the calcium influx triggers processes of cell death and apoptosis. The result is neuronal loss, particularly in the hippocampus, but also in other areas of the cerebral cortex. The process of excitotoxic cell death is exacerbated by the energy failures

Table 9.5 Medical complications in tonic–clonic status epilepticus.

Cerebral	Hypoxic/metabolic cerebral damage
	Seizure-induced cerebral damage
	Cerebral oedema and raised intracranial pressure
	Cerebral venous thrombosis
	Cerebral haemorrhage and infarction
Cardiorespiratory and autonomic	Hypotension
	Hypertension
	Cardiac failure, tachy- and bradydysrhythmia, cardiac arrest, cardiogenic shock
	Respiratory failure
	Disturbances of respiratory rate and rhythm, apnoea
	Pulmonary oedema, hypertension, embolism, pneumonia, aspiration
	Hyperpyrexia
	Sweating, hypersecretion, tracheobronchial obstruction
	Peripheral ischaemia
Metabolic and systemic	Dehydration
	Electrolyte disturbance (especially hyponatraemia, hyperkalaemia, hypoglycaemia)
	Acute renal failure (especially acute tubular necrosis)
	Acute hepatic failure
	Acute pancreatitis
Other	Disseminated intravascular coagulopathy/multiorgan failure
	Rhabdomyolysis
	Fractures
	Infections (especially pulmonary, skin, urinary)
	Thrombophlebitis, dermal injury

inherent in the stage 2 physiological changes, and a vulnerability to cellular damage is usually considered to begin after 1–2 h of continuous seizure activity. The longer the status continues the greater is the risk of damage. For this reason it is important to abolish electrographic changes and not just the motor changes of status. If antiepileptic drug therapy has not controlled both the clinical and electrical manifestations of seizures within 2 h, general anaesthesia should be applied as a method of abolishing all neuronal activity.

The emergency therapy of tonic–clonic status epilepticus: general measures

Cardiorespiratory function

In all patients presenting in status, the protection of cardiorespiratory function takes first priority. It should be assessed, the airway secured and resuscitation carried out if necessary. Hypoxia is usually much worse than appreciated, not least because of the higher metabolic demands of convulsing muscles and increased cerebral activity, and oxygen should always be administered.

Respiratory compromise

This can arise from cardiovascular collapse, high metabolic demands, pulmonary oedema and the respiratory-depressant properties of the drugs used to treat status epilepticus. There should be a low threshold for instituting ventilatory support, and it should be borne in mind that hypoxia is often much greater than initially suspected. The use of subanaesthetic doses of anaesthetic agents without ventilatory support is not recommended. Even as small a dose as 10 mg of intravenous diazepam has been shown to depress respiration in anaesthetic practice (see p. 288). Aspiration pneumonia is common and broad-spectrum antibiotics should be started in any patients requiring assisted ventilation.

Monitoring

Regular neurological observations and measurements of pulse, blood pressure, ECG and temperature should be initiated. Metabolic abnormalities, especially hypoglycaemia, may cause status epilepticus, or develop during its course, and biochemical, blood gas, pH, clotting and haematological measures should be regularly monitored.

Intravenous lines

These should be set up for fluid replacement and drug administration. The drugs should not be mixed and, if two antiepileptic drugs are needed (e.g. phenytoin and diazepam), two intravenous lines should be sited. The lines should be in large veins, as many antiepileptic drugs cause phlebitis and thrombosis at the site of infusion. Arterial lines must never be used for drug administration, because potentially fatal arterial necrosis and spasm can occur.

Emergency investigations

Blood should be drawn for the emergency measurement of blood gases, sugar, renal and liver function, calcium and magnesium levels, full haematological screen (including platelets), blood clotting measures and antiepileptic drug levels. Serum (20 mL) should also be saved for future analysis, especially if the cause of the status epilepticus is uncertain. Other investigations depend on the clinical circumstances.

Intravenous glucose and thiamine

Glucose – 50 mL of a 50% solution – should be given immediately by intravenous injection if hypoglycaemia is suspected. Routine glucose administration in non-hypoglycaemic patients should, however, be avoided because there is some evidence that this can aggravate neuronal damage.

If there is a history of alcoholism or other compromised nutritional state, 250 mg thiamine (e.g. as the high-potency intravenous formulation Pabrinex®, 10 mL of which contains 250 mg) should also be given intravenously. This is particularly important if glucose has been administered, because a glucose infusion increases the risk of Wernicke encephalopathy in susceptible patients. Intravenous high-dose thiamine should be given slowly (e.g. 10 mL of high-potency Pabrinex over 30 min), with facilities for treating the anaphylaxis which is a potentially serious side effect of high-potency thiamine infusions.

Acidosis and other metabolic abnormalities

Lactic acidosis is common and largely caused by convulsive movements and hyperthermia. These can usually be controlled by halting the motor activity by antiepileptic, anaesthetic or paralysing agents. If acidosis is severe, the administration of bicarbonate has been advocated in the hope of preventing shock, and mitigating the effects of hypotension and low cerebral blood flow. In most cases, however, this is unnecessary, and the rapid control of respiration and abolition of motor seizure activity are more effective. Correction of hypoglycaemia and electrolyte and other metabolic abnormalities should be active and rigorous.

Magnesium sulphate

Although magnesium is effective at preventing eclampsia, there is no evidence that increasing magnesium serum concentrations to supranormal levels has any benefit in status epilepticus. However, serum magnesium can be low in people with alcohol problems and patients with acquired immune deficiency syndrome (AIDS), and in these patients intravenous loading with 2–4 g magnesium sulphate over 20 min may help with seizure control and the prevention of arrhythmias. Magnesium is also often given in other cases of refractory status epilepticus.

Pressor therapy

Hypotension can result from the status itself and also from drug treatment, and is a universal problem in severe status. Hypotension increases the risk of cerebral damage, because loss of cerebral autoregulation means that cerebral perfusion becomes directly proportional to systemic blood pressure. Maintenance of blood pressure is, therefore, of paramount importance.

Pressor agents are usually required. Dopamine is the most commonly used, given by continuous intravenous infusion. The dose should be titrated up to achieve the desired haemodynamic and renal responses (usually initially between 2 and 5 μg/kg per min, but this can be increased to >20 μg/kg per min in severe hypotension). Dopamine should be given into a large vein because extravasation causes tissue necrosis. ECG monitoring is required, because conduction defects may occur, and particular care is needed in dosing in the presence of cardiac failure.

Cardiac arrhythmia

Cardiac arrhythmias pose a substantial risk in severe status, caused by autonomic hyperactivity, metabolic derangement, and the infusion of high-dose antiepileptic and anaesthetic drugs. Continuous EEG monitoring is mandatory, and arrhythmias are treated in the conventional manner.

Acute renal or hepatic failure

A number of factors can result in acute renal failure, including myoglobinuria, DIC, hypotension and hypoxia. In the early stages infusion of mannitol and dopamine may be of some benefit. Acute hepatic failure can also have various causes, including hypersensitivity reactions to administered drugs. Care should be taken to avoid these drugs in cases with a prior history of hypersensitivity.

Other physiological changes and medical complications

Some of the complications encountered in tonic–clonic status are listed in Table 9.5. These often need emergency treatment in their own right. Failure to do so can perpetuate the status and worsen outcome. Active treatment is most commonly required for hypoxia, pulmonary oedema and hypertension, cardiac arrhythmias, cardiac failure, hyperpyrexia, rhabdomyolysis and DIC. Rhabdomyolysis can be prevented by artificial ventilation and muscle paralysis.

Establish aetiology

The outcome of status to a great extent depends on the aetiology, and the urgent treatment of causative factors is vital. Computed tomography (CT) or magnetic resonance imaging (MRI) and cerebrospinal fluid (CSF) examination are often necessary, but the choice of investigations depends on the clinical circumstances (see Tables 9.2 and 9.3).

If the status epilepticus has been precipitated by drug withdrawal, the immediate restitution of the withdrawn drug, even at lower doses, will usually rapidly terminate the status epilepticus. Pyridoxine should also be given intravenously to children under the age of 3 years who have a prior history of epilepsy, and to all neonates.

Intensive care and seizure/EEG monitoring

If seizures are continuing in spite of the initial emergency measures, the patient must be transferred to an intensive care setting, where intensive monitoring is desirable, including, for example, intra-arterial blood pressure, capnography, oximetry, central venous pressure and Swan–Ganz monitoring.

Convulsive movements diminish over time in tonic–clonic status and may cease altogether in spite of ongoing epileptic electrographic activity. Such electrographic activity is potentially damaging to the cortical neurons, and anaesthetic therapy is targeted to suppress it by the attainment of the anaesthetic level of burst suppression. Both ongoing epileptic activity and burst suppression require neurophysiological monitoring, which is best provided by a full EEG, carried out regularly or (preferably) continuously. Burst suppression provides an arbitrary physiological target for the titration of barbiturate or anaesthetic therapy, with drug dosing commonly set at a level that aims to produce burst suppression with interburst intervals of between 2 and 30 s.

Raised intracranial pressure and intracranial pressure monitoring

If there is evidence of persisting, severe or progressively elevated intracranial pressure (ICP), monitoring may be required. The need for this is usually determined by the underlying cause rather than the status, and its use is more common in children. If the ICP is critically raised, intermittent positive-pressure ventilation, high-dose corticosteroid therapy (4 mg dexamethasone every 6 h) or mannitol infusion – usually reserved as a temporary measure – can be used to lower the pressure. Neurosurgical decompression is occasionally required.

The emergency therapy of tonic–clonic status epilepticus: drug treatment

In tonic–clonic status epilepticus, as mentioned above, if seizure activity is allowed to persist for more than 1.5–2 h there is a substantial risk of seizure-induced cerebral damage, and this risk rises the longer the seizures continue. For this reason, the drug treatment of tonic–clonic status epilepticus is best divided into stages, with the final stage (anaesthesia) reached within 1.5–2 h of initiating therapy.

The doses of drugs commonly used in status epilepticus are contained in Table 9.6. There have been eight randomized studies of intravenous drug treatment in status epilepticus, studies that have been beset by methodological problems and only limited conclusions can be drawn. These studies have shown the effectiveness of phenytoin, diazepam, lorazepam and valproate. Open studies have produced most of the clinically relevant evidence, but these have not been randomized and the choice of drug regimen is therefore somewhat arbitrary. Nevertheless, a systematic organized approach is important in this emergency situation, and the simple fact of having a protocol has been shown to reduce morbidity and mortality, regardless of the protocol treatment options. The protocol favoured by the author is shown in Figure 9.3, and details of the drugs used are given in Tables 9.6 and 9.7, and on pp. 307–313.

Premonitory stage of status epilepticus

In many cases of status epilepticus, there is a premonitory stage. During this period there is a gradual increase in the frequency of tonic–clonic seizures or of myoclonic jerking. Parenteral drug treatment in this phase will often prevent the development of full-blown status, and the earlier treatment is given the more successful it is. If the patient is at home, antiepileptic drugs should be administered before transfer to hospital, or in the accident and emergency department (A&E) before transfer to the ward. Carers can be trained in the administration of emergency therapy. However, acute parenteral therapy will cause drowsiness or sleep, and occasionally cardiorespiratory collapse, and should therefore be carefully supervised. Initial therapy is the same as for acute seizures. Out-of-hospital therapy can be with either rectal diazepam or buccal or intramuscular midazolam. All are highly effective, and the choice will depend on local circumstances. Rectal diazepam is available in a very convenient formulation with an already prepared syringe and catheter (Stesolid®). Similarly, buccal midazolam is easy and quick to administer. This is currently in most

Stage of early status *(0–30 min)*

Lorazepam 4 mg IV bolus (can be repeated once)

⬇ *(If seizures continue after 30 min)*

Stage of established status *(30–60/90 min)*

Phenobarbital IV infusion of 10 mg/kg at a rate of 100 mg/min
or
Phenytoin IV infusion of 15 mg/kg at a rate of 50 mg/min
or
Fosphenytoin IV infusion of 15 mg PE/kg at a rate of 100 mg PE/min
or
Valproate IV infusion of 25 mg/kg at a rate of 3–6 mg/kg/min

⬇ *(If seizures continue after 30–90 min)*

Stage of refractory status *(> 60/90 min; general anaesthesia)*

Propofol: IV bolus of 2 mg/kg, repeated if necessary, and then followed by a continuous infusion of 5–10 mg/kg/h initially reducing to a dose sufficient to maintain a burst-suppression pattern on the EEG (usually 1–3 mg/kg/h)
or
Thiopental: IV bolus of 100–250 mg given over 20 s with further 50 mg boluses every 2–3 min until seizures are controlled, followed by a continuous IV infusion at a dose sufficient to maintain a burst-suppression pattern on the EEG (usually 3–5 mg/kg/h)
or
Midazolam: IV bolus of 0.1–0.3 mg/kg at a rate not exceeding 4 mg/min initially, followed by a continuous IV infusion at a dose sufficient to maintain a burst-suppression pattern on the EEG (usually 0.05–0.4 mg/kg/h)

When seizures have been controlled for 12 h, the drug dosage should be slowly reduced over a further 12 h. *If seizures recur*, the general anaesthetic agent should be given again for a further 12 h, and then withdrawal attempted again. This cycle may need to be repeated until seizure control is achieved

Figure 9.3 Protocol for the treatment of tonic–clonic status epilepticus in adults. IV, intravenous; PE, phenytoin equivalent. (Note that this is the author's personal protocol, and other published protocols exist with equal claims to effectiveness.)

countries an unlicensed medication, but a convenient formulation exists packaged with a syringe and catheter (Epistatus®). If intravenous therapy can be given in the premonitory stage, lorazepam is the drug of choice (see below).

Stage of early status epilepticus

The early stage of status epilepticus is defined as the first 30 min of status. It is usual to initiate intravenous treatment with a fast-acting benzodiazepine drug.

Intravenous lorazepam is now generally preferred over diazepam as first-line therapy in established status epilepticus. The disadvantage of diazepam is its short

redistribution half-life (<1 h) and large volume of distribution (1–2 L/kg). These properties mean that serum and brain concentrations rapidly fall after initial intravenous dosing, leading to potentially high rates of seizure recurrence. Within 2 h of successful treatment with diazepam, over half the patients with status epilepticus relapse. Repeat boluses of diazepam can lead to significant accumulation and so cannot be recommended. Clonazepam shares many of the pharmacokinetic features of diazepam. It has a similarly rapid brain penetration, short distribution half-life and long elimination half-life. Lorazepam, on the other hand, has a lesser volume of distribution and is less lipid soluble. It enters the brain

Table 9.6 Drugs used in the pre-anaesthetic stages of status epilepticus.

Drug	Route	Adult dose	Paediatric dose
Clonazepam	IV bolus	1–2 mg at 2 mg/min[a]	250–500 μg
Chlormethiazole	IV infusion of 0.8% solution	40–100 mL at 5–15 mL/min, then 0.5–20 mL/min	0.1 mL/kg per min increasing every 2–4 h
Diazepam at 2–5 mg/min[a]	IV bolus Rectal administration	10–20 mg at 2–5 mg/min[a] 10–30 mg[a]	0.25–0.5 mg/kg 0.5–0.75 mg/kg[a]
Fosphenytoin	IV bolus	15–20 mg PE/kg at 150 mg PE/min	
Levetiracetam	IV Bolus	1000–3000 mg at a rate of 1000 mg/15 min	
Lidocaine	IV bolus IV infusion	1.5–2.0 mg/kg at 50 mg/min[a] 3–4 mg/kg per h	
Lorazepam	IV bolus	0.07 mg/kg (usually 4 mg)[a]	0.1 mg/kg
Midazolam	IM or rectally IV bolus IV infusion	5–10 mg[a] 0.1–0.3 mg/kg at 4 mg/min[a] 0.05–0.4 mg/kg per h	0.15–0.3 mg/kg[a]
Paraldehyde	Rectally or IM	5–10 mL (approx 1 g/mL) in equal volume of water[a]	0.07–0.35 mL/kg[a]
Phenobarbital	IV bolus	10–20 mg/kg at a rate not exceeding 100 mg/min	15–20 mg/kg
Phenytoin	IV bolus/infusion	15–20 mg/kg at a rate not exceeding 50 mg/min	20 mg/kg at a rate not exceeding of 1–3 mg/kg per min
Valproate	IV bolus	10–30 mg/kg	20–40 mg/kg

IM, intramuscularly; IV, intravenous; PE, phenytoin equivalent.
[a]Can be repeated.

more slowly, taking up to 30 min to reach peak levels, although therapeutic levels are reached within a few minutes. Its distribution half-life is much longer (2–3 h), and its elimination half-life is shorter (approximately 10–12 h). Its effects are, therefore, longer lasting than those of diazepam, and for this reason lorazepam is the benzodiazepine of choice in status epilepticus. Lorazepam should be given as a bolus that can be repeated once after 10 min, at which time phenytoin should be administered.

Lidocaine as a bolus followed by an infusion has been recommended as an alternative to benzodiazepines in those in whom respiratory depression is a concern, but is not now widely used. The intravenous injection of subanaesthetic doses of propofol has also been tried. In most episodes of status, initial therapy treatment will be highly effective.

In young children, it is customary to give intravenous pyridoxine, in case of an occult deficiency.

Even if seizures cease, 24-hour inpatient observation should follow. In people with no previous history of epilepsy, chronic antiepileptic drug treatment should be introduced and, in those already on maintenance antiepileptic therapy, this should be reviewed.

Stage of established status epilepticus
If seizures have continued for 30 min, in spite of the therapy outlined above, the stage of established status epilepticus is entered.

In the protocol used by the author, there are four alternative first-line treatment options (see Figure 9.3), but each has drawbacks. The author's own current preference is for phenobarbital, but there are many potential advantages to intravenous valproate or intravenous

Table 9.7 Anaesthetics for refractory status epilepticus.

Drug	Adult dose	Comments
Midazolam	0.1–0.3 mg/kg at 4 mg/min bolus followed by infusion at 0.05–0.4 mg/kg per h	Elimination half-life of 1.5 h, but accumulates with prolonged use Tolerance and rebound seizures can be problematic
Thiopental	100–250 mg bolus over 20 s then further 50 mg boluses every 2–3 min until seizures are controlled. Then infusion to maintain burst suppression (3–5 mg/kg per h). Child (1 month to 18 years) initially up to 4 mg/kg by slow intravenous infusion and then up to 8 mg/kg per h by continuous intravenous infusion	Complicated by hypotension. It has saturable pharmacokinetics, and a strong tendency to accumulate. Metabolized to pentobarbital. It can also cause pancreatitis, hepatic disturbance and hypersensitivity reaction
Pentobarbital	10–20 mg/kg at 25 mg/min then 0.5–1 mg/kg per h increasing to 1–3 mg/kg per h	As above
Propofol	2 mg/kg then 5–10 mg/kg per h	Large volume of distribution and short half-life. Rapid recovery. Can be complicated by lipaemia, acidosis and rhabdomyolysis especially in children. Rebound seizures with abrupt withdrawal

levetiracetam – although neither of these latter drugs is licensed for this indication.

Phenobarbital is easier to use, and possibly more effective than phenytoin, but phenytoin may be associated with a lower risk of respiratory depression. Controlled studies have not, however, been carried out, and the relative merits of the two therapies are unclear. Phenytoin is relatively insoluble in water, and its parenteral formulation has a high pH; consequently, it has a number of side effects related to its physicochemical properties. It may crystallize and precipitate in solutions; it may cause thrombophlebitis (particularly with extravasation); its vehicle, propylene glycol, can cause hypotension; and phenytoin is poorly and erratically absorbed after intramuscular injection. Fosphenytoin (3-phosphoryloxymethyl phenytoin disodium) is a water-soluble phenytoin prodrug that has some advantages relating to tolerability over phenytoin. Fosphenytoin is itself inactive, but is metabolized to phenytoin with a half-life of 8–15 min. It can be administered two to three times faster than phenytoin and achieves similar mean serum concentrations, although there is considerable scatter of levels. Cardiac monitoring is still required with fosphenytoin, and the dosing units of the drug are confusing and have caused problems in practice in inexperienced emergency units. There are no controlled trials of fosphenytoin in status epilepticus, and it is

not clear if the potential tolerability advantages of fosphenytoin overcome the potential variability in phenytoin levels and the difficulties in dosage translate, in practice, into a better outcome than that achieved by phenytoin.

The major advantages of valproate and levetiracetam are their seeming lack of cardiovascular depression, the absence of drug-induced hypotension, the lack of interaction and the lack of local irritation at the injection site. However, neither has been subjected to a randomized trial in status epilepticus and the full range of side effects is not yet established.

Subanaesthetic infusions of benzodiazepine drugs were once fashionable in the stage of established status. However, because of drug accumulation (see pp. 289–290), sudden respiratory depression, cardiovascular collapse and/or severe hypotension can occur. For these reasons, continuous benzodiazepine infusions (or repeated bolus injections) at this stage should not be given (the exception is with midazolam – see below). Clomethiazole infusion carries similar risks. Lidocaine infusion is essentially a short-term therapy and so should not be employed at this stage.

The stage of refractory status epilepticus
In most patients, if seizures continue for 60–90 min in spite of the therapy outlined above, full anaesthesia is

required. In some emergency situations (e.g. postoperative status, severe or complicated convulsive status, patient already in intensive care unit [ICU]), anaesthesia can and should be introduced earlier. The prognosis for patients reaching this stage of status epilepticus is much poorer, and there is a moderate risk of mortality and morbidity.

The most commonly used anaesthetics are the intravenous barbiturates thiopental and pentobarbital, and the intravenous non-barbiturate infusional anaesthetics propofol and midazolam. There have been no randomized controlled studies comparing these treatment options, but a meta-analysis suggests no difference in terms of mortality, although pentobarbital was more effective than midazolam at the expense of greater hypotension. Propofol and midazolam have significant pharmacokinetic advantages over the barbiturates. Other anaesthetics that can be used include isoflurane, etomidate and ketamine. Experience with these agents in status is, however, meagre. Ketamine in particular is theoretically an attractive option because it has a strong blocking action at N-methyl-D-aspartate (NMDA) receptors, which might provide neuroprotection.

It is imperative at this stage to be monitoring the patient's EEG, as a patient in a drug-induced coma, with little outward sign of convulsions, can still have ongoing electrographic epileptic activity. The point of therapy is to abolish electrographic activity and the attendant risk of excitotoxic cerebral damage, and EEG monitoring can be the only way to detect such activity. The depth of anaesthesia should be that which abolishes all EEG epileptic activity, and commonly 'burst suppression' is the targeted level of anaesthesia. Burst suppression with interburst intervals of 2–30 s is an acceptable endpoint because it supposedly represents appropriate membrane inactivity, although it can be difficult to achieve, because this degree of anaesthesia commonly leads to hypotension.

All the anaesthetic drugs are given in doses sufficient to induce deep unconsciousness, and therefore assisted respiration, intensive cardiovascular monitoring and the full panoply of intensive care are essential.

Once the patient has been free of seizures for 12–24 h, and provided that there are adequate plasma levels of concomitant antiepileptic medication, the anaesthetic can be slowly tapered. There are some data to suggest that those who are loaded with phenobarbital do better than those who are not. If seizures recur, anaesthesia should be re-established. If one anaesthetic agent is ineffective then it should be substituted by another. In severe cases anaesthesia may be required for weeks or even months,

and it is important to recognize that even prolonged status epilepticus can remit and the patient can recover with slight long-term effects. The process of maintaining a patient under anaesthetic for weeks or months requires great skill, in view of the attendant risks. The ultimate outcome is worse the longer the status continues, but, even after very prolonged attacks, a complete recovery can occur. Much depends on the underlying cause – and the ultimate prognosis is more dependent on this than on the duration of seizures. There is a tendency, especially among anaesthetists, to consider refractory status a terminal condition – a tendency that should be resisted.

In refractory status epilepticus, trials of steroids are often given. In patients in whom immunologically based aetiologies are present, or in those in whom no cause is identified, repeated courses of intravenous IgG are sometimes effective. Intravenous magnesium can be tried.

Additional maintenance antiepileptic therapy

In addition to emergency drug therapy, it is important that maintenance antiepileptic drug treatment should continue via a nasogastric tube. If this is forgotten, seizures will almost inevitably recur when the anaesthesia is lightened.

Failure to respond to treatment

In the great majority of cases, the above measures will control seizures and the status will resolve. If drug treatment fails, there are often complicating factors. Common reasons for the failure to control seizures in status epilepticus are as follows.

Inadequate drug treatment

• Insufficient emergency antiepileptic drug therapy: a particular problem is the administration of intravenous drugs at too low a dose (e.g. phenobarbital or phenytoin).
• Failure to initiate or continue maintenance antiepileptic drug therapy in parallel with the acute emergency therapy will result in a recrudescence of seizures once the effects of the emergency drug treatment have worn off.

Medical factors

• Medical complications can exacerbate seizures.
• A failure to treat (or identify) the underlying cause can result in intractable status. This is particularly the case in acute progressive cerebral disorders and cerebral infections.

Misdiagnosis

• A common problem is the failure to diagnose pseudo-status epilepticus. Indeed, in specialist practice, this condition is more common than true epileptic status. The diagnosis can usually be made easily by clinical observation, once considered, and confirmed by EEG in cases of uncertainty.

Treatment of tonic–clonic status in special circumstances

Drug withdrawal

Status epilepticus can result from antiepileptic drug withdrawal (or too rapid a reduction of dose). This can be the result of injudicious medical advice or poor compliance. In this situation, the rapid reintroduction of the drug often effectively terminates the status epilepticus and obviates the need for the above more elaborate measures. The drug should be given intravenously where possible.

Alcohol withdrawal

Alcohol withdrawal can also result in status epilepticus in the 24–48 h after withdrawal. The withdrawal of opiates, cocaine and other recreational drugs can have the same effect. Traditionally, benzodiazepine, paraldehyde or clomethiazole is given either as treatment or prophylactically. The patients should be referred, on recovery, to units specializing in addiction.

Drug overdose

Status epilepticus can occur during drug overdose. The status is usually treated with midazolam infusion. Other aspects of management are directed at reducing the levels of the offending drug, at controlling complications and general supportive measures.

Post-neurosurgery or post-head injury

Status epilepticus in the immediate post-neurosurgery situation is associated particularly with cerebral oedema and brain swelling, and should be managed by immediate anaesthesia. The same also applies where possible to status epilepticus after severe head injury.

The clinical characteristics and treatment of other forms of status epilepticus

(Table 9.8)

Epilepsia partialis continua

Epilepsia partialis continua (EPC) can be defined as spontaneous regular or irregular clonic twitching of cerebral cortical origin, sometimes aggravated by action or sensory stimuli, confined to one part of the body, and

Table 9.8 Treatment of different types of non-convulsive status epilepticus (NCSE).

Type	Treatment choice	Other drugs that can be used
Typical absence status epilepticus	IV or oral benzodiazepines	Acetazolamide, valproate or chlormethiazole
Complex partial status epilepticus	Oral clobazam	IV lorazepam and phenytoin (or fosphenytoin), levetiracetam, valproate, phenobarbital
Atypical absence status epilepticus	Oral valproate	Oral benzodiazepines (with caution), lamotrigine, topiramate
Tonic status epilepticus	Oral lamotrigine	Methylphenidate, steroids
Myoclonic status epilepticus in coma	Barbiturate anaesthesia (for short trial period)	Steroids, midazolam
Other forms of myoclonic status epilepticus	Oral valproate, benzodiazepines	Levetiracetam
Epilepsia partialis continua	Any oral anticonvulsant	Steroids, immunosuppression
NCSE in the aftermath of tonic–clonic seizures	IV benzodiazepines	IV phenytoin or phenobarbital
Subtle status epilepticus	Anaesthesia	Steroids

IV, intravenous.

continuing for hours, days or weeks. It is a remarkable condition, with highly characteristic features, and has a number of underlying causes (Table 9.9). The clonic jerks in EPC can affect any group of muscles. In some individuals they are confined to a single muscle or muscle group, but in others the distribution is more widespread, and the distribution of the jerks can vary over time. Agonists and antagonists are affected together, and distal muscles are more commonly involved than the proximal musculature. The jerks are spontaneous, and often exacerbated by action, startle or sensory stimuli. They can be single or cluster, and may have a rhythmic quality with a wide range of frequencies and amplitudes. Some jerks recur only every few minutes and others are more frequent. In chronic cases the jerks can continue relentlessly for months or years.

EPC needs to be differentiated from myoclonic dystonia and brain-stem myoclonus. Diagnosis can be difficult; the EEG may show focal abnormalities, but can be normal. EPC can result from structural abnormalities such as stroke, trauma, cerebral infarction, cerebral abscess, neuronal migration disorders and vascular malformation. EPC can be due to a variety of encephalitides, commonly Rasmussen encephalitis, but also subacute panencephalitis and Creutzfeldt–Jakob disease. It is also not uncommon in the autoimmune encephalopathies. Metabolic causes have also been described, including, importantly, hyponatraemia and hyperglycaemia.

Treatment should be largely directed at the underlying cause. The seizures can remit spontaneously in acute cases. In a well-established case, however, EPC can be particularly resistant to therapy, and intravenous antiepileptic therapy, even to the point of anaesthesia, can produce only temporary respite. It is usual to prescribe oral antiepileptic drugs, to prevent secondary generalization, even if the EPC itself is not controlled. Any of the antiepileptic drugs can be used and treatment follows conventional lines. In addition, the oral corticosteroids are sometimes helpful. Where there is an inflammatory or post-infective cause, or in EPC of uncertain cause, courses of high-dose intravenous IgG have been used, sometimes with startling benefit. Plasma exchange has been tried with little effect, as have other immunosuppressive therapies and zidovudine. The long-term outcome depends on the underlying cause, but in many cases the clonic movements continue in spite of medical therapy. Very occasionally, there is resort to surgical therapy, either resective or by multiple subpial transection.

Table 9.9 Causes of epilepsia partialis continua.

Cerebral tumour	Primary (benign/malignant), metastasis
Cerebral infection	Bacterial abscess, tuberculoma, parasitic infection (e.g. cysticercosis), viral encephalitis, meningitis, HIV, Whipple disease
Cerebral inflammatory disorder	Antibody-mediated immunological diseases (NMDA receptor, VGKA), Rasmussen encephalitis, paraneoplastic disease, coeliac disease
Cerebrovascular disease	Cerebral infarction/haemorrhage, arteriovenous malformation, venous thrombosis
Mitochondrial disease	Alpers disease, MERRF, others
Congenital disorders	Cortical dysplasia (many types)
Drugs, toxins and metabolic disorders	Many drugs, toxins and metabolic disturbances

MERRF, myoclonic encephalopathy with ragged red fibres; NMDA, N-methyl-D-aspartate; VGKA, voltage-gated K$^+$ channel antibodies.

Complex partial status epilepticus

This form of non-convulsive status can be defined as a prolonged epileptic episode in which fluctuating or frequently recurring focal electrographic epileptic discharges result in a confusional state. There are highly variable clinical symptoms, and the focal epileptic discharges may arise in temporal or extratemporal cortical regions. Any condition causing complex partial seizures can also cause status, although structural defects in the frontal lobe seem particularly likely to result in episodes of status epilepticus.

Complex partial status epilepticus has to be differentiated from other forms of non-convulsive status epilepticus, postictal states, and other neurological and psychiatric conditions. EEG may be helpful, but the scalp EEG changes can be non-specific and the diagnosis has to be largely clinical. It is this author's view that the condition is overdiagnosed, and the tendency to attribute any confusional state in patients with epilepsy to complex partial status epilepticus should be resisted.

Clinical features

Confusion, which can fluctuate or be fairly continuous, is the leading clinical feature. The severity of the confusion can vary: from profound stupor with little response to external stimuli in some cases, to others in whom subtle abnormalities on cognitive testing are the only sign. Amnesia is usual but not invariable. Associated with the confusion are behavioural changes, speech and language disturbance, and motor and autonomic features. These can be very variable and cause considerable diagnostic difficulty. Periods of complex partial status can last for days or even weeks, although typically an episode will persist for several hours. It is most common in adults, usually with long histories of complex partial epilepsy. Precipitating factors include menstruation, and alcohol and drug withdrawal, but not usually photic stimulation or overbreathing as in typical absence status. The onset and offset are usually less well defined than in absence status, and the response to intravenous therapy more gradual. Complex partial status may typically follow a secondarily generalized tonic–clonic seizure (or cluster of seizures), but is rarely terminated by a generalized convulsion, in contrast to the case in typical absence status. Episodes of complex partial status are usually recurrent, and in a few patients there is a remarkable periodicity. Complex partial status can arise in focal epilepsies of widely varying aetiologies.

The abnormalities on scalp EEG findings may be slight, although the EEG is seldom normal. A whole range of EEG patterns is seen including continuous or frequent spikes or spike–wave paroxysms, which are sometimes widespread or focal, and also episodes of desynchronization. The longer the status proceeds, the less likely is discrete ictal activity to be noticeable.

The prognosis of complex partial status is good. It is not usually life threatening, and resolves with oral or intravenous therapy or is self-limiting. There is, however, a strong tendency for recurrence. Permanent neurological or psychological sequelae are rare, in contrast to the poor prognosis of tonic–clonic status.

Drug treatment of complex partial status epilepticus

How aggressively complex partial status epilepticus needs to be treated is a matter of some controversy. It is the author's view that in most cases there is little risk of cerebral damage due to the seizures, and for this reason intravenous therapy is not needed unless the condition is particularly severe or resistant. Others disagree and treat complex partial status using similar protocols to that described above for tonic–clonic status. There is, however,

no good evidence that aggressive treatment improves the prognosis in this condition, and intravenous medication can result in hypotension, respiratory depression and occasionally cardiorespiratory arrest. In one series of nonconvulsive status epilepticus in elderly people, aggressive treatment carried a worse prognosis than no treatment.

Early recognition is a critical goal. At present, treatment with oral benzodiazepines is usually first-line therapy. Lorazepam or clobazam is the most commonly prescribed drug. In patients who have repetitive attacks of complex partial status epilepticus (a common occurrence), oral clobazam over a period of 2–3 days, given early at home, can abort the status epilepticus, and such strategies should be discussed with the patient and carers. The response to benzodiazepines can be disappointing. Often there is only a slow and partial improvement, in marked contrast to the complete and rapid improvement in absence status epilepticus. In other patients there may be resolution of the electrographic status epilepticus without concomitant clinical improvement. Although the response to benzodiazepines is often not complete, most episodes are self-limiting and will recover spontaneously. Valproate may be an alternative, because intravenous valproate is well tolerated with little respiratory or cardiac depression; trials are urgently needed in this area.

For more persistent or resistant complex partial status epilepticus, intravenous therapy can be used and lorazepam followed by phenytoin (or fosphenytoin) are the traditional drugs of choice. Intravenous valproate or levetiracetam has been shown in small case series to be highly effective. Whether general anaesthesia is ever justified remains a matter for speculation.

Treatment of the underlying cause where this is possible (e.g. encephalitis or metabolic derangement) is of course paramount. The routine maintenance antiepileptic drug regimen should also be manipulated to provide maximum control of seizures.

Absence status epilepticus

Absence status can be best subdivided into various separate syndromes, albeit with overlapping clinical and EEG features. These should all be distinguished from complex partial status, which can take a somewhat similar clinical form. Although this is a tidy classification scheme, there are transitional cases that do not fit easily into any particular category.

Typical absence status epilepticus ('petit-mal' status)

This occurs only in patients with idiopathic generalized epilepsy, usually as part of the subcategory childhood absence epilepsy, in which a history of absence status occurs in about 3–9%. Absence status occurs also in the other syndromes of idiopathic generalized epilepsy, including myoclonic–astatic epilepsy, epilepsy with myoclonic absences, eyelid myoclonia with absences and juvenile absence epilepsy. The attacks can recur and last for hours or occasionally days. The episodes are typically precipitated by factors such as menstruation, withdrawal of medication, hypoglycaemia, hyperventilation, flashing or bright lights, sleep deprivation, fatigue, stress or grief. The principal clinical feature is clouding of consciousness. This can vary from slight clouding to profound stupor. At one extreme, patients have nothing more than slowed ideation and expression, and deficits in activities requiring sustained attention, sequential organization or spatial structuring; amnesia may be slight or even absent. At the other extreme there may be immobility, mutism, simple voluntary actions performed only after repeated requests, long delays in verbal responses, and monosyllabic and hesitant speech. Typically, the patient is in an expressionless, trance-like state with slow responses and a stumbling gait. Motor features occur in about 50% of cases, including myoclonus, atonia, rhythmic eyelid blinking, and quivering of the lips and face. Facial, especially eyelid, myoclonus is common in absence status, but rare in complex partial status. Episodes of absence status are often terminated by a tonic–clonic seizure. The diagnostic electrographic pattern is continuous or almost continuous bilaterally synchronous and symmetrical spike–wave activity, with little or no reactivity to sensory stimuli.

Typical absence status can usually be rapidly and completely abolished by benzodiazepine therapy given as intravenous bolus doses. The usual drugs are diazepam 0.2–0.3 mg/kg, clonazepam 1 mg (0.25–0.5 mg in children) or lorazepam 0.07 mg/kg (0.1 mg/kg in children). The bolus doses can be repeated if required. If this is ineffective, intravenous clomethiazole or valproate may be needed. In childhood absence epilepsy, maintenance therapy with valproate, ethosuximide or other agents is required once the status is controlled. There is little likelihood that absence status induces neuronal damage, and thus aggressive treatment is not warranted.

Atypical absence status
This form of status is common in patients with diffuse cerebral damage and is typically seen as part of the Lennox–Gastaut syndrome. Although the clinical phenomenology of typical and atypical absence status overlaps greatly, there are important differences. The clinical context is very different: typical absence status occurs in patients with childhood absence epilepsy and without intellectual deterioration; atypical absence epilepsy occurs in the epileptic encephalopathies (typically the Lennox–Gastaut syndrome), with other seizure types and in the context of intellectual disability. The episodes of atypical absence status are usually longer and more frequent, with a gradual onset and offset. Atypical absence status is often preceded by changes in motor activity, mood or intellectual ability, for hours or days before the overt seizures develop. This prodromal stage might be due to subclinical status. Atypical absence status tends to fluctuate, and minor motor, myoclonic or more typically tonic seizures interrupt, but do not terminate an episode. Tonic seizures usually last a few minutes but occur in series. In some patients the mental state fluctuates gradually in and out of this ill-defined epileptic state over long periods of time – days or weeks – with little distinction possible between ictal and interictal phases. In contrast to typical absence status, tonic–clonic seizures seldom occur at the beginning or end of the status episode, and atypical absence status often responds poorly to injection of a benzodiazepine. Indeed, antiepileptic drug therapy may have little effect, and the condition fluctuates, apparently uninfluenced by external factors. Atypical absence status is more likely to occur if the patient is drowsy or under-stimulated, and it is thus important not to over-medicate patients with the Lennox–Gastaut syndrome. The EEG during atypical absence status may show continuous irregular slow (2 Hz) spike–wave, or hypsarrhythmia, or more discrete ictal patterns.

In contrast to typical absence status epilepticus, this condition is usually poorly responsive to intravenous benzodiazepines, which should, in any case, be given cautiously, because they can induce tonic status epilepticus in susceptible patients. Oral rather than intravenous treatment is usually more appropriate, and the drugs of choice are valproate, lamotrigine, clonazepam, clobazam, levetiracetam and topiramate. Barbiturates, carbamazepine, gabapentin, phenytoin, pregabalin, tiagabine and vigabatrin can worsen the episode.

New absence status of late life
This curious syndrome presents in late adult life. The leading symptom is confusion, although the other features of absence status can occur. Many patients have a history of absence epilepsy in early life that has been in long remission. Many cases are misdiagnosed as dementia or cerebrovascular disease, but the abrupt onset

should suggest the possibility of absence status, and the diagnosis is easily confirmed by EEG. In most cases, psychotropic drug (particularly benzodiazepine) toxicity or withdrawal seems to be the antecedent cause of the episode. The condition is rapidly alleviated by intravenous lorazepam (4 mg) or other benzodiazepines, and tends not to recur. Long-term antiepileptic drug treatment is not usually required.

Autonomic status epilepticus

This is a form of status epilepticus that occurs typically in Panayiotopoulos syndrome (see p. 26). The exact prevalence of this syndrome is unclear, and estimates have ranged from 0% to 6% of all children with epilepsy. The seizures consist of episodes of nausea, retching and vomiting, and deviation of the eyes. There may or may not be altered awareness. Other autonomic features occur including incontinence of urine, pallor, hyperventilation and headache. The EEG shows occipital spiking or runs of 3 Hz spike–wave and there is also often evidence of photosensitivity. About half of the seizures last longer than 30 min and so are categorized as 'status epilepticus'. The prognosis of the syndrome is excellent and at least 50% of patients have only a single attack, and most require no treatment. Intravenous benzodiazepine, rectal diazepam or buccal midazolam can be used to terminate an attack.

Tonic status epilepticus

Tonic status epilepticus occurs in patients with syndromes such as the Lennox–Gastaut syndrome. The tonic seizures are usually short-lived but are rapidly repeated and a series can persist for days. Tonic status epilepticus is poorly responsive to conventional treatment, and can be dramatically worsened by benzodiazepines, which should be used with care. Sedating medication can worsen all seizure types in the Lennox–Gastaut syndrome, and thus should be avoided. Lamotrigine, adrenocorticotrophic hormone (ACTH) and corticosteroids are reported sometimes to be effective.

Myoclonic status epilepticus in coma

This diagnosis is made in patients who have suffered severe brain injury (e.g. cerebral anoxia after cardiac arrest) and are in deep coma, sometimes with subtle myoclonic twitching, in whom the EEG shows PLEDs or bilateral synchronous epileptiform discharges (BPEDs), periodic discharges, encephalopathic triphasic patterns or burst suppression patterns. It occurs in up to 8% of patients in coma. To what extent this is really an 'epileptic' state, or simply a sign of a severely damaged brain, is arguable, but most European neurologists accept the latter proposition and that the EEG changes simply indicate underlying widespread cortical damage or dysfunction. It is often an agonal event with an extremely poor prognosis, although survival can occur especially if the initial insult was primarily hypoxia related. Survivors may be left with Lance–Adams-type action myoclonus. Whether antiepileptic treatment influences the course of this condition is quite unclear. Some authorities recommend aggressive antiepileptic therapy, and others none at all. It is this author's practice to recommend aggressive anti-status therapy, including anaesthesia, for a 12- to 24-hour period, but at this stage, in the absence of any improvement, the antiepileptic therapy should be withdrawn. Barbiturate or non-barbituate infusional anaesthetic drugs are given.

Other forms of myoclonic status epilepticus

Myoclonic status in the progressive myoclonic epilepsies and in primary generalized epilepsy does not usually require intravenous therapy, although if needed an intravenous benzodiazepine can be given. The preferred therapy is with oral valproate, benzodiazepine, levetiracetam or piracetam.

Subtle status epilepticus

This term is best reserved, in the author's view, to the form of electrographic non-convulsive status epilepticus that sometimes occurs in the aftermath of a convulsive seizure. The patient is often stuporose or confused, and often misdiagnosed as being in a prolonged post-ictal state. The EEG may show rhythmic slow activity or patterns similar to that of myoclonic status epilepticus in coma (see above). In contrast to the situation in myoclonic status epilepticus in coma, this state undoubtedly represents seizure activity and the recommended treatment is with intravenous benzodiazepines.

Simple partial status epilepticus

Simple partial motor status epilepticus is known as epilepsia partialis continua and its treatment is discussed above. Other forms of prolonged simple partial seizures are rare. Any condition causing simple partial seizures can also result in status, although, as is the case with complex partial status, prolonged simple partial seizures are also quite characteristic of some of the benign partial epilepsy syndromes of childhood, particularly the occipital and rolandic epilepsy syndromes. Emergency administration of benzodiazepines is traditionally given, and the principles of treatment are similar to those of complex partial status epilepticus.

Other forms of generalized non-convulsive status epilepticus

Episodes of non-convulsive status in various conditions are not easily classified as either absence status or complex partial status, although their clinical forms are very similar. This applies particularly to the rare childhood epilepsy syndromes. Episodes of non-convulsive status are a particularly characteristic feature of the ring chromosome 20 syndrome. Generally speaking, treatment follows the same lines as that of atypical absence status epilepticus.

Antiepileptic drugs used in status epilepticus

Many of the main-line antiepileptic drugs have been used in status epilepticus. The potential for use of the newer agents has been only partly explored, and both topiramate and levetiracetam, for example, show promise in experimental models and in preliminary reports on human status. Among the anaesthetic agents ketamine has the potential advantage of antiglutaminergic action, which might confer neuroprotectant properties, but it has not been extensively used. Lacosamide (previously known as harkeroside) is a novel agent, the use of which in status epilepticus has been specifically investigated. Salient properties of the antiepileptic drugs most commonly used parenterally are briefly listed below.

Clomethiazole

Clomethiazole had previously been widely employed at the stage of established status epilepticus, although its use is now largely abandoned. It is given by intravenous bolus followed by a continuous infusion. The drug is rapidly redistributed and has a very rapid and short-lived initial action. Dosage can be initially titrated against response, on a moment-by-moment basis, a unique property among the drugs used in status. The danger of clomethiazole is that it accumulates on prolonged use, with the risk of sudden cardiorespiratory collapse, hypotension and sedation. There is also a danger of respiratory arrest and hypotension if the maximum rate of injection is exceeded. Other side effects include cardiac rhythm disturbances,

vomiting and thrombophlebitis, and there is a tendency for seizure recurrence on discontinuing therapy. Prolonged therapy carries the risk of fluid overload and electrolyte disturbance. Despite its widespread usage, there is limited published experience in status, particularly in children. Hepatic disease reduces the metabolism and elimination of the drug, and prolonged contact with plastic tubing (e.g. in drip sets) results in substantial resorption.

Usual preparation

This is a 0.8% (8 mg/mL) solution of clomethiazole edisylate in 500 mL of 4% dextrose.

Usual dosage

Intravenous infusion of 40–100 mL (320–800 mg), at a rate of 5–15 mL/min, followed by a continuous infusion, with dosage titrated according to response (usually 1–4 mL/min, range 0.5–20 mL/min) (adults), or initially 0.1 mL/kg per min (0.8 mg/kg per min), increasing progressively every 2–4 h as required (children).

Clonazepam

Clonazepam is an alternative to diazepam at the stage of early status epilepticus, and there is little to choose between the two drugs. It has a similar onset of action and a longer duration of action (half-life, 22–33 h), and may have a lower incidence of late relapse. There is wide experience with the drug in adults and children, although not in neonates, and the drug has proven efficacy in tonic–clonic, partial and absence status. Clonazepam accumulates on prolonged infusion, with the resulting risk of respiratory arrest, hypotension and sedation – a side-effect profile very similar to that of diazepam (see below). The drug has a negative inotropic action, and as with diazepam thrombophlebitis may occur. There is also a danger of sudden collapse if the recommended rate of injection is exceeded. A continuous infusion of clonazepam is not now recommended because of the dangers of accumulation, and respiratory and cardiovascular collapse.

Usual preparation

A 1 mL ampoule containing 1 mg of clonazepam.

Usual dosage

Either a 1–2 mg bolus injection over 30 s (adults) or 250–500 µg (children), which can be repeated up to four times. The 1 mL ampoule of clonazepam is mixed with 1 mL of water for injection (provided as diluent) *immediately* before administration. The rate of injection should not exceed 1 mg in 30 s. The drug can also be given more slowly in a 5% dextrose or 0.9% sodium chloride solution (1–2 mg in 250 mL).

Diazepam

Diazepam is useful in the premonitory stage or the stage of epilepsy status epilepticus. There is extensive clinical experience in adults, children and newborns, and the drug has well-proven efficacy in many types of status, a rapid onset of action, and well-studied pharmacology and pharmacokinetics. It can be given by rectal administration, and the rectal tubule is a convenient preparation. Diazepam used to be used as a long-term infusion, but this practice is now largely abandoned because of the risk of accumulation.

There are a number of disadvantages to the use of diazepam. First, although it has a rapid onset of action, it is highly lipid soluble and thus has a short duration of action – usually <1 h – after a single injection. This means that there is a strong tendency for seizure relapse after initial control. For this reason, lorazepam is often used in its place at the stage of early status epilepticus. Second, diazepam accumulates on repeated injections or after continuous infusion, and this accumulation carries a high risk of sudden respiratory depression, sedation and hypotension. Midazolam is the only benzodiazepine now recommended for use in prolonged infusion. A third problem, shared with the other benzodiazpines, is the cardiorespiratory depressant effect of diazepam. The respiratory effect of diazepam can be pronounced (see p. 288) and the fall in ventilatory capacity is likely to be exacerbated by ongoing seizures in which respiration is already compromised. Hypotension is common, and a mean fall in blood pressure of 10 mmHg was noted in healthy individuals in one study after a 10 mg intravenous injection. Mild sedation is common, too, with parenteral diazepam. In occasional patients, very low doses of diazepam result in severe respiratory depression, and facilities for resuscitation should be available whenever the drug is administered intravenously. Finally, tolerance to the effects develops rapidly, often within 12 h, which limits its long-term use. Other disadvantages are its dependency on hepatic metabolism and its metabolism to an active metabolite, which can complicate prolonged therapy. Diazepam has a tendency to precipitate from concentrated solutions and to interact with other drugs, and is absorbed onto plastic on prolonged contact. The Diazemuls® preparation (or similar preparation) should always be used for intravenous administration, because this minimizes the risk of thrombophlebitis.

As a result of the risks of accumulation, respiratory and cardiovascular depression and tolerance, the drug should be used in short-term therapy only (a bolus dose given once or twice) and long-term infusions are not now recommended.

Usual preparation

Intravenous formulation: diazepam emulsion (Diazemuls®), 1 mL ampoule containing 5 mg/mL, or intravenous solution 2 mL ampoule containing 5 mg/mL. Rectal formulation: 2.5 mL rectal tube (Stesolid), containing 2 mg/mL, or using the intravenous solution 2 mL ampoule containing 5 mg/mL.

Usual dosage

Intravenous bolus (undiluted) 10–20 mg (adults) or 0.25–0.5 mg/kg (children), at a rate not exceeding 2–5 mg/min. The bolus dosing can be repeated. Rectal administration 10–30 mg (adults) or 0.5–0.75 mg/kg (children), which can be repeated.

Fosphenytoin

Fosphenytoin is a prodrug of phenytoin, and is a drug of choice at the stage of established status epilepticus. It is converted in the plasma into phenytoin by widely distributed phosphatase enzymes. The half-life of conversion is about 15 min, and conversion is not affected by age, hepatic status or the presence of other drugs. Fosphenytoin is soluble in water and prepared in a tris (tris[hydroxymethyl]aminomethane) buffer; it thus causes less thrombophlebitis than phenytoin when given intravenously. It can also be administered intramuscularly as prophylaxis in acute epilepsy, but absorption is too slow for its use by intramuscular administration in status epilepticus. Fosphenytoin itself is inert, and its action in status is entirely due to the derived phenytoin. When fosphenytoin is infused at 100 mg phenytoin equivalents (PE)/min, the mean rate at which free phenytoin levels are reached in the serum is similar to that achieved by a phenytoin infusion of 50 mg/min, although there is considerable individual scatter in the levels reached. Fosphenytoin can therefore be administered twice as fast as phenytoin, with equivalent risks of hypotension, cardiac arrhythmias and respiratory depression. Its rate of antiepileptic action is also similar. The faster administration and the lower incidence of local side effects are the main advantages of fosphenytoin over phenytoin. A disadvantage is the confusing units in which the dose is expressed, and fatal mistakes in dosing in A&E have been made. Fosphenytoin is more expensive than phenytoin, but cost-effectiveness studies have shown that the two drugs have purported to show equivalent value.

Usual preparation

Fosphenytoin is formulated in a tris buffer at physiological pH. Phials of 50 mg PE are available for mixture with dextrose or saline.

Usual dosage

The dosage of the drug is expressed in PEs (thus, 15 mg PE of fosphenytoin is the same as 15 mg phenytoin). It is administered at a dose of 15 mg PE/kg at a rate of between 100 and 150 mg PE/min (100 mg PE/min is, in the author's experience, safer, so the average adult dose of 1000 mg PE is administered in 10 min). The drug is currently not recommended for children aged <5 years. For older children the dose in milligrams PE per minute is the same as for adults.

Isoflurane

Inhalational anaesthesia is a rare option in the treatment of refractory status epilepticus status. However, when it is chosen, isoflurane is the drug of choice. It has advantages over other inhalational anaesthetics such as halothane or enflurane: lower solubility, less hepatotoxicity or nephrotoxicity, less effect on cardiac output, fewer cardiac arrhythmias, less hypotension, less effect on cerebral blood flow and autoregulation, less increase in intracranial pressure, less convulsant effect and linear kinetics. It has a very rapid onset of action and recovery, and no tendency to accumulate. Although hypotension is common it is generally mild. There is no hepatic metabolism, and the drug is unaffected by hepatic or renal disease. There is, however, little published experience in status epilepticus or of long-term use, and the side-effect profile in this situation is not really known. Another major disadvantage is the logistical problems caused by the use of an anaesthetic system in the ICU situation. A scavenging apparatus is required, together with the other usual ICU paraphernalia of assisted ventilation, intensive care and cardiorespiratory monitoring.

Usual preparation

Almost pure (99.9%) liquid, for use in a correctly calibrated vaporizer via an anaesthetic system.

Usual dosage

Inhalation of isoflurane at doses producing end-tidal concentrations of 0.8–2%, with the dose titrated to maintain a burst-suppression pattern on the EEG.

Lidocaine

Lidocaine is a second-line drug for use in the stage of early status epilepticus only. It is given as a bolus injection or short intravenous infusion. The clinical effects and pharmacokinetics have been extensively studied in patients of all ages, and the drug is highly effective. The main disadvantage of lidocaine is that its antiepileptic effects are short-lived, and seizures are controlled for a matter of hours only. Lidocaine is thus useful only while more definitive antiepileptic drug treatment is administered. The risk of drug accumulation is low, and the incidence of respiratory or cerebral depression and hypotension is lower than with other antiepileptics. The drug has been claimed to be particularly valuable in patients with respiratory disease. Other disadvantages include a possible proconvulsant effect at high levels, an active metabolite that may accumulate on prolonged therapy, the need for cardiac monitoring, because cardiac rhythm disturbances are common, and the dependency of the clearance of lidocaine on hepatic blood flow.

Usual preparation

A 5 mL ready-prepared syringe containing lidocaine 20 mg/mL (2%) or a 10 ml ready-prepared syringe containing lidocaine 10 mg/ml (1%) (i.e. both syringes contain 100 mg). Lidocaine is also available as a 5 mL vial containing 20 mg/mL (2%) (i.e. 100 mg) lidocaine or a 5 mL vial containing 200 mg/mL (20%) (i.e. 1000 mg) lidocaine, and as ready-made 0.1% (1 mg/mL) and 0.2% (2 mg/mL) infusions (in 500 mL containers in 5% dextrose).

Usual dosage

Intravenous bolus injections of 1.5–2.0 mg/kg (usually 100 mg in adults), at a rate of injection not exceeding 50 mg/min. The bolus injection can be repeated once if necessary. A continuous infusion can be given at a rate of 3–4 mg/kg per h (usually of 0.2% solution in 5% dextrose, for no more than 12 h) or 3–6 mg/kg per h (neonates).

Lorazepam

Lorazepam is the drug of choice in the stage of early status epilepticus, given by intravenous bolus injection.

A single injection is highly effective, and the drug has a longer initial duration of action and a smaller risk of cardiorespiratory depression than diazepam. There is little risk of drug accumulation, and also a lower risk of hypotension. The duration of action of lorazepam after a single initial infection is about 12 h. However, the main disadvantage of lorazepam is a stronger tendency for tolerance to develop, so it is usable only as initial therapy, and longer-term maintenance antiepileptic drugs must be given in addition. There is a large clinical experience in adults, children and newborns, with well-proven efficacy in tonic–clonic and partial status, and the pharmacology and pharmacokinetics of the drug are well characterized. Lorazepam is a stable compound that is not likely to precipitate in solution, and is relatively unaffected by hepatic or renal disease. It has the disadvantage of not being available in many countries.

Usual preparation

A 1 mL ampoule containing 4 mg/mL for intravenous injection.

Usual dosage

Intravenous bolus of 0.07 mg/kg (usually 4 mg), repeated after 10 min if necessary (adults) and bolus of 0.1 mg/kg (children). The rate of injection is not crucial.

Levetiracetam

Intravenous levetiracetam is not licensed currently for use in status epilepticus, although there are now substantial numbers of patients reported in open studies of many different types of status epilepticus. The drug can be used in the established stage of tonic–clonic status epilepticus, and in this situation has the major advantages of lack of any cardiorespiratory depressant effect and the absence of drug-induced hypotension. As a result of these advantages, it is possible that levetiracetam (or valproate for similar reasons) will soon become the drug of first choice in the therapy of tonic–clonic status epilepticus in the established stage. It would be helpful to have a randomized clinical trial because there are currently no controlled data. Adverse events reported after intravenous administration of levetiracetam include dizziness, somnolence, fatigue and headache, and are similar to those after oral administration.

Usual preparation

A 5 mL ampoule containing 100 mg/mL levetiracetam.

Usual dosage

Intravenously, 1000–3000 mg (adults) in 0.9% saline (1000 mg/100 mL saline) infused at a rate of 1000 mg per 15 min.

Midazolam

Midazolam is another benzodiazepine, and it can be used: (1) in the premonitory stage or stage of early status epilepticus or (2) as an anaesthetic in the stage of refractory status epilepticus. It is a water-soluble compound with a ring structure that closes when in contact with serum to convert it into a highly lipophilic structure. Its solubility in water provides one major advantage over diazepam, i.e. it can be rapidly absorbed by intramuscular injection or by intranasal or buccal administration. It is therefore useful in situations in which intravenous administration is difficult or ill-advised. In early status, blinded comparisons of buccal midazolam and rectal diazepam show no differences in efficacy or speed of action. Although there is a danger of accumulation on prolonged or repeated therapy, this tendency is less marked than with diazepam. Occasionally severe cardiorespiratory depression occurs after intramuscular administration, and other adverse effects include hypotension, apnoea, sedation and thrombophlebitis. Similar to diazepam, the drug is short acting, and there is a strong tendency for seizures to relapse after initial control. As with diazepam, its metabolism is altered by hepatic disease and its half-life is significantly prolonged in hepatic disease or in elderly people.

The use of midazolam as an intravenous anaesthetic in status epilepticus has become fashionable in recent years, in spite of an absence of controlled data. It is the only widely used benzodiazepine that can be given by continuous intravenous infusion without a risk of drug accumulation. It carries a lower risk of hypotension than pentobarbital or thiopental, but the rate of rebound seizures on drug reduction is greater. In many ICUs, it is now the drug of choice in refractory status epilepticus.

Usual preparation

A 5 mL ampoule containing 2 mg/mL midazolam hydrochloride.

Usual dosage

Intramuscularly or rectally, 5–10 mg (adults) and 0.15–0.3 mg/kg (children). This can be repeated once after 15 min. Buccal instillation of 10 mg can be given by a syringe and catheter in children or adults. For purposes of anaesthesia, an intravenous bolus of 0.1–0.3 mg/kg, at a rate not exceeding 4 mg/min, which can be repeated once after 15 min, is given, followed by an intravenous infusion at a rate of 0.05–0.4 mg/kg per h.

Paraldehyde

Paraldehyde still has a minor role in the premonitory stage given rectally, as an alternative to the benzodiazepines in situations where facilities for resuscitation are not available. Paraldehyde is rapidly and completely absorbed after intramuscular injection or rectal administration. The risk of drug accumulation, hypotension or cardiorespiratory arrest is small, and seizures do not often recur after control has been obtained. Paraldehyde has been used for many years in status and, although there is wide experience in patients of all ages in status, no modern pharmacokinetic or clinical studies have been carried out. Toxicity is unusual provided that the solution is freshly made, used immediately and correctly diluted. The use of decomposed or inadequately diluted intravenous solutions is dangerous, causing precipitation, microembolism, thrombosis or cardiorespiratory collapse. The intramuscular injection of paraldehdye is painful, and can cause sterile abscess and sciatic nerve damage if wrongly placed. Other side effects include cardiorespiratory depression, sedation, and metabolic or lactic acidosis. The drug rapidly binds to plastic, and glass tubing and syringes are advisable unless injected immediately upon drawing the solution up. The drug should not be exposed to light. The half-life of paraldehyde is markedly increased by hepatic disease.

Usual preparation

Ampoules containing 5 mL paraldehyde (equivalent to approximately 5 g) in darkened glass.

Usual dosage

Paraldehdye can be given rectally (or intramuscularly), 5–10 mL diluted by the same volume of water for injection (adults) or 0.07–0.35 mL/kg (children). This dose can be repeated after 15–30 min.

Pentobarbital

Pentobarbital is an alternative to thiopental as barbiturate anaesthesia in the stage of refractory status epilepticus. It shares many of the characteristics of thiopental, but has the advantages of a shorter elimination half-life than thiopental, non-saturatable kinetics and no active metabolite. It is a stable compound and is unreactive with plastic. There is a surprising dearth of published information about its value, in spite of widespread use. Indeed, published trials have shown a uniformly poor outcome.

Respiratory depression and sedation are invariable, and hypotension and cardiorespiratory dysfunction are common. Decerebrate posturing and flaccid paralysis occur during induction of anaesthesia, and a flaccid weakness can persist for weeks in survivors. There is a tendency for seizures to recur when the drug is withdrawn. It requires intensive care, artificial ventilatory support, and EEG and cardiovascular monitoring. Blood-level monitoring is usually advised, although there is in fact only an inconsistent relationship between serum levels and seizure control.

Usual preparation

This is 100 mg in a 2 mL injection vial, formulated in propylene glycol 40% and ethyl alcohol 10%.

Usual dosage

Intravenous loading dose of 10–20 mg/kg, at a rate not exceeding 25 mg/min, followed by a continuous infusion of 0.5–1.0 mg/kg per h, increasing if necessary to 1–3 mg/kg per h. Additional 5–20 mg/kg boluses can be given if breakthrough seizures occur. The dose should be tapered 12 h after the last seizure by 0.5–1 mg/kg per h every 4–6 h (depending on blood level).

Phenobarbital

Phenobarbital is the drug of first choice at the stage of established status epilepticus. It is a reliable antiepileptic drug, with well-proven effectiveness in tonic–clonic and partial status, and there is extensive clinical experience in adults, children and neonates. Phenobarbital has a stronger anticonvulsant action than other barbiturates and an additional potential cerebral protective action. It has a rapid onset and long-lasting action, and can be administered much faster than can phenytoin. Its safety at high doses has been established, and the drug can be continued as chronic therapy. The disadvantages of the drug relate to prolonged use, where, because of the long elimination half-life, there is a risk of drug accumulation and inevitable sedation, respiratory depression and hypotension. Marked autoinduction may also occur.

Usual preparation

A 1 mL ampoule containing phenobarbital sodium 200 mg/mL in propylene glycol (90%) and water for injection (10%).

Usual dosage

Intravenous loading dose of 10 mg/kg at a rate of 100 mg/min (usual adult dose 600–800 mg), followed by maintenance dose of 1–4 mg/kg (adults), or intravenous loading dose of 15–20 mg/kg, followed by maintenance dose of 3–4 mg/kg (children and neonates). Higher doses can be given, with monitoring of blood concentrations.

Phenytoin

Phenytoin is a drug of choice and a highly effective medication for the stage of established status epilepticus. Extensive clinical experience has been gained in adults, children and neonates, and phenytoin has proven efficacy in tonic–clonic and partial status. The drug has a prolonged action, with a relatively small risk of respiratory or cerebral depression, and no tendency for tachyphylaxis. Its main disadvantages are the time necessary to infuse the drug and its delayed onset of action. Fosphenytoin is a prodrug of phenytoin that can be administered more quickly. The pharmacokinetics of phenytoin are problematic, with zero-order kinetics at conventional doses and wide variation between individuals. Toxic side effects include cardiac rhythm disturbances, thrombophlebitis and hypotension. The risk of cardiac side effects is greatly increased if the recommended rate of injection is exceeded, and cardiac monitoring is advisable during phenytoin infusion. There is a risk of precipitation if phenytoin is diluted in solutions other than 0.9% saline or if mixed with other drugs.

Usual preparation

A 5 mL ampoule containing 250 mg stabilized in propylene glycol, ethanol and water (alternatives exist, e.g. phenytoin in tris buffer or in infusion bottles of 750 mg in 500 mL of osmotic saline).

Usual dosage

In adults, a 15–18 mg/kg intravenous infusion. This can be given via the side arm of a drip or, preferably, directly via an infusion pump. The rate of infusion should not exceed 50 mg/min (20 mg/min in elderly people). In children a 20 mg/kg intravenous infusion is usually given, at a rate not exceeding 25 mg/min. The drug should never be given by intramuscular injection.

Propofol

Propofol is the anaesthetic agent of choice for non-barbiturate infusional anaesthesia in the stage of refractory status epilepticus. It is an excellent anaesthetic with very good pharmacokinetic properties. In status, it has a very rapid onset of action and rapid recovery. There are few haemodynamic side effects, and the drug has been used in all ages. There is, however, only limited published

experience of its use in status, or indeed of prolonged infusions. Unlike isoflurane, it is metabolized in the liver and affected by severe hepatic disease. As with all anaesthetics, its use requires assisted ventilation, intensive care and intensive care monitoring. A particular risk is the propofol infusion syndrome, which is a term used to describe the occurrence of hyperkalaemia, lipaemia, metabolic acidosis, myocardial failure, renal failure and rhabdomyolysis. It occurs usually on long-term infusion (>48 h) but has been reported even after only 5 h of infusion. It is much more common in young children (and indeed for this reason the use of propofol is relatively contraindicated in children). The syndrome is often fatal. It may be caused by drug-induced impairment of oxidation of chains of fatty acids and inhibition of oxidative phosphorylation in the mitochondria, especially in the presence of high catecholamine and cortisol levels. Involuntary movements (without EEG change) can occur, and should not be confused with seizure activity. Rebound seizures are a problem when it is discontinued too rapidly, and a decremental rate of 1 mg/kg every 2 h is recommended when the drug is to be withdrawn.

Usual preparation

A 20 mL ampoule containing 10 mg/mL (i.e. 200 mg) as an emulsion.

Usual dosage

A 2 mg/kg bolus, repeated if necessary, and then followed by a continuous infusion of 5–10 mg/kg per h initially, reducing to 1–3 mg/kg per h.

Thiopental

Thiopental is, in most countries, the usual choice for barbiturate anaesthesia in the stage of refractory status epilepticus. It is a highly effective antiepileptic drug, with additional potential cerebral protective action. It reduces ICP and cerebral blood flow, and has a very rapid onset of action. Its principal metabolite is pentobarbital. The drug has a number of pharmacokinetic disadvantages including saturable kinetics and a strong tendency to accumulate. Indeed, severe sedation commonly persists for days after a thiopental infusion has been withdrawn because of the lipid accumulation and slow clearance. Blood-level monitoring of the parent drug and its active metabolite (pentobarbital) is advisable on prolonged therapy. There is often some tachyphylaxis owing to its sedative, and to a lesser extent its anticonvulsant, properties. Respiratory depression and sedation are inevitable, and hypotension is common. Other less common side effects include pancreatitis, hepatic dysfunction and spasm at the injection site. Full ICU facilities with artificial ventilatory support and intensive EEG and cardiovascular monitoring are needed. It can react with co-medication and with plastic giving sets, and is unstable when exposed to air. Autoinduction occurs, and hepatic disease prolongs the elimination of thiopental. Although it is extensively used in the treatment of status epilepticus, this is only on the basis of anecdotal published case series.

Usual preparation

Injection of thiopental sodium 2.5 g with 100 mL, and 5 g with 200 mL diluent (to make 100 and 200 mL of a 2.5% solution). It is also available as 500 mg and 1 g vials to make 2.5% solutions.

Usual dosage

Intravenous 100–250 mg bolus given over 20 s, with further 50 mg boluses every 2–3 min until seizures are controlled, followed by a continuous intravenous infusion to maintain a burst-suppression pattern on the EEG (usually 3–5 mg/kg per h). The dose should be lowered if systolic blood pressure falls below 90 mmHg despite cardiovascular support.

Valproate

In recent years there has been much interest in the use of valproate in status epilepticus, and it is possible that the drug will assume the role of drug of first choice in the established stage of tonic–clonic status epilepticus. It has been shown to be rapidly effective by bolus intravenous injection in a number of open case series in various types of status epilepticus. It appears to have remarkably few side effects given by intravenous infusion, even at high dosage. It shares with levetiracetam the great advantages over phenytoin or phenobarbital that there is no risk of drug-induced hypotension or respiratory depression. It can also be infused rapidly (within 5–10 min in adults). In adults, a dose of 25 mg/kg produces levels that are generally therapeutic (>100 mg/L). Potential side effects such as prolonged bleeding time, hepatic dysfunction, pancreatitis and hyperammonaemia have not been adequately assessed in large studies. Valproate should be avoided in patients with hepatic or mitochondrial disease.

Usual preparation

Injection of 400 mg valproate powder with vial of 4 mL ampoule of water for injection (100 mg/mL).

Usual dosage

This is 25 mg/kg in adults and 30–40 mg/kg in children. The rate of injection should be between 3 and 6 mg/kg per min.

10 The Surgical Therapy of Epilepsy

The concept of resecting abnormal cortical tissue to abolish epilepsy was developed in the second half of the nineteenth century, and was linked to the advances in clinical cerebral localization. The basic principles have hardly changed since, and the improvements in the surgical treatment of epilepsy in the past century have been largely in the technical rather than the theoretical field. The developments have been highly dependent on applied investigatory technologies of EEG and imaging and those of surgical method.

The first resective surgery (a cortical resection for partial epilepsy based on clinical localization) was performed in the 1880s by William Macewen in Glasgow and Sir Victor Horsley in London, following improvements in anaesthetics and surgical instrumentation. Surgical treatment remained a therapeutic curiosity, however, until the late 1930s, when the introduction of EEG provided a seemingly objective method of localization, which, combined with the localization on the basis of clinical observation, allowed a greater number of patients to undergo resection. This 'electroclinical' localization of the 'epileptic focus' became and remains the cornerstone of epilepsy surgery.

Until this time, surgery was largely confined to resection of the central cortex, because it was here that clinical localization was most accurate. After the advent of EEG, temporal lobe epilepsy became a focus of attention, and the first temporal lobectomy was carried out in the 1940s. The standard operation with removal of the hippocampus, popularized (but probably not devised) by Penfield, was first carried out in 1951. Intracranial depth EEG was introduced in 1944 and EEG-video telemetry in the mid-1960s. Temporal lobe epilepsy remains the most surgically remediable form of epilepsy.

Imaging at this stage was confined to skull radiology and air encephalography. Signs such as asymmetrical dilatation of the horns of the lateral ventricles or changes in middle fossa curvature were relied on to suggest hippocampal sclerosis (both signs now thoroughly discredited), and air encephalography and angiography were used to diagnose tumours and vascular malformations. Computed tomography (CT) was introduced in 1971 and allowed the visualization of vascular and mass lesions. In 1982 the first magnetic resonance imaging (MRI) of a patient with epilepsy was reported. Since then, the use of MRI has simplified presurgical investigation and improved patient selection. Hippocampal sclerosis and cortical dysplasia, which are largely invisible to CT or other forms of X-ray imaging, are readily identified by MRI. As a result, there has been a considerable increase in the proportion of patients for whom resective surgery has become a realistic option. Surgical technique has also improved through technological advance. The first stereotactic atlas was published in 1957, the use of the operative microscope became widespread in the late 1960s and MRI has provided audit feedback in resective neurosurgery. Neuroanaesthesia has also improved progressively, allowing more targeted surgery with less morbidity.

In spite of these developments, epilepsy remains an essentially 'medical' condition and only a small minority of patients with epilepsy can be helped by surgical therapy, perhaps 2% of those with medically refractory partial epilepsy. On this basis, one can estimate that about 100–250 cases per million people in a population would benefit from epilepsy surgery, with the addition of about 10–25 new patients per million people per year.

Epilepsy surgery

Epilepsy surgery is defined as surgery carried out specifically to control epileptic seizures. This includes operations on tumours and vascular lesions where epilepsy is the primary indication for surgery. There is clearly an overlap with lesional surgery carried out for other primary reasons, if the lesion is causing epilepsy and, even if the operation influences the epilepsy, such operations are not

Handbook of Epilepsy Treatment, 3rd Edition. By Simon Shorvon.
Published 2010 by Blackwell Publishing Ltd.

generally included in epilepsy surgery statistics. The distinction is not always clear cut, however, and the control of epilepsy can be an important additional consideration in the decision to undertake surgery. The term 'epilepsy surgery' also implies a particular mindset and a specific approach to presurgical assessment that is discussed further below.

There are five main types of surgical approach:
1 Focal resection for hippocampal sclerosis and other lesions in the mesial temporal lobe
2 Focal resections for other overt lesions (lesionectomies) in temporal neocortex or other cortical areas
3 Non-lesional focal resections (where there is no lesion on imaging, but epileptic tissue is localized by functional methods and/or on clinical grounds)
4 Hemispherectomy, hemispherotomy and other large multilobar resections
5 Functional procedures – multiple subpial transection, corpus callosectomy, focal ablation, focal stimulation, vagal nerve stimulation.

The most common therapeutic operations now are the insertion of a vagal nerve stimulator and temporal lobectomy for hippocampal sclerosis and other mesial temporal lobe lesions. Focal resections and lesionectomies are also frequently carried out. Non-lesional resections and other functional procedures account for less than 10% of operations.

Presurgical assessment – general points

Selection of patients
As a general rule, surgical treatment should be at least considered in any patient with partial seizures that are intractable to medical therapy. When surgery is to be contemplated, the patient should be referred to an experienced epilepsy surgery team for presurgical evaluation. The evaluation will depend on the type of surgery being proposed, but usually the presurgical assessment has the aims listed in Table 10.1.

Presurgical assessment requires specialist knowledge and a specific approach to investigation that are not usually available outside a tertiary centre. This process is usually emotionally demanding and time-consuming for the patient, and this must be made clear at the outset. Not infrequently, surgery will prove not to be possible, and this rejection can be devastating for a person who has made a considerable emotional investment in the process. The decision to proceed with surgery is, in view of its risks and uncertainties, often difficult, and the balance of

Table 10.1 Aims of presurgical assessment for epilepsy surgery.

To confirm that the patient has epilepsy and that the seizures are medically intractable

To define the outcome goals of the chosen surgical procedure (e.g. seizure freedom [usually]) and estimate the chances of attaining this successful outcome

To define the likely gains in terms of quality of life if surgery is carried out

To determine the risks of carrying out the surgical procedure, e.g. in terms of mortality, neurological morbidity, psychological and social effects; also the risks of not operating

To determine that the person is medically fit for surgery

To counsel the patient appropriately about the outcome and risks

risks and benefits seldom clear cut. The decision must always be an individual one, and one made by the patient; the doctor's role is to provide information, notably on the risk of adverse effects and the chance of seizure freedom, and to advise on this basis. The decision should be a considered choice on the basis of the information provided. The patient must feel confident that sufficient information has been given, and that this information is accurate and unbiased. Surgery should never be performed if the patient is reluctant or undecided.

The specific investigations and operations are covered in subsequent sections. However, a few general points can be made here.

Medically intractable epilepsy
The definition of 'medically intractable' is arbitrary and, strictly speaking, epilepsy can be defined as intractable only in retrospect. For pragmatic reasons, in the author's usual practice, epilepsy is regarded as sufficiently intractable to contemplate surgery if it has been continuously active for 5 years (or less in severe epilepsy) in spite of adequate trials of therapy with three or more mainline antiepileptic drugs, and if seizures are frequent (more than one a month). The chances of further medical therapy completely controlling seizures after 5 years of intractability, thus defined, depend on the skills of the treating physician, but are generally less than 30% with

currently available drugs (although it should not be forgotten that newer drugs may be developed which might control the seizures).

Others have used different criteria. A recent trend has been to define intractability earlier – after 2 or 3 years of failure to respond to medical therapy – based on studies showing that an early failure of treatment generally predicts later intractability. However, common clinical experience shows that in some patients seizures are initially uncontrolled by drugs but they do respond later. For this reason, it seems to this author at least that, in most cases, a 2- to 3-year history of epilepsy is too short a period to recommend proceeding to surgical therapy.

These criteria are guidelines only, and there will be patients in whom epilepsy surgery is appropriate, and yet who do not fulfil these criteria, e.g. some patients with lesional epilepsy may be operated upon after a single seizure. The merits of each case should be considered individually, and this requires skill and experience.

Estimating the seizure outcome after surgery and the risks of surgery

The purpose of the presurgical evaluation is to provide an estimate of outcome in terms of seizure control and surgical risk. The estimate should be based both on the literature and where possible on the audited record of the surgical unit. The estimate of outcome and risk depends on the nature of the epilepsy, the nature of the surgery being offered and other factors (see below). Estimates are usually given in percentage terms. A common example is the 50–70% chance of freedom from seizures after a modified anterior temporal lobectomy in an uncomplicated case of mesial temporal epilepsy. The estimates of risk and outcome should be given in writing to the patient, who must be given time for careful consideration and who should also be offered the opportunity for discussion and counselling. The patient's family or carers should usually be included in the discussion, and it must be clear that the patient fully comprehends the risks.

One risk, poorly studied, is the possibility that resective surgery lowers 'cerebral reserve' and that, over time, this reduction in reserve capacity will lead to late deterioration. Certainly, one encounters patients who years after surgery have deteriorated intellectually, but there are no formal studies of this important issue.

Quality-of-life gain

The prediction of the extent of the expected quality-of-life gain due to surgery is a key part of the presurgical assessment. Surgery should be offered only to those whose quality of life is seriously compromised by the occurrence of seizures and in whom the expected outcome of surgery is likely to result in major overall improvement in the quality of life. This may seem obvious, but it is in fact often difficult to decide. The focus of this assessment should be broader than simple seizure control. There are patients who have had surgery that successfully controls seizures but who regret having had the operation, and whose lives have shown little improvement. Frequent seizures, e.g. mild seizures, simple partial seizures or seizures occurring only at night, are not necessarily disabling. In some situations, even severe seizures are not the key determinant of quality of life, e.g. in patients with multiple disabling features. Emotional factors are important, and surgery that is successful in controlling seizures will not automatically alleviate other negative lifestyle aspects, even if these have been moulded by the epilepsy. Social structures and interpersonal relationships may be predicated on a lifetime of seizures, and their sudden cure by surgery may result in changes in personal circumstances that can be hard to adjust to (this has been termed 'the burden of normality'). Skilful counselling is vital in this area.

Non-epileptic seizures

Sometimes, a patient referred for surgery, on investigation, turns out to have non-epileptic seizures, either alone or in combination with genuine epileptic attacks. Generally speaking, non-epileptic attacks, even in combination with genuine attacks, are a contraindication for surgery. Therapy should be directed at the physical or psychological causes that underpin these attacks. If surgery is carried out in patients with a combination of attacks, the psychogenic attacks frequently worsen even if the genuine attacks are relieved. Once non-epileptic attacks have been successfully alleviated by psychological therapies, the question of surgery can be revisited. Decisions about surgical treatment in this area should be made only in a specialist setting.

Learning disability, behavioural disorder and psychosis

Learning disability (a full-scale IQ <70) is a complicating factor when considering surgical therapy, for a number of reasons. First, it often indicates widespread cerebral dysfunction and resective surgery is less likely to control seizures even if a single lesion is demonstrable. Second, in multiply handicapped individuals, epilepsy may not be the most important aspect of disability, and control of seizures will not necessarily lead to major gains in quality of life. Third, fully informed consent can sometimes not be obtained, and consent by proxy (from relatives) should be accepted only after careful deliberation. The ethical issues surrounding informed consent are extremely important, and can be difficult. Finally, 'cerebral reserve' may be lower in people with learning disability. On the other hand, many patients with learning disability are severely handicapped by severe epilepsy and have the potential for great benefit from surgery. Expert evaluation of these issues is necessary for all affected individuals, and the risk–benefit equation needs careful formulation and discussion with the patient and carers.

Surgery is generally also contraindicated in individuals who show severely dysfunctional behaviour. It should not be contemplated if it is likely that the patient will not be able to tolerate the intensive investigation or hospitalization required for epilepsy surgery, or make informed and considered judgements about the potential risks and benefits of epilepsy surgery, or be able to exploit the opportunities afforded by successful surgery.

The presence of a chronic interictal psychosis is also generally a contraindication to surgery, because the psychosis can worsen dramatically after surgery. Decisions about surgical treatment should not be made by severely depressed patients. Psychosis and depression may also prevent informed consent. Again, individual decisions in this situation require a detailed assessment by an experienced practitioner.

Medical fitness and age

Some patients have added risks due to general medical problems, e.g. cervical, spinal or vascular disease. Surgery should be contemplated only in those who can withstand prolonged anaesthesia.

Surgery is not commonly carried out in those aged >50 years, for a number of reasons: in the older patient, lifestyle is often adapted well to the epilepsy and may be difficult to change; the risks of surgery may be greater; in the ageing brain the adverse consequences can be more severe; and the reduction in cerebral reserve can be more critical in older age groups. Age, however, is only one factor, and some elderly patients do spectacularly well after epilepsy surgery. The key assessment is the potential for quality-of-life gain, whatever the patient's age.

The risk of continuing epilepsy

Another consideration that weighs in the balance when deciding about epilepsy surgery is the risk of 'not operating' and thus consigning the person to ongoing epilepsy. In patients with continuing seizures, the epilepsy carries a variety of risks, which are described in an earlier section of this book (see pp. 76–81). From the perspective of epilepsy surgery, the following are the most important.

Accidents and death

Epilepsy carries a significant risk of accidents and even of death (see pp. 76–78). These risks are greatest in those with tonic–clonic seizures (unfortunately also the seizure type that responds generally less well to epilepsy surgery). The risk of death due largely to sudden unexpected death in epilepsy (SUDEP) in patients who undergo presurgical evaluation, but who do not have surgery or are waiting for surgery, is about 1 per 100 cases per year.

Psychological and social consequences of epilepsy

Epilepsy has many adverse psychological and social consequences (described elsewhere in this book) and the loss of opportunity that continuing epilepsy presents, and the limitations and restrictions that it imposes, should not be underestimated.

Secondary epileptogenesis

In experimental animal models, 'kindling' and the development of mirror focus provide indisputable evidence of secondary epileptogenesis. It seems likely in humans too that the many physiological and chemical changes, and changes in gene expression, that occur in chronic epilepsy might well lead to a worsening of the epilepsy.

Progression of the disease

In some patients, medically refractory epilepsy (particularly partial epilepsy of limbic origin) produces progressive problems and mental deterioration – including psychiatric and behavioural change (including psychosis), cognitive deficit (especially on memory) and worsening seizures. Thankfully such a progression is uncommon, but if starting is another reason for the serious consideration of surgical therapy. In children, too, there is evidence to show that frequent seizures can interfere with normal growth and development of the immature brain.

The timing of epilepsy surgery

In recent years there has been a vogue for recommending surgery at an early stage in epilepsy, especially in children. This is to minimize the impact of the seizure disorder on education and social development, to minimize the potential for morbidity or death due to epileptic seizures, to prevent the possibility of secondary epileptogenesis (either through injury or 'kindling') and the possibility of progressive intellectual or behavioural decline, and to minimize the cognitive and psychological impact of epilepsy. Uncontrolled seizures also jeopardize the chance of an independent lifestyle, and children with intractable epilepsy are likely to be excluded from normal educational, social and vocational opportunities.

Approach to investigation

There are a number of investigatory modalities used in assessing suitability for epilepsy surgery: interictal scalp EEG, ictal scalp EEG, intracranial EEG, magnetoencephalography, MRI, neuropsychological tests and functional imaging with single photon emission computed tomography (SPECT), positron emission tomography (PET) and functional MRI (fMRI) (Table 10.2). The use of these should be protocol driven, and tests should be performed to answer specific questions. Their role and value depend on the type of surgery being performed (see below), but the following general points apply to all resective surgery and underpin investigation in all forms of epilepsy surgery.

Table 10.2 The approach to presurgical investigation taken at the National Hospital for Neurology and Neurosurgery, London.

Medical history and examination	All patients
Psychiatric assessment	All patients
24-channel scalp EEG (and review of previous EEG)	All patients
Seizure recordings using video-EEG telemetry	95% of patients
MRI at 1.5 T T1-weighted thin slice volumetric, T2 and FLAIR acquisitions	All patients
Regional measurement of hippocampal volume and of T2 signal intensity	All patients undergoing investigation with a view to hippocampal surgery; >50% of patients with extrahippocampal lesions to determine outcome and guide surgical planning
Other MRI techniques are used, selected from the following: MR angiography, diffusion imaging, perfusion imaging, MR spectroscopy, fMRI, three-dimensional reconstruction and rendering of the cortical surface, surface area/volume measurements. Co-registration with EEG, angiographic, SPECT or PET	All patients with normal MRI ('MRI-negative cases') being investigated with a view to resective surgery. In selected patients, techniques are selected to answer specific questions. MRS used mainly in hippocampal epilepsy, and other tests in extrahippocampal epilepsy. Use of diffusion scanning, perfusion scanning, surface area/volume measurements fMRI and fMRI–EEG is still confined largely to research
Other neuroimaging techniques (CT, plain skull radiography, angiography)	Selected patients
Neuropsychological assessment of general intellectual ability, language and memory	All patients
Other neuropsychological tests	Selected patients to address specific questions. Used mainly in extrahippocampal epilepsy
Sodium amytal test	10% of patients (see text for indications)
Intracranial EEG	15% of patients (see text for indications)
Functional imaging using HMPAO–SPECT or ^{18}FDG-PET	15% of patients (see text for indications)
Other functional imaging investigations (ligand or receptor PET, MEG, SISCOM), TMS	Use still confined largely to research
Individual counselling	All patients

See text for abbreviations.

The concept of the epileptogenic zone

The approach to resective surgery for epilepsy can, since the time of Horsley, be summarized as follows: in many cases of epilepsy, the seizures originate in a small area of brain (the epileptic focus), and surgery aims to resect this epileptogenic tissue, sufficient in extent to lead to the resolution of the seizures. Unfortunately, this is a simplistic view – a phrenological approach to brain function – and often patently incorrect. A clear-cut and restricted 'focus' of epileptic brain tissue does exist in some cases, particularly in epilepsy due to small extratemporal neocortical lesions. However, many seizures are in fact sustained by quite widespread and complex neuronal networks and circuits. In such cases, the concept of a discrete focus is both naïve and untenable.

It is as a response to this problem that the concept of the epileptogenic zone has gained currency, but this concept is also fraught with difficulty and inconsistency. This term is defined as the anatomical area necessary for initiating seizures and the removal or disconnection of which results in the abolition of seizures. The presurgical evaluation of a patient, therefore (it is argued), aims to define the anatomical boundaries of the epileptogenic zone and, having done so, the feasibility and risks of resection.

Unfortunately, there are no preoperative clinical or laboratory tests that can totally reliably define the area in any individual patient. It is only possible to ascertain whether an 'epileptogenic zone' was successfully resected after years of postoperative freedom from seizures – and even then without knowing how much unnecessary resection of additional brain tissue was carried out. The concept of the 'epileptogenic zone' is therefore a circular one dependent on retrospective assessment; this is unsatisfactory, and in the author's opinion, adds little to that of the epileptic focus. The concept, however, has one virtue – it emphasizes what has been known for more than half a century, that the amount of brain resection necessary often extends beyond the lesion visualized on neuroimaging.

This latter area is often known as the irritative zone. The irritative zone can also, conversely, extend beyond the epileptogenic zone, and it is common for residual tissue left after surgery to exhibit active spiking on electrocorticography (ECoG). Furthermore, the apparent extent of the irritative zone will vary with different types of EEG investigation.

On ictal recordings the electrographic onset of a seizure is sometimes known as the ictal onset zone. This area provides a rough indication of where to target surgery, but again its value depends on the extent to which the epileptic network is localized, or more diffuse, and its detection is highly dependent on the method of investigation employed.

It has been shown pragmatically that the incomplete resection of structurally abnormal areas of brain tissue often fails to control seizures, but even complete excision does not always result in seizure control. The chance of success depends on the aetiology of the lesion – the resection of most types of cortical dysplasia, for example, has a much lower success rate than that of mesial temporal sclerosis. The reasons are complex. Subtle anatomical changes may be present beyond the resolution of neuroimaging. Also, complex neuronal networks can spread well beyond the anatomical or even pathological defects.

The complexity of seizure generation is well demonstrated in mesial temporal lobe epilepsy. Here there is good experimental and clinical evidence that the seizures involve a network that extends well beyond the mesial temporal lobe, yet resection of the hippocampus, which will remove only part of this network, is often successful in controlling seizures (although auras often remain – further evidence that the 'focus' of the epilepsy cannot be simply the abnormal hippocampus). Furthermore, the presence of residual spiking in the brain tissue adjacent to the resection (detected on peroperative ECoG) is not predictive of surgical outcome, and many patients with residual spiking will be rendered completely seizure free.

In contrast to the situation in mesial temporal lobe epilepsy where restricted resections are often adequate, in neocortical areas, the bigger the resection the more likely is seizure control (a 'more is better' surgical approach proposed many times since the introduction of epilepsy surgery). Nevertheless, even in apparently well-localized, non-lesional, frontal epilepsy, resection of large areas of frontal cortex will stop seizures in only a relatively small proportion of patients.

The principle of concordance of investigations

An observation fundamental to presurgical assessment is that resective surgery is more likely to be successful if the findings from the different modalities of presurgical investigations are concordant, i.e. if each points to a similar localization of the epilepsy. Conversely, if results are discordant, resective surgery is likely to be less successful. It follows that all patients require multimodal investigation aimed at defining the seizure localization. This is of course a highly simplistic concept, laughable at a theoretical level, but one in practice that has clinical utility. There are four main components of investigation – radiological, neurophysiological, psychological and clinical. Different centres use different methods of investigation in these four areas (see below), and attribute different weight to the findings, but all four modalities should be carried out in most patients being worked up for surgery. It follows also that incomplete or unfocused investigation has a higher failure rate. It is for these reasons that presurgical evaluation is best carried out in a designated centre with multidisciplinary experience.

The importance of aetiology

As pointed out above, a key determinant of surgical outcome, independent of electroclinical localization, is the underlying aetiology. This is why MRI has proved so important in the surgical work-up. Indeed, because of this, MRI should be the starting point of all investigations. Resective surgery is best for those with well-localized lesions shown on MRI, especially those with unilateral mesial temporal lobe sclerosis, small cavernomas, or benign or low-grade tumours. The demonstration of aetiology is also of prognostic importance in other types of surgery, e.g. for hemispherectomy and corpus callosectomy.

MRI as a screening test and MRI-negative cases

Before the introduction of MRI many cases of epilepsy (including virtually all cases of hippocampal sclerosis) were 'non-lesional', in the sense that no lesion could be detected preoperatively. The nature and extent of the surgery in these cases depended on clinicoelectrographic localization, and thus on scalp and invasive EEG. It was realized even then that, if no pathology was found in the pathological examination of the excised specimen, the prognosis for seizure control was likely to be poor.

The advent of MRI has radically altered the clinical approach, because preoperative MRI can identify most structural lesions, including many that are hidden from other modalities. The total dependency on EEG for localization has been lost, and the requirement for invasive EEG has been reduced. It has been shown that, if MRI shows no lesion preoperatively, a so-called MRI-negative epilepsy, the chances of successful surgery are diminished, even after intensive work-up using other modalities. In routine practice, therefore, MRI has become in effect a screening test for further surgical evaluation and has now displaced EEG in this role. The question of surgery in MRI-negative cases is discussed further below.

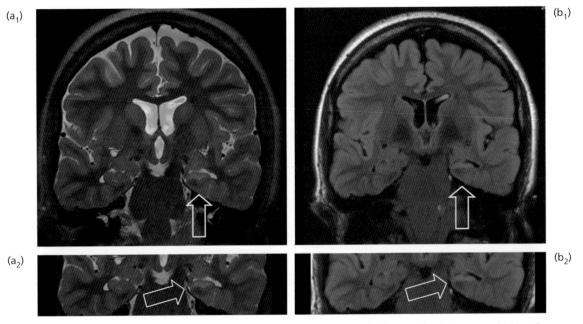

Figure 10.1 A typical example of unilateral left MTS, showing a loss of hippocampal volume, a signal increase and a loss of internal anatomical structure on the pathological side. (a1) and (a2), STIR; (b1) and (b2), FLAIR.

Surgery in epilepsy arising in the mesial temporal lobe

Pathology of mesial temporal lobe epilepsy

The most common pathology causing temporal lobe epilepsy (TLE) is hippocampal sclerosis (more accurately known as mesial temporal sclerosis).

The pathophysiology of hippocampal sclerosis, and the potentially causative role of febrile seizures in early childhood, is described on pp. 54–55.

Mesial TLE can also be caused by tumours (in about 10–15% of all cases of surgically treated mesial temporal lobe epilepsy). The most common are low-grade gliomas, oligodendrogliomas and other astrocytic or glial tumours. Cortical dysplasia of various types is also associated with hippocampal sclerosis, even if the dysplasia does not seemingly itself involve the hippocampus. This accounts for a further 15–25% of cases. Trauma, cavernous haemangioma (cavernoma) and other vascular disease, and cerebral infections (meningitis or encephalitis) can also result in TLE. The last two categories carry a generally poorer surgical prognosis by virtue of the more widespread and often bitemporal epileptogenic changes.

Which patients should be evaluated?

The general rules mentioned above apply. Usually, a patient will be referred with a history of temporal lobe seizures and MRI showing a hippocampal lesion (most commonly hippocampal sclerosis). The process of preoperative evaluation should follow the following standard protocol.

Clinical history and examination

A detailed history of the seizure disorder, its prior treatment and its causation must be obtained. Hippocampal sclerosis usually causes simple and complex partial seizures of mesial temporal lobe type (see pp. 13–15). Additional secondary generalized tonic–clonic seizures are typically absent or infrequent, and indeed a history of secondarily generalized seizures is associated with poorer outcome after temporal lobe surgery. Other seizure types are not to be expected in hippocampal epilepsy, and their presence indicates an epileptogenic zone that extends beyond the mesial temporal lobe structures. A history of childhood febrile convulsions (especially if prolonged or focal) is very strongly associated with hippocampal sclerosis. The outcome of hippocampal surgery is better if such a history is present (and that of surgery for extrahippocampal epilepsy is worse). The presence of a family history was initially thought to worsen surgical outcome, but recent study has thrown doubt on this.

A detailed epilepsy history should include the aspects listed in Table 10.3. The aetiology of the epilepsy can often be ascertained from the history and enquiry should be directed towards this. The clinical history may provide clues to the localization, and discordance between the clinical and investigatory localization should warn against surgery (Table 10.4).

There are usually no signs on clinical examination, and indeed, if motor or cognitive signs (other than memory defects – see below) are present, this implies extrahippocampal damage. The examination should be meticulously recorded to document preoperative deficit as a baseline for comparison with postoperative findings.

The patient's medical status and general suitability for a long anaesthetic and intracranial surgery should be assessed.

Psychiatric assessment

A detailed neuropsychiatric evaluation is a vital part of the presurgical assessment and should be carried out routinely in the early stages of the assessment process. The structured clinical interview schedule can be backed up by the use of rating scales which might include: Neurobehavioural Inventory, State–Trait Anxiety Inventory, Beck Depression Inventory, Subjective Handicap of Epilepsy Scale, Quality of Life in Epilepsy

Table 10.3 The epilepsy history.

The observable features of the seizures
The aura and seizure manifestations as experienced by the patient
Postictal features
Lateralizing features
Seizure precipitants
Temporal evolution of the seizures and their pattern over time
Seizure frequency and timing
Family history
Treatment history and response to individual therapies

Table 10.4 Clinical ictal features that predict side of seizure onset.

Ictal feature	Side of onset
Common signs that are reliable	
Unilateral dystonic or tonic posturing	Contralateral to seizure onset
Unilateral automatisms	Ipsilateral to seizure onset
Clonic jerks	Contralateral to seizure onset
Ictal speech	Seizure onset in non-dominant hemisphere
Postictal dysphasia	Seizure onset in dominant hemisphere
Postictal hemiparesis (Todd paresis)	Contralateral to seizure onset
Less reliable (or rare) signs	
Ictal blinking[a]	Ipsilateral to seizure onset
Ictal spitting[a]	Seizure onset in non-dominant hemisphere
Postictal nose wiping[a]	Ipsilateral to seizure onset
Head turning at onset of seizure (non-forced version)	Ipsilateral to seizure onset
Forced head version before secondary generalization	Contralateral to seizure onset
Ictal vomiting[a,b]	Seizure onset in non-dominant hemisphere

[a]Uncommon occurrences, where reliability is uncertain.
[b]Applies to ictal vomiting, which is rare, but not to postictal vomiting, which is common.

Scale, and the Minnesota Multiphasic Personality Inventory. The evaluation has four purposes:

1 To identify the presence of psychiatric contraindications to surgery. Usually, surgery should not be performed in patients with ongoing interictal psychosis or a history of interictal psychosis, severe personality disorder or psychopathy, co-morbid non-epileptic seizures, or ongoing alcohol or drug abuse. Peri-ictal psychosis is often considered to be a factor weighing on the side of epilepsy surgery, although outcome is not always good in the author's experience. A history of severe depression or obsessive–compulsive disorder is also a relative contraindication to surgery.

2 To estimate the ability of the person to withstand the long process of surgical evaluation and any adverse consequences of surgery. Psychosocial and family support

is often needed postoperatively, and surgery should not be offered to vulnerable individuals in the absence of such support.

3 To confirm that the patient is able to provide informed consent for the procedure and is able to understand the potential risks and benefits of surgery and is able to evaluate these.

4 To estimate the potential for psychological and psychiatric quality-of-life gains postoperatively, if seizure control is achieved. This requires judgement and experience, and the epilepsy rating scales can be helpful adjuncts. The patient should be encouraged to focus on this issue.

Psychiatry is, however, not an exact science, and the predictive value of premorbid psychiatric features is not fully established. This is a crucial deficiency, and high-quality research data in this area are largely lacking.

Magnetic resonance imaging

MRI is undertaken in all patients undergoing evaluation for TLE surgery (Table 10.5). Indeed, it is now the primary screening test for entry into a programme of presurgical evaluation. The imaging must be of an appropriate quality and tailored to the visualization of mesial temporal pathologies. Substandard MRI, for example, with wide inter-slice intervals or sequences with poor grey–white differentiation, frequently fails to detect hippocampal sclerosis, which is then shown on better targeted imaging. For presurgical assessment in our own unit, the minimum MRI dataset applied, using high-quality 1.5-tesla scanning, is as follows:

• A volume acquisition T1-weighted coronal dataset that covers the whole brain in slices of 1.0 or 1.5 mm thickness (a sequence that provides approximately cubic voxels which can be used for reformatting in any orientation, quantitation of hippocampal volume and other morphological measures, three-dimensional reconstruction and surface rendering)

• An oblique inversion recovery sequence, heavily T1 weighted and oriented perpendicularly to the long axis of the hippocampus (a sequence that provides good hippocampal anatomical definition and contrast)

• An oblique T2-weighted sequence oriented perpendicularly to the long axis of the hippocampus (a sequence that provides the basis for regional hippocampal T2 intensity measurement)

• FLAIR (fluid attenuation inversion recovery) or fast-FLAIR (sequences that increase the sensitivity of MRI to hippocampal sclerosis and other lesions).

Table 10.5 MRI techniques in assessing temporal lobe epilepsy.

Technique	Objective	Comment
Structural MRI	For assessing anatomy and detecting structure lesions	Enormous value. Fully validated. Sensitivity varies with magnet strength and sequences (see text)
Structural MRI	For determining pathological nature of lesion	Valuable, but not infallible
MR angiography	For assessing vasculature in arteriovenous and venous anomalies	Validated but generally less sensitive that conventional angiography
Diffusion imaging, perfusion imaging	For assessing lesional size and nature	Of limited value in assessment of temporal lobe epilepsy (and note that seizure activity can be mistaken for a structural abnormality)
MR spectroscopy	For assessing nature of lesion	Generally of very limited usefulness in temporal lobe epilepsy
MR tractography	For assessing position of major white matter tracts	Unvalidated and of very limited use in temporal lobe epilepsy. Can help predict the risk of a visual field defect after surgery
Co-registered MRI and EEG	For localizing spike discharges	Unvalidated. Of little utility in temporal lobe epilepsy
Functional MRI,	For localizing function	Value in lateralizing (but not localizing) speech function. Memory function may be possible to assess in the future
Three-dimensional reconstruction and rendering of the cortical surface	For detecting subtle cortical dysplasia	Claims made in the past have not been substantiated
Surface area and volume measurements of other brain structures	For assessing extent of abnormalities	Unvalidated as a method of assessing extent of epileptogenic zone and predicting surgical outcome

This MRI approach can demonstrate hippocampal sclerosis with high specificity and sensitivity (Figure 10.2). The primary MRI signs of hippocampal sclerosis are loss of volume on T1-weighted imaging and increased T2-weighted signal (the latter sign being less constant than the former). Other much less reliable signs are the loss of grey–white differentiation and loss of internal structure of the hippocampus. However, care must be taken not to misinterpret the MRI signs. On occasions, hippocampal atrophy is the result, not the cause, of epilepsy (e.g. after status epilepticus or in lesional cortical epilepsies). A swollen hippocampus on one side due to tumour can lead to the mistaken diagnosis of an atrophic contralateral hippocampus. Increased hippocampal T2 signal is a relatively non-specific sign that occurs also in patients with hippocampal tumour, vascular or developmental abnormalities, and in traumatic or postinfective lesions. Seizure activity, during or immediately before the scan, can occasionally also produce transiently increased T2 signal. In addition, in a sizeable number of patients, MRI will demonstrate more than one potentially causative lesion (so-called 'dual pathology' – see below).

Measurement of the volume of the hippocampus (hippocampal volumetry) and quantification of hippocampal T2 values are also routinely undertaken in patients being assessed for hippocampal surgery (Figure 10.3). These measurements provide objective information about the

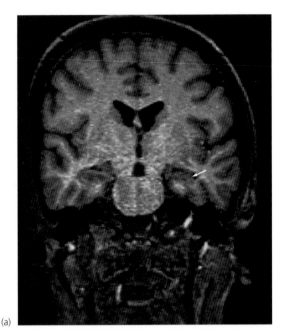
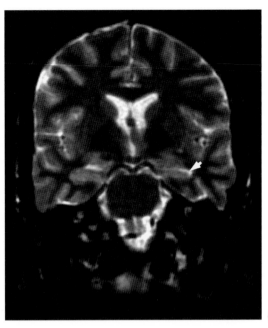

(a)　　　　　　　　　　　　　　　　　　　　　　　　　　　　　　　　　　　　　(b)

Figure 10.2 MRI in temporal lobe epilepsy, showing: (a) left-sided hippocampal atrophy (arrowed), with low intensity within the hippocampus on T1-weighted image. (b) T2-weighted image at same location reveals minor signal-intensity increase of hippocampus on left (arrowed). It is interesting to note in this case that there are only relatively subtle T2-weighted changes despite atrophy of >50% on volumetry.

severity of the hippocampal sclerosis and the detection of bilateral damage.

Hippocampal volumetry is also used in many patients with extrahippocampal lesions, because coexisting hippocampal atrophy worsens the prognosis in extrahippocampal lesional epilepsy and assists in deciding whether to include hippocampal resection during extrahippocampal surgery.

Scanning at 3 T is now also widely available, and arguably can increase the perspicacity of hippocampal lesions, via different sequences (e.g. the Propeller sequence). There is, however, with increased magnet strength, the risk of over-interpretation and the attribution of abnormality where none actually exists. This seems to be a particular problem in the interpretation of epilepsy MRI, not helped by lack of control data and also the inability to differentiate casual from consequential lesions.

Other techniques are used in selected cases (Table 10.5). Each is designed to address a particular issues, and interpretation of the tests requires a good understanding of the clinical context. The importance of tailoring the MRI examination to address specific questions cannot be overemphasized, and in this sense MRI differs from CT. However, it must also be recognized that most techniques are still in the research phase, and with the exceptions of structural MRI and angiography have not been validated in terms of specificity or sensitivity or predictive value.

Other forms of neuroimaging

CT still has a role in detecting small calcified lesions (e.g. small low-grade tumours in cysticrosis) which can be overlooked on MRI, and also where MRI is contraindicated (e.g. patients with pacemakers, aneurysm clips, metal plates, other metal implants). MRI is relatively (but not absolutely) contraindicated in patients with vagal nerve stimulators, but CT can be safely used. Plain skull radiography is now largely redundant. Conventional angiography is still used, mainly to determine the anatomical features of blood supply to vascular malformations and venous malformations, MR angiography is also used to determine the position of the major vessels before depth electrode placement. The angiographic findings can be co-registered with other neuroimaging techniques to guide the positioning of electrodes.

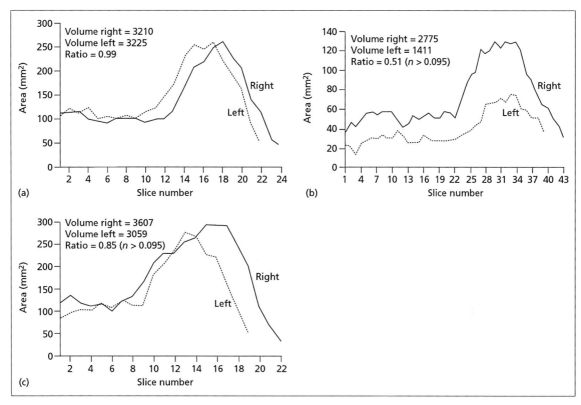

Figure 10.3 Three graphs showing regional hippocampal volume measure on the MRI. In the graphs, the cross-sectional areas of the hippocampus are measured from successive slices of volumetric T1-weighted coronal MR images of the hippocampus covering the whole anterior to posterior extent of the hippocampus and amygdala. The MRI slices are spaced 1.5 mm apart. (a) Normal hippocampus; (b) gross generalized hippocampal atrophy; (c) focal anterior hippocampal atrophy.

Interictal scalp EEG

The interictal scalp EEG was, before MRI and video-telemetry, the gold standard test for identifying candidates for temporal lobectomy – and as far as can be judged because, of course, the range of patients being operated upon has changed, the outcome of surgery in those days was not significantly inferior to that of today. The presence of anterior or mid-temporal spikes (or other epileptiform abnormalities) is common in TLE, and an important element of 'concordance' (Figure 10.4).

Unilateral interictal spikes

When these are present, and when the MRI shows hippocampal atrophy and other tests are concordant, the interictal EEG provides almost as much information of the ictal recording, and many authorities doubt that ictal recording (long-term recording) is necessary in this situation. This is important, because avoiding

EEG-telemetry would greatly simplify and render less costly the process of presurgical evaluation. Furthermore, concordance of MRI and interictal EEG predicts surgical outcome after temporal lobectomy. In one series, 84 patients with unilateral hippocampal atrophy who underwent temporal lobectomy showed an excellent outcome (92% seizure free or virtually seizure free at 24 months) even if ictal recordings were discordant or non-localizing.

In other situations, however, anterior temporal interictal abnormalities can be falsely localizing and can occur in foci in lateral temporal and frontal, parietal and occipital regions. Thus, ictal recordings still remain necessary in most cases undergoing epilepsy surgery evaluations.

Bilateral independent interictal spikes

Some cases of unilateral TLE exhibit bilateral independent temporal spike on the interictal EEG. If 80% or

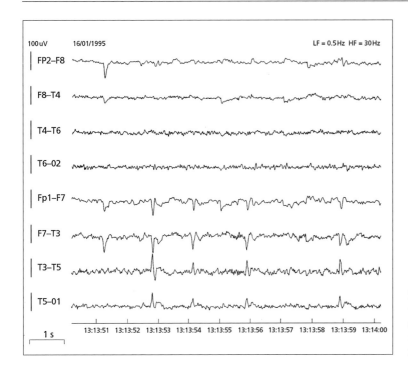

Figure 10.4 EEG showing lateralized temporal sharp waves with phase reversal seen in the left mid-temporal region (T3). This is a common interictal finding in mesial temporal lobe epilepsy.

more of the spikes are on the atrophic side, epilepsy can be reliably assumed to be arising in the atrophic hippocampus and the surgical outcome after resection is significantly better than in cases with less than 90% preponderance.

Focal slow activity

Lateralized temporal delta activity was found to have a similar lateralizing value to temporal spikes in a group of 141 patients who had undergone temporal lobe resection and whose MR scans were normal or showed mesial temporal lobe sclerosis. In this study, lateralized slow activity had a favourable surgical outcome regardless of the laterality or topography of spikes and other 'epileptiform' patterns. Temporal intermittent rhythmic delta activity (TIRDA) is also highly predictive of unilateral TLE.

Ictal scalp EEG and video-EEG telemetry

The ictal scalp EEG recording of a complex partial seizure remains a fundamental part of the presurgical evaluation. Long recordings are usually performed with concurrent video (video-EEG telemetry). To catch seizures, recordings may need to be continued for days or even weeks. In unilateral hippocampal sclerosis, a clear-cut ictal unilateral temporal/sphenoidal rhythmic discharge of 5 Hz

or faster within the first 30 s of the ictal recording occurs in about 50–60% of patients (Figure 10.5), and this is reliably localizing in about 90% of these cases (thus, in a small number of cases, the ictal EEG mislocalizes the epilepsy, owing to rapid undetected contralateral propagation, which is important not to forget). About 30% of patients show no lateralizing or localizing features in the scalp ictal recordings. Similar figures apply to other mesial temporal lesions (e.g. cavernoma, glioma and dysembryoplastic neuroepithelial tumour [DNET]).

Typically, the EEG in seizures in mesial temporal epilepsy exhibit rhythmic activity, distinct from the background rhythms, which increases in frequency with simultaneous development of phase reversals across the anterior temporal electrodes and then postictal δ slowing in the same region. In a study of 706 seizures in 110 patients, the presence of ≥5 Hz unilateral temporal/sphenoidal rhythm within the first 30 s in 57 patients correctly predicted an ipsilateral temporal depth onset in 82% of cases. The seizure pattern in lateral temporal or extratemporal seizures is somewhat different (see below).

Video-telemetry allows detailed scrutiny of the clinical features of the seizure, and certain signs are reliable indicators of the side of onset of the seizure (Table 10.4). In one study, unilateral clonic jerks or dystonic or tonic

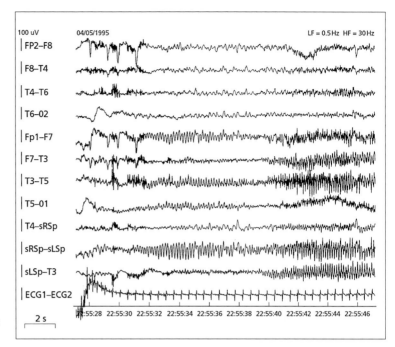

Figure 10.5 EEG showing typical temporal lobe seizure with rhythmic lateralized epileptiform activity in the left temporal leads.

posturing was a strong lateralizing sign of a contralateral epileptic focus (predictive value between 86% and 100%), unilateral automatisms predicted an ipsilateral seizure focus in 80% of patients and ictal speech preservation indicated seizure focus in the non-dominant hemisphere in 80%. Other signs are less reliable, such as ictal spitting, vomiting, unilateral eye blinking and nose wiping. Postictal hemiparesis or dysphasia is a reliable sign. Clinical signs in 262 seizures recorded in 59 patients with TLE lateralized 46% of seizures. The combination of ictal scalp EEG with ictal behaviour lateralized 80% of seizures in 95% of patients (95%), and the combined lateralization was concordant with the side of operation in 33 of 34 patients with a good postoperative outcome.

About 5% of patients with TLE show additional generalized spike-and-slow-wave discharges. These imply a genetically lowered seizure threshold, and their presence worsens postsurgical outcome.

Intracranial ictal EEG in TLE

In some centres, intracranial EEG recordings used to be carried out on almost all patients with TLE being evaluated for epilepsy surgery (Figures 10.6 and 10.7). With the advent of MRI this practice seems now to be obsolete in most cases; indeed in our unit it is applied in less than 10% of mesial temporal cases. Depth EEG does record

from otherwise functionally inaccessible cortex, but the EEG data come from only a small area around the electrode (≤1 cm core) and, unless the electrodes are placed logically to address specific questions, results can be misleading.

In the work-up for surgery of TLE, intracranial EEG is used in six main clinical situations:

1 To determine from which temporal lobe seizures are arising in patients with MRI evidence of bilateral hippocampal sclerosis (see below)

2 To determine the location of the seizure foci in patients in whom imaging shows 'dual pathology', and where the scalp EEG is inconclusive (see below)

3 To lateralize the seizure discharge in patients with discordant MRI and ictal or interictal EEG (see below)

4 To lateralize seizure onset in patients with a unilateral hippocampal lesion on MRI but where ictal scalp EEG suggests bilateral seizure onsets (see below)

5 In cases suggestive of mesial TLE, but with a normal MRI ('MRI-negative' cases – see below)

6 In lesional TLE, EEG is required only in the following circumstances:

  – non-localizing or discordant ictal scalp recordings

  – to assess the need to remove the hippocampus and mesial structures in patients with temporal lobe lesions adjacent to the mesial structures

– need for cortical stimulation for brain mapping with lesions overlying, or adjacent to, eloquent cortex

– in cortical dysplasia, to help define the epileptogenic zone.

Depth electrodes

Electrodes are usually placed bitemporally, and in other sites as determined by the questions being addressed. There is a 1–2% risk of haemorrhage or infection from each electrode placement, and the overall risk of the procedure increases with the number of electrodes inserted. There is no place for the insertion of multiple electrodes without a prior idea about the most likely sites of seizure onset and without tailoring the placement to the clinical questions being addressed.

In patients requiring depth EEG, a substantial number have findings that exclude surgery. Even where surgery can be offered, the chances of seizure freedom are often lower than in patients in whom depth EEG is not needed.

In other words, the yield of successful surgery is relatively small and it is important that this is fully appreciated before embarking on depth recordings.

Flexible rather than rigid depth electrodes are now generally used. They usually carry 4–18 contacts along their length, usually spaced 5–10 mm apart, and are made of MRI-compatible material (stainless steel, platinum or nichrome). They are usually inserted guided by frameless stereotaxy. In mesial TLE, the electrodes can be placed longitudinally (via an occipital insertion) but, due to risks of visual damage, most are now placed transversely through the lateral temporal lobe. Accuracy of placement is vital and precision is possible using modern computer-assisted MRI-based stereotaxy.

Risks of depth electrodes

Overall, in a retrospective survey of 115 patients, clinically significant complications occurred in 4.3% of patients.

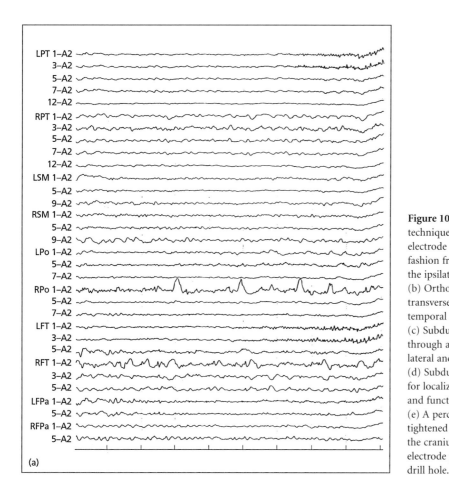

(a)

Figure 10.6 Diagrams of invasive EEG techniques: (a) longitudinal depth electrode inserted in an anteroposterior fashion from the occipital lobe toward the ipsilateral hippocampus.
(b) Orthogonal depth electrodes inserted transversely from lateral to medial temporal lobe at various locations.
(c) Subdural strip electrodes inserted through a temporal burr hole to study lateral and medial temporal neocortex.
(d) Subdural grid electrode implanted for localization of the epileptogenic zone and functional topographic mapping.
(e) A percutaneous epidural screw tightened into a twist drill hole through the cranium and an epidural peg electrode placed in another twist drill hole.

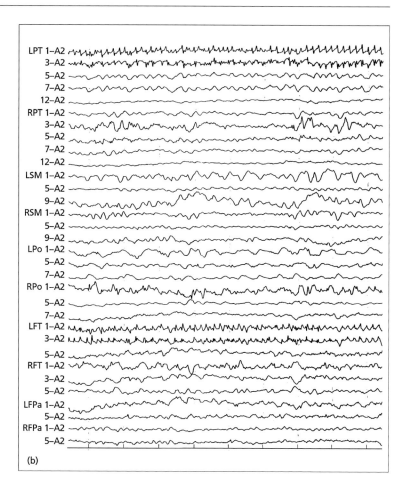

Figure 10.6 *Continued*

The risk includes haemorrhage, and a clinically significant haemorrhage occurs in 1–3% of electrode placements. The more electrodes placed, the greater the risk of haemorrhage. Some centres will not place electrodes in patients on valproate therapy because of the risk of haemorrhage.

Infection occurs in 0.5–5% of insertions and can sometimes prompt the early removal of electrodes. Infection is usually easily treated. Prophylactic antibiotic cover is sometimes given, but not routinely in most centres.

It is also of note that there have been reports in the literature of transmission of Creutzfeldt–Jakob disease through reused depth electrodes and, for this reason, single-use disposable electrodes are now used.

Pathological studies have shown gliosis, cystic degeneration and microbial abscesses after depth electrode placement. But none has shown any significant functional deficits caused by uncomplicated electrode placement. These included a detailed neuropsychometric study of depth electrode implantation into an unaffected hippocampus of the speech-dominant hemisphere, which shows no effect on verbal memory. Although microscopic haemorrhagic change is often seem pathologically along the track of a depth electrode, there is no evidence of epileptogenesis caused by depth electrode placement.

Other forms of invasive EEG

Sometimes depth electrode placement is combined with the implantation of subdural strips for seizures originating from mesial temporal lobe structures. The need for this depends on the clinical situation. The complication rate is higher, with greater risks of haemorrhage and meningitis. In one study, permanent neurological complications occurred in 0.7% and transient complications in 2.9%, in 279 invasive diagnostic

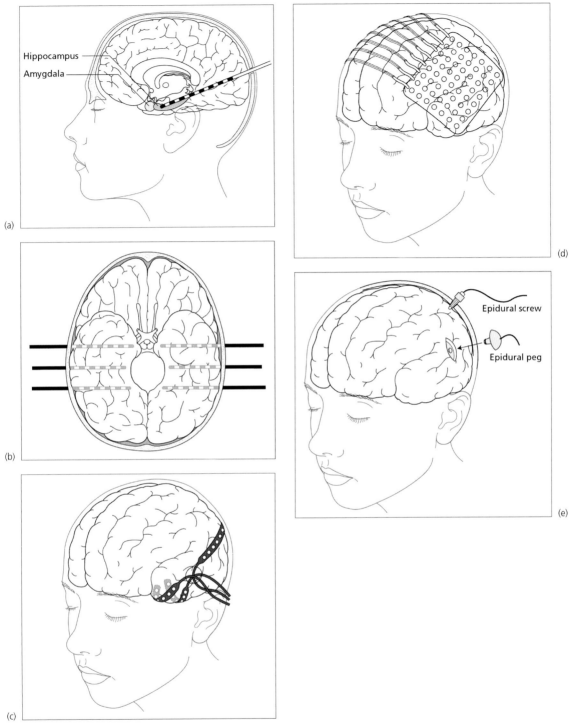

Figure 10.7 Depth EEG in temporal lobe epilepsy: one typical mesial temporal seizure onset pattern is seen in these continuous EEG segments as low-voltage fast discharge in LPT 1,3 (left depth electrode contacts at tip). Simultaneous seizure onset of similar morphology is identified in distal contacts of left temporal subdural strip (LFT 1,3) overlying the entorrhinal cortex. Electrode contacts are labelled from distal (1) to proximal. LPT, RPT, left and right hippocampal depth electrodes; LSM, RSM, supplementary motor subdural strips; LPo, RPo, LFT, RFT, LFPa, RFPa, left and right frontopolar, frontotemporal and frontoparietal subdural strips. Full scale, 1000 μV; each division, 1 s.

procedures using various combinations of strip, grid and depth electrodes. Others have found higher rates of complication, notably infection (in up to 15% of cases). In one study of 198 cases with subdural grid electrodes, complications occurred in 52 patients, including infection (12.1%), transient neurological deficit (11.1%), epidural haematoma (2.5%), increased intracranial pressure (2.5%) and infarction (1.5%). One patient died during grid insertion. Cerebrospinal fluid (CSF) leaks are another problem, occurring particularly in children.

Other forms of EEG used in evaluating TLE

Sphenoidal recordings, which were previously widely used, are now generally considered no better than recording from superficial sphenoidal electrodes, although they avoid the significant morbidity of sphenoidal electrode placement (pain, infection, bruising).

Foramen ovale electrode placement, in which the electrode tip is inserted through the foramen ovale to lie medial to the hippocampus, is a form of extracerebral intracranial electrode placement. It is a straightforward technique and does not require a craniotomy or stereotactic equipment. However, this technique is now rarely employed because it has a significant complication rate, including facial pain, meningitis and vascular damage to the brain stem. There is probably little place for this in modern practice.

Common problems in assessing TLE

With high-quality MRI and EEG, certain specific issues worth are further comment:

Are ictal recordings always required?

In the past, it had been the rule that ictal recordings were required in all patients with TLE. Evidence now suggests that ictal recordings add little in one important category of patients with TLE: those with clear-cut MRI unilateral abnormalities, a concordant clinical history/psychometry, concordant lateralized interictal EEG and in whom there is no question of non-epileptic attacks. Thus, it is now current practice in some centres not to require ictal recordings in these patients. However, if there are any discordant or complicating features, seizures should be recorded.

Bilateral hippocampal sclerosis, demonstrated by MRI

Significant bilateral pathological changes, albeit asymmetrical, in hippocampal structures are found in at least a third of patients with hippocampal sclerosis. With the use of absolute volumetry and quantification of T2 measures, such bilateral sclerosis can now be detected radiographically. Bilateral changes occur most often in patients with a history of previous encephalitis or meningitis and, in such cases, seizures usually arise independently from both temporal lobes, and the chances of a good surgical outcome are poor. The presence of two clinical seizure types is even more suggestive of bilateral epileptogenesis. The scalp ictal and interictal EEGs are much less reliable in bilateral than in unilateral hippocampal sclerosis. One study reported discordant ictal scalp EEG lateralization in almost 20% of patients with asymmetrical bilateral hippocampal sclerosis. If surgery is to be considered, most patients with bilateral hippocampal sclerosis require depth EEG. With clear-cut bilateral hippocampal atrophy, even after invasive EEG, surgery is usually not feasible because of bilateral epileptogenesis and also because of the risks of surgery to memory function.

Bitemporal EEG changes

As emphasized above, in the absence of bilateral hippocampal abnormalities on MRI, bilateral interictal temporal spikes on scalp EEG do not necessarily indicate bilateral epileptogenesis or less good surgical outcome. Between 40% and 70% of patients with bilateral independent interictal spikes on scalp EEG have unilateral seizures on depth EEG.

In most centres, it is considered that patients with bitemporal independent interictal spikes on scalp EEG do not require depth EEG if the ratio of spikes over the affected side compared with the unaffected side is 8 : 1 or higher, and/or if surface recorded seizures arise over one temporal lobe and are concordant with MRI, neuropsychological and other data.

Conversely, bilateral ictal onsets on scalp EEG should be taken as strong evidence of bilateral temporal epileptogenesis. Depth EEG is required in these patients if temporal lobectomy is to be considered. The usual policy in this situation is to record five or more seizures. If 80% or more arise in one temporal lobe, surgery can be offered with a good chance of improvement (but with a small chance only of seizure freedom). Surgical outcome is good, particularly if other complementary tests strongly favour the resected side. It is also important to recognize that apparent bitemporal epileptogenesis may well be due to extratemporal seizure onset with bitemporal seizure spread. This is not infrequent in patients with parietal or occipital lobe epilepsies, in whom the onset of seizures may be difficult to identify on scalp EEG. Depth EEG with additional electrode placements may be helpful in this setting.

Hippocampal sclerosis with another pathology (dual pathology)

The term 'dual pathology' is used to define the presence of hippocampal atrophy and a second potentially epileptic pathology (dysplasia or tumour). Between 5% and 15% of patients with hippocampal sclerosis have evidence of additional pathology (mostly cortical dysplasia) and about 15% of extrahippocampal lesions have coincident hippocampal sclerosis (Figure 10.8). In one study hippocampal sclerosis was found in 30% of patients with porencephalic cysts, 20% of those with cortical dysgenesis, 9% of those with vascular abnormalities and 2% of those with tumours. These are important to diagnose, because hippocampal resection alone in the presence of additional pathologies has a generally poor outcome.

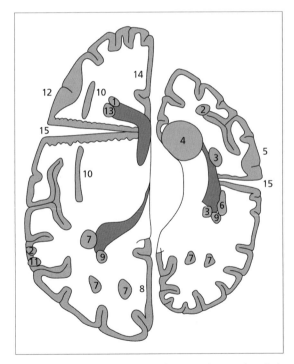

Figure 10.8 Diagram showing the location of areas of cortical dysgenesis in 15 patients with dual pathology from a series of 100 patients with hippocampal sclerosis (cases 1, 3, 4, 6, 9 and 13, subependymal heterotopia; cases 2 and 11, gyral abnormalities; case 8, focal cortical dysplasia; cases 5 and 12, macrogyria; cases 7 and 14, tuberous sclerosis; case 10, band heterotopia; case 15 schizencephaly).

Patients with dual pathology will often require invasive monitoring.

'MRI-negative' patients

A few patients are encountered with typical TLE in whom the MRI is normal. In such patients it is important to check that the MRI is of high enough quality, because poorly performed MRI will miss many cases of hippocampal sclerosis. Intensive EEG, including depth EEG, is almost always required in patients with normal MRI, but the fact of a normal MRI reduces the chance of a good surgical outcome, with perhaps 30% or less of patients becoming free from seizures even if invasive recording demonstrates apparently localized seizure onset. There may also be a place for PET and SPECT (see below), although, in MRI-negative adult TLE, these techniques alone are seldom sensitive enough to localize the onset of seizures.

Discordant MRI and ictal EEG

In occasional patients with hippocampal sclerosis demonstrable by MRI, the ictal EEG lateralizes to the contralateral side. In most of these cases, the EEG is falsely lateralizing (due, usually, to rapid undetected contralateral propagation) and, with concordant clinical and other data, resection of the MRI abnormality results in seizure control in most patients. This is particularly the case in patients with very severe hippocampal sclerosis ('burned-out' hippocampus). Currently, although resection of the MRI abnormality usually has a good outcome in terms of seizure control, invasive EEG is still advised.

Neuropsychology

Neuropsychometric evaluation is a vital part of presurgical assessment, and it is shocking to encounter patients in whom this has been omitted. In mesial TLE, the minimum battery includes measures of intelligence, frontal executive skills, memory, attention, visuospatial skills and language. The dominant (usually left) temporal lobe mediates memory for verbal material such as names, word lists, stories or number sequences, and the non-dominant (usually right) temporal lobe mediates memory for material that cannot be verbalized readily, such as faces, places, music or abstract designs. Bilateral lesions can cause global memory deficits. Core neuropsychology has two main functions:

1 To identify dysfunctioning cortex: if neuropsychological findings point to dysfunction that is discordant or more wide ranging than the damage seen on MRI or from the EEG findings, the epileptogenic zone may extend beyond the damaged hippocampus and the outcome of surgery will generally be unfavourable. Broadly speaking, an overall IQ <70 usually indicates widespread cerebral dysfunction and is a relative contraindication to surgery. A discrepancy between verbal and non-verbal memory and learning tests also indicates lateralized dysfunction, which should be concordant with the side of the hippocampal sclerosis.

2 To assess the risk of amnesia as a consequence of temporal lobe resection: the better the preoperative verbal memory or learning abilities, the worse will be the memory outcome after dominant temporal lobectomy. Conversely, a poor verbal memory does not usually worsen after surgery, because poor verbal memory preoperatively implies that hippocampal memory function is already damaged. A similar but less striking pattern is encountered with regard to non-verbal memory and the non-dominant temporal lobe. Bilateral hippocampal dysfunction should be suspected if both verbal and non-verbal memory tests are affected, and surgery in this situation carries the risk of severe amnesia, even if the preoperative memory scores are low on the side to be operated upon.

Intracarotid amytal test (Wada test, sodium amytal test)

This procedure consists of the intra-arterial injection of a fast-acting barbiturate (usually sodium amobarbital) into the internal carotid artery, usually through a groin catheter. This barbiturate is absorbed into the injected hemisphere and 'anaesthetizes' it for a short period of time (5–8 min). During this time, neuropsychological tests are performed to test the ability of the contralateral (unanaesthetized) hemisphere in isolation. The injection is then performed on the other side and the tests repeated. The injection is made by a radiologist who has performed an arterial angiogram before the test to verify that there is no serious vascular anomaly and to predict the drug distribution. In most institutions an EEG is performed during the test, to confirm the lateralized effect of the drug. The test is invasive, and carries a risk of inducing focal cerebral spasm and infarction in about 1 in 200 cases.

The neuropsychological tests applied are basic language and memory tests. The memory testing consists of showing new material while only one hemisphere is functional, and testing memory for that material later, when the drug effects have worn off and both hemispheres are back to baseline functioning. Speech tests are simple and usually include naming, serial or automatic speech.

The test has two main purposes:

1 To assess language dominance: this may be necessary in left-handed individuals, or in others if the routine psychological testing suggests that speech is lateralized unexpectedly, or is bilaterally represented – a not infrequent situation in epilepsy.

2 To confirm that resective surgery (imitated by the transient anaesthesia) will not result in severe memory disturbance. If a patient 'fails' the amytal, surgery is usually not carried out, on the basis that the risk of amnesia is too great.

Wada tests are also used in some centres for lateralizing seizure onset and for assessing the degree of postoperative memory loss. Their value in these situations is controversial.

In the past, the amytal test was performed in some centres on all patients being assessed for temporal lobe resection. However, in current practice, the test is increasingly being abandoned in favour of less invasive options. Functional MRI has already replaced the sodium amytal test to lateralize language dominance in uncomplicated cases, although, where language is bilaterally represented, fMRI is currently too inconsistent to be relied on. It is worth noting that, even in cases where fMRI can lateralize language, it cannot localize it, and fMRI is not currently sensitive enough to map language or to replace invasive cortical mapping for this purpose. Attempts are also being made to develop fMRI tests of memory function, although currently these are too unreliable for use for clinical purposes.

Finally, it is surprising to note that the predictive value of the amytal test for amnesia has never been formally validated, and there is an increasing feeling among psychologists that conventional neuropsychological testing provides reliable enough prediction without the need to resort to this test. Furthermore, the test–re-test reliability of the test, in the small number of patients who have repeat amytal tests, has been shown to be relatively poor.

Currently, amytal testing is used in about 5% of all cases being assessed for temporal lobe surgery in the author's own unit, and its use is reserved to identify risks of amnesia in patients who already demonstrate significant memory deficits and in whom neuropsychological findings are complex or contradictory, and to lateralize language in patients in whom atypical or bilateral representation is suspected.

Functional imaging using SPECT and PET

The use of functional imaging techniques varies from centre to centre, and there is little agreement about the necessity of these investigations in mesial temporal lobe surgery.

SPECT is the most commonly used and the most generally useful functional imaging method. Interictal SPECT can show low-perfusion areas in the temporal lobe, although the value of the test has been shown to be limited by a low sensitivity of 44% and a false-positive rate of 7%.

Ictal SPECT (obtained by injecting the ligand during a seizure) demonstrates hyperperfusion in the area of the epileptic focus. Certainly, perfusion changes do occur in mesial temporal lobe complex partial seizures and the pattern has been well studied. During the initial phases of the seizure the whole temporal lobe is hyperperfused, and in the immediate postictal phase the mesial temporal structures remain hyperperfused, although the lateral temporal structures are hypoperfused. Within 2–15 min postictally, there is hypoperfusion of the whole temporal lobe, and a return to normal is seen in 10–30 min. SPECT can demonstrate these changes, and the sensitivity of the test is said by some authorities to be as high as 97%. The sensitivity of ictal SPECT localization during simple partial seizures is much lower. Timing is obviously crucial and, if the injection is in the postictal period, false lateralizing results will be obtained. Also, ictal activity not infrequently switches sides during a seizure and, if this switch occurs early, there is the chance that the ictal SPECT would falsely lateralize the seizure, with the hyperperfusion reflecting the propagated activity.

A recent development has been the comparison of ictal and interictal SPECT signals, and the resulting 'subtraction ictal SPECT' can be co-registered to MRI (this method is known as SISCOM). Abnormalities demonstrated using this method have been shown to predict surgical outcome, but it is unclear how much this adds to more conventional investigatory methods in temporal lobe surgery.

The use of interictal 2-[^{18}F]fluoro-2-deoxyglucose PET (^{18}FDG-PET) for detecting temporal lobe seizure foci (which appear interictally as hypometabolic areas) has been well studied. The test has a sensitivity of 84% and a specificity of 86%, and it is interesting to note that the area of interictal hypoperfusion tends to be concordant with, but smaller than, the areas of hypermetabolism. Interictal ^{18}FDG-PET and ictal SPECT are both sensitive techniques for the detection of the epileptic focus, but ictal SPECT is probably more sensitive and specific than interictal ^{18}FDG-PET, easier to interpret and less expensive. For this reason, in most centres, PET is not routinely used, in TLE at least, although it can contribute to the investigation of patients with complex or discordant results on other modalities. Ictal PET is generally not feasible for practical reasons.

The outcome of mesial temporal lobe surgery
Seizure outcome

It is important not to take an over-optimistic view of temporal lobectomy, or to give the impression that the operation guarantees long-term seizure control (Table 10.6). The short-term outcome of temporal lobectomy has been carefully studied, but there is a lack of longer-term information (in spite of the fact that the operation has been performed now for over 50 years). At 1 year after surgery, in published studies, 'seizure freedom' rates have generally ranged between 50 and 80% (median 70%) and, at 5 years, rates have ranged between 50 and 70%. 'Seizure freedom' in these studies includes patients who continue to have auras (or other 'non-disabling' seizures) or seizures occurring only on drug withdrawal, and the rates for true 'complete seizure freedom' are lower. Furthermore, the quoted 5-year rates include patients who had been free from seizures for a year or more at the time of follow-up – only 50–55% of quoted patients had been seizure free for the whole of the 5-year period. Longer-term data are largely lacking, but one study showed a 7% drop – from 52% to 45% – in seizure freedom rates from 5 years to 10 years after surgery. The proportion of 'seizure-free' patients has increased by about 5–10% since the widespread use of MRI due to its impact on patient selection. If seizures are continuing at a point 12 months after surgery, the chance of remission in the next 5 years is only about 10%.

Table 10.6 Outcome of temporal lobectomy for hippocampal sclerosis.

Seizure outcome (%)	Seizure freedom	50–70
	Improvement	10–30
	No change	10–20
Mortality rate (%)	Operative mortality	0.5
	Late mortality	4
Morbidity rate (%)	Serious operative morbidity	<5
	Long-term physical morbidity (excluding hemianopia)[a]	<5
	Long-term psychiatric morbidity[a]	Not known

[a]See text.

A further 10–30% of patients, even if not completely free from seizures, achieve at least a 75% reduction in seizures in the year after surgery. The longer-term outcome of these patients has not been reported. Only 10–20% of patients do not experience any improvement after surgery, although in one series 18% of patients who had been operated on had at least monthly seizures at a point 5 years after the surgery.

Generalized tonic–clonic seizures occurring in the first few weeks after surgery are generally considered to be of little prognostic significance to the long-term outcome, and may reflect the acute trauma of surgery. Similarly partial seizures may continue for a few months and then fade away (so-called run-down seizures). About 1% of patients develop recurrent convulsive seizures several years after surgery. These seizures are probably due to the surgical procedure and are usually readily controlled medically, but it is important that patients are warned about this before surgery.

The factors predicting outcome have been studied in only an imprecise manner. Difficulties in studying this include the need for prolonged follow-up to determine outcome accurately, the variation in the battery of investigations and the criteria used to determine which patients are operated on. Moreover, many different outcome classification systems are used, some standardized, some idiosyncratic. The following are the only findings that were consistently made:
• In hippocampal sclerosis, the outcome of temporal lobectomy is best if there is a history of febrile seizures and the absence of a history of secondarily generalized seizures.
• In TLE, outcome is worse if the investigations are 'discordant' or if the MRI is normal.
• Aetiology is important and the outcome for surgery on hippocampal sclerosis is better than that on neuromigrational defects, central nervous system (CNS) infections or vascular lesions.
• Complete hippocampal resection has a better outcome than partial resection.

None of the other factors, including various clinical, EEG and investigatory features, have been shown to reliably predict outcome. Extensive atrophy on MRI in extrahippocampal regions (e.g. in the parahippocampal gyrus or temporal lobe) may, however, lead to a worse outcome after temporal lobectomy but this aspect needs further study.

Immediate neurological complications and morbidity

Temporal lobectomy has a number of potential complications. The most common neurological deficit is a superior quadrantanopia, due to damage to the optic radiation, which loops through the posterior temporal lobe. Published rates for any field defect have varied between 2 and 50%, but in recent years, with modified operations, a functionally significant field defect has been found in less than 5% of cases. This is an important complication from the driving point of view, and in the UK a visual field cut that exceeds 15° will prevent licensing.

The risk of hemiplegia after temporal lobe surgery is about 1–2%, and is usually due to damage to the anterior choroidal artery and the pial vessels that lie on the surface of the midbrain, mesial to the hippocampus. Selective hippocampectomy is a technically more difficult operation, and the risk of hemiplegia is slightly greater (up to 4%).

A transient mild dysphasia is not uncommon with dominant temporal lobe resections, and especially after invasive EEG, but a permanent dysphasia should occur in less than 1% of operated cases. Other risks of surgery include third nerve palsy, meningitis, bone or scalp infection, vascular spasm, subdural haematoma or empyema, cerebellar haemorrhage, acute hydrocephalus and pneumocephalus.

The overall risk of serious permanent neurological complications of temporal lobectomy (excluding quadrantanopia) in an experienced centre is of the order of 2–3%, and the mortality rate of surgery for temporal lobectomy for hippocampal sclerosis is less than 0.5%. These risks must be carefully explained to the patient before surgery, if possible in writing.

It should not be forgotten, however, that uncontrolled epilepsy itself carries greater potential risks, e.g. the annual mortality rate in people with severe intractable epilepsy is up to 1 per 100 and is particularly high in patients experiencing convulsive attacks. The mortality rate of the operation depends on aetiology, and resective surgery on large arteriovenous malformations (AVMs), for example, carries a significant mortality and morbidity.

Outcome in relation to memory

A temporal lobectomy involves the resection of much of the temporal lobe tissue thought to be involved in memory and learning – although it may not be an exaggeration to say that the mechanism and exact neural substrate of memory are almost totally unknown. It is not surprising therefore that postoperative memory deficits, detectable on neuropsychological testing, are common. What is perhaps more remarkable is that these are generally remarkably mild, and a marked deterioration in memory should be a rare complication if patients

Table 10.7 Factors influencing memory outcome after temporal lobe surgery for epilepsy.

Age	Poorer outcome after age of 50 years
Preoperative IQ	Patients with a higher IQ do less well
Preoperative memory deficits	The better the preoperative memory, the more likely a negative effect on functional memory
Dominant vs non-dominant resections	Dominant resections have a generally greater negative effect on functional memory than non-dominant resections
Unilateral hippocampal atrophy	The more atrophic the resected hippocampus, the less the effect resection has on memory
Bilateral hippocampal damage	Unilateral resections in the presence of bilateral hippocampal damage carry a significant risk of severe amnesia
Cortical dysplasia	Resections for cortical dysplasia have a poorer memory outcome than resections for hippocampal sclerosis
Extent of surgical resection	Large dominant resections may cause more deficits in memory than smaller dominant resections, but the evidence is conflicting
Seizure outcome after surgery	There is a better outcome in terms of memory function for those who are seizure free after surgery
Affect, attention, psychiatric status	These can greatly impact on memory function, and are often more important functionally than even moderate changes in psychometric test results

are prudently selected. Indeed, memory and intellectual function can actually improve after surgery owing presumably to better seizure control and the need for fewer antiepileptic drugs. A profound amnesia occurs in less than 1% of cases in modern practice. The memory defects after temporal lobectomy involve verbal memory and learning in dominant lobe (usually left-sided) surgery, and non-verbal memory and learning deficits in non-dominant lobe surgery. The former type of memory deficiency is much more noticeable in daily life than the latter, and can be the cause of more disability. The selective amygdalo-hippocampectomy was introduced to minimize memory disturbance, but in practice the rates of memory deficit seem to be broadly similar to those in more extensive surgery.

The underlying pathology, particularly the preoperative status of the hippocampus targeted for removal, is an important predictive factor. Hippocampal MRI volumetry is a vital test in this regard. In cases where there is unilateral hippocampal sclerosis with significant MRI volume loss, postsurgical memory deficit is usually minimal, perhaps because the target hippocampus is already so damaged that it performs little useful function in relation to memory. At the other extreme, if a normal

sized hippocampus is to be removed as an adjunct to lesionectomy, some loss in memory function is inevitable.

Lesional mesial temporal lobe surgery overall carries more risk to memory than surgery for hippocampal sclerosis. If the temporal lobe pathologies have been present since childhood, the risk of surgery to memory is also less, presumably as a result of brain plasticity and the reassignment of cerebral function away from the epileptic focus during the child's development. Resections of cortical dysplasia seem to have a worse memory outcome than resections of hippocampal sclerosis. Other factors influencing memory are shown in Table 10.7.

Psychiatric outcome

Postoperative psychiatric disturbance is perhaps the biggest risk after temporal lobe surgery. Epilepsy surgery is not usually considered to be a form of psychosurgery and thus does not require the complex oversight and careful ethical regulatory framework that govern surgery for psychological disorders. Nevertheless, in the author's opinion, careful and extensive counselling is vital about the potential psychiatric aspects, yet is often not provided.

Psychosis and depressive illness

Unfortunately, there is still uncertainty about the extent of this problem. In early series, the incidence of schizophreniform illness after temporal lobectomy was about 15%, but in recent studies the incidence of new psychosis after temporal lobe surgery is much lower – <5%. This is because a preoperative chronic psychosis is now usually considered a contraindication to temporal lobe surgery, whereas in the past surgery was carried out more often in psychotic patients (sometimes in the hope that the psychosis would improve). A depressive illness after surgery is more common, occurring in about 35% of patients in the first year after surgery. The rate may be higher after non-dominant resections. The rates of psychiatric disease are significantly higher in those who are not seizure free after surgery, and these patients – with postoperative seizures and psychotic illness – pose a grave problem for postoperative rehabilitation.

Other organic mental disorders

These are very poorly studied, and may well be quite common after temporal lobe surgery. Large resections of brain tissue will inevitably have psychological consequences, but the studies in TLE have been confined largely to memory, depression and psychoses. It is remarkable how little systematic study there has been of other effects, despite the fact that the limbic system subserves many aspects of emotional life. A range of potential organic mental disorders and psychological syndromes has been almost completely ignored and where there is information it is often anecdotal at best.

It is not uncommon to find changes in sexual function after temporal lobe surgery. At an anecdotal level, the most common change is diminution of libido and sometimes also male erectile dysfunction. More commonly described in the literature, but less common in practice, is the occurrence of sudden hypersexuality after temporal lobe surgery, which can on occasions result in serious social disturbance. An extreme example is the Klüver–Bucy syndrome, which is a consequence of temporal lobectomy where there is bilateral temporal lobe disease, and comprises hypersexuality, visual agnosia, strong orally directed tendencies, overeating and hypermetamorphosis.

Temporal lobectomy can also have a marked effect on emotional responses. It is not uncommon to hear a patient describe some degree of flattening of affect and lack of emotional colouring – and occasionally these effects can be severe. In one study, 'emotional–motivational blunting' was found in almost half of 53 temporal lobectomy patients in the first year after temporal lobe surgery. In another study, emotional disturbances of varying types occurred in 38.9% of 90 patients after temporal lobectomy. In a further study of 44 patients, temporal lobe surgery exacerbated the 'interictal dysphoric syndrome' in 39%. This is a frequently observable trait in patients with TLE comprising a constellation of symptoms including depression, anergia, irritability, pain, insomnia, euphoric mode, fear and anxiety.

A range of other psychiatric complications has been reported after epilepsy surgery, but almost all at an anecdotal level, and the extent of this problem is not well studied. In one retrospective chart review of 325 anterior temporal lobectomies and 125 extratemporal cases, 7 patients were found to have developed undifferentiated somatoform disorder after anterior temporal lobectomy, 1 patient pain and body dysmorphia, 1 patient another pain disorder and 1 patient body dysmorphia alone, but none was found after extratemporal surgeries. Nine of these ten cases followed a right anterior temporal lobectomy.

Reduced cerebral reserve

Another worrying prospect is that temporal lobe resection will reduce 'cerebral reserve' and thus render the patient susceptible to the development of psychological or cognitive decline in the longer term. Certainly, at an anecdotal level, a number of patients, years after a temporal lobectomy, undergo significant decline and develop a rather typical syndrome of increasing vagueness, circumstantiality, loss of social skills and loss of cognitive sharpness. There are no long-term studies in this area and this is a deficiency that needs to be addressed.

Psychosocial outcome

After successful surgery, a major readjustment is needed to a life without epilepsy. This can be difficult and painful, as is the realization that the problems of life are not automatically resolved. There is often a sense of anticlimax, at least in the first 12 months after surgery. Furthermore, if the operation fails, disappointment and depression are almost inevitable. Seizure freedom will not immediately reverse years of social isolation, a lack of self-confidence or a strong sense of identity, or missed educational or career opportunities. Becoming seizure free can alter interpersonal relationships, which might have been based on dependence or a 'sick role'. Appropriate preoperative counselling can help to prepare people, and in some cases a structured postoperative rehabilitation programme can be helpful.

However, when freedom from seizures is obtained, and where patients have been carefully selected, the temporal lobectomy can have an extraordinarily positive effect, allowing the patient, often for the first time, to engage in all aspects of life with confidence and unencumbered by the constant fear of seizures. This can be profoundly beneficial.

Different surgical approaches to temporal lobe surgery

As a result of the rate of complications, surgical techniques have been modified to try to avoid some of the adverse effects.

The standard temporal lobectomy extends for 4–5 cm behind the temporal pole in the dominant temporal lobe (Figure 10.9) and up to 6 cm in the non-dominant temporal lobe, sparing the posterior part of the superior temporal gyrus. Most of the hippocampus, the amygdala and some surrounding mesial structures are removed. Modified temporal lobectomies have also been devised, and in the most common type only 3 cm of the temporal tip is removed, providing good access to the amygdala and hippocampal formation, which are then resected in their entirety. This is now the most common operation performed.

The selective amygdalo-hippocampectomy can be carried out stereotactically (Figure 10.10) through the middle temporal gyrus or occipital cortex, or by an approach along the sylvian fissure. This preserves much of the lateral cortex. However, there is little convincing evidence that the selective amygdalo-hippocampectomy actually has a better outcome with regard to memory function or cognition and, as the surgery is technically more difficult to perform, the rates of vascular distur-

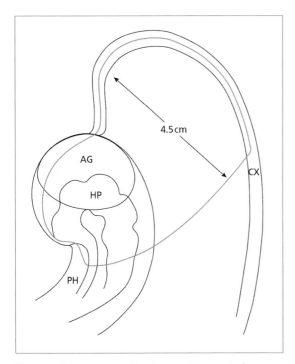

Figure 10.9 Diagram showing the operative extent of a standard temporal lobectomy. Transverse plane showing the habitual extent of temporal resections (cortical and limbic) in the dominant hemisphere. AG, amygdala; CX, neocortex; HP, hippocampus; PH, parahippocampus; grey line, extent of resection.

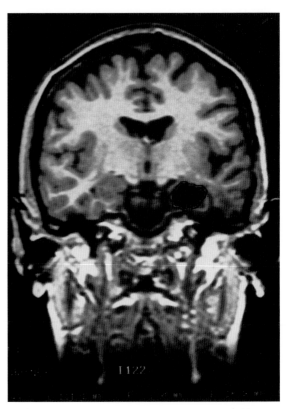

Figure 10.10 Postoperative MRI after stereotactic amygdalohippocampectomy via a lateral temporal neocortical approach. The coronal postoperative MR image demonstrates the focal mesial resection that is possible with this technique, while sacrificing the minimum of temporal lobe neocortex, and shows complete resection of the mesial temporal structures.

bance and hemiplegia are higher than in temporal lobectomy. The selective operations do have a lower risk of dysphasia or visual field defect. Furthermore, the rates of long-term seizure freedom, although not adequately studied, appear at an anecdotal level to be slightly less good than after standard or modified temporal lobectomy.

A recent development has been the use of radiosurgery with the gamma knife to ablate mesial temporal lobe structures, which is performed on an outpatient basis. Preliminary experience is promising, but anxieties remain about the risk of deterioration as a result of late progressive radiation-induced necrosis. Conflicting results are reported. In a European study of 21 patients given a dose of 24 Gy, 65% were seizure free at 2 years, and no serious long-term neurological deficits, apart from visual field deficits, were recorded. A report from the Cleveland Clinic of five patients treated with 20 Gy showed, however, that none achieved seizure freedom and all required subsequent surgery. Gamma knife surgery must at present be considered an experimental procedure, but shows promise and is likely to be increasingly used. The use of the 'proton pencil beam' is another technique currently in development.

Follow-up is essential of all patients after epilepsy surgery, and a protocol for follow-up is shown in Table 10.8.

Surgery in epilepsy arising in extratemporal regions and the temporal neocortex

The presurgical assessment of extratemporal epilepsies poses somewhat different problems to those of mesial

Table 10.8 Follow-up protocol for patients without complications after successful temporal lobe epilepsy surgery.

Neurosurgical follow-up	6 weeks, 1 year, and then annually
Neurological follow-up	3, 6, 9, 12 months, then annually
Psychiatry	1, 6, 12 months, and then annually
Psychology	3, 12 months
Field testing	6 months
MRI	3 months
Counselling	3, 12 months

This is based on the protocol used by the author.

TLE for a number of reasons. It is more difficult to define the boundary of the resection. In mesial TLE, a standard resection is carried out (usually of the hippocampus, parahippocampal gyrus, uncus and basolateral amygdala). In neocortical epilepsy, there is no such standard procedure. Each case has to be tailored to the individual epilepsy. MRI has made lesion detection relatively easy, but often the resections have to include more than just the lesion to terminate the seizures. Aetiology is, however, of paramount important and the outcome of surgery will depend more on the aetiology of the lesion than is the case in the surgery of mesial TLE. The lesions most commonly treated by epilepsy surgery are small, slow-growing or benign tumours, small AVMs and cavernomas. Large AVMs also cause epilepsy, but surgical therapy carries significant risks and should generally be avoided.

Aetiologies
Tumours

Epilepsy occurs in approximately 50% of patients with intracerebral neoplasms (see pp. 59–60); with a higher frequency in the more benign tumours – in the Montreal series, seizures occurred in 70% of patients with astrocytomas, in 92% of patients with oligodendrogliomas and in 37% of patients with glioblastomas. The surgical management of malignant, rapidly growing tumours depends on oncological factors rather than epilepsy. For small benign tumours, however, surgery is sometimes indicated with the primary aim of controlling epilepsy.

The primary aim of the treatment should be the complete removal of the lesion, but this is often not possible without causing neurological deficit, and much depends on the cerebral location of the lesion. If complete removal of the lesion cannot be achieved without added risk and morbidity, incomplete lesion removal may, albeit less often, provide satisfactory results. Many of the tumours associated with medically intractable epilepsy are indolent, with no tendency to progress, and in these cases adjuvant tumour therapy does not appear to be necessary.

The seizure outcome after surgery for tumours will depend on a number of different factors. The first is the pathological nature of the tumour. In the Montreal series of 108 patients with astrocytomas and other low-grade primary intracranial neoplasms, 70% became seizure free or had a marked reduction in seizures. Seizure control after surgery for malignant astrocytomas was much less good. The seizure outcome after resective surgery for gangliogliomas and DNETs was either complete or almost complete in 90% of patients. The extent of resection is another important factor and, if the lesion is complex and influenced by the pathology and the extent of the removal of a complete lesion, resection is associated with a much higher chance of a seizure-free outcome than incomplete removal of the lesion – the exception is for DNETs where incomplete resection is often very successful (presumably reflecting the fact that seizures are generated within the lesion, not around its perimeter). Surgical ECoG is sometimes carried out after lesion resection, and has some role in predicting outcome – patients with no post-resection spikes had a better prognosis than patients with residual spikes

Gliomas in patients presenting with epilepsy: the role of surgery and radiotherapy

Not uncommonly, gliomas are identified on CT or MRI in patients who have presented with new-onset seizures with no other neurological signs. The management of these cases crucially depends on the histological grade of the glioma. In patients aged <50 years, MRI is now sufficiently reliable to predict this with a >90% degree of accuracy (CT is less reliable), but the rate of diagnostic error on MRI and CT is greater in older patients. On MRI, low-grade gliomas (grades I and II) are generally non-enhancing whereas high-grade gliomas (grades III and IV) usually enhance markedly and have an irregular outline, necrotic centre and vasogenic oedema. However, low-grade gliomas have a strong tendency to 'transform' to become more malignant over time, sometimes after many years of quiescence. This transformation is unpredictable, and because of this the surgical management of low-grade tumours can be difficult and contentious.

The author's usual practice with regard to the management of an MRI-defined low-grade glioma presenting with epilepsy is as follows:
- In patients aged >50 years: biopsy is usually carried out (in view of the greater risk of diagnostic error).
- In patients aged <50 years in whom MRI suggests a low-grade glioma: biopsy with a view to resection is advised only if the tumour is small and in a location where resection is feasible. In other cases, biopsy and/or resection is usually deferred and the lesion is assessed by serial scanning – initially at 3 months and then at 6- and 12-monthly intervals. Serial scanning is continued as long as the MRI appearances to not change.
- In patients in whom new clinical signs develop, or in whom serial MRI shows changing size or new enhancement even in the absence of new signs, biopsy is advised, with a view to resection.

- When resection is performed, it should be as complete as possible without causing neurological deficit.
- Radiotherapy is usually reserved for those with evidence of malignant transformation, or occasionally in patients whose epilepsy is wholly intractable and in whom resection is not possible.
- The epilepsy is treated initially medically, along conventional lines. If the seizures persist or are severe enough to warrant surgical intervention, epilepsy surgery is considered (see below).

In patients with MRI findings suggestive of high-grade gliomas, and in all patients with increasing neurological signs and/or signs of increased intracranial pressure, urgent surgical referral with a view to tumour resection is advised. The resection should be as extensive as possible, and the surgery is usually followed by immediate radiotherapy. Adjunctive chemotherapy is sometimes advised in glioblastomas, and currently oral temozolomide is the most commonly used agent. More experimental approaches using biodegradable polymers containing carmustine (BCNU) inserted into the resection cavity are also under investigation.

In patients with gliomas, a multidisciplinary approach to treatment should be taken, with neurological, oncological and neurosurgical input. The patient should be fully involved in what are often difficult decisions, and fully informed of the potential risks and benefits of the various treatment options.

Benign tumours: the role of epilepsy surgery

The beneficial effect of epilepsy surgery in patients with medically refractory partial seizures associated with small benign tumours is well established. In well-selected cases, about 50–80% can expect to be seizure free after surgery, and seizures are reduced in most other cases. The outcome of the surgical treatment of tumoral epilepsy is influenced largely by the underlying pathology (often possible to determine only after surgery) and how complete the resection of the lesion is. Seizure-free rates of 70% or so are reported in patients with low-grade astrocytomas (completely resected) but rates are lower in more malignant tumours. Total excision of gangliogliomas and DNETs relieves seizures in 80% of cases. Seizure-free rates are generally less if the resection is incomplete, although this does not apply in the case of DNETs, in which epileptogenesis is often intrinsic to the tumour.

The necessity to investigate the extent of surrounding epileptogenicity in the resective surgery of tumours by EEG, where complete lesional resection is possible, has not been clearly established, but most patients undergo ancillary epilepsy-related investigations (see below). Exactly what these add to surgical outcome is, however, unclear, and in most cases extensive EEG or functional testing is not required. The main exception to this rule is the not uncommon situation in which extrahippocampal lesions are associated with hippocampal sclerosis, which occurs especially when the tumour is situated in the temporal lobe. Resection of the lesion alone in these cases has a lower chance of seizure control, and hippocampectomy is often carried out together with the lesionectomy. Hippocampal resection should generally not be performed if the hippocampus shows no radiological signs of atrophy, especially in the dominant temporal lobe, because resection of healthy hippocampal tissue is associated with a significant loss of memory skills. The other complications and outcome are similar to those in hippocampal sclerosis.

Hypothalamic hamartoma

The surgery of hypothalamic hamartoma also requires special mention. These lesions are a cause of severe epilepsy and characteristically of gelastic epilepsy (see pp. 59–60). The lesions are sometimes divided into two categories – parahypothalamic and intrahypothalamic – with precocious puberty and endocrine disturbance more prominent in the former and epilepsy in the latter. The lesions are intrinsically epileptogenic and it is for this reason that resective surgery may be particularly beneficial.

The detection of hypothalamic harmatomas requires carefully performed MRI. Large lesions are easily seen, but small lesions are often overlooked, particularly when confined to the tuber cinereum. High-quality T1-weighted images produce the best visualization, although the lesions are often isodense on T1- and T2-weighted images. The EEG is usually non-localizing, and has limited value.

Resective surgery or radiosurgery can be very effective. Overall, complete seizure remission can be expected in about 50% of cases (2-year follow-up) with improvement in another 35%. Early surgery also may prevent learning disability, behavioural disturbance and precocious puberty, as well as evolution into intractable epilepsy. Better results are obtained in smaller lesions. Surgical complications include severe endocrine disturbances and amnestic syndromes.

Various approaches have been attempted, including thermocoagulation, stereotactic (gamma knife) radiosurgery, and open or stereotactic resection via transcallosal and other approaches. The choice of procedure depends to some extent on the size and location of the lesion.

Surgical resection may be best for larger or pedunculated lesions. For lesions confined to the hypothalamus, stereotactic radiosurgery is probably the treatment of choice. Lesions expanding into the third ventricle, but limited to one side of the hypothalamus, can be resected via an endoscopic approach. The choice of approach ultimately depends on the experience of the surgeon.

Arteriovenous malformations

Epilepsy is the presenting symptom in 20–40% of cases of cerebral AVMs, and is present in over 60%. The effect on epilepsy of surgical resection of the AVM depends largely on its size and location.

The complete resection of a small AVM, particularly if sited in the temporal lobe, will frequently control seizures completely. However, the resection of large AVMs, which anyway is often incomplete, has little chance of controlling epilepsy and should not usually be performed for this purpose – indeed surgery for large AVMs carries significant risk and should generally be avoided where possible. Stereotactic radiosurgery is an accepted alternative therapy for small lesions in which the nidus measures <2.5–3 cm in diameter, particularly if located deep in the brain. This technique induces endothelial proliferation and ultimately causes obliteration of the lumen over a period of 1–2 years. Stereotactic radiosurgery is non-invasive and can be administered on an outpatient basis. The pathological changes induced by radiation, and thus also the clinical benefits, take months to develop. Studies have shown that stereotactic radiosurgery will obliterate all lesions with a diameter <2 cm within 3 years after treatment but only 50% of lesions with a diameter >2.5 cm. In open studies epilepsy has been shown to improve in over two-thirds of cases after radiosurgery, and seizures are improved even before complete occlusion of the nidus. In one series of 160 AVMs, 48 patients had epilepsy. At 2-year follow-up, 38% of these cases were seizure free, 22% had improved seizure control and 6% were worse.

Endovascular embolization is also available for the treatment of cerebral AVMs and increasingly is the preferred primary therapy for most AVMs. It can be used also as a prelude to surgery. However, it often does not achieve permanent obliteration of the malformation as a result of the high rate of recanalization. It can also induce acute haemodynamic changes in the treated region, and multiple procedures may be required to complete the treatment. The complication rate for this procedure has been estimated to be about a 1.5% risk of severe deficit, a 1–2% risk of death, a 10% risk of haemorrhage (including 3% first-time haemorrhage) and a 3% risk of new-onset seizures.

The seizure outcome after surgery for AVMs has differed in different series, but generally speaking seizures will remit or improve after successful AVM surgery in about 50%, and surgical treatment in some series, but not others, was no better in terms of seizure control than medical treatment. Seizure control after surgery is probably better in those with a short seizure history, those with generalized tonic–clonic rather than partial seizures, those with deep-seated locations and those in whom complete resection was possible. Radiotherapy may in itself improve epilepsy. There is also anecdotal evidence of markedly improved seizure control after gamma knife surgery for small AVMs, for example. Embolization as a treatment modality, excellent for the prevention of haemorrhage, is generally considered to have no effect on the frequency or severity of epilepsy due to AVMs.

Cavernous haemangiomas (cavernomas)

Cavernomas (see p. 65) are vascular malformations consisting of closely clustered enlarged capillary channels ('caverns') with a single layer of endothelium without normal intervening brain parenchyma or mature vessel wall elements, ranging in size from a few millimetres to several centimetres. The characteristic lesion on MRI is of mixed signal intensity with a central reticulated core, surrounded by a dark ring. The latter is presumed to be haemosiderin deposition from a prior haemorrhage (Figure 10.11).

There is a risk of haemorrhage from these lesions of between 0.5 and 2% per year. Thus, although the per-annum risk of haemorrhage is lower than that of AVMs, the cumulative lifetime risk for younger patients is not insubstantial. It is generally acknowledged that such a risk is higher for patients with documented previous haemorrhage. Haemorrhage is, however, under low pressure and often not as catastrophic as an arterial haemorrhage.

The effect of complete resection of a cavernoma on seizure control has been investigated by a number of authors. In a meta-analysis of retrospective surgical results of 268 supratentorial cavernous haemangiomas, it was found that 84% of patients were seizure free and 8% were improved, with no change in only 6% and 2% becoming worse. Of the 82% who were seizure free after surgery, 50% were not taking antiepileptic drugs. Such retrospective surgical series can be misleading, due to selection bias, and more recent experience suggests that

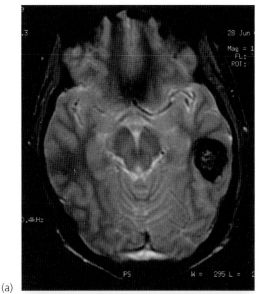

(a)

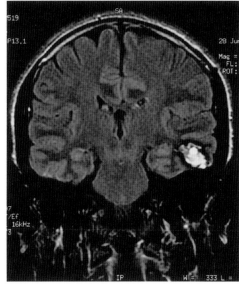

(b)

Figure 10.11 (a) MRI of a left temporal cavernous angioma causing complex partial seizures in a 27-year-old man. The scan shows the typical appearances of a hypointense haemosiderin halo with a mixed-signal core on a T2-weighted image. (b) Same cavernoma on a T1-weighted coronal view.

overall results are not as good as this. One recent series revealed a seizure freedom rate of only 42%, which is more in accord with the author's personal experience. What is clear is that lesionectomy should be carried out where possible with corticectomy, especially of surrounding cortex stained with haemosiderin. The outcome of surgery is best in those with a short seizure history.

Focused radiosurgery (e.g. with the gamma knife) can also be used to treat cavernomas. However, if the lesion is surgically accessible and the risk of surgical morbidity low, surgery is the preferred option, because it offers a better chance of controlling seizures and less risk of re-bleeding, which has been shown to be as high as 33% in one study after radiosurgery. After radiosurgery, in one multicentre study, 53% of patients became seizure free, 4% experienced only auras, 20% had a significant decrease in seizure frequency and 26% were unchanged. Location was an important variable, with those in the mesial temporal region having a poorer outcome.

Cavernomas are sometimes multiple, and surgical resection of individual lesions in such cases is advisable only if epilepsy can be clearly localized or the risk of haemorrhage is thought to be particularly high. Surgical resection for epilepsy in familial cavernoma is possible where there is a single accessible lesion, but generally the lesions are multiple and develop over time, and surgery to individual lesions is of limited value.

Cerebral infections
Encephalitis or meningitis
In general, surgical therapy for chronic postmeningitic or postencephalitic epilepsy carries a poor outcome for seizure control. Even if an apparently single lesion is uncovered on imaging (e.g. apparently unilateral hippocampal atrophy after herpes simplex encephalitis) there is usually more subtle widespread diffuse damage in other areas of the brain, and localized resection will fail to control seizures. This may be because the boundaries of the destructive process in postinfective lesions are seldom sharply defined, and it is these boundary areas that contribute most to epileptogenesis.

Acute brain abscess
The same applies to epilepsy after acute brain abscess (Figure 10.12). Although surgery is usually carried out in the acute phase, the optimal surgical management of a brain abscess depends on the type of infecting organism and the immunological state of the patient. Various procedures are utilized, including continuous tube drainage, stereotactic or open aspiration, marsupialization of the abscess and craniotomy with complete excision. Unfortunately, epilepsy follows a brain abscess, whether or not surgically treated, in between 40 and 80% of cases, and is often severe and intractable. Surgical

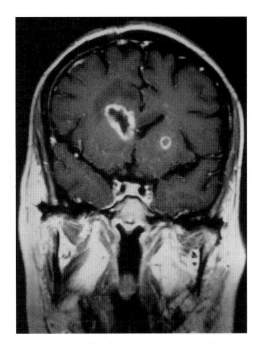

Figure 10.12 Aspergillus abscesses in a 38-year-old immunocompromised man.

resection of the cavity in an attempt to control the seizures can be attempted, but the results are generally disappointing. Corpus callosotomy (see below) is sometimes used in severe intractable seizures after a frontal brain abscess.

Neurocysticercosis
Neurocysticercosis (see pp. 62–63) with a solitary or small number of cerebral lesions is a self-limiting infestation with a pattern of spontaneous resolution (Figure 10.13). Resection of persisting calcified lesions to control seizures is hardly ever required.

The main debate about surgical intervention for neurocysticercosis has revolved around the need for biopsy for diagnostic purposes, especially in patients in endemic areas presenting with seizures and a solitary enhancing CT lesion. Assuming that there are no other clinical features, over 90% of these lesions turn out to be due to neurocysticercosis, and biopsy is now largely abandoned. The epilepsy is usually treated medically with antiepileptic drugs, and imaging is repeated at 12–16 weeks. If there is no resolution, or if the lesion has increased in size, diagnosis should be reconsidered and anticysticercal therapy instituted. Stereotactic or

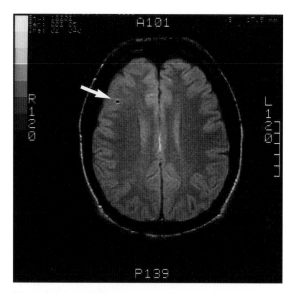

Figure 10.13 A calcified degenerated cysticercal cyst in a 36-year-old right-handed man with seizures since age 15 years, including sensations of heat or cold and forced head turning to the left, with no loss of consciousness or postictal confusion. Axial proton-density MRI shows the small lesion with low signal intensity in the right frontal lobe (arrowed).

image-guided excision should be reserved for lesions that enlarge or persist.

Surgical excision is also indicated where cysts exert a local mass effect or cause raised intracranial pressure, for subarachnoid cysts refractory to albendazole, cysts in the parasellar region and large racemose cysts. These forms do not present with epilepsy.

Tuberculosis

Tuberculoma (see pp. 63–64) is one of the most common lesions causing focal epilepsy in some parts of the developing world, and in immunocompromised patients (e.g. with HIV infection). Medical treatment with antituberculous drugs is the therapy of choice. A stereotactic biopsy is sometimes necessary to establish the diagnosis (usually to differentiate tuberculoma from neurocysticercosis). Occasionally excision of the residual cerebral lesion is necessary to control chronic intractable seizures.

Rasmussen chronic encephalitis

This is a syndrome of uncertain pathogenesis, but which has the histological appearances of a chronic encephalitis. It presents as intractable focal epilepsy, often with periods

of epilepsia partialis continua (EPC), and progressive neurological deficit including hemiplegia, aphasia and hemianopia. Wide lobar excision or hemispherectomy will be curative if the lesion is completely excised without causing unacceptable neurological deficit.

Trauma

As is the case in postinfectious epilepsy, the physiological changes causing refractory seizures after closed head trauma are often widespread and ill-defined. The MRI lesions do not necessarily correlate well with the extent of the histological changes, and limited surgical resection is often ineffective. In open trauma (including depressed fracture with dural breach), emergency débridement of the lesion will often prevent or reduce the intensity of subsequent epilepsy and should be carried out wherever possible. The wide débridement of established chronic lesions, including the resection of haemosiderin-lined cavities, will also sometimes improve chronic refractory epilepsy, although in general the results of surgery are disappointing, even where the damage appears to be relatively circumscribed. In penetrating head injury, surgery to remove bone fragments is also important to prevent abscess formation, which can cause severe epilepsy. Abscess development can be very delayed after penetrating head injury, and cases presenting 10–15 years after the injury have been reported.

Presurgical assessment

Small indolent lesions, such as cavernomas, indolent gliomas and DNETs, are readily recognized on neuroimaging and increasingly such patients are undergoing limited lesional resections (lesionectomy) with the primary aim to control seizures. Presurgical assessment is usually triggered by scanning with MRI or CT, which demonstrates the visible lesion.

The discovery of an intracerebral lesion in a patient with epilepsy does not inevitably mean that the lesion is causing the epilepsy, and the main purposes of the presurgical evaluation for epilepsy surgery are to confirm that the lesion is responsible for the epilepsy, to define the extent of the epileptogenic areas and to determine the risk of neurological deficit should resective surgery be undertaken.

The extent of resection is a key factor in lesional epilepsy. For most lesions, incomplete resection has a low chance of controlling seizures, whatever EEG or other investigations show. This should not be contemplated except as a last resort if the purpose of surgery is to control seizures, although it is often carried out for oncological reasons or to lower the risk of haemorrhage from AVMs. Only in the case of DNETs does incomplete resection seem routinely to control seizures.

Clinical assessment

The clinical features of partial seizures are a reliable indicator of the anatomical localization of seizure onset, and so a comprehensive seizure description is vital in deciding whether the seizure onset co-locates with the lesion. The most useful seizures, from the point of view of localization, are simple partial seizures or the auras or initial phenomena of complex partial seizures. This 'clinical localization' is of fundamental importance, and discordant findings are associated with much poorer surgical outcome.

Generalized epilepsy worsens outcome, and lesionectomy rarely controls epilepsy in childhood epilepsy syndromes (e.g. the Lennox–Gastaut syndrome or West syndrome) even where these are associated with obvious lesions.

Magnetic resonance imaging

MRI should be carried out in all cases, whether or not a lesion has been demonstrated by CT. Particular MRI characteristics help to identify the underlying pathology, but the histological or pathological features of a lesion cannot be predicted with absolute accuracy. If MRI shows a cortically based homogenous tumour with sharply defined borders, little or no surrounding oedema, and little or no contrast enhancement, the tumour is likely to be benign (Figure 10.14), although exceptions occur. Some lesions may have characteristic distinguishing features, e.g. DNETs, gangliogliomas, cavernomas, tuberculomas, neurocysticercosis, hypothalamic hamartomas, AVMs, and the lesions in tuberous sclerosis or the Sturge–Weber syndrome.

Assessment (and particularly volumetric measurements) of the hippocampi should now be routine in lesional epilepsy in order to characterize the possible extent of the epileptogenic zone(s), especially given the propensity of chronic epileptic lesions to cause secondary hippocampal sclerosis (dual pathology).

Interictal scalp EEG

In the presence of a neocortical lesion, interictal scalp EEG can be unreliable. The spatial distribution of an EEG focus coincides exactly with lesion localization in less than a third of patients, and can indeed be widely discrepant (Figure 10.15). This is due to the rapid and wide propagation of seizure discharges in neocortical regions.

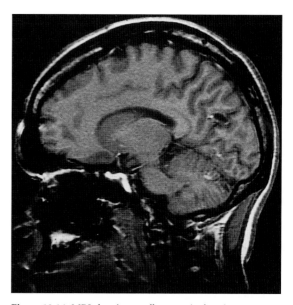

Figure 10.14 MRI showing small parasagittal parieto-occipital lesion (biopsy-proven oligodendroglioma) in a patient with brief complex partial seizures characterized by visual disturbance, arrest of activity and loss of awareness.

The site of the lesion also influences the interictal EEG. In lesional parietal or occipital lobe epilepsy, for example, only a minority of lesions show interictal spikes well correlated to the site of the lesion. In one series, only 1 of 11 patients with parietal lesions showed a focal EEG onset concordant with the parietal lesion, whereas 2 of the patients showed an ictal onset ipsilateral to the lesion and 8 showed no focal changes at ictal onset. Despite the high rate of discordance between the side of lesion and the ictal onset, 10 of the patients underwent lesionectomy and all had a good outcome. Even large lesions may sometimes be associated with scalp EEG changes that predominate over the contralateral side, and there are well-documented cases of scalp EEG recordings showing ictal onset on the side contralateral to a known gross focal cerebral lesion, in patients in whom depth recordings subsequently documented seizures arising from the lesion and in whom resection of the lesion resulted in seizure freedom. Lesions in the temporal neocortex are more often associated with concordant EEG data. Bilateral changes occur in many patients with unilateral hemispherical lesions, particularly in lesional frontal lobe epilepsy, The nature of the lesion is important. In cortical dysplasia the interictal EEG is often widely distributed. In tumours and infective lesions it has more specificity

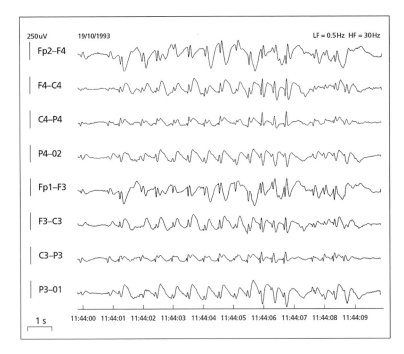

Figure 10.15 EEG showing the interictal EEG from the patient illustrated in Figure 10.14 showing widespread bilateral slow spike-and-wave discharges; findings widely discordant with the known causative lesion.

but still often lacks reliability, and there are few data to indicate which neurophysiological factors should influence the extent of resection.

Ictal scalp EEG

Ictal recordings (with video-EEG telemetry) are more informative than interictal EEG, but still lack critical reliability (Figures 10.16 and 10.17). However, in cases where clinico-EEG data correlate well with the visible lesion, the data are usually sufficient to proceed to surgery without invasive monitoring or other investigations. Some claim that concordant ictal fast activity particularly predicts a good surgical outcome. However, the potential for misleading or multifocal scalp EEG changes in patients with surgically resectable focal structural lesions should be recognized in planning investigative strategies, and surgery should certainly not be rejected merely because of discordant scalp electrographic findings.

The difference in localizing value of ictal EEG in extra-temporal versus temporal epilepsy was well shown in one series of 486 ictal EEGs in 72 patients with epilepsy arising in mesial temporal, neocortical temporal, mesial frontal, dorsolateral frontal, parietal and occipital regions. The ictal scalp EEG was localized in 72% of cases, more often in temporal versus extratemporal cases, with 57% of localized onsets originating from the mesial temporal,

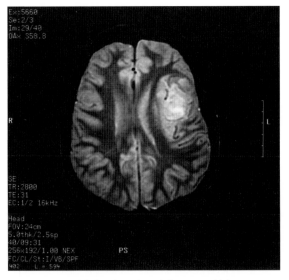

Figure 10.16 MRI showing a large left temporal lobe structural abnormality.

lateral frontal and parietal lobe regions. Lateralized onsets were seen more frequently in neocortical TLE and generalized onsets were seen more frequently in mesial frontal lobe epilepsy and occipital lobe epilepsy, with

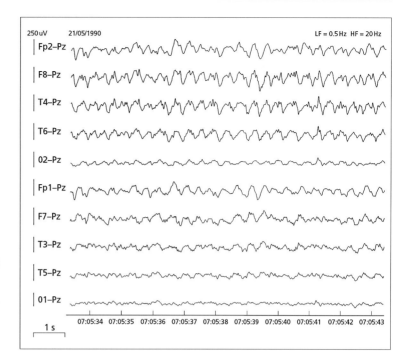

Figure 10.17 Ictal EEG from the patient whose scan is shown in Figure 10.16, showing widespread rhythmic activity over the right hemisphere, and irregular slowing over the left temporal region (the site of the known large structural lesion).

more false localization/lateralization occurring in occipital and parietal seizures.

The ictal scalp EEG does have limitations. In simple partial seizures (and also complex partial seizures arising from the mesial frontal lobe), the ictal EEG is often normal. In some cases of frontal lobe, and occasionally occipital lobe seizures, the ictal pattern is of generalized spike–wave activity. In young children with focal brain lesions, the ictal EEG can be especially unreliable. In one series of 50 children with severe refractory lesional epilepsy, in whom 30–100% of preoperative epileptiform discharges were generalized or contralateral, 72% patients were rendered seizure free after resective surgery.

Intracranial EEG

The use of intracranial EEG in extrahippocampal lesional epilepsy varies from centre to centre, as do the techniques employed. Intracranial EEG is needed in patients with lesional extrahippocampal epilepsy for the following reasons:
• Non-localizing or discordant ictal scalp recordings suggest that the lesion might not be responsible for the seizures.
• It is necessary to decide whether or not to carry out hippocampal resection in patients with lesions adjacent to it, who are at risk of memory decline after surgery.

• It is necessary to define the margins of the epileptogenic zone to guide the extent of resection (although other strategies such as ECoG, and radiological or pathological evaluation of margins may be used). The epileptogenicity of cortical dysplasia and post-traumatic lesions, in particular, tend to extend beyond the radiologically demonstrable lesion.
• For cortical stimulation for brain mapping with lesions overlying or adjacent to the eloquent cortex (see below).

Depth electrodes subdural strip electrodes, subdural grid electrodes and epidural electrodes are all used for invasive EEG (see Figure 10.7), and indeed the techniques are often combined. The recording type is tailored to the individual patient and the neurophysiological question being addressed. Each technique has advantages and disadvantages, and all carry significant morbidity. The usefulness depends on the nature and site of the lesion. Formal studies have shown surprisingly little value from depth recordings. All also have the problem that the area of brain sampled around an electrode is very small (<1 mm) and so, if the electrodes are placed even a small distance away from an epileptic focus, they have little value.

Interictal epileptic discharges on depth EEG are of less value than interictal discharges from the scalp. However, widespread discharges extending beyond the limits of any resection would predict a poor surgical outcome, even if the region of ictal onset were resected. Conversely, patients with focal discharges only within the area of surgical resection generally do well after surgery. In occipital or parietal lesions in particular depth EEG is often non-localizing.

The ictal EEG in extratemporal epilepsy can take several forms, differing from that of mesial TLE, of which the most common is low-voltage fast activity. However, there is no consistent correlation between the type of ictal pattern and the surgical outcome. The focus can be small and discrete or much larger (sometimes occupying a region with shifting foci from seizure to seizure). Surgical outcome does not seem always to depend on how widespread the ictal foci are, and the seizure characteristics may be primarily dependent on anatomical location and network connections. The concept of epilepsy as a highly focal phenomenon, with spread similar to the ripples in a pond, is clearly simplistic and many epilepsies are subserved by large neural networks – and this fact mitigates against the value of highly focalized depth recordings.

Cortical mapping and cortical stimulation

Cortical mapping of functionally important cortex is a vital function where neurosurgical procedures are planned in sensory, motor or speech areas, and is required to identify eloquent areas and thus avoid postsurgical neurological deficit. The mapping can be done preoperatively with subdural electrodes or operatively by direct cortical stimulation with a bipolar stimulating electrode. The cortical functions of greatest concern are those subserving hand motor, sensory or language function over the motor and sensory strip, and superior temporal language regions.

Preoperatively, stimulation of subdural electrodes placed on the cortical surface (and co-registered with MRI) allows detailed studies of cortical function to be carried out. The clinical effects of electrical stimulation are observed from each cortical contact. Ictal and interictal EEGs can be recorded at the same time. Mapping is important because lesions commonly alter or distort the normal topography of the cerebral cortex and vascular landmarks.

Acute intraoperative mapping can be carried out under local anaesthetic in a conscious patient, using a hand-held device at the end of which are two stimulating electrodes. Time is shorter and so less elaborate functional tasks can be evaluated than in chronic longer-term preoperative mapping. Subdural grids of electrodes have

also been used for recording cortical somatosensory-evoked potentials from peripheral nerve stimulation, to locate the somatosensory cortex.

It has been proposed that fMRI has the potential to replace cortical mapping in the identification of the primary motor areas, but currently fMRI cannot localize speech or language areas with anything like sufficient accuracy to be practically useful.

Electrical stimulation can be used to locate the epileptogenic zone by finding areas of low after-discharge threshold. In the past, stimulation was also used to identify seizure loci by trying to reproduce a seizure by stimulation, but this was unreliable because of secondary activation of epileptogenic cortex remote from the area stimulated electrically. A recent development has been to use a very small single-pulse electrical stimulation (up to 8 mA, 1 ms in duration) to identify epileptogenic cortex, with promising early results, and this technique may prove to be a sensitive way of mapping epileptogenic areas.

Neuropsychology

A battery of standard neuropsychological tests, aimed at lateralizing and localizing the area(s) of functional abnormality, are also routinely used in the preoperative evaluation. However, the value of the tests for localizing lesions is limited, and neuropsychological testing has much less value in extratemporal epilepsy than in TLE. The evaluation of frontal lobe functioning in epilepsy includes tests of problem-solving, fluency, susceptibility to interference, planning and motor skills, but are relatively non-specific and, apart from language-oriented tests, are non-lateralizing. The value of psychometric assessment of parietal and occipital lobe dysfunction in epilepsy is even more limited, perhaps because the abnormalities are too subtle to be detected by existing neuropsychological tests.

In a recent study, neuropsychological findings were congruent with the lateralization of the lesion in 56% but incongruent in 14%; furthermore, localization corresponded with the lobe of the lesion in 26% but was misleading in 30%. Neuropsychology also helps to predict postoperative deficit, but its value is generally less in extratemporal than in temporal lobe surgery.

SPECT and PET

SPECT is usually carried out with ^{99m}Tc-labelled hexamethyl-propyleneamine oxime ([^{99m}Tc]HMPAO). It should be injected as close to the onset of the seizure as possible, and its uptake in the brain begins about 30 s after the injection; to be valuable in extratemporal epilepsy, it has been suggested that the injection has to be complete at least 10-15 s before the end of the seizure. About 40% of simple partial seizures show no change on ictal SPECT and the best results are in complex partial seizures. It has been claimed by some authorities that the sensitivity of ictal SPECT in extratemporal epilepsy is as high as 90% but this is greater than the author's own clinical experience. However, it is clear that ictal SPECT is far more useful than interictal SPECT. In extratemporal lesional epilepsy, if subtraction ictal SPECT co-registered on MRI (SISCOM) localizes a seizure accurately enough, and with concordance with other modalities, then about 40% of patients can expect to be seizure free after surgery and a further 40% to have a favourable surgical outcome. In one study, SISCOM localization was concordant with the site of the surgical excision in 52.8%, non-concordant in 13.9% and non-localizing in 33.3% of cases.

Interictal or peri-ictal PET using [18]FDG-PET is included routinely in the presurgical evaluation protocols of many epilepsy surgery programmes. However, PET findings, characterized by the increased or decreased uptake of [18]FDG, reflect the neuronal activity not only at the site of the ictal onset but also in areas of ictal spread and postictal depression. Interictal PET has been shown to be more sensitive than MRI in detecting foci of gliotic tissue with decreased metabolic uptake of [18]FDG, but gliotic tissue does not necessarily correlate with an epileptogenic region. Only a third of patients with extratemporal seizures have relevant hypometabolic abnormalities concordant with an abnormal EEG focus, and these regions of hypometabolic activity are frequently widely distributed and poorly localized.

Electrocorticography

Intraoperative EEG recording directly from the cortex (ECoG) can be used to identify and resect epileptogenic tissue surrounding a lesion, and has been used for at least 50 years. Its value, however, still remains controversial. In one study of patients with low-grade gliomas and intractable epilepsy who underwent ECoG during surgery and in whom resection was guided by ECoG, 41% of the adults and 85% of the children were rendered seizure free. Others have found that ECoG has no predictive value and does not assist surgery. Perhaps surprisingly, the complete resection of all spiking areas identified at corticography seems by no means always to succeed in stopping seizures, nor does incomplete resection always fail.

Cortical dysplasia (malformations of cortical development)

Cortical dysplasia is an important cause of medically intractable seizures; MRI detects dysplasia in 5–10% of patients with refractory epilepsy and up to 15% of children with refractory epilepsy and learning disability. Cortical dysplasia accounts for less than 10% of epilepsy surgery resections in adults but over 50% of operated children (67% in children operated on in the first year of life and 75% in infants).

The presurgical assessment has a different emphasis from that of other conditions. Multimodal investigation is needed, but the rate of 'concordance' is much lower. Success depends on complete resection – more than in other conditions, possibly partly because the lesions themselves, not the surrounding adjacent tissue, are epileptogenic. The boundaries of the lesions are, however, often ill-defined and extend pathologically well beyond the edge of the MRI-defined abnormality. In at least 20% of operated cases, histologically proven dysplasia is found on examination of tissue removed at surgery in patients with refractory epilepsy, in spite of a normal conventional MRI. Perhaps because of this, there has been a tendency to attribute subtle variations in MRI to cortical dysplasia. There is a risk of over-interpretation, and caution in determining what is normal and abnormal, and some authors have clearly overstated the significance of both minor pathological changes and minor changes on MRI. What is 'abnormal' in terms of imaging and histology can be difficult to be certain about.

The success of surgery depends on identifying the extent of the dysplasia and a complete resection. Presurgical assessment of cortical dysplasia must be multimodal and aimed at identifying the dysplasia and its limits. The clinical history and the MRI may be helpful in defining the general region of abnormality. A striking feature of studies of surgical outcome is the lack of the predictive utility of EEG. Interictal scalp EEG often shows widespread, generalized or multifocal interictal spiking, and ictal EEG is often poorly localized (being helpful in less than 50% of cases). Indeed, even in those with clear-cut MRI lesions, ictal EEG is localized in less than 60%, and often ictal onsets appear to be discordant with MRI lesions. The lack of specificity of EEG, conversely, means that some patients have good outcomes after resective surgery even if the interictal and ictal scalp EEGs show widespread changes (Figure 10.18).

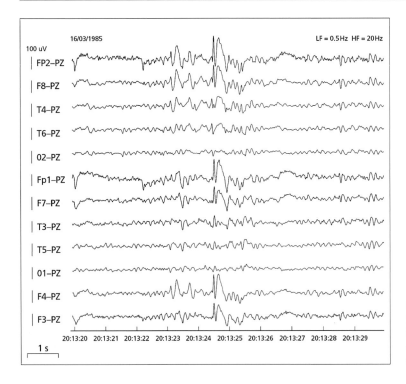

Figure 10.18 EEG showing widespread bilateral anteriorly predominant interictal spikes recorded from a patient with an area of localized macrogyria in the left motor cortex.

Intracranial recordings are often applied, but the onset of seizures is often diffuse and sometimes widely so. The surgical outcome in most series does not seem to correlate well with intracranial EEG findings. ECoG is widely used to guide resections peroperatively but the results from different studies are contradictory, and ECoG is unhelpful in at least half the cases. Interictal PET can identify brain malformations that are invisible to MRI but are histologically verified at surgery. In paediatric practice PET may have a clinical role, revealing abnormalities that are otherwise difficult to detect, and leading to successful surgical intervention, particularly in young children undergoing large excisions for overwhelming epilepsy. PET is said to localize the abnormalities (at least broadly) in over 80% of cases. MRI is normal in at least 30% of operated cases in which the histology shows dysplasia. Ictal SPECT is not as reliable in cortical dysplasia as in other pathologies, and is localizing in only about 60% of cases of extratemporal epilepsy due to cortical dysplasia as it is in hippocampal epilepsy.

In a recent review, the accuracy of investigations in cortical dysplasia was said to be: interictal scalp electroencephalography (EEG) 50%; ictal scalp EEG 65%; MRI 66%; [18]FDG-PET 81%; and SPECT 57%. Intracranial electrodes are used in about 50% of patients with cortical dysplasia.

Given the uncertainties of the different investigatory modalities, it is perhaps not surprising that the effects of surgery are unpredictable, and often disappointing. This uncertainty must be conveyed to the patient. Making prognostic predictions in terms of percentage chances (as is usually done, for example, before surgery for hippocampal sclerosis) is often done (30% chance of seizure freedom is a typical prediction) but, given the variation between patient and the relatively small number of operated cases, such predictions often seem to be based on little concrete evidence.

The best outcome follows complete resection of focal cortical dysplasia (Taylor dysplasia), with short-term (1-year) seizure-free rates of about 50–60% of cases, and there are few data about longer-term outcome. Resection of small areas of subcortical heterotopia also alleviates epilepsy in a reasonable number of cases. Other types of dysplasia, however, fare worse, and the comparatively poor outcome of all types of dysplastic lesion must reflect widespread epileptogenesis that extends beyond the margins of the lesions visible on conventional MRI.

Furthermore, brain anatomy is often abnormal in patients with cortical dysplasia, cortical mapping shows aberrant location of functional cortex, and surgical morbidity can be greater than is the case in surgery for other cortical lesions. In focal cortical dysplasia and subcortical heterotopia, a good outcome requires at least the complete resection of the visible lesion. In one series a seizure-free outcome was achieved in 60% with complete resection compared with 27% of those with incomplete resection. Of these, 89% had a lesion detected by MRI. The seizure-free rate was 81.6% for those who had complete resection and 25% for those with partial resection. Patients with dysplasia in the temporal lobe were more often seizure free (68.3%) than those with extratemporal resections (50.0%).

It is also likely that, the larger the resection, the better the chances of seizure control, although studies on this point are few. Resective surgery for more widespread lesions such as polymicrogyria, schizencephaly, periventricular heterotopia or lissencephaly is almost never successful and not recommended,

Surgery where no lesion is apparent on neuroimaging ('MRI-negative cases')

Before the advent of MRI many cases of epilepsy (including virtually all cases of hippocampal sclerosis and cortical dysgenesis) were considered 'non-lesional'. The nature and extent of the surgery in these cases depended heavily on scalp and invasive EEG. It was realized, even then, that if no pathology was found in the operated specimen the prognosis for seizure control was poor. Often, however, small lesions were found and the prognosis was good.

Since the advent of MRI the situation has radically altered, because many of these previously occult lesions can be clearly demonstrated preoperatively. Where the MRI is normal the chances of finding a 'lesion' in operated tissue are greatly reduced. The outcome is poor if the surgical specimen is normal, but better if an abnormality is found (and cortical dysplasia is the usual finding in this situation). Surgery therefore must be considered a treatment of last resort. It should be offered only to patients with severe epilepsy, and usually only to patients experiencing secondarily generalized tonic–clonic seizures (on the basis that these carry greater risk if left untreated). It would be unusual to operate on individuals with partial seizures only, unless they were particularly handicapping.

The presurgical assessment needs to be tailored to individual cases, but a number of general principles apply:

• MRI studies should be of adequate quality. It is important to stress that a patient should not be considered MRI negative unless a detailed MRI examination has been made, applying appropriate sequences and techniques. A critical approach is needed. Many patients with apparently normal MR scans using inappropriate examinations show clear lesions when scanned using the epilepsy-oriented MRI protocols; this is especially true of patients harbouring such lesions as hippocampal atrophy, small vascular lesions or tumours, or cortical dysplasia. These 'pseudo-MRI-negative' cases emphasize the importance of a tailored MRI approach. Good quality structural scans are crucial, and these can sometimes be supplemented by other more experimental scanning techniques (see Table 10.5) but with care taken to avoid over-interpretation.

• If MRI is truly normal, multimodal functional investigations are an absolute requirement. These should always include ictal scalp recordings and neuropsychometric assessment, and invasive EEG, SPECT and/or PET is also usually carried out. The interictal EEG is seldom helpful in localization. Ictal scalp EEG will help to define where invasive EEG monitoring should be undertaken, and seldom will invasive EEG be contemplated if the scalp ictal EEG shows no localizing features. Although invasive EEG is often conceived as a gold standard, it should also be realized that only small areas of cortical tissue are sampled around implanted electrodes; the scalp EEG surveys a bigger territory. Invasive EEG should never be undertaken blindly (a 'fishing expedition'), and electrode placement should address specific questions and be guided by other clinical or investigatory findings. In one series ictal scalp EEG, ictal SPECT and interictal PET allowed surgery to be carried out in 41 MRI-negative cases, of whom 39% were free from seizures at 1 year, and the ictal scalp EEG predicted good outcome more often than the other tests (70% vs 43% vs 33%, respectively). In another study only 5 of 40 MRI-negative cases were found after intensive investigation to have localized lesions, and only 3 could be offered surgery.

• The bigger the resection, the better the outcome. In young children in particular, large resections carry less functional penalty because brain plasticity allows reallocation of function during subsequent development. Thus, in young children with devastating epilepsy, large-scale resections, guided, for example, by interictal PET hypoperfusion, are considered appropriate even where no lesion or focal EEG disturbance is present. It has also become clear, however, that operating on adults without MRI changes, even in the presence of a clear-cut EEG focus and even after a wide resection (e.g. a frontal lobectomy for epilepsy originating in anterior frontal regions), carries a generally poor prognosis, and fewer than 30% of patients can expect any great improvement in seizure frequency.

Hemispherectomy, hemispherotomy and other large resections

The term 'hemispherectomy' is used here to cover a variety of operations in which one cerebral hemisphere is excised or disconnected from the other. These are operations carried out in children or adolescents (and occasionally adults) with medically refractory seizures due to severe unilateral hemisphere damage. The operations are nowadays carried out only to improve the control of epilepsy, although originally hemispherectomy was performed as a form of tumoral surgery.

Preoperative assessment

The suitability of any individual for hemispherectomy depends upon the aetiology, clinical features, neurological examination, scalp EEG and results of neuroimaging. The assessment aims to examine the diseased hemisphere, and also the status of the 'good' hemisphere.

Aetiology

The usual aetiologies in patients undergoing hemispherectomy are shown in Table 10.9. It is imperative to ascertain that the cerebral damage is wholly or very largely confined to one hemisphere. Even where the

Table 10.9 Approximate frequencies of underlying aetiologies treated by hemispherectomy.

Rasmussen chronic encephalitis	35%
Perinatal insult (usually vascular, leading to unilateral porencephaly)	30%
Hemimegencephaly	10%
Migrational disorder	5%
Sturge–Weber disease	5%
Viral or bacterial infection	5%
Cerebral trauma	5%
Postnatal cerebrovascular event	5%

primary pathology is unilateral, e.g. after a vascular or traumatic event, secondary bihemispherical damage can result from prolonged anoxia or coma. The results of surgery where there is bilateral damage are far less good.

Seizures

Only patients with severe epilepsy, intractable to medical therapy, should be considered for this operation. Most patients going forward for hemispherectomy will have multiple seizure types and frequent (more than five) seizures each day. The seizures must have a focal onset in the damaged hemisphere. The condition in which focal motor seizures are most frequently seen is EPC, usually secondary to Rasmussen encephalitis. Commonly, combinations of secondarily generalized tonic–clonic seizures, drop attacks and focal motor seizures coexist. Complex partial seizures are not common in the types of pathology for which hemispherectomy is appropriate.

Neurological status

The great majority of suitable candidates for hemispherectomy have a preoperative fixed hemiplegia, reflecting the severity of the hemispherical damage. This can be associated with other signs, such as hemianopia or hemisensory loss, and most patients have some degree of learning disability and psychomotor retardation.

The operation is almost always carried out only where the hemiparesis is severe enough to impair the performance of individual finger movements. The preoperative ability to perform gross movements of the fingers, or at other major joints (e.g. shoulder, elbow, hip, knee), is not a contraindication to surgery. These movements are not usually worse after a hemispherectomy, nor is a pre-existing spastic gait, although there may be a transient worsening for several weeks after the operation. Lesser degrees of disability will deteriorate postoperatively. Occasionally patients with lesser defects are offered hemispherectomy, if they have a progressive disorder that, it is deemed, will inevitably lead to hemiplegia. In such children social and intellectual development will be accelerated with the improved seizure control resulting from the operation, so that early hemispherectomy can be considered despite the inevitable worsening of motor function that will be caused by the operation. Hemianopia is usually but not always complete in the cases being considered. Its absence should not be considered an absolute contraindication to hemispherectomy, although the operation will inevitably result in a complete hemianopia – but this deficit is not usually severely disabling.

The presence or absence of sensory loss is not usually a consideration in deciding whether or not to proceed to surgery, because hemispherectomy rarely results in any marked change in sensory function.

The degree of intellectual impairment of patients suitable for hemispherectomy will vary, and is a good index of the functional status of the 'good' hemisphere. Severe psychomotor retardation should be interpreted as reflecting bilateral cerebral damage, and in this situation the outcome of hemispherectomy will be less good. Pathologies present early in life are generally associated with better preservation of function as a result of brain plasticity.

Finally, if this operation is performed on the language-dominant hemisphere, permanent aphasia will result unless language functions can be transferred to the other side of the brain by processes of cortical plasticity and development. These processes are age dependent. It is possible to carry out dominant hemispherectomy before the age of 5 years without any impairment of language functions. Recovery of language after dominant hemispherectomy after the age of 5 years is, however, rarely complete although some transfer of language functions is possible until the early teens. Language lateralization in older children can be confirmed preoperatively by the intracarotid amytal test.

EEG

Interictal scalp EEG is usually sufficient, and invasive EEG is not usually required, in the preoperative assessment for hemispherectomy. Ideally, the EEG should show low-amplitude slow activity and epileptic discharges confined to the affected hemisphere, but this is not always the case (Figure 10.19). Sometimes the damaged hemisphere is incapable of generating sufficiently strong electrical signals to be detectable on scalp EEG, and discharges appear to be of higher amplitude on the side of the normal hemisphere. In about 50% of cases, secondary or independent epileptiform abnormalities occur in the 'good' hemisphere. Although these raise the possibility of bilateral damage, they are not an absolute contraindication to the operation. Even apparently independent epileptic spikes originating from the 'good' hemisphere usually disappear after hemispherectomy.

MRI and CT

The appearances depend on the aetiology. Often unilateral hemispherical atrophy is present, with increased skull thickness, enlarged sulci and ventricles, and a small cerebral peduncle (Figure 10.20). Calcification, porencephaly, hemimegalencephaly, signal change, dysgenesis or other lesions can be demonstrated on radiology.

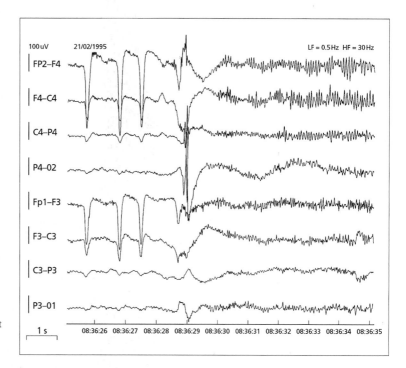

Figure 10.19 Ictal scalp EEG from the patient whose MRI is shown in Figure 10.20. Note the rhythmic activity evident over both hemispheres but of higher amplitude over the normal hemisphere.

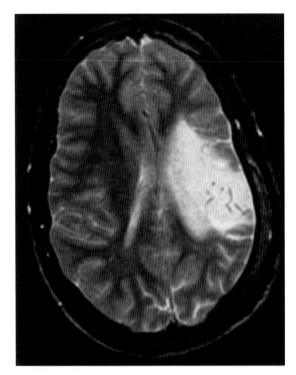

Figure 10.20 Preoperative MRI in a patient subsequently undergoing a left hemispherectomy showing the consequences of cerebral infarction, occurring in early childhood, leading to medically intractable seizures.

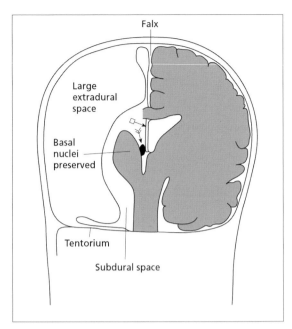

Figure 10.21 Diagram showing the extent of the resection in a modified hemispherectomy. The arrows show the muscle plug and the foramen of Monro.

The contralateral hemisphere should show no major lesions.

Surgical techniques and surgical outcome
Type of operation
The original surgical operation (the so-called 'anatomical hemispherectomy') has been shown in recent years to have serious late postoperative complications (see below). It has, therefore, been largely abandoned, and a variety of new surgical techniques has been developed. The anatomical hemispherectomy consisted of the complete removal of the affected cerebral hemisphere with or without the basal ganglia, either en bloc or in fragments. The modified hemispherectomy links this operation with procedures to eliminate communication of CSF with the hemispherectomy cavity by creating a largely extradural cavity and obstructing the foramen of Monro with a piece of muscle (Figure 10.21). The operations of hemidecortication and hemicorticectomy consist of excision of the cortex with the preservation of as much white matter as possible. The functional hemispherectomy consists of a subtotal anatomical hemispherectomy with complete physiological disconnection. The technique involves a large central removal including parasagittal tissue and exposure of the whole length of the corpus callosum. All fibres entering the corpus callosum are then interrupted by undercutting, from within, the lateral ventricle in a parasagittal plane. The residual frontal and parieto-occipital lobes are disconnected by aspiration of white and grey matter in the posterior frontal region to the level of the sphenoid wing, and in the parieto-occipital region down to the tentorium. A large temporal lobectomy, including excision of medial structures, is finally carried out. The hemispherotomy and peri-insular hemispherotomy are variations on this principle, allowing cortical disconnection via alternative surgical routes.

The choice of surgical method depends on the experience and preference of the surgeon, but functional hemispherectomy and hemispherotomy are now widely preferred to the anatomical hemispherectomy because of the smaller risks of morbidity.

Early surgical morbidity
Fatal complications include brain swelling, blood loss and tentorial herniation, and the overall mortality of

hemispherectomy, which is often carried out in very young children, is in the region of 2–10%. This is partly due to the anatomical anomalies and the high vascularity of the abnormal hemisphere, with abnormal drainage. The duration of surgery is also a factor in morbidity in very young children. Early morbidity includes haemorrhage and infection. Early hydrocephalus develops in 5–40% of cases and will require CSF shunting. Transient worsening of motor or speech function occurs but usually resolves.

Late surgical morbidity

The traditional anatomical hemispherectomy is associated with two specific late complications – superficial cerebral haemosiderosis and late hydrocephalus. Superficial cerebral haemosiderosis results in a gradual neurological deterioration evident at a mean of 8 years after surgery. The pathological findings are obstructive hydrocephalus due to aqueduct stenosis, gliosis and ependymitis, and the hemispherectomy cavity becomes lined with a membrane similar to that found in a chronic subdural haematoma. The fluid in the ventricle is brownish and of 'machine oil' appearance. This complication is due to chronic bleeding into the subdural hemispherectomy cavity, and occurs in at least 30–50% of cases, leading eventually to disability and death. Late hydrocephalus is presumably produced by a similar mechanism. Patients who have had the operation require regular brain scans for early warning of these complications. The newer operations, and in particular the functional operations, are not followed by these disastrous complications.

Outcome for seizure control and behaviour

Hemispherectomy is a very effective operation in carefully selected patients. Complete seizure control is expected in about 70–80%, and an improvement in seizures of at least 80% in over 90% suitably selected and competently operated cases. Even in carefully selected cases, however, 5% of operated patients will show no worthwhile benefit. Aetiology is an important determinant of outcome, with patients with the Sturge–Weber syndrome having the highest seizure-free rates and those with extensive cortical dysplasias (including hemimegencephaly) the lowest.

The primary indication of the operation is to control seizures. Secondary gains in terms of behaviour and psychosocial development usually also occur. Severely abnormal behaviour patterns are common in the sorts of children with severe epilepsy who undergo surgery.

Typically taking the form of aggression and regressive behaviour, these are often a consequence of repeated seizures, subclinical EEG activity and drug treatment. A remarkable improvement can be expected postoperatively in children whose seizures have been controlled, and there are also gains in social development and intellectual function. Children whose seizures are controlled almost always integrate better into their family and school, and demonstrate greatly improved abilities to learn and concentrate. The intellectual deterioration that is inevitable without the operation is usually halted. Some children will develop to the stage where independent living and work are possible.

Other large resections

A basic principle of the surgery of extratemporal neocortical epilepsy is that, the wider the excision around an epileptic focus, the more likely is complete seizure control to be achieved. This 'more-is-better' philosophy has characterized the surgical approach to epilepsy in non-eloquent cortical regions, e.g. a large frontal lobectomy can be carried out with no gross deficit and only an approximately 3% risk of hemiparesis. The inferior central region, over the face area, can be resected without sensory or motor deficit, presumably due to bilateral cortical representation, although resections in the hand or leg areas of the cortex do result in monoplegia. Similarly, a large resection of the non-dominant parietal lobe can be carried out with minor sensory deficit only. Dominant parietal resections carry a risk of profound sensory loss and apraxia. These large lobar resections are less common now because the MRI localization of structural disease has allowed more precise surgical planning.

Sturge–Weber syndrome

In selected cases, resective surgery in this syndrome can have an excellent result. This should be carried out as early as is feasible in view of the danger of progressive neurological impairment caused by episodes of status epilepticus in this condition (see p. 49). Hemispherectomy can be carried out in patients with extensive lesions, and lesionectomy or lobectomy in smaller lesions. Corpus callosotomy has been used as a palliative procedure, but where possible resective surgery is preferable. MRI is the main presurgical investigation, and neither preoperative EEG nor corticography has much influence on surgical procedure or outcome. The outcome after appropriate resective surgery is good, with at least 80% seizure control. The outcome for behaviour and intellectual development is also improved by early surgery.

Corpus callosectomy (corpus callosum section, corpus callosotomy)

This operation, the transection of the corpus callosum, can be carried out in a one- or a two-stage procedure. Although first performed in 1940, even now neither the precise physiological rationale for the surgery nor its indications are clearly defined. It was originally proposed that section of the corpus callosum would prevent the rapid spread of epileptic activity from one hemisphere to the other, but in fact seizure activity can propagate widely via non-callosal pathways. It is simplistic to assume that the operation prevents secondary generalization, but it does have a desynchronizing effect on epileptic activity and can inhibit seizures, although exactly how or why is unclear. In recent years the number of patients undergoing callosectomy has declined to a very low level.

Indications

The operation, which is primarily a palliative rather than a curative procedure, is now primarily reserved for:
• patients with severe secondarily generalized epilepsy manifest by frequent drop attacks causing injury
• patients in whom medical therapy is ineffective and where other surgical procedures are not possible
• where it is thought possible to lessen the frequency of generalized seizures by the disruption of seizure spread.

The procedure is therefore mostly considered in patients with tonic or atonic seizures, many of whom have additional seizure types and moderate or severe learning disability; many have the Lennox–Gastaut syndrome. However, it has also been shown to have an effect in complex partial seizures, some myoclonic seizures and tonic–clonic seizures.

It can also be used in combination with resective surgery, and the operation can have a particular role, combined with frontal lobe resection, in patients with severe frontal lobe damage after trauma or an abscess.

As will be clear, most patients undergo surgery on the basis of the clinical manifestations of the epilepsy, rather than the EEG or pathophysiological findings. There seems little way of selecting out those patients who will do well from those who will not, and this lack of predictability, combined with its generally disappointing effects and its potential hazards, renders the corpus callosectomy a last-ditch operation now only infrequently carried out. Vagal nerve stimulation carries far less risk, and many patients who would previously have been considered for corpus callosectomy are currently referred instead, initially at least, for vagal nerve stimulation.

Preoperative assessment

EEG, MRI and psychometric assessment are usually carried out. Patients with lateralized EEG findings have been consistently found to have a better outcome than those with purely generalized changes, but almost all candidates for the operation have bilateral synchronous epileptic discharges in addition. The outcome of those with a focal area of damage on MRI is probably better than for those with normal MRI or diffuse generalized changes.

Operative procedure

In most centres corpus callosectomy is carried out as a two-stage procedure. In the first stage the anterior two-thirds of the corpus callosum are sectioned (Figure 10.22), sparing the splenium. If this is ineffective, the section can be completed at a second operation. Occasionally a posterior section is carried out first, in those with clearly posterior epilepsy. The two-stage procedure has a lower morbidity. Actual surgical technique varies and improvements in recent times have lowered the rate of complications. ECoG is sometimes used to guide the extent of the first-stage resection. A recent development has been the use of focused radiosurgery with the gamma knife to carry out an anterior callosal section, and this may become the method of choice.

Outcome

The operation must be considered a palliative procedure, intended to reduce seizure severity and in particular to reduce injuries due to falls. No patient should undergo the procedure on the assumption that epileptic seizures will stop completely. Short-term freedom from seizures does occur in about 5–10% of cases, but there is a strong tendency to relapse over months or years. Nevertheless, the number of generalized seizures or seizures with falls are usually reduced by the operation (albeit sometimes with an increase in the number of partial seizures).

Both the one- and the two-stage operation carry significant risks of neurological deficit. Hemiparesis can be due to traction peroperatively or to vascular infarction caused by damage to the pericallosal arteries or venous thrombosis. A transient and highly distinctive disconnection syndrome with mutism, urinary incontinence and bilateral leg weakness is a not uncommon consequence of a one-stage complete callosal section. It is present in the immediate postoperative period and usually resolves after a matter of weeks, although in 5% of cases it can be

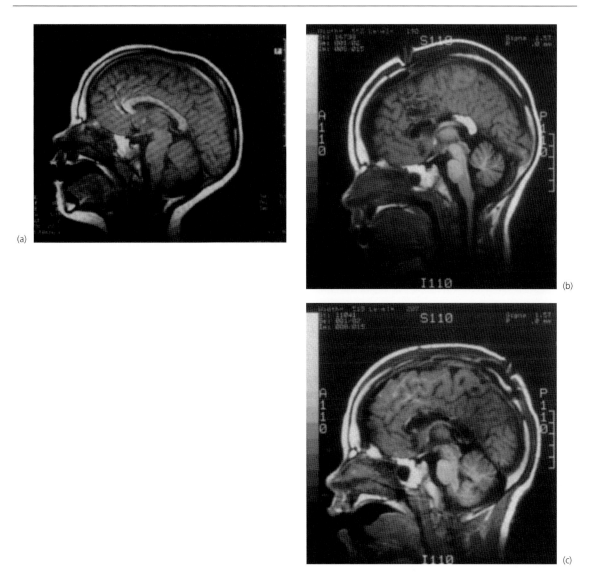

Figure 10.22 MRI showing sagittal cuts through the corpus callosum in a 9-year-old patient. (a) Preoperative; (b) after anterior two-thirds corpus callosotomy; and (c) after callosotomy completion.

permanent; the pathophysiology of this effect is not clear. A posterior disconnection syndrome in which complex motor tasks become impossible occurs in about 5% of cases after a one-stage procedure. After the completed transection, most patients will exhibit elements of a 'split-brain' profile on neuropsychological testing (and intensive studies of this phenomenon are published), although remarkably this causes little disability in everyday living. Other recorded complications include extra-

dural haematoma, air embolism, infection, and an increase in the frequency or intensity of partial seizures or the appearance of new hemiclonic seizures. Callosectomy does not seem to affect overall behaviour or personality. Overall, the risks of permanent severe sequelae (those reducing quality of life) after corpus callosum section, either neurological or neuropsychological, are of the order of 5–10%, and there is a mortality rate of about 1–5%.

Multiple subpial transection

This operation is also referred to as the Morrell procedure. Parallel rows of 4- to 5-mm deep cortical incisions are ploughed, perpendicular to the cortical surface, in epileptogenic cortex. This is done on the theoretical basis that the transections sever horizontal cortical connections and thus disrupt the lateral recruitment of neurons, which is essential for the production of synchronized epileptic discharges (Figure 10.23). At the same time normal function is preserved, because this is supported largely by vertically oriented afferent and efferent connections. There are many critics of this theory, and it is not clear whether or not this is a valid explanation of the post-operative consequences, or whether the damage to the cortex caused by the procedure itself reduces seizures.

The procedure has, theoretically, one major advantage – it can be used when the epileptogenic zone involves eloquent brain cortex, in which resection would result in significant neurological deficit. It has thus been principally applied to patients with epileptic foci in language, or primary sensory or motor cortex. In many cases it has been combined with a resection of a lesion in or adjacent to the eloquent cortex.

Typically, this is carried out in patients with focal motor seizures or EPC due to Rasmussen encephalitis, cortical dysplasia or lesions in the central region, or in those with the Landau–Kleffner syndrome. Multiple subpial transection has been successfully carried out in the Broca area, the pre-central and post-central gyrus, and the Wernicke area, without noticeable loss of function.

The procedure has been the subject of only a rather limited evaluation, and its true role is yet to be defined. A meta-analysis of data in 211 patients from 6 centres has been published: 53% underwent the procedure without resection. In those in whom it was combined with resection, a short-term excellent result (≥95% reduction in seizures) was observed in 87% of those with generalized seizures and 68% of those with simple and complex partial seizures; in those who underwent the procedure without resection the figures were 71%, 62% and 63%, respectively. Neurological deficits occurred postoperatively in 23% of those underwent surgery with resection and 19% of those who had multiple subpial transection alone. These results are certainly encouraging, but most patients were followed for a short time and there is only limited information about long-term seizure control. It is clear that there is a substantial relapse rate after

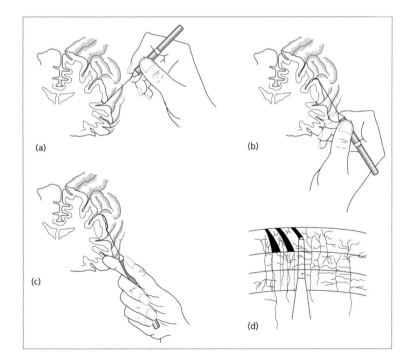

(a)

(b)

(c)

(d)

Figure 10.23 Diagram showing the technique of multiple subpial transection. (a) After a tiny incision is created in the pia, a hook is inserted down one gyral edge. (b) It is then swept across the full width of the gyrus. (c) The hook is brought back to its starting point such that the tip is just visible under the pia as it crosses the gyrus. (d) The procedure is repeated at intervals of <5 mm along the gyrus, leaving thin but visible scars. Thus, the transverse fibres only are sectioned, preserving the columnar organization.

initial improvement. It has been attempted in Rasmussen encephalitis without long-term benefit and in refractory focal status epilepticus. In many centres, the procedure has fallen from favour and is reserved for patients with severe frequent seizures arising from the eloquent cortex, in whom all alternative strategies have been exhausted.

The operation has in addition a particular role in the Landau–Kleffner syndrome. In one series of 24 patients (13 undergoing the procedure without additional lesion resection), all had the classic Landau–Kleffner syndrome and continuous spike–wave in slow-wave sleep from a unilateral perisylvian focus. At a follow-up of at least 2 years, two-thirds were able to form complex sentences. Other reports have been less promising, and the problem of evaluating outcome in this condition is its fluctuating course and the tendency for spontaneous improvement.

The acute operative morbidity is due to cerebral oedema, which is maximal in the third to fourth postoperative day. Transient loss of function is expected in this period, but this usually resolves. There is a risk of haemorrhage and other complications, and a complication rate of about 15% is to be expected. In the surgical series, 7% of patients are left with permanent severe deficit. The long-term morbidity of this operation in routine surgical practice has not been clearly established, but the few series that are published all purport to show minimal long-term deficits. Despite this, the use of this operative approach seems to be declining.

Vagal nerve stimulation

In 1997 vagal nerve stimulation was approved by the US Food and Drug Administration (FDA) for use as adjunctive therapy for adults and adolescents aged >12 years whose partial-onset seizures are refractory to antiepileptic medications. Vagal nerve stimulation was then also approved in European Union countries for use in reducing the frequency of seizures in patients of any age whose epileptic disorder is dominated by partial seizures (with and without secondary generalization) or generalized seizures. Its use has grown rapidly in the past 5 years, and it is now the most common epilepsy surgery procedure carried out in the UK. By June 2008 over 45 000 patients had been implanted with vagal nerve stimulation worldwide. There is no clear idea how vagal nerve stimulation influences epileptic seizures (which are, after all, a cortical phenomenon) but there is considerable experimental and clinical data now confirming

that there is an observable, albeit usually extremely modest, effect.

The operative procedure and stimulator parameters

The operation comprises the implantation of a stimulator below the skin in the chest wall with bipolar electrodes wrapped around the left vagus nerve (Figure 10.24). The latest version of the stimulator box is a hermetically sealed titanium generator weighing 16 g, and measuring $45 \times 33 \times 6.9$ mm. The operation takes only 1–2 h to perform and is often carried out as a day case. It is a relatively minor procedure, lacking the inherent risks of intracranial surgery, hence its immediate attraction to physicians and patients alike.

The stimulation parameters can be set via a programming wand beaming radiofrequency signals to the generator. The wand is further used to perform diagnostic checks of wand–generator communications, lead impedance, programmed current and an estimate of the remaining generator battery life. Once implanted, the stimulation parameters are slowly ramped up during the first 12 months after implantation. The ramp-up procedure and settings are tailored according to individual response and side effects (Table 10.10). Patients can also trigger the stimulator at any time by applying a magnet to the skin over the generator. The generator in the current models

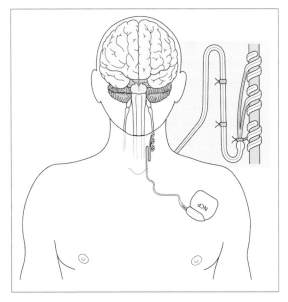

Figure 10.24 Schematic drawing show the placement of the vagus nerve stimulator and the bipolar stimulating lead.

Table 10.10 Available stimulation parameter settings in vagus nerve stimulation (Model 103 vagus nerve stimulation therapy).

Stimulation parameter	Available settings
Output current	0–3.5 mA in 0.25-mA steps, ± 10%, >1 month
Signal frequency	1, 2, 5, 10, 15, 20, 25, 30 Hz ± 6%
Pulse width	130, 250, 500, 750, 1000 μs ± 10%
Signal on time	7, 14, 21, 30, 60 s ± 7 s
Signal off time	0.2, 0.3, 0.5, 0.8, 1.1, 1.8, 3 min, and 5–180 min (5–6 min in 5-min steps; 60–180 min in 30-min steps) +4.4/−8.4 s or ±1% whichever is greater

From Schachter SC. Vagal nerve stimulation. In: Shorvon SD, Perucca E, Engel J (eds), *The Treatment of Epilepsy*, 3rd edn. Oxford: Wiley-Blackwell, 2009: 1017–1024.

should provide between 6 and 11 years of operation, after which it can be replaced, which involves only a minor procedure performed under local anaesthesia.

Efficacy of vagal nerve stimulation

The effectiveness and safety of vagal nerve stimulation were investigated in clinical trials in a manner identical to that applied to new antiepileptic drugs. This was a copybook example of a regulatory trial programme, the only example in epilepsy surgery, and was highly successful.

Single-blind pilot studies in patients with refractory partial seizures were followed by two pivotal, multicentre, double-blind, randomized, parallel, group-controlled trials, with vagal nerve stimulation added as adjunctive therapy. Two different vagal nerve stimulation protocols – high stimulation (30 Hz, 30 s on, 5 min off, 500 ms pulse width) and low stimulation (1 Hz, 30 s on, 90–180 min off, 130 ms pulse width) – were compared, the low stimulation protocol acting as an 'active control'. Individuals were monitored over a 12- to 16-week prospective baseline period, and then randomized to high- or low-stimulation groups. Over the next 2 weeks those in the high-stimulation group had their generator output current increased to as high a level as was tolerated, and those in the low-stimulation group had the current increased until stimulation could be just perceived.

Efficacy was then assessed during the remaining 12 weeks of the treatment phase. The patient characteristics were similar to those in antiepileptic drug trials.

In both studies the primary efficacy analysis was the percentage change in seizure frequency during treatment compared with baseline. In one trial the mean reduction in the high- and low-stimulation groups was 24.5 and 6.1%, respectively, and this difference was significant at a level of $P = 0.01$. In the second the mean percentage decreases in seizure frequency during treatment compared with baseline were 28% and 15% for the high- and low-stimulation groups, a statistically significant result at a level of $P = 0.039$. Secondary efficacy measures in both studies showed statistically significant effects in favour of high stimulation. In the first study 31% of patients in the high-stimulation group had a reduction in seizures of at least 50% compared with 13% of patients in the low-stimulation group ($P = 0.02$). In the second study 11% of patients in the high-stimulation group had a reduction in seizure frequency of at least 75% vs 2% for patients in the low-stimulation group ($P = 0.01$). On the basis of these results, the device was licensed for use. A study was then carried out in 60 children aged 3–18 years with pharmacoresistant epilepsy. After 6 months of vagal nerve stimulation treatment ($n = 55$), the median reduction in seizure frequency was 31%. The corresponding figures at 12 and 18 months were 34% ($n = 51$) and 42% ($n = 46$), respectively. Other studies, some controlled, have shown progressive (but modest) falls in seizure rates over the longer term and a progressive decrease in the number of antiepileptic drugs needed as co-therapy. Studies have also been carried out in generalized epilepsy, in the Lennox–Gastaut syndrome, in elderly people, in children with epileptic encephalopathy, and in those with learning disability. In all these studies positive effects were noted.

Safety and tolerability of vagal nerve stimulation

Perioperative complications include infection, left vocal fold paralysis, lower facial muscle paresis, pain and fluid accumulation over the generator requiring aspiration.

The rates of side effects in the first double-blind study are shown in Table 10.11. Dyspnoea and hoarseness of the voice were the only adverse events that were reported significantly more often with high stimulation than with low stimulation. Longer-term effects were studied in a cohort of 444 patients in the long-term extensions of the clinical trials. Of these, 97% continued with vagal nerve stimulation for at least 1 year, 85% for 2 years and 72% for

Table 10.11 Adverse events among patients treated with low or high vagal nerve stimulation (randomized double-blind study).

Adverse event	Low stimulation ($n= 103$) Number (%)	High stimulation ($n= 95$) Number (%)
Voice alteration	31 (30.1)	63 (66.3)
Cough	44 (42.7)	43 (45.3)
Pharyngitis	26 (25.2)	33 (34.7)
Pain	31 (30.1)	27 (28.4)
Dyspnoea	11 (10.7)	24 (25.3)
Headache	24 (23.3)	23 (24.2)
Dyspepsia	13 (12.6)	17 (17.9)
Vomiting	14 (13.6)	17 (17.9)
Paraesthesia	26 (25.2)	17 (17.9)
Nausea	21 (20.4)	14 (14.7)
Accidental injury	13 (12.6)	12 (12.6)
Fever	19 (18.4)	11 (11.6)
Infection	12 (11.7)	11 (11.6)

Only adverse events that occurred in more than 10% of high-stimulation patients are listed.

3 years. The most common side effects were: at 12 months, hoarseness (29%) and paraesthesias (12%); at 24 months hoarseness (19%) and cough (6%); and at 36 months shortness of breath. No excess mortality was recorded. One anxiety has been the question of vagally induced cardiac arrhythmia, and there have been increasing numbers of reports of stimulation-induced asystole and other cardiac arrhythmias. Effects on cardiac function are routinely tested peroperatively, during implantation (a brief stimulation at 1.0 mA, 500 ms and 20 Hz) and, if this induces asytole, the device is not implanted. The published rate of SUDEP in treated patients is 4.1 per 1000 person-years, which is said on rather weak grounds not to be in excess of that expected in a matched population.

Chronic stimulation can also mildly impair swallowing and increase the risk of aspiration in vulnerable individuals. Other side effects recorded include posture-dependent stimulation of the phrenic nerve and worsening of pre-existing obstructive sleep apnoea.

There are other practical issues. MRI at 3 T is advised against in those with an implanted vagal nerve stimulator, and 1.5 T scanning should be carried out with the stimulator turned off and with other precautions in place. The use of short-wave diathermy, microwave diathermy or therapeutic ultrasound diathermy should be avoided.

Another significant problem is that, although the stimulator box can be removed, the wires wrapped around the vagal nerve cannot, and so are in place permanently.

The long-term effects of this on the nerve are not known. Furthermore, if infection or inflammation occurs, the removal of the wires leads to a high rate of nerve damage, and one of the author's patients developed permanent recurrent laryngeal palsy, which required surgical reconstruction of the vocal folds to restore intelligible speech.

Quality-of-life measures have demonstrated apparent improvements in energy, memory, daytime sleepiness, social aspects, mental effects and fear of seizures, and these effects occur whether or not seizures have been improved. The common sedative side effects of new drugs do not occur, and this is of course a very important difference and a major attraction of the procedure to patients. Vagal nerve stimulation also has an antidepressant action, and is licensed for use in refractory depression in some countries.

Clinical role for vagal nerve stimulation

There seems to be no doubt that vagal nerve stimulation can exert a slight antiepileptic action. No patient should be given the impression that full seizure control will be achieved, because this is a rare event. Many patients do, however, experience some apparent improvement.

Vagal nerve stimulation has the advantage of not being a drug, and so patients can escape the cognitive and CNS side effects associated with all conventional antiepileptic medication. Furthermore, the stimulator can be simply implanted with low surgical morbidity – and certainly none of the risks of intracranial surgery. However, the effectiveness of the procedure has not, in the opinion of many, lived up to the promise apparent from the clinical trials. Few patients have gained seizure freedom from the technique, and there often appears to be little or no effect at all. The problem of assessing the procedure is compounded by both the large number of possible variations in stimulation parameters that can be tried, and the suggestion that effects on seizure frequency may be delayed and become observable months or even years after the initiation of therapy.

The epilepsy indications for the procedure are not fully explored, but currently it can be offered to any patient in whom seizures have failed to respond to conventional medical therapy, and in whom resective surgical therapy is not appropriate. There is no clear evidence that one seizure type does better than any other, although the use of vagal nerve stimulation in generalized epilepsy is currently evinced only by open, uncontrolled studies. Assessment is complicated as psychogenic non-epileptic seizures can improve strikingly with this procedure.

The usual initial target parameters are shown in Table 10.12. Programming is started a few weeks after

Table 10.12 Usual initial target stimulation parameters for vagal nerve stimulation in patients with epilepsy.

Stimulation parameter	Setting
Output current	1.5 mA
Signal frequency	20–30 Hz
Pulse width	250–500 ms
Signal on time	30 s
Signal off time	5 min

implantation. The ramping up of stimulation parameters is typically performed at outpatient follow-up visits, by a specially trained nurse, every 1–2 weeks over the next few months. The current is usually increased by 0.25 mA increments, or more, to the maximum tolerated settings or until ≥50% reduction in seizure frequency. If side effects occur, the current can be reduced by 0.25 mA decrements or the bandwidth lessened. If seizures have not improved after 9 months of stimulation, the 'off time' is usually decreased from 5 min to 3 min. Further reduction to 1.8 and 0.2 min can be tried (with an associated decrease of 'on time' to 7 s – 'rapid cycle'). If this fails to improve seizures within 12–18 months, it is usual to turn the device off and remove the stimulator box.

The patient can override stimulation patterns with the magnet, which can be used to trigger stimulation or to suppress programmed activity. The sense of empowerment this conveys to patients over their epilepsy may be one reason for the observed benefits of the therapy.

The initial cost of vagal nerve stimulation is high, much higher than the initial costs of pharmacotherapy, and attempts have been made to demonstrate long-term cost-effectiveness.

Other functional surgical procedures

Both stereotactic ablation and deep-brain stimulation (DBS) have been used, in small numbers of patients, in an attempt to control or modify seizures since the 1930s. Targets have included the amygdala, various thalamic nuclei, the fields of Forel, the anterior commissure, the fornix and the posterior limb of the internal capsule. The results of these operations in the past were often poor, and this type of functional surgery had until recently been largely abandoned. However, there has been a recent resurgence of interest in DBS, encouraged by the improved anatomical precision of stereotaxy made possible by MRI, better surgical instrumentation and stimulation technol-

ogy, and also the success of these procedures in other conditions such as Parkinson disease and in pain.

Targets that are most favoured include the caudate nucleus, the centromedian nucleus of the thalamus, the anterior thalamic nucleus, the mamillary bodies and the subthalamic nucleus. Direct stimulation of the epileptic focus, in both the neocortex and the hippocampus, has also been attempted. All these approaches have had encouraging results in animal experimentation, and there are small human case reports and small series.

Pioneering double-blind studies in small numbers of patients with severe epilepsy have been reported. In six of nine patients, stimulation of the subthalamic nuclear resulted in a >80% reduction in seizures and, in a study of five patients, stimulation of the anterior thalamus produced an average 54% seizure reduction after a mean follow-up of 15 months. A recent multicentre, double-blind, randomized controlled trial of bilateral stimulation of the anterior nuclei of thalamus was conducted in focal epilepsy (SANTE trial): 110 patients were included, and in the last month of the blinded phase the stimulated group had a ≥50% reduction in seizures. At 24 months of follow-up, there was a 56% median reduction in seizure frequency, 54% of patients had a seizure reduction of at least 50% and 14 patients were seizure free for at least 6 months. Five deaths occurred, none from implantation or stimulation. It was concluded by the researchers that the anterior thalamus is useful for some people with medically refractory partial and secondarily generalized seizures. Centromedian nucleus stimulation has also shown promising results with stimulation settings in the range 60–130 Hz, 2.5–5.0 V, 0.2–1.0 ms duration for 1 min in every 5 min. A >50% reduction in seizures occurred in an open investigation of amygdalo-hippocampal stimulation in three patients. However, well-controlled and blinded studies of cerebellar stimulation and hippocampal stimulation have shown no benefit. Another study was recently completed using the NeuroPace RNS system. This device is chronically implanted around the seizure focus, where it continuously monitors brain electrical activity, identifies the onset of a seizure, and delivers a brief electrical stimulation with the intention of suppressing the seizure. The study demonstrated a statistically significant reduction in seizure frequency in the treatment group (responsive stimulation active) of 29% compared with the sham stimulation group (responsive stimulation inactive) of 14%. In the long-term extension period of the trial, 47% of patients experienced a ≥50% reduction in their seizure frequency. DBS carries risks, notably of infection and haemorrhage (a rate of about

5%), and as yet none of these techniques is in routine clinical usage in any major centre.

A related technique is transcranial magnetic stimulation (TMS), which has been used to treat myoclonus and partial seizures. Anecdotal case reports are encouraging, and in one open study eight of nine patients with myoclonus showed a seizure reduction of 39%. However, a study of 24 patients with frequent partial and secondarily generalized seizures treated with low-frequency, repetitive TMS on 5 consecutive days resulted in a mean reduction of only 16% in seizures, which was not significant.

Gamma knife or proton pencil beam surgery is also under investigation for use in focal ablations and other forms of functional surgery. In addition there is research interest in the possibility of stem-cell and neural transplantation, and in the possibility of stereotactic drug implantation. These techniques can be applied to the seizure focus, the 'trigger site' of seizures or to propagation pathways. Seizure-stimulated drug release directly into the seizure focus is also being explored. None of these procedures is yet at a stage where surgery in routine clinical practice is possible.

A note of caution is needed, however, when considering functional surgical approaches to epilepsy. Over the past century various functional procedures have been conducted, usually without proper evaluation, which are now considered worthless (Table 10.13). The current vogue for

Table 10.13 A lesson from history – 'functional operations' still being performed for epilepsy, 1900–1930.

Trepanation
Trephination
Carotid artery occlusion
Bilateral vertebral artery occlusion
Cervical sympathectomy
Castration
Circumcision
Hysterectomy/oopherectomy
Adrenalectomy
Dural splitting
Colectomy and other bowel resections
Arterialization of internal jugular vein

Table 10.14 The characteristics of level 1 and level 2 epilepsy centres.

	Level 1 centres	Level 2 centres
Patients	Adults	Adults and children (in some centres)
Type of surgery	Anterior temporal lobectomy	A full range of epilepsy surgical procedures
General facilities	Full range of neurological and neurosurgical facilities, and neurosurgical intensive care unit	As for level 1
MRI facilities	1.5 T with facilities for thin slice volumetric imaging	As for level 1, with additional facilities where possible for fMRI, MRS and post-processing
Other neuroimaging facilities	CT and angiography	As for level 1, with access to other procedures such as PET, SPECT, SISCOM
Neuropsychological facilities	Routine neuropsychology and facilities for Wada testing	As for level 1
EEG facilities	Routine scalp EEG, video telemetry and corticography	As for level 1, with additional facilities for intracranial recording and stimulation
Staffing	Access to: neurology, neurosurgery, clinical neurophysiology, neuroradiology, neuropsychiatry, neurorehabilitation, neuropathology, counselling, full technical support	As for level 1, with additional paediatric specialities if paediatric surgery is being performed
Audit	An audit of surgical volume and results should be available where possible	As for level 1

See text for abbreviations.

functional surgery (including vagal nerve stimulation) requires careful evaluation to avoid similar mistakes.

The organization of epilepsy surgery care: the epilepsy surgery centre

It should be clear that epilepsy surgery is a specialized field of endeavor that requires, for almost every patient, input from specialists in different non-surgical areas, e.g. neurology, neurophysiology, neuroradiology, neuropaediatrics, neurorehabilitation, neuropsychology and psychiatry. The input is needed to select suitable patients for surgery, to counsel patients adequately about the potential risks and benefits of surgery, and to follow up patients after surgery. A full range of necessary facilities and expertise is likely to be available only in designated centres, and standards for such centres have been defined by the ILAE Commission on Neurosurgery.

It has been proposed that there should be two levels of epilepsy surgery centre: basic epilepsy surgery centres (level 1) and reference epilepsy surgery centres (level 2). Both should be sited within a comprehensive neuroscience centre, and the typical characteristics of each level are shown in Table 10.14. In the age of clinical governance and audit, it is inevitable as well as desirable that epilepsy surgery services are organized in such a formal and regulated fashion.

Pharmacopoeia

Handbook of Epilepsy Treatment, 3rd Edition. By Simon Shorvon.
Published 2010 by Blackwell Publishing Ltd.

Antiepileptic drugs – indications in epilepsy

Drug	Therapeutic indications in epilepsy	Commonly used as first-line drug
Acetazolamide	All seizure types. Catamenial epilepsy	No
Carbamazepine	Monotherapy and adjunctive therapy in partial and generalized seizures (excluding absence, tonic and myoclonic seizures), and in childhood epilepsy syndromes. Adults and children	Yes
Clobazam	Adjunctive and monotherapy in epilepsy. Also for intermittent therapy, one-off prophylactic therapy. Adults and children	No
Clonazepam	Monotherapy and adjunctive therapy in partial and generalized seizures (including absence and myoclonus) and also the Lennox–Gastaut syndrome, neonatal seizures, infantile spasms and status epilepticus. Adults and children	No
Eslicarbazepine acetate	Adjunctive therapy in refractory partial-onset seizures. Adults only	No
Ethosuximide	Monotherapy or adjunctive therapy for generalized absence seizures. Adults and children	No
Felbamate	Refractory partial and secondarily generalized epilepsy and the Lennox–Gastaut syndrome as last resort therapy	No
Gabapentin	Partial or secondarily generalized epilepsy: adjunctive therapy in adults and children aged ≥6 years. Monotherapy in adults and children aged ≥12 years (Europe; not licensed for monotherapy in the USA)	No
Lacosamide	Adjunctive therapy of partial-onset seizures. Adults only	No
Lamotrigine	Adjunctive or monotherapy of partial seizures and generalized seizures, and seizures associated with the Lennox–Gastaut syndrome in those aged ≥13 years. Adjunctive therapy of partial seizures and generalized seizures and monotherapy of typical absence seizures in those aged 2–12 years	Yes
Levetiracetam	Adjunctive therapy in partial-onset seizures in adults and children aged >1 month, and in myoclonic and tonic–clonic seizures in juvenile myoclonic epilepsy, aged ≥12 years. Monotherapy in partial seizures with or without secondarily generalized seizures in patients aged ≥16 years	Yes
Oxcarbazepine	Monotherapy and adjunctive therapy in partial-onset seizures and generalized tonic–clonic seizures. Adults and chldren aged ≥6 years	Yes
Phenobarbital	Monotherapy and adjunctive therapy in partial or generalized seizures (including absence and myoclonus) in adults and children. Also, status epilepticus, the Lennox–Gastaut syndrome, other childhood epilepsy syndromes, febrile convulsions, neonatal seizures	Yes – in some countries
Phenytoin	Monotherapy and adjunctive therapy in partial-onset seizures and generalized tonic–clonic seizures. Also status epilepticus. Adults and children	Yes – in some countries
Piracetam	Myoclonus, especially in progressive myoclonic epilepsies. Adults and children	No
Pregabalin	Adjunctive therapy in partial-onset seizures. Adults only	No
Primidone	Monotherapy and adjunctive therapy in partial-onset seizures and generalized tonic clonic seizures. Adults and children.	No

(Continued)

Antiepileptic drugs – indications in epilepsy (*Continued*)

Drug	Therapeutic indications in epilepsy	Commonly used as first-line drug
Rufinamide	Adjunctive therapy in the Lennox–Gastaut syndrome, aged ≥4 years	No
Tiagabine	Adjunctive therapy in partial and secondarily generalized seizures in patients aged ≥12 years	No
Topiramate	Adjunctive therapy for partial-onset seizures and for the Lennox–Gastaut syndrome aged ≥2 years. Monotherapy for partial-onset and generalized seizures; aged ≥6 years	Yes
Valproate	Monotherapy and adjunctive therapy in partial-onset and generalized seizures, including myoclonus and absence, and for the seizures associated with the Lennox–Gastaut syndrome. Idiopathic generalized epilepsy, febrile convulsions, other childhood epilepsy syndromes. Adults and children	Yes
Vigabatrin	West syndrome. Also, adjunctive therapy in partial-onset seizures where other therapy has been ineffective and the risk vs benefit ratio is appropriate. Adults and children	No
Zonisamide	Adjunctive therapy in partial-onset seizures in adults aged ≥18 years (in Europe and the USA). Monotherapy and adjunctive therapy in children and adults for a broad range of epilepsy (in Japan and Asia)	No

Antiepileptic drugs – dose, average adult values

Drug	Initial dose (mg/day)	Drug initiation: usual dose increment (mg/day) stepped up every 2 weeks	Usual initial maintenance dose on monotherapy (mg/day)	Usual maximum dose in monotherapy (mg/day)	Dosing intervals (per day)	Drug reduction: usual dose decrement (mg/day) stepped down every 2–4 weeks	Doses can be affected by co-medication
Acetazolamide	250 mg	250	250–750	750	1–2	250	
Carbamazepine[a]	100–200	200	400–1600	2400	2–3	200	Yes
Clobazam	10	10	10–30	30	1–2	10	No
Clonazepam	0.25	0.25–0.5	0.5–4	4	1–2	0.5	No
Eslicarbazepine acetate	400	200–400	800–1200	1200	1	400	Yes
Ethosuximide	250	250	750–1500	1500	2–3	250	Yes
Felbamate	1200	1200	1200–3600	3600	2–3	600	Yes
Gabapentin	300–400	300–400	900–3600	3600	2–3	300–400	No
Lacosamide	50	50	200–400	400	2	50	No
Lamotrigine	12.5–25	50	100–400	600	2	50–100	Yes
Levetiracetam	125–250	250–500	750–4000	4000	2	250–500	Occasionally
Oxcarbazepine	300	300	900–2400	3000	2	300	Yes
Phenobarbital	30	15–30	30–120	180	1	15–30	Yes
Phenytoin	200	25–100	200–450	500	1–2	50	Yes
Piracetam	4800	2400	1200–32 000	32 000	2–3	2400	No
Pregabalin	50	50	150–400	600	2–3	50	No
Primidone	62.5–125	125–250	250–1000	1500	1–2	125–250	Yes
Rufinamide	400	400	1200–3200	3200	2	400	Yes
Tiagabine	15	4–5	30–45	56–60	2–3	4–5	Yes
Topiramate	25–50	25–50	75–300	600	2	50	Yes
Valproate	200–500	200–500	500–2000	3000	2–3	200–500	Yes
Vigabatrin	500	500	1000–3000	4000	2	500	No
Zonisamide	50	50	200–400	600	1–2	50	Yes

[a]Values are for the slow-release formulation, which is the formulation of choice, particularly at high doses.
Note that values in this table are based on the author's own practice, and may vary from those published elsewhere.

Antiepileptic drugs – dose, interactions

Drug	Is dose commonly affect by co-medication?	Is dose affected by renal or hepatic disease?	Does this drug commonly affect doses of other drugs in co-medication?	Does this drug affect the contraceptive pill?	Is serum level monitoring useful in defining dose?	Target range of serum levels (adults)
Acetazolamide	No	Avoid in renal and hepatic disease	No	No	Not useful	
Carbamazepine	Yes	Severe hepatic disease	Yes	Yes	Very useful	20–50 µmol/L (10,11-epoxide – <9 µmol/L)
Clobazam	No	Severe hepatic disease	No	No	Not useful	
Clonazepam	No	Severe hepatic disease	No	No	Not useful	
Eslicarbazepine acetate	Yes	Moderate renal disease	Yes	Yes	Utility not established	
Ethosuximide	Yes	Hepatic disease and severe renal disease	No	No	Very useful	300–700 µmol/L
Felbamate	Yes	Renal disease. Avoid in hepatic disease	Yes	Yes	Potentially useful	30–60 mg/L
Gabapentin	No	Severe renal disease	No	No	Not useful	
Lacosamide	No	No	No	No	Utility not established	
Lamotrigine	Yes	Avoid in hepatic disease	No	No	Useful	2–20 mg/L
Levetiracetam	Occasionally	Renal disease	No	No	Not useful	
Oxcarbazepine	Yes	Severe renal disease	Yes	Yes	Useful (measures of MHD derivative)	50–140 µmol/L (MHD derivative)
Phenobarbital	Yes	Severe hepatic and renal disease	Yes	Yes	Very useful	50–130 µmol/L
Phenytoin	Yes	Severe hepatic disease	Yes	Yes	Very useful	40–80 µmol/L
Piracetam	No	Severe renal disease	No	No	Not useful	
Pregabalin	No	Renal disease	No	No	Not useful	
Primidone	Yes	Severe hepatic and renal disease	Yes	Yes	Very useful (measures of derived phenobarbital)	50–130 µmol/L (derived phenobarbital)
Rufinamide	Yes	Insufficient data in hepatic disease	Yes	Yes	Utility not established	
Tiagabine	Yes	Hepatic disease	No	No	Utility not established	
Topiramate	Yes	Renal disease	Slight	Yes	Potentially useful	10–60 µmol/L
Valproate	Yes	Avoid in hepatic disease	Yes	No	Useful	300–700 µmol/L
Vigabatrin	No	Renal disease	Slight	No	Not useful	
Zonisamide	Yes	Avoid in severe renal disease	No	No	Potentially useful	30–140 µmol/L

Antiepileptic drugs – dose, in children

Drug	Children – average initial dose	Children – average maintenance dose
Acetazolamide	10 mg/kg per day	30 mg/kg/day
Carbamazepine	<1 year, 50 mg/day 1–5 years: 100 mg/day 5–10 years: 200 mg/day 10–15 years: 100 mg/day	<1 year: 100–200 mg/day 1–5 years: 200–400 mg/day 5–10 years: 400–600 mg/day 10–15 years: 600–1000 mg/day
Clobazam	0.25 mg/kg per day	0.25–1.5 mg/kg per day
Clonazepam	<1 year: 0.25 mg/day 1–5 years: 0.25 mg/day 5–12 years: 0.25 mg/day	<1 year: 1 mg/day 1–5 years: 1–2 mg/day 5–12 years: 1–3 mg/day
Eslicarbazepine acetate	–	–
Ethosuximide	10–15 mg/kg per day	20–40 mg/kg per day
Felbamate	15 mg/kg per day	45–80 mg/kg per day
Gabapentin	10–15 mg/kg per day/kg	3–4 years: 40 mg/kg per day 5–12 years: 25–35 mg/kg per day >12 years: as for adults
Lacosamide	–	–
Lamotrigine	2–12 years: 0.3 mg/kg per day (monotherapy) 0.15 mg/kg per day (with valproate co-medication) 0.6 mg/kg per day (with co-medication with enzyme inducing drugs)	2–12 years: 1–10 mg/kg per day (monotherapy) 1–5 mg/kg per day (with valproate co-medication) 5–15 mg/kg per day (with co-medication with enzyme inducing drugs)
Levetiracetam	10–20 mg/kg per day	20–60 mg/kg per day
Oxcarbazepine	4–5 mg/kg per day	20–45 mg/kg per day
Phenobarbital	Neonates: 1–2 mg/day 1 month–12 years: 1–1.5 mg/kg per day, >12 years: 15 mg/day	Neonates: 3–4 mg/day 1 month–12 years: 3–8 mg/kg per day >12 years: 30–180 mg/day
Phenytoin	1 month–12 years: 1.5–2.5 mg/kg per day >12 years: 50 mg/day	1 month–12 years: 2.5–7.5 mg/kg per day >12 years: 75–150 mg/day
Piracetam	–	–
Pregabalin	–	–
Primidone	1–2 mg/kg per day	10–20 mg/kg per day
Rufinamide	<30 kg: 200 mg	<30 kg not receiving valproate: 1000 mg/day <30 kg receiving valproate: 600 mg/day
Tiagabine		
Topiramate	0.5–1 mg/kg per day	5–9 mg/kg per day
Valproate	Neonates, 20 mg/kg 1 month–12 years: 10–15 mg/kg	Neonates, 20 mg/kg 1 month–12 years: 25–30 mg/kg (up to 60 mg/kg in infantile spasms)
Vigabatrin	10–15 kg, 125 mg/day 15–30 kg: 250 mg/day >30 kg: 500 mg/day	10–15 kg, 40 mg/kg per day or 500–1000 mg/day 15–30 kg, 1000–1500 mg/day >30 kg, 1500–3000 mg/day
Zonisamide	2–4 mg/kg per day	4–8 mg/kg per day

Antiepileptic drugs – summary of side effects

Drug	Common side effects	Risk of hypersensitivity
Acetazolamide	Acidosis, drowsiness, anorexia, irritability, nausea and vomiting, loss of appetite, weight loss, enuresis, headache, thirst, dizziness, hyperventilation, flushing, loss of libido, renal stones. Severe hypersensitivity affecting skin and blood	Yes – marked risk
Carbamazepine	Drowsiness, fatigue, dizziness, ataxia, diplopia, blurring of vision, sedation, headache, insomnia, gastrointestinal disturbance, tremor, weight gain, impotence, effects on behaviour and mood, hepatic disturbance, rash and other skin reactions, bone marrow dyscrasia, leucopenia, hyponatraemia, water retention, endocrine effects, effects on cardiac conduction, effects on immunoglobulins	Yes
Clobazam	Drowsiness, sedation, asthenia, ataxia, weakness and hypotonia, diplopia, mood and behavioural change, dependency, withdrawal symptoms	Slight
Clonazepam	Drowsiness, sedation, asthenia, ataxia, weakness and hypotonia, diplopia, mood and behavioural change, drooling and hypersalivation, dependency, withdrawal symptoms	Slight
Eslicarbazepine acetate	Headache, dizziness, somnolence, nausea, diplopia, vomiting, blurred vision, vertigo, fatigue, constipation and diarrhoea. Others as with oxcarbazepine, but probably less hyponatremia	None to date
Ethosuximide	Gastrointestinal symptoms, drowsiness, ataxia, diplopia, headache, dizziness, hiccups, sedation, behavioural disturbances, acute psychotic reactions, extrapyramidal symptoms, blood dyscrasia, rash, lupus-like syndrome, severe hypersensitivity	Yes – marked risk
Felbamate	Severe hepatic disturbance and aplastic anaemia, insomnia, weight loss, gastrointestinal symptoms, fatigue, dizziness, lethargy, behavioural change, ataxia, visual disturbance, mood change, psychotic reaction, rash, neurological symptoms	Yes – marked risk
Gabapentin	Drowsiness, dizziness, ataxia, headache, tremor fatigue, weight gain, exacerbation of non-convulsive generalized seizures	Slight
Lacosamide	Dizziness, headache, nausea, diplopia, ataxia, memory impairment, somnolence, tremor, vertigo, constipation, pruritus, asthenia, fatigue	None to date
Lamotrigine	Rash (sometimes severe), blood dyscrasia, headache, ataxia, asthenia, diplopia, nausea, vomiting, dizziness, somnolence, insomnia, depression, behavoral effects, psychosis, tremor	Yes – marked risk
Levetiracetam	Somnolence, asthenia, infection, dizziness, headache, irritability, aggression, behavioural and mood changes, emotional lability, depersonalization, psychosis, nervousness, seizure exacerbation, rhinitis, cough, vomiting	Slight
Oxcarbazepine	Somnolence, headache, dizziness, diplopia, ataxia, rash, hyponatraemia, weight gain, alopecia, nausea, gastrointestinal disturbance	Yes
Phenobarbital	Sedation, ataxia, dizziness, insomnia, hyperkinesis (children), dysarthria, mood changes (especially depression), behaviour change, aggressiveness, cognitive dysfunction, impotence, reduced libido, folate deficiency and megablastic anaemia, vitamin K and vitamin D deficiency, osteomalacia, Dupuytren contracture, frozen shoulder, shoulder–hand syndrome, connective tissue abnormalities, rash. Risk of dependency. Potential for abuse	Slight

Antiepileptic drugs – summary of side effects (*Continued*)

Drug	Common side effects	Risk of hypersensitivity
Phenytoin	Ataxia, dizziness, lethargy, sedation, headaches, dyskinesia, acute encephalopathy (phenytoin intoxication), hypersensitivity, rash, fever, blood dyscrasia, gingival hyperplasia, folate deficiency, megaloblastic anaemia, vitamin K deficiency, decreased immunoglobulins, mood changes, depression, coarsened facies, hirsutism, peripheral neuropathy, osteomalacia and osteoporosis, hypocalcaemia, hormonal dysfunction, loss of libido, hepatitis, coagulation defects	Yes
Piracetam	Dizziness, insomnia, nausea, gastrointestinal discomfort, hyperkinesis, weight gain, tremulousness, agitation, drowsiness, rash	No
Pregabalin	Weight gain, somnolence, dizziness, ataxia, asthenia, tremor, blurred vision, double vision, amnesia, depression, insomnia, nervousness, anxiety, cognitive effects and confusion	No
Primidone	As for phenobarbital. Also dizziness and nausea on initiation of therapy	Slight
Rufinamide	Headache, dizziness, somnolence, fatigue, nausea, diplopia, blurred vision, ataxia	None to date
Tiagabine	Dizziness, tiredness, nervousness, tremor, diarrhoea, nausea, headache, confusion, psychosis, flu-like symptoms, ataxia, depression, word-finding difficulties, encephalopathy, non-convulsive status epilepticus	No
Topiramate	Dizziness, ataxia, headache, paraesthesia, tremor, somnolence, cognitive dysfunction, confusion, agitation, amnesia, depression, emotional lability, nausea, diarrhoea, diplopia, weight loss	No
Valproate	Nausea, vomiting, hyperammonaemia and other metabolic effects, endocrine effects, severe hepatic toxicity, pancreatitis, drowsiness, cognitive disturbance, aggressiveness, tremor, weakness, encephalopathy, thrombocytopenia, neutropenia, aplastic anaemia, hair thinning and hair loss, weight gain, polycystic ovarian syndrome	Yes
Vigabatrin	Mood change, depression, psychosis, aggression, confusion, weight gain, insomnia, changes in muscle tone in children, tremor and diplopia. Irreversible visual field constriction	No
Zonisamide	Somnolence, ataxia, dizziness, fatigue, nausea, vomiting, irritability, anorexia, impaired concentration, mental slowing, itching, diplopia, insomnia, abdominal pain, depression, skin rashes, hypersensitivity. Significant risk of renal calculi, metabolic acidosis, weight loss, and oligohidrosis. Risk of heat stroke	Yes

Antiepileptic drugs – summary of metabolism

Drug	Major metabolic pathways	Hepatic enzymes involved in metabolism	Inhibitor or induce of hepatic enzymes	Drug interactions	Active metabolite
Acetazolamide	None	No	No	No	No
Carbamazepine	Epoxidation and hydroxylation, and then conjugation	CYP3A4, CYP2C8, CYP1A2 and then UGT (15%)	Induces CYP2B6, CYP2C9, CYP2C19, CYP3A, CYP1A2, UGT1A4	Common	Carbamazepine epoxide
Clobazam	Desmethylation and hydroxylation and then conjugation	CYO3A4	Slight effects only	Minor only	*N*-Desmethylclobazam
Clonazepam	Reduction, hydroxylation and acetylation	CYP3A4	Slight effects only	Minor only	No
Eslicarbazepine acetate	Hydrolysis and conjugation	No	Inhibits CYP2C9	Common	Eslicarbazepine
Ethosuximide	Hepatic oxidation then conjugation	CYP3A4	No	Common	No
Felbamate	Hydroxylation and conjunction	CYP3A4 CYP2E1, UDPGT (10%)	Induces CYP3A4, inhibits CYP2C19	Common	No
Gabapentin	None	No	No	No	No
Lacosamide	*O*-Desmethylation	CYP2C19	Inhibits CYP2C19	Some drug interactions	No
Lamotrigine	Only phase 2 glucuronidation	UGT14A (>80%)	Induces UGT1A4	Common	No
Levetiracetam	Hydrolysis in many body tissues	No	No	Minor only	No
Oxcarbazepine	Reduction to MHD, then conjugation	Aldo-ketoreductase enzymes (not via CYP enzymes), UDPGT (60%)	Inhibits CYP2C19, induces CYP3A, UGT1A4	Some	MHD
Phenobarbital	Oxidation, glucosidation and hydroxylation, then conjugation	CYP2C9, CYP2C19, CYP2E1	Induces CYP2B6, CYP2C9, CYPC19, CYP3A, UGT1A4	Common	No
Phenytoin	Oxidation, hydroxylation , and glucosidation.	CYP2C9, CYP2C19, CYP3A4 UDPGT1A	Induces CYP2B6, CYP2C9, CYP2C19, CYP3A4, UGT1A4	Common	No
Piracetam	None	No	No	No	No
Pregabalin	None	No	No	No	No

Antiepileptic drugs – summary of metabolism (*Continued*)

Drug	Major metabolic pathways	Hepatic enzymes involved in metabolism	Inhibitor or induce of hepatic enzymes	Drug interactions	Active metabolite
Primidone	Metabolism to phenobarbital, and then biotransformation as for phenobarbital	As per phenobarbital	As per phenobarbital	Common	Phenobarbital
Rufinamide	Hydrolysis	Carboxylesterase enzymes, (not via CYP enzymes)	Induces CYP 3A4	Common	No
Tiagabine	Oxidation then conjugation	CYP3A4	No	Common	No
Topiramate	No[a] (in polytherapy: hydoxylation or hydrolysis and then conjugation)	Not in monotherapy	Inducer of CYP3A4, inhibits CYP2C19	Some drug interactions	No
Valproate	Oxidation, epoxidation, reduction and then conjunction	CYP2C9, CYP2C19, CYP2B6, UGT1A4	Inhibits CYP2C9, UGT1A4 (and a very weak inhibitor of CYP2C19 and CYP3A4)	Common	No
Vigabatrin	None	No	No	No	No
Zonisamide	Reduction, *N*-acetylation and conjunction	CYP3A4	No	Common	No

[a]In monotherapy. In polytherapy, some hepatic metabolism.
CYP, cytochrome P450 enzyme; UGT, uridine glucuronyl transferase enzyme.

Antiepileptic drugs – summary of pharmacokinetic values (typical adult values)

Drug	Oral bioavailability (%)	Time to peak levels (h)	Volume of distribution (L/kg)	Elimination half life (h)	Plasma clearance[b] (L/kg per h)	Protein binding (%)
Acetazolamide	<90	1–3	0.2	10–12	Insufficient data	90–95
Carbamazepine	75–85	4–8	0.8–2	5–26[d]	0.133[d]	75
Clobazam	90	1–4	0.9–1.8	10–30[e] 50[f]	0.021–0.038[f]	83
Clonazepam	80	1–4	3	20–55	0.09	86
Eslicarbazepine acetate[c]	<100	2–3	2.7	13–20	0.055	30
Ethosuximide	<100	4	0.65	40–70[d]	0.010–0.015[d]	<10
Felbamate	<100	1–4	0.75	11–25[d]	0.027–0.032[d]	20–25
Gabapentin	<65[g]	2–3	0.65–1.04	5–9	0.120–0.130	0
Lacosamide	<100	2–4	0.5–0.8	12–16	Insufficient data	<15
Lamotrigine	<100	1–3	0.9–1.31	12–60[d]	0.044–0.08[d]	55
Levetiracetam	<100	0.5–2	0.5–0.7	6–8	0.036	0
Oxcarbazepine	<100	4–6[a]	0.7–0.8[a]	8–10[a]	0.04–0.05[d]	38[a]
Phenobarbital	80–100	0.5–4	0.36–0.73	75–120	0.006–0.009[d]	45–60
Phenytoin	95	4–12	0.5–0.8	7–42[d]	0.003–0.02[d]	80–95
Piracetam	<100	0.5–0.7	0.6	5–6	Insufficient data	0
Pregabalin	>90	1	0.56	5–7	0.042–0.06	0
Primidone	<100	0.27–3.2	0.64–0.72	3.3–22.4[d]	0.035–0.052[d]	25
Rufinamide	<85	4–6	0.8	8–12[d]	0.09[d]	30
Tiagabine	<100	1–2	1.0	5–9[d]	0.109[d]	96
Topiramate	<100	2–4	0.6–1.0	19–25[d]	0.022–0.036[d]	13–17
Valproate	<100	0.5–2	0.13–0.30	13–16[d]	0.010–0.115[d]	70–95
Vigabatrin	<100	0.5–2	0.8	4–7	0.102–0.114	0
Zonisamide	<100	2.4–4.6	1.1–1.7	49–69[d]	0.0089–0.001[d]	40–50

[a]Figures refer to MHD derivative (the active metabolite of oxcarbazepine).
[b]Values given for monotherapy in most cases.
[c]Figures refer to eslicarbazepine (the active metabolite of eslicarbazepine acetate).
[d]Depend on co-medication.
[e]Clobazam.
[f]Desmethylclobazam.
[g]Dose dependant absorption.

Antiepileptic drugs – modes of action

Drug	Mechanism of action
Acetazolamide	Carbonic anhydrase inhibition
Carbamazepine	Inhibition of sodium channel conductance. Also action on monoamine, acetylcholine and NMDA receptors
Clobazam	GABA$_A$-receptor agonist
Clonazepam	GABA$_A$-receptor agonist
Eslicarbazepine acetate	Inhibition of voltage-dependent sodium conductance.
Ethosuximide	Inhibition of calcium T-channel conductance
Felbamate	Inhibition of NMDA receptor (glycine recognition site) and sodium channel conductance
Gabapentin	Action on α_2–δ subunit of the voltage-gated calcium channel
Lacosamide	Inhibition of sodium channel conductance
Lamotrigine	Inhibition of sodium channel conductance
Levetiracetam	Action via binding to SV2A protein
Oxcarbazepine	Inhibition of sodium channel conductance. Also effects on potassium conductance, N-type calcium channels, NMDA receptors
Phenobarbital	GABA$_A$ receptor agonist. Also depresses glutamate excitability, and affects sodium, potassium and calcium conductance
Phenytoin	Inhibition of sodium channel conductance
Piracetam	Probably via binding to the SV2A protein. Other properties include enhancement of oxidative glycolysis, anticholinergic effects, rheological effects
Pregabalin	Action on α_2–δ subunit of the voltage-gated calcium channel. Also reduces release of glutamate and other excitatory neurotransmitters
Primidone	As for phenobarbital – GABA$_A$-receptor agonist. Also depresses glutamate excitability, and affects sodium, potassium and calcium conductance
Rufinamide	Inhibition of sodium channel conductance
Tiagabine	Inhibition of postsynaptic GABA reuptake
Topiramate	Inhibition of sodium channel conductance, potentiation of GABA-mediated inhibition at the GABA$_A$ receptor, reduction of AMPA receptor activity, inhibition of high-voltage calcium channels, carbonic anhydrase activity
Valproate	Effects on GABA and glutaminergic activity, calcium (T) conductance and potassium conductance
Vigabatrin	Inhibition of GABA transaminase activity
Zonisamide	Inhibition of sodium channel conductance, T-type calcium currents, benzodiazepine GABA$_A$ receptor excitatory glutaminergic transmission, carbonic anhydrase

AMPA, α-amino-3-hydroxyl-5-methyl-4-isoxazole-propionate; GABA, γ-aminobutyric acid; NMDA, N-methyl-D-aspartate; SV2A, synaptic vesicle glycoprotein 2A.

Further Reading

The purpose of this section is to provide guidance for further reading on the topics in this book. This is not intended to be a comprehensive list of citations (in the age of PubMed, this seems not really necessary), but simply a selection of recent reviews, key articles and important summary papers. Where data are cited in the text, the source is also included here. The list should be sufficient for the interested reader to follow up any aspect of particular interest.

The key text is the sister book, *The Treatment of Epilepsy*, 3rd edn (Shorvon SD, Perucca E, Engel J Jr. Oxford: Blackwell Publishing Ltd, 2009). Most of the chapters in the book have comprehensive citation lists and these are an invaluable source for further study, and are separately listed here. Some text in this book is taken with permission from these chapters in the book. Other textbooks that provide comprehensive citations are also listed below. The citations to articles in the scientific journals are biased towards recently published papers.

Chapters 1–6

Chapters from: Shorvon SD, Perucca E, Engel J Jr, eds (2009). *The Treatment of Epilepsy*. Oxford: Blackwell Publishing Ltd

Gurnett CA, Dodson WE. Definitions and classification of epilepsy, pp. 3–30.

Forsgren L. Hesdorffer D. Epidemiology and prognosis of epilepsy, pp. 21–32.

Shorvon S. Aetiology of epilepsy, 33–54.

Cook M. Differential diagnosis of epilepsy, pp. 55–66.

Avanzini G. Franceschetti S. Mechanisms of epileptogenesis, pp. 67–80.

White S. Antiepileptic drug discovery, pp. 81–90.

Walker M, Surges R, Fisher F. Mechanisms of antiepileptic drug action, pp. 91–108.

Löscher W, Schmidt D. Mechanisms of tolerance and drug resistance, pp. 109–120.

Perucca E. General principles of medical management, pp. 121–140.

Hart YM. Management of newly diagnosed epilepsy, pp. 141–152.

Shorvon SD. Management of chronic active epilepsy in adults, pp. 153–162.

Kwan P, Leung H. Management of epilepsy in remission, pp. 163–170.

Chiron C. Management of epilepsy in infants, pp. 171–178.

Ferrie CD. Childhood epilepsy syndromes, pp. 179–194.

Livingston JH. Management of epilepsies associated with specific diseases in children, pp. 195–202.

Arif J, Mendiratta A, Hirsch L. Management of epilepsy in the elderly, pp. 203–218.

Brodtkorb E. Management of epilepsy in people with learning disabilities, pp. 219–230.

Walker MC, Shorvon SD. Emergency treatment of seizures and status epilepticus, pp. 231–248.

Dichter M, Temkin NR. Traumatic brain injury and other risks, pp. 249–258.

Singh G. Management of medical co-morbidity associated with epilepsy, pp. 259–272.

Elliott B, Amarouche M, Shorvon SD. Psychiatric features of epilepsy and their management, pp. 273–289.

Zaccara G, Balestrieri F, Ragazzoni A. Management of side-effects of antiepileptic drugs, pp. 289–300.

Kossoff EH, Jennifer L, Dorward JL. Ketogenic diets, pp. 301–310.

Whitmarsh T. Non-pharmacological, complementary and alternative treatments for epilepsy, pp. 311–322.

Tomson T. Reproductive aspects of epilepsy treatment, pp. 323–334.

Linklater A, Patsika P, Usiskin S. Epilepsy counselling, pp. 335–340.

Zara F. Genetic counselling in epilepsy, pp. 341–360.

Spina E. Drug interactions, pp. 361–378.

Birkbeck G. Medical treatment of epilepsy in situations with limited resources, pp. 379–388.

Books

Arzimanoglou A, Guerrini R, Aicardi J. *Aicardi's Epilepsy in Children*, 3rd edn. Philadelphia: Lippincott, Williams & Wilkins, 2003.

Clarke C, Howard R, Rossor M, Shorvon SD (eds), *Neurology: A Queen Square textbook*. Oxford: Wiley-Blackwell, 2009.

Handbook of Epilepsy Treatment, 3rd Edition. By Simon Shorvon. Published 2010 by Blackwell Publishing Ltd.

Davis LE, Kennedy PGE. *Infectious Diseases of the Nervous System*. Oxford: Butterworth Heinemann, 2000.

Engel J, Pedley TA, eds. *Epilepsy: A comprehensive textbook*, 3rd edn. New York: Raven Press, 2008.

Lennox WG. *Epilepsy and Related Disorders*. Boston: Little Brown, 1969.

Murphy PA. *Treating Epilepsy Naturally*. Chicago: Keats Publishing, 2001.

Panayiotopoulos CP. *A Clinical Guide to Epileptic Syndromes and Their Treatment*. New York: Springer-Verlag, 2007.

Panayiotopoulos CP. *Atlas of Epilepsies*. New York: Springer-Verlag, 2010.

Panayiotopoulos CP. *The Epilepsies: Seizures, syndromes and management*. Chipping Norton: Bladon Medical Publishing, 2005.

Roger J, Bureau M, Dravet C, Dreifuss F, Perret A, Wolf P, eds. *Epileptic Syndromes in Infancy, Childhood and Adolescence*, 2nd edn. London: John Libbey & Co., 1992.

Shorvon SD, Pedley TA, eds. *Blue Book of Neurology: The epilepsies*, 3rd edn. Philadelphia: Saunders, 2009.

Wallace SJ, Farrell K, eds. *Epilepsy in Children*. London: Arnold, 2004.

Journal articles/chapters in books

Adab N, Kini U, Vinten J, et al. The long term outcome of children born to mothers with epilepsy. *J Neurol Neurosurg Psych* 2004; **75**: 1575–1583.

Adab N, Tudur SC, Vinten J, et al. *Common Antiepileptic Drugs in Pregnancy in Women with Epilepsy (Cochrane review)*. Cochrane Library, Chichester: John Wiley & Sons Ltd, 2004.

Ahmed SN, Siddiqi ZA. Antiepileptic drugs and liver disease. *Seizure* 2006; **15**: 156–164.

Alper K, Schwartz KA, Kolts RL, et al. Seizure incidence in psychopharmacological clinical trials: an analysis of Food and Drug Administration (FDA) summary basis of approval reports. *Biol Psychiatry* 2007; **62**: 345–354.

Alvarez N. Discontinuance of antiepileptic medications in patients with developmental disability and diagnosis of epilepsy. *Am J Ment Ret* 1989; **93**: 593–599.

Amarouche M. *Organic Mental Disorders (other than memory disorders, depression and psychosis) after Temporal Lobe Epilepsy Surgery. Occurrence, diagnostic schemes, classification and design of future studies*. London: Rockefeller Medical Library, UCL Institute of Neurology and the National Hospital for Neurology and Neurosurgery, 2008: 23–39.

American Academy of Pediatrics Committee on Quality Improvement, Subcommittee on Febrile Seizures. Practice parameter: long-term treatment of the child with simple febrile seizures. *Pediatrics* 1999; **103**: 1307–1309.

Anhoury S, Brown RJ, Krishnamoorthy ES, et al. Psychiatric outcome after temporal lobectomy: a predictive study. *Epilepsia* 2000; **41**: 1608–1615.

Annegers JF, Hauser WA, Beghi E, Nicolosi A, Kurland LT. The risk of unprovoked seizures after encephalitis and meningitis. *Neurology* 1988; **38**: 1407–1410.

Annegers JF, Hauser WA, Elveback LR. Remission of seizures and relapse in patients with epilepsy. *Epilepsia* 1979; **30**: 729–737.

Annegers JF, Hauser WA, Shirts SB, Kurland LT. Factors prognostic of unprovoked seizures after febrile convulsions. *N Engl J Med* 1987; **316**: 493–498.

Anonymous. Proposal for revised clinical and electroencephalographic classification of epileptic seizures. From the Commission Classification and Terminology of the International League Against Epilepsy. *Epilepsia* 1981; **22**: 489–501.

Anonymous. Proposal for revised classification of epilepsies and epileptic syndromes. Commission on Classification and Terminology of the International League Against Epilepsy. *Epilepsia* 1989; **30**: 389–399.

Arzimanoglou AA, Andermann F, Aicardi J, et al. Sturge–Weber syndrome: indications and results of surgery in 20 patients. *Neurology* 2000; **55**: 1472–1479.

Baulac S, Gourfinkel-An I, Nabbout R, et al. Fever, genes, and epilepsy. *Lancet Neurol* 2004; **3**: 421–430.

Baulac S, Huberfeld G, Gourfinkel-An I, et al. First genetic evidence of GABA$_A$ receptor dysfunction in epilepsy: a mutation in the γ2-subunit gene. *Nat Genet* 2001; **28**: 46–48.

Becker AJ, Blümcke I, Urbach H, Hans V, Majores M. Molecular neuropathology of epilepsy-associated glioneuronal malformations. *J Neuropathol Exp Neurol* 2006; **65**: 99–108.

Beghi E. The management of a first seizure. Still a major debate. *Epilepsia* 2008; **49**(suppl 1): 1–61.

Berg AT, Vickrey GB, Langfitt JT, et al. Reduction of AEDs in postsurgical patients who attain remission. *Epilepsia* 2006; **47**: 64–71.

Bergamasco B, Benna P, Ferrero P, Gavinelli R. Neonatal hypoxia and epileptic risk: a clinical prospective study. *Epilepsia* 1984; **25**: 131–136.

Bergey GK. Initial treatment of epilepsy: special issues in treating the elderly. *Neurology* 2004; **63**(10 suppl 4): S40–48.

Berkovic SF, Harkin L, McMahon JM, et al. De-novo mutations of the sodium channel gene SCN1A in alleged vaccine encephalopathy: a retrospective study. *Lancet Neurol* 2006; **5**: 488–492.

Berkovic SF, Heron SE, Giordano L, et al. Benign familial neonatal-infantile seizures: characterization of a new sodium channelopathy. *Ann Neurol* 2004; **55**: 550–557.

Bharucha NE, Raven RH, Nambiar VK. Review of seizures and status epilepticus in HIV and tuberculosis with preliminary view of Bombay hospital experience. *Epilepsia* 2009; **50**(suppl 12): 64–66.

Birbeck G, Chomba E, Ddumba E, Kauye F, Mielke J. Lack of appropriate treatment for people with comorbid HIV/AIDS and epilepsy in sub-Saharan Africa. *Epilepsia* 2007; **48**: 1424–1425.

Bjørnaes H, Stabell KE, Heminghyt E, et al. Resective surgery for intractable focal epilepsy in patients with low IQ: predictors for seizure control and outcome with respect to seizures and neuropsychological and psychosocial functioning. *Epilepsia* 2004; **45**: 131–139.

Blandford M, Tsuboi T, Vogel F. Genetic counseling in the epilepsies. *Hum Genet* 1987; **76**: 303–331.

Blumenfeld H, Klein JP, Schridde U, et al. Early treatment suppresses the development of spike–wave epilepsy in a rat model. *Epilepsia* 2008; **49**: 400–409.

Boling W, Andermann F, Reutens D, et al. Surgery for temporal lobe epilepsy in older patients. *J Neurosurg* 2001; **95**: 242–248.

Bough KJ, Rho JM. Anticonvulsant mechanisms of the ketogenic diet. *Epilepsia* 2007; **48**: 43–58.

Brodie MJ, Overstall PW, Giorgi L. Multicentre, double-blind, randomised comparison between lamotrigine and carbamazepine in elderly patients with newly diagnosed epilepsy. The UK Lamotrigine Elderly Study Group. *Epilepsy Res* 1999; **37**: 81–87.

Brodtkorb E. The diversity of epilepsy in adults with severe developmental disabilities: age at seizure onset and other prognostic factors. *Seizure* 1994; **3**: 277–285.

Brodtkorb E, Mula M. Optimizing therapy of seizures in adult patients with psychiatric comorbidity. *Neurology* 2006; **67**(suppl 4): 39–44.

Brodtkorb E, Aamo T, Henriksen O, et al. Rectal diazepam: pitfalls of excessive use in refractory epilepsy. *Epilepsy Res* 1999; **35**: 123–133.

Brodtkorb E, Sand T, Strandjord RE. Neuroleptic and antiepileptic treatment in the mentally retarded. *Seizure* 1993; **2**: 205–211.

Brown S. Deterioration. *Epilepsia* 2006; **47**(suppl 2): 19–23.

Buist NRM, Dulac O, Bottiglieri T, et al. Metabolic evaluation of infantile epilepsy: summary recommendations of the Amalfi group. *J Child Neurol* 2002; **17**: 3S98–102.

Burn J, Dennis M, Bamford J, Sandercock P, Wade D, Warlow C. Epileptic seizures after a first stroke: the Oxfordshire Community Stroke Project. *BMJ* 1997; **315**: 1582–1587.

Callaghan BC, Anand K, Hesdorffer D, Hauser WA, French JA. Likelihood of seizure remission in an adult population with refractory epilepsy. *Ann Neurol* 2007; **62**: 382–389.

Canitano R, Luchetti A, Zappella M. Epilepsy, electroencephalographic abnormalities, and regression in children with autism. *J Child Neurol* 2005; **20**: 27–31.

Caraballo R, Cerósimo R, Fejerman N. Panayiotopoulos syndrome: a prospective study of 192 patients. *Epilepsia* 2007; **48**: 1054–1061.

Caraballo R, Cerósimo R, Fejerman N. Childhood occipital epilepsy of Gastaut: a study of 33 patients. *Epilepsia* 2008; **49**: 288–297.

Caraballo RH, Cersosimo RO, Sakr D, et al. Ketogenic diet in patients with myoclonic-astatic epilepsy. *Epileptic Disord* 2006; **8**: 151–155.

Carpio A, Escobar A, Hauser WA. Cysticercosis and epilepsy: a critical review. *Epilepsia* 1998; **39**: 1025–1040.

Carter JA, Neville BG, White S, et al. Increased prevalence of epilepsy associated with severe falciparum malaria in children. *Epilepsia* 2004; **45**: 978–981.

Cascino GD. Epilepsy and brain tumors: implications for treatment. *Epilepsia* 1990; **31**(suppl 3): S37–S44.

Castilla-Guerra L, del Carmen Fernández-Moreno M, López-Chozas JM, Fernández-Bolaños R. Electrolytes disturbances and seizures. *Epilepsia* 2006; **47**: 1990–1998.

Cavalleri GL, Walley NM, Soranzo N, et al. A multicenter study of BRD2 as a risk factor for juvenile myoclonic epilepsy. *Epilepsia* 2007; **48**: 706–712.

Chadwick D. Does withdrawal of different antiepileptic drugs have different effects on seizure recurrence? Further results from the MRC Antiepileptic Drug Withdrawal Study. *Brain* 1999; **122**: 441–448.

Chadwick D, Smith D. The misdiagnosis of epilepsy. *BMJ* 2002; **324**: 495–496.

Cheuk DKL, Wong V. Acupuncture for epilepsy. *Cochrane Database Syst Rev* 2006; (**2**): CD005062.

Chevrie JJ, Aicardi J. Convulsive disorders in the first year of life: aetiologic factors. *Epilepsia* 1977; **18**: 489–498.

Chong JY, Rowland LP, Utiger RD. Hashimoto encephalopathy: syndrome or myth? *Arch Neurol* 2003; **60**: 164–171.

Choulika S, Grabowski E, Holmes LB. Is antenatal vitamin K prophylaxis needed for pregnant women taking anticonvulsants? *Am J Obstet Gynecol* 2004; **190**: 882–883.

Christensen J, Vestergaard M, Mortensen PB, et al. Epilepsy and risk of suicide: a population-based case-control study. *Lancet Neurol* 2007; **6**: 693–698.

Cimaz R, Meroni PL, Shoenfeld Y. Epilepsy as part of systemic lupus erythematosus and systemic antiphospholipid syndrome (Hughes syndrome). *Lupus* 2006; **15**: 191–197.

Cleary P, Shorvon S, Tallis R. Late-onset seizures as a predictor of subsequent stroke. *Lancet* 2004; **363**: 1184–1186.

Cockerell OC, Johnson AJ, Goodridge DMG, Sander JWAS, Shorvon SD. Remission of epilepsy: results from the National General Practice Study of Epilepsy. *Lancet* 1995; **346**: 140–144.

Cockerell OC, Johnson AJ, Goodridge DMG, Sander JWAS, Shorvon SD. Prognosis of epilepsy: a review and further analysis of the first nine years of the British National General Practice Study of Epilepsy, a prospective population-based study. *Epilepsia* 1997; **38**: 31–46.

Colledge NR, Wilson JA, Macintyre CC, et al. The prevalence and characteristics of dizziness in an elderly community. *Age Ageing* 1994; **23**: 117–120.

Comi AM. Sturge–Weber syndrome and epilepsy: an argument for aggressive seizure management in these patients. *Expert Rev Neurother* 2007; **7**: 951–956.

Commission on Classification and Terminology of the International League Against Epilepsy. Proposal for revised clinical and electroencephalographic classification of epileptic seizures. *Epilepsia* 1981; **22**: 489–501.

Commission on Classification and Terminology of the International League Against Epilepsy. Proposal for revised classification of epilepsies and epileptic syndromes. *Epilepsia* 1989; **30**: 389–399.

Conry JA. Pharmacological treatment of catastrophic epilepsies. *Epilepsia* 2004; **45**(suppl 5): 12–16.

Cossette P, Liu L, Brisebois K, et al. Mutation of GABRA1 in an autosomal dominant form of juvenile myoclonic epilepsy. *Nat Genet* 2002; **31**: 184–189.

Crawford PM, West CR, Shaw MDM, Chadwick DW. Cerebral arteriovenous malformations and epilepsy: factors in the development of epilepsy. *Epilepsia* 1986; **27**: 270–275.

Cross JH. Neurocutaneous syndromes and epilepsy-issues in diagnosis and management. *Epilepsia* 2005; **46**(suppl 10): 17–23.

D'Ambrosio R, Perucca E. Epilepsy after head injury. *Curr Opin Neurol* 2004; **17**: 731–735.

D'Ambrosio R, Fairbanks JP, Fender JS, Born DE, Doyle DL, Miller JW. Post-traumatic epilepsy following fluid percussion injury in the rat. *Brain* 2004; **127**: 304–314.

D'Ambrosio R, Fender JS, Fairbanks JP, et al. Progression from frontal-parietal to mesial-temporal epilepsy after fluid percussion injury in the rat. *Brain* 2005; **128**: 174–188.

Daumas-Duport C, Scheithauer BW, Chodkiewicz JP, Laws ER Jr, Vedrenne C. Dysembryoplastic neuroepithelial tumor: a surgically curable tumor of young patients with intractable partial seizures. Report of thirty-nine cases. *Neurosurgery* 1988; **23**: 545–556.

de Koning TJ, Klomp LW. Serine-deficiency syndromes. *Curr Opin Neurol* 2004; **17**: 197–204.

De Smet PAGM, D'Arcy PF. Drug interactions with herbal and other non-orthodox drugs. In: Wellington PJ, D'Arcy PF (eds), *Drug Interactions*. Heidelberg: Springer-Verlag, 1996.

Delgado MR, Riela AR, Mills J, et al. Discontinuation of antiepileptic drug treatment after two seizure free years in children with cerebral palsy. *Pediatrics* 1996; **97**: 192–197.

Deonna T, Roulet E. Autistic spectrum disorder: evaluating a possible or causal role of epilepsy. *Epilepsia* 2006; **47**(suppl 2): 79–82.

Desai J. Perspectives on interactions between anti-epileptic drugs and anti-microbial agents. *Epilepsia* 2008; **49**(suppl 6): 47–49.

Devlin RJ, Henry JA. Clinical review: major consequences of illicit drug consumption. *Crit Care* 2008; **12**: 202.

Di Martino A, Tuchman RF. Antiepileptic drugs: affective use in autism spectrum disorders. *Pediatr Neurol* 2001; **25**: 199–207.

Ding D, Hong Z, Chen GS, et al. Primary care treatment of epilepsy with phenobarbital in rural China: Cost-outcome analysis from the WHO/ILAE/IBE global campaign against epilepsy demonstration project. *Epilepsia* 2008; **49**: 535–539.

Dravet C, Bureau M, Oguni H, Fukuyama Y, Cokar O. Severe myoclonic epilepsy in infancy: Dravet syndrome. *Adv Neurol* 2005; **95**: 71–102.

Dreifuss FE. Fatal liver failure in children on valproate. *Lancet* 1987; **i**: 47–48.

Dreifuss FE, Langer DH, Moline KA, et al. Valproic acid hepatic fatalities. II. US experience since 1984. *Neurology* 1989; **139**: 201–207.

Eisermann MM, DeLaRaillere A, Dellatolas G, et al. Infantile spasms in Down syndrome: effects of delayed anticonvulsive treatment *Epilepsy Res* 2003; **55**: 21–27.

Elliott B, Joyce EM, Shorvon SD. Delusions, illusions and hallucinations in epilepsy: 1. elementary phenomena. *Epilepsy Res* 2009; **85**: 162–171.

Elliott B, Joyce EM, Shorvon SD. Delusions, illusions and hallucinations in epilepsy: 2. complex phenomena and psychosis. *Epilepsy Res* 2009; **85**: 172–186.

Engel J Jr. Report of the ILAE classification core group. *Epilepsia* 2006; **47**: 1558–1568.

Engelhard HH, Stelea A, Cochran EJ. Oligodendroglioma: pathology and molecular biology. *Surg Neurol* 2002; **58**: 111–117.

Eriksen HR, Ellertsen B, Gronningsaeter H, Nakken KO, Loyning Y, Ursin H. Physical exercise in women with intractable epilepsy. *Epilepsia* 1994; **35**: 1246–1264.

Eriksson KJ, Koivikko MJ. Prevalence, classification, and severity of epilepsy and epileptic syndromes in children. *Epilepsia* 1997; **38**: 1275–1282.

Escayg A, MacDonald BT, Baulac S, et al. Mutations of SCN1A, encoding a neuronal sodium channel, in two families with GEFS+. *Nat Genet* 2000; **24**: 343–345.

Ettinger AB, Reed ML, Goldberg JF, et al. Prevalence of bipolar symptoms in epilepsy vs other chronic health disorders. *Neurology* 2005; **65**: 535–540.

EURAP study group. Seizure control and treatment in pregnancy. Observations from the EURAP epilepsy and pregnancy registry. *Neurology* 2006; **66**: 354–360.

Fejerman N, Caraballo R, Tenembaum SN. Atypical evolutions of benign localization-related epilepsies in children: are they predictable? *Epilepsia* 2000; **41**: 380–390.

Ferraro TN, Buono RJ. Polygenic epilepsy. *Adv Neurol* 2006; **97**: 389–398.

Ferraro TN, Dlugos DJ, Buono RJ. Role of genetics in the diagnosis and treatment of epilepsy. *Expert Rev Neurother* 2006; **6**: 1789–1802.

First Seizure Trial Group. Randomized clinical trial on the efficacy of antiepileptic drugs in reducing the risk of relapse after a first unprovoked tonic clonic seizure. *Neurology* 1993; **43**: 478–483.

Forsgren L. Prevalence of epilepsy in adults in northern Sweden. *Epilepsia* 1992; **33**: 450–458.

Freeman JL, Coleman LT, Wellard RM, et al. MR imaging and spectroscopic study of epileptogenic hypothalamic hamartomas: analysis of 72 cases. *Am J Neuroradiol* 2004; **25**: 450–462.

Freitag H, Tuxhorn I. Cognitive function in preschool children after epilepsy surgery: rationale for early intervention. *Epilepsia* 2005; **46**: 561–567.

French JA, Kanner AM, Bautista A, et al. Efficacy and tolerability of the new antiepileptic drugs, I: treatment of new onset epilepsy: report of the Treatment and Technology Assessment Subcommittee and the Quality Standards Subcommittee of the American Academy of Neurology and the American Epilepsy Society. *Neurology* 2004; **62**: 1252–1260.

French JA, Kanner AM, Bautista A, et al. Efficacy and tolerability of the new antiepileptic drugs, II: treatment of refractory epilepsy: report of the Treatment and Technology Assessment Subcommittee and the Quality Standards Subcommittee of the American Academy of Neurology and the American Epilepsy Society. *Neurology* 2004; **62**: 1261–1273.

Frey LC. Epidemiology of posttraumatic epilepsy: a critical review. *Epilepsia* 2003; **44**(suppl 10): 11–17.

Fried S, Kozer E, Nulman I, et al. Malformation rates in children of women with untreated epilepsy. A meta-analysis. *Drug Saf* 2004; **27**: 197–202.

Frucht MM, Quigg M, Schwaner C, Fountain NB. Distribution of seizure precipitants among epilepsy syndromes. *Epilepsia* 2000; **41**: 1534–1539.

Fujiwara T. Clinical spectrum of mutations in SCN1A gene: severe myoclonic epilepsy in infancy and related epilepsies. *Epilepsy Res* 2006; **70**(suppl 1): S223–230.

Gaggero R, Devescovi R, Zaccone A, Ravera G. Epilepsy associated with infantile hemiparesis: predictors of long-term evolution. *Brain Dev* 2001; **23**: 12–17.

Gambardella A, Andermann F, Shorvon S, Le Piane E, Aguglia U. Limited chronic focal encephalitis: another variant of Rasmussen syndrome? *Neurology* 2008; **70**: 374–377.

Garcia HH, Modi M. Helminthic parasites and seizures. *Epilepsia* 2008; **49**(suppl 6): 25–32.

Gayatri NA, Livingston JH. Aggravation of epilepsy by anti-epileptic drugs. *Dev Med Child Neurol* 2006; **48**: 394–398.

Gidal BE, Tamura T, Hammer A, Vuong A. (2005) Blood homocysteine, folate and vitamin B-12 concentrations in patients with epilepsy receiving lamotrigine or sodium valproate for initial monotherapy. *Epilepsy Res* 2005; **64**: 161–166.

Gilliam FG, Barry JJ, Hermann BP, et al. Rapid detection of major depression in epilepsy: a multicentre study. *Lancet Neurol* 2006; **5**: 399–405.

Gilliam FG, Fessler AJ, Baker G, et al. Systematic screening allows reduction of adverse antiepileptic drug effects. A randomised trial. *Neurology* 2004; **62**: 23–27.

Glauser T, Ben-Menachem E, Bourgeois B. ILAE treatment guidelines: evidence-based analysis of antiepileptic drug efficacy and effectiveness as initial monotherapy for epileptic seizures and syndromes. *Epilepsia* 2006; **47**: 1094–1120.

Gloor P, Olivier A, Quesney LF, et al. The role of the limbic system in experiential phenomena of temporal lobe epilepsy. *Ann Neurol* 1982; **12**: 129–144.

Goldstein LH. Effectiveness of psychological interventions for people with poorly controlled epilepsy. *J Neurol Neurosurg Psychiatry* 1997; **63**: 137–142.

Goodkin HP, Yeh JL, Kapur J. Status epilepticus increases the intracellular accumulation of GABA$_A$ receptors. *J Neurosci* 2005; **25**: 5511–5520.

Goodridge DMG, Shorvon SD. Epileptic seizures in a population of 6000. II. Treatment and prognosis. *BMJ* 1983; **287**: 645–647.

Gopaul KP, Crook MA. The inborn errors of sialic acid metabolism and their laboratory investigation. *Clin Lab* 2006; **52**: 155–169.

Gourfinkel-An I, Baulac S, Nabbout R, et al. Monogenic idiopathic epilepsies. *Lancet Neurol* 2004; **3**: 209–218.

Grivas A, Schramm J, Kral T, et al. Surgical treatment for refractory temporal lobe epilepsy in the elderly: seizure outcome and neuropsychological sequels compared with a younger cohort. *Epilepsia* 2006; **47**: 1364–1372.

Grote CL, Slyke PV, Hoeppner J-AB. Language outcome following multiple subpial transaction for Landau-Kleffner syndrome. *Brain* 1999; **122**: 561–566.

Guarnieri R, Araujo D, Carlotti CG Jr, et al. Suppression of obsessive-compulsive symptoms after epilepsy surgery. *Epilepsy Behav* 2005; **7**: 316–319.

Guerrini R, Marini C. Genetic malformations of cortical development. *Exp Brain Res* 2006; **173**: 322–333.

Guerrini R, Bonanni P, Patrignani A, et al. Autosomal dominant cortical myoclonus and epilepsy (ADCME) with complex partial and generalized seizures: a newly recognized epilepsy syndrome with linkage to chromosome 2p11.1–q12.2. *Brain* 2001; **124**: 2459–2475.

Guerrini R, Carrozzo R, Rinaldi R, Bonanni P. Angelman syndrome: etiology, clinical features, diagnosis, and management of symptoms. *Paediatr Drugs* 2003; **5**: 647–661.

Guerrini R, Dobyns WB, Barkovich AJ. Abnormal development of the human cerebral cortex: genetics, functional consequences and treatment options. *Trends Neurosci* 2008; **31**: 154–162.

Hadjipanayis A, Hadjichristodoulou C, Youroukos S. Epilepsy in patients with cerebral palsy. *Dev Med Child Neurol* 1997; **39**: 659–663.

Hägg S, Spigset O. Anticonvulsant use during lactation. *Drug Saf* 2000; **22**: 425–440.

Harkin LA, McMahon JM, Iona X, et al. The spectrum of SCN1A-related infantile epileptic encephalopathies. *Brain* 2007; **130**: 843–852.

Hart YM, Sander JWAS, Johnson AL, Shorvon SD, for the NGPSE (National General Practice Study of Epilepsy). Recurrence after a first seizure. *Lancet* 1990; **336**: 1271–1274.

Harvey AS, Freeman JL. Epilepsy in hypothalamic hamartoma: clinical and EEG features. *Semin Pediatr Neurol* 2007; **14**: 60–64.

Hauser WA, Kurland LT. The epidemiology of epilepsy in Rochester, Minnesota, 1935 through 1967. *Epilepsia* 1975; **16**: 1–66.

Hauser WA, Annegers JF, Kurland LT. Prevalence of epilepsy in Rochester, Minnesota: 1940–1980. *Epilepsia* 1991; **32**: 429–445.

Hauser WA, Annegers JF, Kurland LT. Incidence of epilepsy and unprovoked seizures in Rochester, Minnesota: 1935–1984. *Epilepsia* 1993; **34**: 453–468.

Hauser WA, Rich SS, Lee JRJ, Annegers JF, Anderson VE. Risk of recurrent seizures after two unprovoked seizures. *N Engl J Med* 1998; **338**: 429–434.

Henderson CB, Filloux FM, Alder SC, et al. Efficacy of the keto-genic diet as a treatment option for epilepsy: meta-analysis. *J Child Neurol* 2006; **21**: 193–198.

Herlenius E, Heron SE, Grinton BE, et al. SCN2A mutations and benign familial neonatal-infantile seizures: the phenotypic spectrum. *Epilepsia* 2007; **48**: 1138–1142.

Heron SE, Crossland KM, Andermann E, et al. Sodium-channel defects in benign familial neonatal-infantile seizures. *Lancet* 2002; **360**: 851–852.

Hillbom M, Pieninkeroinen I, Leone M. Seizures in alcohol-dependent patients: epidemiology, pathophysiology and management. *CNS Drugs* 2003; **17**: 1013–1030.

Hirsch LJ, Arif H, Buchsbaum R, et al. Effect of age and co-medication on levetiracetam pharmacokinetics and tolerability. *Epilepsia* 2007; **48**: 1351–1359.

Huber B, Hauser I, Horstmann V. Long-term course of epilepsy in a large cohort of intellectually disabled patients. *Seizure* 2007; **16**: 35–42.

Huf RL, Mamelak A, Kneedy-Cayem K. Vagus nerve stimulation therapy: 2-year prospective open-label study of 40 subjects with refractory epilepsy and low IQ who are living in long-term care facilities. *Epilepsy Behav* 2005; **6**: 417–423.

Hung SI, Chung WH, Jee SH, et al. Genetic susceptibility to carbamazepine-induced cutaneous adverse drug reactions. *Pharmacogenet Genomics* 2006; **16**: 297–306.

Huppke P, Köhler K, Brockmann K, et al. Treatment of epilepsy in Rett syndrome. *Eur J Paediatr Neurol* 2007; **11**: 10–16.

Hurana DS, Salganicoff L, Melvin JJ, et al. Epilepsy and respira-tory chain defects in children with mitochondrial encepha-lopathies. *Neuropediatrics* 2008; **39**: 8–13.

Inoue Y, Fujiwara T, Matsuda K, et al. Ring chromosome 20 and nonconvulsive status epilepticus. A new epileptic syndrome. *Brain* 1997; **120**: 939–953.

Irwin K, Bird V, Lees J, et al. Multiple subpial transection in Landau-Kleffner syndrome. *Dev Med Child Neurol* 1991; **43**: 248–252.

Isojärvi JIT, Taboll E, Herzog AG. Effect of antiepileptic drugs on reproductive endocrine function in individuals with epi-lepsy. *CNS Drugs* 2005; **19**: 207–223.

Isojärvi JI, Turkka J, Pakarinen AJ, Kotila M, Rättyä J, Myllylä VV. Thyroid function in men taking carbamazepine, oxcar-bazepine, or valproate for epilepsy. *Epilepsia* 2001; **42**: 930–934.

Jansen FE, van Huffelen AC, Algra A, van Nieuwenhuizen O. Epilepsy surgery in tuberous sclerosis: a systematic review. *Epilepsia* 2007; **48**: 1477–1484.

Jarrar RG, Buchhalter JR, Raffael C. Long-term outcome of epilepsy surgery in patients with tuberous sclerosis. *Neurology* 2004; **62**: 479–481.

Jeavons PM, Harper JR, Bower BD. Long-term prognosis in infantile spasms: a follow-up report on 112 cases. *Dev Med Child Neurol* 1970; **12**: 413–421.

Jentarra G, Snyder SL, Narayanan V. Genetic aspects of neuro-cutaneous disorders. *Semin Pediatr Neurol* 2006; **13**: 43–47.

Joensuu T, Lehesjoki AE, Kopra O. Molecular background of EPM1-Unverricht-Lundborg disease. *Epilepsia* 2008; **49**: 557–563.

Jozwiak S, Domanska-Pakiela D, Kotulska K, Kaczorowska M. Treatment before seizures: new indications for antiepileptic therapy in children with tuberous sclerosis complex. *Epilepsia* 2007; **48**: 1632.

Kälviäinen R, Khyuppenen J, Koskenkorva P, Eriksson K, Vanninen R, Mervaala E. Clinical picture of EPM1-Unverricht-Lundborg disease. *Epilepsia* 2008; **49**: 549–556.

Kammersgaard LP, Olsen TS. Poststroke epilepsy in the Copenhagen stroke study: incidence and predictors. *J Stroke Cerebrovasc Dis* 2005; **14**: 210–214.

Kanemoto K, Kawasaki J, Kawai I. Postictal psychosis: a comparison with acute interictal and chronic psychoses. *Epilepsia* 1996; **37**: 551–556.

Kanner AM, Barry JJ. Is the psychopathology of epilepsy different from that of nonepileptic patients? *Epilepsy Behav* 2001; **2**: 170–186.

Kanner AM, Soto A, Gross-Kanner H. Prevalence and clinical characteristics of postictal psychiatric symptoms in partial epilepsy. *Neurology* 2004; **62**: 708–713.

Kanner AM, Stagno S, Kotagal P, et al. Postictal psychiatric events during prolonged video-electroencephalographic monitoring studies. *Arch Neurol* 1996; **53**: 258–263.

Kaplowitz N. Idiosyncratic drug hepatotoxicity. *Nature Reviews* 2005; **4**: 489–499.

Karceski S, Morrell MJ, Carpenter D. Treatment of epilepsy in adults: expert opinion, 2005. *Epilepsy Behav* 2005; **7**(suppl 1): S1–64; quiz S5–7.

Katz O, Levy A, Wiznitzer A, Sheiner E. Pregnancy and perinatal outcome in epileptic women: a population-based study. *J Matern Fetal Neonatal Med* 2006; **19**: 21–25.

Kaufman DW, Kelly JP, Anderson T, et al. Evaluation of case reports of aplastic anemia among patients treated with felbamate. *Epilepsia* 1997; **38**: 1265–1269.

Kelly K, Stephen LJ, Brodie MJ. Pharmacological outcomes in people with mental retardation and epilepsy. *Epilepsy Behav* 2004; **5**: 67–71.

Kilaru S, Bergyuist AGC. Current treatment of myoclonic astatic epilepsy: clinical experience at the Children's Hospital of Philadelphia. *Epilepsia* 2007; **48**: 1703–1707.

Kim DW, Kim KK, Chu K, et al. Surgical treatment of delayed epilepsy in hemiconvulsion-hemiplegia-epilepsy syndrome. *Neurology* 2008; **70**: 2116–2122.

Kim HL, Donnelly JH, Tournay AE, Book TM, Filipek P. Absence of seizures despite high prevalence of epileptiform EEG abnormalities in children with autism monitored in a tertiary care center. *Epilepsia* 2006; **47**: 394–398.

Kim SH, Lee JW, Choi KG, Chung HW, Lee HW. A 6-month longitudinal study of bone mineral density with antiepileptic drug monotherapy. *Epilepsy Behav* 2007; **10**: 291–295.

Kinirons P, McCarthy M, Doherty CP, Delanty N. Predicting drug-resistant patients who respond to add-on therapy with levetiracetam. *Seizure* 2006; **15**: 387–392.

Kloster R, Larsson PG, Lossius R, et al. The effect of acupuncture in chronic intractable epilepsy. *Seizure* 1999; **8**: 170–174.

Knudsen FU, Paerregaard A, Andersen R, Andresen J. Long term outcome of prophylaxis for febrile convulsions. *Arch Dis Child* 1996; **74**: 13–18.

Koenig SA, Buesing D, Longin E, et al. Valproic acid induced hepatopathy: nine new fatalities in Germany from 1994 to 2003. *Epilepsia* 2006; **47**: 2027–2031.

Kossoff EH, McGrogan JR. Worldwide use of the ketogenic diet. *Epilepsia* 2005; **46**: 280–289.

Kossoff EH, Laux LC, Blackford R, et al. When do seizures improve with the ketogenic diet? *Epilepsia* 2008; **49**: 329–333.

Kossoff EH, McGrogan JR, Bluml RM, et al. A modified Atkins diet is effective for the treatment of intractable pediatric epilepsy. *Epilepsia* 2006; **47**: 421–424.

Kossoff EH, Rowley H, Sinha SR, Vining EPG. A prospective study of the modified Atkins diet for intractable epilepsy in adults. *Epilepsia* 2008; **49**: 316–319.

Kossoff EH, Thiele EA, Pfeifer HH, et al. Tuberous sclerosis complex and the ketogenic diet. *Epilepsia* 2005; **46**: 1684–1686.

Kossoff EH, Vining EP, Pillas DJ, et al. Hemispherectomy for intractable unihemispheric epilepsy etiology vs outcome. *Neurology* 2003; **61**: 887–890.

Kossoff EH, Zupec-Kania BA, Amark PE, et al. Optimal clinical management of children receiving the ketogenic diet: recommendations of the international ketogenic diet study group. *Epilepsia* 2009; **50**: 304–317.

Koszewski W. Epilepsy following brain abscess. The evaluation of possible risk factors with emphasis on new concept of epileptic focus formation. *Acta Neurochir* 1991; **113**: 110–117.

Kotagal P, Rothner AD. Epilepsy in the setting of neurocutaneous syndromes. *Epilepsia* 1993; **34**(suppl 3): S71–78.

Koutroumanidis M, Koepp MJ, Richardson MP, et al. The variants of reading epilepsy. A clinical and video-EEG study of 17 patients with reading-induced seizures. *Brain* 1998; **121**(Pt 8): 1409–1427.

Kuhn KU, Quednow BB, Thiel M, et al. Antidepressive treatment in patients with temporal lobe epilepsy and major depression: a prospective study with three different antidepressants. *Epilepsy Behav* 2003; **4**: 674–679.

Kulaksizoglu IB, Bebek N, Baykan B, et al. Obsessive–compulsive disorder after epilepsy surgery. *Epilepsy Behav* 2004; **5**: 113–118.

Kutluay E, McCague K, D'Souza J, et al. Safety and tolerability of oxcarbazepine in elderly patients with epilepsy. *Epilepsy Behav* 2003; **4**: 175–180.

Kwan P, Brodie MJ. Early identification of refractory epilepsy. *N Engl J Med* 2000; **342**: 314–319.

Lackner TE, Cloyd JC, Thomas LW, et al. Antiepileptic drug use in nursing home residents: effect of age, gender, and co-medication on patterns of use. *Epilepsia* 1998; **39**: 1083–1087.

Lancman ME, Morris HH 3rd. Epilepsy after central nervous system infection: clinical characteristics and outcome after epilepsy surgery. *Epilepsy Res* 1996; **25**: 285–290.

Landau WM, Kleffner FR. Syndrome of acquired aphasia with convulsive disorder in children. *Neurology* 1957; **7**: 523–530.

Landolt H. Serial electroencephalographic investigation during psychotic episodes in epileptic patients and during schizophrenic attacks. In: Lorentz de Haas AM (ed.), *Lectures on Epilepsy*. Amsterdam: Elsevier, 1958: 91–133.

Lang B, Dale RC, Vincent A. New autoantibody mediated disorders of the central nervous system. *Curr Opin Neurol* 2003; **16**: 351–357.

Lee AY, Kim MJ, Chey WY, et al. Genetic polymorphism of cytochrome P4502C9 in diphenylhydantoin-induced cutaneous adverse drug reactions. *Eur J Clin Pharmacol* 2004; **60**: 155–159.

Lefevre F, Aronson N. Ketogenic diet for the treatment of refractory epilepsy in children: a systematic review of efficacy. *Pediatrics* 2000; **105**: e46.

Lempert T, Bauer M, Schmidt D. Syncope: a videometric analysis of 56 episodes of transient cerebral hypoxia. *Ann Neurol* 1994; **36**: 233–237.

Lentz SR, Haynes WG. Homocysteine: is it a clinically important cardiovascular risk factor? *Cleveland Clin J Med* 2004; **71**: 729–734.

Leone M, Tonini C, Bogliun G, et al. Chronic alcohol use and first symptomatic epileptic seizures. *J Neurol Neurosurg Psychiatry* 2002; **73**: 495–499.

Lerche H, Biervert C, Alekov AK, et al. A reduced K$^+$ current due to a novel mutation in KCNQ2 causes neonatal convulsions. *Ann Neurol* 1999; **46**: 305–312.

Lhatoo SD, Johnson AL, Goodridge DM, MacDonald BK, Sander JWAS, Shorvon SD. Mortality in epilepsy in the first 11–14 years after diagnosis: multivariate analysis of a long-term, prospective, population-based cohort. *Ann Neurol* 2001; **49**: 336–344.

Lindqvist G, Malmgren H. Organic mental disorders as hypothetical pathogenetic processes. *Acta Psychiatr Scand Suppl* 1993; **373**: 5–17.

Lonjou C, Thomas L, Borot N, et al. A marker for Stevens-Johnson syndrome: ethnicity matters. *Pharmacogenomics J* 2006; **6**: 265–268.

Lonn E, Yusuf S, Arnold MJ, et al. Homocysteine lowering with folic acid and B vitamins in vascular disease. *N Engl J Med* 2006; **354**: 1567–1577.

Löscher W, Potschka H. Drug resistance in brain diseases and the role of drug efflux transporters. *Nat Rev Neurosci* 2005; **6**: 591–602.

Löscher W, Schmidt D. Experimental and clinical evidence for loss of effect (tolerance) during prolonged treatment with antiepileptic drugs. *Epilepsia* 2006; **47**: 1253–1284.

Lowenstein D, Messing R. Epilepsy genetics: yet more exciting news. *Ann Neurol* 2007; **62**: 549–545.

Luciano AL, Shorvon SD. Results of treatment changes in patients with apparently drug-resistant chronic epilepsy. *Ann Neurol* 2007; **62**: 375–381.

Luef G, Abraham I, Trinka E, et al. Hyperandrogenism, postprandial hyperinsulinism and the risk of PCOS in a cross sectional study of women with epilepsy treated with valproate. *Epilepsy Res* 2002; **48**: 91–102.

McBride AE, Shih TT, Hirsch LJ. Video-EEG monitoring in the elderly: a review of 94 patients. *Epilepsia* 2002; **43**: 165–169.

MacDonald BK, Cockerell OC, Sander JWAS, Shorvon SD. The incidence and lifetime prevalence of neurological disorders in a prospective community-based study in the UK. *Brain* 2000; **123**: 665–676.

MacDonald BK, Johnson AL, Goodridge DM, Cockerell OC, Sander JW, Shorvon SD. Factors predicting prognosis of epilepsy after presentation with seizures. *Ann Neurol* 2000; **48**: 833–841.

McIntosh AM, Kalnins RM, Mitchell LA, Fabinyi GC, Briellmann RS, Berkovic SF. Temporal lobectomy: long-term seizure outcome, late recurrence and risks for seizure recurrence. *Brain* 2004; **127**: 2018–2030.

McIntosh S, Da Costa D, Kenny RA. Outcome of an integrated approach to the investigation of dizziness, falls and syncope in elderly patients referred to a 'syncope' clinic. *Age Ageing* 1993; **22**: 53–58.

McLachlan RS, Chovaz CJ, Blume WT, et al. Temporal lobectomy for intractable epilepsy in patients over age 45 years. *Neurology* 1992; **42**: 662–665.

McLendon RE, Provenzale J. Glioneuronal tumors of the central nervous system. *Brain Tumor Pathol* 2002; **19**: 51–58.

Malmgren K, Olsson I, Engman E, et al. Seizure outcome after resective epilepsy surgery in patients with low IQ. *Brain* 2008; **131**: 535–542.

Malmgren K, Starmark JE, Ekstedt G, et al. Nonorganic and organic psychiatric disorders in patients after epilepsy surgery. *Epilepsy Behav* 2002; **3**: 67–75.

Manford M, Hart YM, Sander JW, Shorvon SD. The National General Practice Study of Epilepsy. The syndromic classification of the International League Against Epilepsy applied to epilepsy in a general population. *Arch Neurol* 1992; **49**: 801–80.

Marcotte L, Crino PB. The neurobiology of the tuberous sclerosis complex. *Neuromolecular Med* 2006; **8**: 531–546.

Marson A, Jacoby A, Johnson A, Kim L, Gamble C, Chadwick D, on behalf of the Medical Research Council MESS Study Group. Immediate versus deferred antiepileptic drug treatment for early epilepsy and single seizures: a randomized controlled trial. *Lancet* 2005; **365**: 2007–2013.

Marson AG, Al-Kharusi AM, Alwaidh M, et al. The SANAD study of effectiveness of valproate, lamotrigine, or topiramate for generalized and unclassifiable epilepsy: an unblinded randomized controlled trial. *Lancet* 2007; **369**: 1016–1026.

Marson AG, Kadir ZA, Hutton JL, Chadwick DW. The new antiepileptic drugs: a systematic review of their efficacy and tolerability. *Epilepsia* 1997; **38**: 859–880.

Martinez CC, Pyzik PL, Kossoff EH. Discontinuing the ketogenic diet in seizure free children: recurrence and risk factors. *Epilepsia* 2007; **48**: 187–190.

Masuko AH, Castro AA, Santos GR, et al. Intermittent diazepam and continuous phenobarbitone to treat recurrences of febrile seizures: a systematic review with meta-analysis. *Arq Neuropsiquiatria* 2003; **61**: 897–901.

Mayberg HS, Lozano AM, Voon V, et al. Deep brain stimulation for treatment-resistant depression. *Neuron* 2005; **45**: 651–660.

Medical Research Council Antiepileptic Drug Withdrawal Study Group. Randomized study of antiepileptic drug withdrawal in patients in remission. *Lancet* 1991; **337**: 1175–1180.

Medical Research Council Antiepileptic Drug Withdrawal Study Group. Prognostic index for recurrence of seizures after remission of epilepsy. *BMJ* 1993; **306**: 1374–1378.

Menéndez M. Down syndrome, Alzheimer's disease and seizures. *Brain Dev* 2005; **27**: 246–252.

Meo R, Bilo L, Striano S, et al. Transient global amnesia of epileptic origin accompanied by fever. *Seizure* 1995; **4**: 311–317.

Meremikwu M, Oyo-Ita A. Paracetamol for treating fever in children. *Cochrane Database Syst Rev* 2002; (**2**): CD003676.

Messenheimer J, Mullens EL, Giorgi L, Young F. Safety review of adult clinical trial experience with lamotrigine. *Drug Saf* 1998; **18**: 281–296.

Michelucci R, Poza JJ, Sofia V, et al. Autosomal dominant lateral temporal epilepsy: clinical spectrum, new epitempin mutations, and genetic heterogeneity in seven European families. *Epilepsia* 2003; **44**: 1289–1297.

Mignat C. Clinically significant drug interactions with new immunosuppressive agents. *Drug Saf* 1997; **16**: 267–278.

Mikati MA, Saab R, Fayad MN, Choueiri RN. Efficacy of intravenous immunoglobulins in Landau-Kleffner syndrome. *Pediatr Neurol* 2002; **26**: 298–300.

Mills PB, Struys E, Jakobs C, et al. Mutations in Antiquitin in individuals with pyridoxine–dependent seizures. *Nat Med* 2006; **12**: 307–309.

Misra UK, Tan CT, Kalita J. Viral encephalitis and epilepsy. *Epilepsia* 2008; **49**(suppl 6): 13–18.

Modi G, Modi M, Martinus I, Saffer D. New-onset seizures associated with HIV infection. *Neurology* 2000; **55**: 1558–1561.

Mohanraj R, Brodie MJ. Diagnosing refractory epilepsy: response to sequential treatment schedules. *Eur J Neurol* 2006; **13**: 277–282.

Monaco F, Cavanna A, Magli E, et al. Obsessionality, obsessive–compulsive disorder, and temporal lobe epilepsy. *Epilepsy Behav* 2005; **7**: 491–496.

Moran NF, Fish DR, Kitchen N, Shorvon S, Kendall BE, Stevens JM. Supratentorial cavernous haemangiomas and epilepsy: a review of the literature and case series. *J Neurol Neurosurg Psychiatry* 1999; **66**: 561–568.

Moran NF, Poole K, Bell G, et al. Epilepsy in the United Kingdom: seizure frequency and severity, anti-epileptic drug utilization and impact on life in 1652 people with epilepsy. *Seizure* 2004; **13**: 425–433.

Morrow JI, Russell A, Gutherie E, et al. Malformation risks of anti-epileptic drugs in pregnancy: a prospective study from the UK Epilepsy and Pregnancy Register. *J Neurol Neurosurg Psychiatry* 2006; **77**: 193–198.

Morse RP. Rasmussen encephalitis. *Arch Neurol* 2004; **61**: 592–594.

Mturi N, Musumba CO, Wamola BM, Ogutu BR, Newton CR. Cerebral malaria: optimising management. *CNS Drugs* 2003; **17**: 153–165.

Mula M, Jauch R, Cavanna A, et al. Clinical and psychopathological definition of the interictal dysphoric disorder of epilepsy. *Epilepsia* 2008; **49**: 650–656.

Mula M, Trimble MR, Sander JW. Are psychiatric adverse events of antiepileptic drugs a unique entity? A study on topiramate and levetiracetam. *Epilepsia* 2007; **48**: 2322–2326.

Mulley JC, Scheffer IE, Harkin LA, Berkovic SF, Dibbens LM. Susceptibility genes for complex epilepsy. *Hum Mol Genet* 2005; **14**(Spec No. 2): R243–249.

Murali J, Prabhakar S. Bacterial meningitis and epilepsy. *Epilepsia* 2008; **49**(suppl 6): 8–12.

Musicco M, Beghi E, Solair A, Viani F, for the First Seizure Trial Group (FIRST Group). Treatment of first tonic–clonic seizure does not improve the prognosis of epilepsy. *Neurology* 1997; **49**: 991–998.

National Institute for Health and Clinical Excellence. *The Diagnosis and Management of the Epilepsies in Adults and Children in Primary and Secondary Care*. London: NICE, 2004. Available at: www.nice.org.uk/pdf/fullguideline.pdf.

Neal EG, Chaffe HM, Schwartz RH, et al. The ketogenic diet in the treatment of epilepsy in children: a randomised, controlled trial. *Lancet Neurol* 2008; **7**: 500–506.

Nelson KB, Ellenberg JH. Predisposing and causative factors in childhood epilepsy. *Epilepsia* 1987; **28**(suppl 1): S16–24.

Norris JW, Hachinski VC. Misdiagnosis of stroke. *Lancet* 1982; **i**: 328–331.

Nsour WM, Lau CB, Wong IC. Review on phytotherapy in epilepsy. *Seizure* 2000; **9**: 96–107.

O'Brien MD, Guillebaud J. Contraception for women with epilepsy. *Epilepsia* 2006; **47**: 1419–1422.

Oguni H, Tanaka T, Hayashi K, et al. The treatment and long-term prognosis of myoclonic-astatic epilepsy of early childhood. *Neuropediatrics* 2002; **33**: 122–132.

Ogunmekan AO, Hwang PA. A randomized, double-blind, placebo-controlled, clinical trial of D-alpha-tocopheryl acetate (vitamin E), as add-on therapy, for epilepsy in children. *Epilepsia* 1989; **30**: 84–89.

Olafsson E, Ludvigsson P, Gudmundsson G, Hesdorffer D, Kjartansson O, Hauser WA. Incidence of unprovoked seizures and epilepsy in Iceland and assessment of the epilepsy syndrome classification: a prospective study. *Lancet Neurol* 2005; **4**: 627–634.

Pacia SV, Devinsky O. Clozapine-related seizures: experience with 5629 patients. *Neurology* 1994; **44**: 2247–2249.

Pack AM. The association between antiepileptic drugs and bone disease. *Epilepsy Curr* 2003; **3**: 91–95.

Pack AM, Morrell MJ, Marcus R, et al. Bone mass and turnover in women with epilepsy on antiepileptic drug monotherapy. *Ann Neurol* 2005; **57**: 781–786.

Pal DK, Evgrafov OV, Tabares P, Zhang F, Durner M, Greenberg DA. BRD2 (RING3) is a probable major susceptibility gene for common juvenile myoclonic epilepsy. *Am J Hum Genet* 2003; **73**: 261–270.

Panayiotopoulos CP. Benign childhood epileptic syndromes with occipital spikes: new classification proposed by the International League Against Epilepsy. *J Child Neurol* 2000; **15**: 548–552.

Panayiotopoulos CP, Michael M, Sanders S, Valeta T, Koutroumanidis M. Benign childhood focal epilepsies: assessment of established and newly recognized syndromes. *Brain* 2008; **131**(Pt 9): 2264–2286.

Pang T, Atefy R, Sheen V. Malformations of cortical development. *Neurologist* 2008; **14**: 181–191.

Park YD. The effects of vagus nerve stimulation therapy on patients with intractable seizures and either Landau-Kleffner syndrome or autism. *Epilepsy Behav* 2003; **4**: 286–290.

Parra J, Kalitzin SN, Lopes da Silva FH. Photosensitivity and visually induced seizures. *Curr Opin Neurol* 2005; **18**: 155–159.

Passero S, Rocchi R, Rossi S, Ulivelli M, Vatti G. Seizures after spontaneous supratentorial intracerebral hemorrhage. *Epilepsia* 2002; **43**: 1175–1180.

Patsalos PN, Berry DJ, Bourgeois BF, et al. Antiepileptic drugs-best practice guidelines for therapeutic drug monitoring: a position paper by the subcommission on therapeutic drug monitoring, ILAE Commission on Therapeutic Strategies. *Epilepsia* 2008; **49**: 1239–1276.

Pelc K, Boyd SG, Cheron G, Dan B. Epilepsy in Angelman syndrome. *Seizure* 2008; **17**: 211–217.

Penry JK, Porter RJ, Dreifuss RE. Simultaneous recording of absence seizures with video tape and electroencephalography. A study of 374 seizures in 48 patients. *Brain* 1975; **98**: 427–440.

Perucca E, Kwan P. Overtreatment in epilepsy: how it occurs and how it can be avoided. *CNS Drugs* 2005; **19**: 897–908.

Perucca E. Pharmacoresistance in epilepsy. How should it be defined? *CNS Drugs* 1998; **10**: 171–179.

Perucca E. Birth defects after prenatal exposure to antiepileptic drugs. *Lancet Neurol* 2005; **4**: 781–786.

Perucca E. Clinical pharmacokinetics of new-generation antiepileptic drugs at the extremes of age. *Clin Pharmacokinet* 2006; **45**: 351–363.

Perucca E, Tomson T. Prenatal exposure to antiepileptic drugs. *Lancet* 2006; **367**: 1467–1469.

Perucca E, Albani F, Capovilla G, et al. Recommendations of the Italian League Against Epilepsy Working Group on Generic Products of Antiepileptic Drugs. *Epilepsia* 2006; **46**(suppl 5): 16–20.

Perucca E, Beghi E, Dulac O, et al. Assessing risk to benefit ratio in antiepileptic drug therapy. *Epilepsy Res* 2000; **41**: 107–139.

Perucca E, Berlowitz D, Birnbaum A, et al. Pharmacological and clinical aspects of antiepileptic drugs use in the elderly. *Epilepsy Res* 2006; **68**(suppl 1): 49–63.

Perucca E, Dulac O, Shorvon S, Tomson T. Harnessing the clinical potential of antiepileptic drug therapy: Dosage optimisation. *CNS Drugs* 2001; **15**: 609–621.

Perucca E, Gram L, Avanzini G, Dulac O. Antiepileptic drugs as a cause of worsening of seizures. *Epilepsia* 1998; **39**: 5–17.

Peyrière H, Dereure O, Breton H, et al. Variability in the clinical pattern of cutaneous side-effects of drugs with systemic symptoms: does a DRESS syndrome really exist? *Therapeutics* 2006; **155**: 422–428.

Pinto D, Kasteleijn-Nolst Trenité DG, Cordell HJ, et al. Explorative two-locus linkage analysis suggests a multiplicative interaction between the 7q32 and 16p13 myoclonic seizures-related photosensitivity loci. *Genet Epidemiol* 2007; **31**: 42–45.

Pitkänen A, Kharatishvili I, Karhunen H, et al. Epileptogenesis in experimental models. *Epilepsia* 2007; **48**(suppl 2): 13–20.

Pugh MJ, Cramer J, Knoefel J, et al. Potentially inappropriate antiepileptic drugs for elderly patients with epilepsy. *J Am Geriatr Soc* 2004; **52**: 417–422.

Rajashekhar V. Solitary cerebral cysticercus granuloma. *Epilepsia* 2003; **44**(suppl 1): 25–28.

Rajshekhar V, Jeyaseelan L. Seizure outcome in patients with a solitary cerebral cysticercus granuloma. *Neurology* 2004; **62**: 2236–2240.

Ramaratnam S, Sridharan K. Yoga for epilepsy (Cochrane Review). In: *The Cochrane Library*, Issue 2. Oxford: Update Software, 2001.

Ranganathan LN, Ramaratnam S. Vitamins for epilepsy. *Cochrane Database Syst Rev* 2005; (**2**): CD004304.

Rantakallio P, von Wendt L. A prospective comparative study of the aetiology of cerebral palsy and epilepsy in a one-year birth cohort from Northern Finland. *Acta Paediatr Scand* 1986; **75**: 586–592.

Rantala H, Tarkka R, Uhari MA. Meta-analytic review of the preventive treatment of recurrences of febrile seizures. *J Pediatr* 1997; **131**: 922–955.

Raspall-Chaure M, Neville BG, Scott RC. The medical management of the epilepsies in children: conceptual and practical considerations. *Lancet Neurol* 2008; **7**: 57–69.

Rating D, Wolf C, Bast T, for the Sulthiame Study Group. Sulthiame as monotherapy in children with benign childhood epilepsy with centrotemporal spikes: a 6-month randomized, double-blind, placebo-controlled study. *Epilepsia* 2000; **41**; 1284–1288.

Rättyä J, Turkka J, Pakarinen AJ, et al. Reproductive effects of valproate, carbamazepine, and oxcarbazepine in men with epilepsy. *Neurology* 2001; **56**: 31–36.

Rosanoff MJ, Ottman R. Penetrance of LGI1 mutations in autosomal dominant partial epilepsy with auditory features. *Neurology* 2008; **71**: 567–571.

Rowan AJ, Ramsay RE, Collins JF, et al. New onset geriatric epilepsy: a randomized study of gabapentin, lamotrigine, and carbamazepine. *Neurology* 2005; **64**: 1868–1873.

Rugg-Gunn FJ, Simister RJ, Squirrell M, Holdright DR, Duncan JS. Cardiac arrhythmias in focal epilepsy: a prospective long-term study. *Lancet* 2004; **364**: 2212–2219.

Sadler RM. The syndrome of mesial temporal lobe epilepsy with hippocampal sclerosis: clinical features and differential diagnosis. *Adv Neurol* 2006; **97**: 27–37.

Satishchandra P. Hot-water epilepsy. *Epilepsia* 2003; **44**(suppl 1): 29–32.

Satishchandra P, Sinha S. Seizures in HIV-seropositive individuals: NINHAMS experience and review. *Epilepsia* 2008; **49**(suppl 6): 33–41.

Scheffer IE. Autosomal dominant nocturnal frontal lobe epilepsy. *Epilepsia* 2000; **41**: 1059–1060.

Scheffer IE, Bhatia KP, Lopes-Cendes I, et al. Autosomal dominant frontal epilepsy misdiagnosed as sleep disorder. *Lancet* 1994; **343**: 515–517.

Scheffer IE, Harkin LA, Grinton BE, et al. Temporal lobe epilepsy and GEFS+ phenotypes associated with SCN1B mutations. *Brain* 2007; **130**(Pt 1): 100–109.

Scheller J. Role for complementary and alternative treatments in epilepsy. *Arch Neurol* 2005; **62**: 1471–1472.

Schmidt D, Löscher W. Drug resistance in epilepsy: putative neurobiologic and clinical mechanisms. *Epilepsia* 2005; **46**: 858–877.

Schmidt D, Baumgartner C, Loescher W. Seizure occurrence after planned discontinuation of antiepileptic drugs in seizure free patients after epilepsy surgery: a review of current clinical experience. *Epilepsia* 2004; **45**: 179–186.

Sedel F, Gourfinkel-An I, Lyon-Caen O, Baulac M, Saudubray JM, Navarro V. Epilepsy and inborn errors of metabolism in adults: a diagnostic approach. *J Inherit Metab Dis* 2007; **30**: 846–854.

Sheth RD, Harden CL. Screening for bone health in epilepsy. *Epilepsia* 2007; **48**: 39–41.

Shorvon SD. The temporal aspects of prognosis in epilepsy. *J Neurol Neurosurg Psychiatry* 1984; **47**: 1157–1165.

Shorvon S. The treatment of chronic epilepsy: a review of recent studies of clinical efficacy and side-effects. *Curr Opin Neurol* 2007; **20**: 159–163.

Shorvon S, Berg A. Pertussis vaccination and epilepsy – an erratic history, new research and the mismatch between science and social policy. *Epilepsia* 2008; **49**: 219–225.

Shorvon S, Luciano AL. Prognosis of chronic and newly diagnosed epilepsy: revisiting temporal aspects. *Curr Opin Neurol* 2007; **20**: 208–212.

Shorvon SD, Sander JWAS. Temporal patterns of remission and relapse of seizures in patients with epilepsy. In: Schmidt D, Morselli PL, eds. *Intractable Epilepsy: Experimental and Clinical Aspects*. New York: Raven Press, 1986: 13–24.

Shorvon SD, Chadwick D, Galbraith AW, Reynolds EH. One drug for epilepsy. *BMJ* 1978; **1**: 474–476.

Shorvon SD, Tallis RC, Wallace HK. Antiepileptic drugs: coprescription of proconvulsant drugs and oral contraceptives: a national study of antiepileptic drug prescribing practice. *J Neurol Neurosurg Psychiatry* 2002; **72**: 114–115.

Shostak S, Ottman R. Ethical, legal, and social dimensions of epilepsy genetics. *Epilepsia* 2006; **47**: 1595–1602.

Silva ML, Cieuta C, Guerrini R, Plouin P, Livet MO, Dulac O. Early clinical and EEG features of infantile spasms in Down syndrome. *Epilepsia* 1996; **37**: 977–982.

Singh G, Driever PH, Sander JW. Cancer risk in people with epilepsy: the role of antiepileptic drugs. *Brain* 2005; **128**: 7–17.

Singh G, Prabhakar S. The effects of antimicrobial and antiepileptic treatment on the outcome of epilepsy associated with central nervous system (CNS) infections. *Epilepsia* 2008; **49**(suppl 6): 42–6.

Singh R, Gardner RJ, Crossland KM, Scheffer IE, Berkovic SF. Chromosomal abnormalities and epilepsy: a review for clinicians and gene hunters. *Epilepsia* 2002; **43**: 127–140.

Singh R, Scheffer IE, Crossland K, Berkovic SF. Generalized epilepsy with febrile seizures plus: a common childhood-onset genetic epilepsy syndrome. *Ann Neurol* 1999; **45**: 75–81.

Sinha S, Satishchandra P, Nalini A, et al. New-onset seizures among HIV infected drug naïve patients from south India. *Neurology Asia* 2005; **10**: 29–33.

Sinha S, Satishchandra P, Santosh V, Gayatri N, Shankar SK. Neuronal ceroid lipofuscinosis: a clinicopathological study. *Seizure* 2004; **13**: 235–240.

Sirven JI, Malamut BL, O'Connor MJ, et al. Temporal lobectomy outcome in older versus younger adults. *Neurology* 2000; **54**: 2166–2170.

Specchio LM, Beghi E. Should antiepileptic drugs be withdrawn from seizure free patients? *CNS Drugs* 2004; **18**: 201–212.

Spina E, Perucca E. Clinical significance of pharmacokinetic interactions between antiepileptic and psychotropic drugs. *Epilepsia* 2002; **43**(suppl 2): 37–44.

Stafstrom CE, Spencer S. The ketogenic diet: a therapy in search of an explanation. *Neurology* 2000; **54**: 282–283.

Stephani U. Typical semiology of benign childhood epilepsy with centrotemporal spikes (BCECTS). *Epileptic Disord* 2000; **2**: S3–S4.

Sterman MB, Egner T. Foundation and practice of neurofeedback for the treatment of epilepsy. *Appl Psychophysiol Biofeedback* 2006; **31**: 21–35.

Striano P, Orefice G, Brescia Morra V, et al. Epileptic seizures in multiple sclerosis: clinical and EEG correlations. *Neurol Sci* 2003; **24**: 322–328.

Stromberger C, Bodamer OA, Stockler-Ipsiroglu S. Clinical characteristics and diagnostic clues in inborn errors of creatine metabolism. *J Inherit Metab Dis* 2003; **26**: 299–308.

Suzuki T, Delgado-Escueta AV, Aguan K, et al. Mutations in EFHC1 cause juvenile myoclonic epilepsy. *Nat Genet* 2004; **36**: 842–849.

Swink TD, Vining EPG, Freeman JM. The ketogenic diet: 1997. *Adv Pediatr* 1997; **44**: 297–329.

Takeda Y, Inoue Y, Tottori T, et al. Acute psychosis during intracranial EEG monitoring: close relationship between psychotic symptoms and discharges in amygdala. *Epilepsia* 2001; **42**: 719–724.

Tanaka M, Olsen RW, Medina MT, et al. Hyperglycosylation and reduced GABA currents of mutated GABRB3 polypeptide in remitting childhood absence epilepsy. *Am J Hum Genet* 2008; **82**: 1249–1261.

Tatum WOT, Ross J, Cole AJ. Epileptic pseudodementia. *Neurology* 1998; **50**: 1472–1475.

Teasell R, Bayona N, Lippert C, Villamere J, Hellings C. Posttraumatic seizure disorder following acquired brain injury. *Brain Injury* 2007; **21**: 201–214.

Tellez-Zenteno JF, Patten SB, Jette N, et al. Psychiatric comorbidity in epilepsy: a population-based analysis. *Epilepsia* 2007; **48**: 2336–2344.

Temkin NR. Antiepileptogenesis and seizure prevention trials with antiepileptic drugs: meta-analysis of controlled trials. *Epilepsia* 2001; **42**: 515–524.

Temkin NR. Risk factors for posttraumatic seizures in adults. *Epilepsia* 2003; **44**(suppl 10): 18–20.

Temkin NR, Anderson GD, Winn HR, et al. Magnesium sulfate for neuroprotection after traumatic brain injury: a randomised controlled trial. *Lancet Neurol* 2007; **6**: 29–38.

Temkin NR, Dikmen SS, Anderson GD, et al. Valproate therapy for prevention of posttraumatic seizures: a randomized trial. *J Neurosurg* 1999; **91**: 593–600.

Temkin NR, Dikmen SS, Wilensky AJ, Keihm J, Chabal S, Winn HR. A randomized, double-blind study of phenytoin for the prevention of post-traumatic seizures. *N Engl J Med* 1990; **323**: 497–502.

Tennis P, Stern RS. Risk of serious cutaneous disorders after initiation of use of phenytoin, carbamazepine, or sodium valproate: a record linkage study. *Neurology* 1997; **49**: 542–546.

Tergau F, Naumann U, Paulus W, Steinhoff B. Low-frequency repetitive transcranial magnetic stimulation improves intractable epilepsy. *Lancet* 1999; **353**: 2209.

Theodore WH, Fisher RS. Brain stimulation for epilepsy. *Lancet Neurology* 2004; **3**: 111–118.

Theodore WH, Porter RJ, Albert P, et al. The secondarily generalized tonic–clonic seizure: a videotape analysis. *Neurology* 1994; **44**: 1403–1407.

Thio LL, Wong M, Yamada KA. Ketone bodies do not directly alter excitatory or inhibitory hippocampal synaptic transmission. *Neurology* 2000; **54**: 325–331.

Tomson T. Gender aspects of pharmacokinetics of new and old AEDs. Pregnancy and breast-feeding. *Ther Drug Monit* 2005; **6**: 718–721.

Tomson T, Battino D. Pharmacokinetics and therapeutic drug monitoring of newer antiepileptic drugs during pregnancy and the puerperium. *Clin Pharmacokinet* 2007; **46**: 209–219.

Tomson T, Hiilesmaa V. Epilepsy in pregnancy. *BMJ* 2007; **335**: 769–773.

Tomson T, Battino D, French J, et al. Antiepileptic drug exposure and major congenital malformations: the role of pregnancy registries. *Epilepsy Behav* 2007; **11**: 277–282.

Tomson T, Palm R, Källén K, et al. Pharmacokinetics of levetiracetam during pregnancy, delivery, in the neonatal period, and lactation. *Epilepsia* 2007; **48**: 1111–1116.

Torta R, Keller R. Behavioral, psychotic, and anxiety disorders in epilepsy: etiology, clinical features, and therapeutic implications. *Epilepsia* 1999; **40**(suppl 10): S2–20.

Trenité DG. Photosensitivity, visually sensitive seizures and epilepsies. *Epilepsy Res* 2006; **70**(suppl 1): S269–279.

Tsuru MM, Mizuguchi M, Momoi MY. Effect of high-dose intravenous corticosteroid therapy in Landau-Kleffner syndrome. *Pediatr Neurol* 2000; **22**: 145–147.

Tuchman R, Rapin I. Epilepsy in autism. *Lancet Neurol* 2002; **1**: 352–358.

Vajda FJE, Hitchcock A, Graham J, et al. Seizure control in antiepileptic drug-treated pregnancy. *Epilepsia* 2008; **49**: 172–176.

Van der Berg BJ, Yerushalmy J. Studies on convulsive disorders in young children. I. Incidence of febrile and nonfebrile convulsions by age and other factors. *Pediatr Res* 1969; **3**: 298–304.

Verrotti A, Greco R, Altobelli E, et al. Centro-temporal spikes in non-epileptic children: a long-term follow up. *J Paediatr Child Health* 1999; **35**: 60–62.

Verrotti A, Manco R, Matricardi S, et al. Antiepileptic drugs and visual function. *Pediatr Neurol* 2007; **36**: 353–360.

Viinikainen K, Heinonen S, Eriksson K, Kälviäinen R. Fertility in women with active epilepsy. *Neurology* 2007; **69**: 2107–2108.

Vincent A, Bien CG. Temporal lobe seizures, amnesia and autoantibodies – identifying a potentially reversible form of non-paraneoplastic limbic encephalitis. *Epileptic Disord* 2005; **7**: 177–179.

Walczak T. Do antiepileptic drugs play a role in sudden unexpected death in epilepsy? *Drug Saf* 2003; **26**: 673–683.

Walker DG, Kaye AH. Low grade glial neoplasms. *J Clin Neurosci* 2003; **10**: 1–13.

Walker JE, Kozlowski GP. Neurofeedback treatment of epilepsy. *Child Adolesc Psychiatr Clin N Am* 2005; **14**: 163–176.

Wallace H, Shorvon S, Tallis R. Age-specific incidence and prevalence rates of treated epilepsy in an unselected population of 2,052,922 and age-specific fertility rates of women with epilepsy. *Lancet* 1998; **352**: 1970–1973.

Wallace SJ. Epilepsy in cerebral palsy. *Dev Med Child Neurol* 2001; **43**: 713–717.

Wang D, Pascual JM, Yang H, et al. Glut–1 deficiency syndrome: clinical, genetic, and therapeutic aspects. *Ann Neurol* 2005; **57**: 111–118.

Wang HS, Kuo MF, Chou ML, et al. Pyridoxal phosphate is better than pyridoxine for controlling idiopathic intractable epilepsy. *Arch Dis Child* 2005; **90**: 512–515.

Wasserman S, Iyengar R, Chaplin WF, et al. Levetiracetam versus placebo in childhood and adolescent autism: a double-blind placebo-controlled study. *Int Clin Psychopharm* 2006; **21**: 363–367.

Weiner HL, Ferraris N, Lajoie J, et al. Epilepsy surgery for children with tuberous sclerosis complex. *J Child Neurol* 2004; **19**: 687–689.

Wheless JW, Clarke DF, Carpenter D. Treatment of pediatric epilepsy: expert opinion, 2005. *J Child Neurol* 2005; **20**(suppl 1): S1–S56.

Wong LJ, Naviaux RK, Brunetti-Pierri N, et al. Molecular and clinical genetics of mitochondrial diseases due to POLG mutations. *Hum Mutat* 2008 [Epub ahead of print].

Yamatogi Y, Ohtahara S. Early-infantile epileptic encephalopathy with suppression-bursts, Ohtahara syndrome; its overview referring to our 16 cases. *Brain Dev* 2002; **24**: 13–23.

Yaqub BA. Electroclinical seizures in Lennox–Gastaut syndrome. *Epilepsia* 1993; **34**: 120–12.

You SJ, Kang HC, Ko TS, et al. Comparison of corpus callostomy and vagus nerve stimulation in children with Lennox–Gastaut syndrome. *Brain Dev* 2008; **30**: 195–199.

Zaccara G, Franciotta D, Perucca E. Idiosyncratic adverse reactions to antiepileptic drugs. *Epilepsia* 2007; **48**: 1223–1244.

Zaccara G, Gangemi PF, Cincotta M. Central nervous system adverse effects of new antiepileptic drugs. A meta-analysis of placebo-controlled studies. *Seizure* 2008; **17**: 405–421.

Zafeiriou DI, Kontopoulos EE, Tsikoulas I. Characteristics and prognosis of epilepsy in children with cerebral palsy. *J Child Neurol* 1999; **14**: 289–294.

Zeng LH, Xu L, Gutmann DH, Wong M. Rapamycin prevents epilepsy in a mouse model of tuberous sclerosis complex. *Ann Neurol* 2008; **63**: 444–453.

Chapters 7–8

Chapters from: Shorvon SD, Perucca E, Engel J Jr, eds. *The Treatment of Epilepsy.* Oxford: Blackwell Publishing Ltd, 2009

Somerville ER, Michell A. Gabapentin, pp. 519–526.

Sachdeo R. Lacosamide, pp. 527–534.

Matsuo F, Riaz A. Lamotrigine, pp. 535–558.

French JA, Tonner F. Levetiracetam, pp. 559–574.

Faught E, Limdi N. Oxcarbazepine, pp. 575–584.

Michelucci R, Pasini E, Tassinari CA. Phenobarbital, primidone and other barbiturates, pp. 585–604.

Eadie E. Phenytoin, pp. 605–618.

Shorvon SD. Piracetam, pp. 619–626.

Rheims S, Ryvlin P. Pregabalin, pp. 627–636.

Mansbach H, Baulac M. Retigabine, pp. 637–646.

Biton V. Rufinamide, pp. 647–656.

Eriksson K, Keränen T. Stiripentol, pp. 657–662.

Kälviäinen R. Tiagabine, pp. 663–672.

Cross J, Riney C. Topiramate, pp. 673–984.

Bourgeois B. Valproate, pp. 685–698.

Krämer G, Wohlrab G. Vigabatrin, pp. 699–712.

Wroe S. Zonisamide, pp. 713–720.

Meierkord H, Holtkamp M. Other drugs rarely used, pp. 721–733.

Patsalos P, Sander J. Antiepileptic drugs in early clinical development, pp. 733–742.

Books

Engel J, Pedley TA, eds. *Epilepsy: A comprehensive Textbook*. 3rd edn New York: Raven Press, 2007.

Levy R, Mattson RH, Meldrum BS, and Perucca E, eds. *Antiepileptic Drugs*, 5th edn. Philadelphia: Lippincott, Williams & Wilkins, 2002.

Journal articles/chapters in books

Adab N, Kini U, Vinten J, et al. The longer term outcome of children born to mothers with epilepsy. *J Neurol Neurosurg Psychiatry* 2004; **75**: 1575–1583.

Äikiä M, Jutila L, Salmenperä T, Mervaala E, Kälviäinen R. Comparison of the cognitive effects of tiagabine and carbamazepine as monotherapy in newly diagnosed adult patients with partial epilepsy: pooled analysis of two long-term, randomized, follow-up studies. *Epilepsia* 2006; **47**: 1121–1127.

Aldenkamp AP, Arends J, Bootsma HP, et al. Randomized double-blind parallel-group study comparing cognitive effects of a low-dose lamotrigine with valproate and placebo in healthy volunteers. *Epilepsia* 2002; **43**: 19–26.

Alvestad S, Lydersen S, Brodtkorb E. Cross-reactivity pattern of rash from current aromatic antiepileptic drugs. *Epilepsy Res* 2008; **80**: 194–200.

Anderson GD. Children versus adults: pharmacokinetic and adverse-effect differences. *Epilepsia* 2002; **43**(suppl 3): 53–59.

Anhut H, Ashman P, Feuerstein TJ, Sauermann W, Saunders M, Schmidt B. Gabapentin (Neurontin) as add-on therapy in patients with partial seizures: a double-blind, placebo-controlled study. The International Gabapentin Study Group. *Epilepsia* 1994; **35**: 795–801.

Arroyo S. Rufinamide. *Neurotherapeutics* 2007; **4**: 155–162.

Arroyo S, Anhut H, Kugler AR, et al. Pregabalin add-on treatment: a randomized, double-blind, placebo-controlled, dose-response study in adults with partial seizures. *Epilepsia* 2004; **45**: 20–27.

Asconapé JJ, Penry JK, Dreifuss FE, Riela A, Mirza W. Valproate-associated pancreatitis. *Epilepsia* 1993; **34**: 177–183.

Askmark H, Wiholm B. Epidemiology of adverse drug reactions to carbamazepine as seen in a spontaneous reporting system. *Acta Neurol Scand* 1990; **81**: 131–140.

Banu SH, Jahan M, Koli UK, Ferdousi S, Khan NZ, Neville B. Side effects of phenobarbital and carbamazepine in childhood epilepsy: randomised controlled trial. *BMJ* 2007; **334**: 1207.

Barcs G, Walker EB, Elger CE, et al. Oxcarbazepine placebo-controlled, dose-ranging trial in refractory partial epilepsy. *Epilepsia* 2000; **41**: 1597–1607.

Baruzzi A, Albani F, Riva R. Oxcarbazepine: pharmacokinetic interactions and their clinical relevance. *Epilepsia* 1994; **35**(suppl 3): S14–S19.

Battino D, Tomson T. Management of epilepsy during pregnancy. *Drugs* 2007; **67**: 2727–2746.

Battino D, Croci D, Rossini A, Messina S, Mamoli D, Perucca E. Topiramate pharmacokinetics in children and adults with epilepsy: a case-matched comparison based on therapeutic drug monitoring data. *Clin Pharmacokinet* 2005; **44**: 407–416.

Beenen LF, Lindeboom J, Kasteleijn-Nolst Trenite DG, et al. Comparative double-blind clinical trial of phenytoin and sodium valproate as anticonvulsant prophylaxis after craniotomy: efficacy, tolerability and cognitive effects. *J Neurol Neurosurg Psychiatry* 1999; **67**: 474–480.

Ben-Menachem E. International experience with tiagabine add-on therapy. *Epilepsia* 1995; **36**: 14–21.

Ben-Menachem E. Pregabalin pharmacology and its relevance to clinical practice. *Epilepsia* 2004; **45**: 13–18.

Ben-Menachem E, Falter U. Efficacy and tolerability of levetiracetam 3000 mg/d in patients with refractory partial seizures: a multicenter, double-blind, responder-selected study evaluating monotherapy. European Levetiracetam Study Group. *Epilepsia* 2000; **41**: 1276–1283.

Ben-Menachem E, Abou-Khalil B, Biton V, Doty P, Jatuzis D, Rudd GD. Efficacy and safety of oral lacosamide as adjunctive therapy in adults with partial-onset seizures. *Epilepsia* 2007; **48**: 1308–1317.

Berkovic SF, Knowlton RC, Leroy RF, Schiemann J, Falter U. Placebo-controlled study of levetiracetam in idiopathic generalized epilepsy. *Neurology* 2007; **69**: 1751–1760.

Beydoun A, Sachdeo RC, Rosenfeld WE, et al. Oxcarbazepine monotherapy for partial onset seizures: a multicenter, double-blind, clinical trial. *Neurology* 2000; **54**: 2245–2251.

Bialer M. Pharmacokinetics and interactions of new antiepileptic drugs: an overview. *Ther Drug Monit* 2005; **27**: 722–726.

Bialer M. New antiepileptic drugs that are second generation to existing antiepileptic drugs. *Expert Opin Invest Drugs* 2006; **15**: 637–647.

Bialer M. Extended-release formulations for the treatment of epilepsy. *CNS Drugs* 2007; **21**: 765–774.

Bill PA, Vigonius U, Pohlmann H, et al. A double-blind controlled clinical trial of oxcarbazepine versus phenytoin in adults with previously untreated epilepsy. *Epilepsy Res* 1997; **27**: 195–204.

Biton V, Fountain N, Rosenow F, et al. Safety and tolerability of lacosamide: a summary of adverse events in epilepsy clinical trials. Paper presented at: 8th European Congress on Epileptology; September 21–25, 2008; Berlin, Germany.

Biton V, Mirza W, Montouris G, et al. Weight change associated with valproate and lamotrigine monotherapy in patients with epilepsy. *Neurology* 2001; **56**: 172–177.

Biton V, Montouris GD, Ritter F, et al. A randomized, placebo-controlled study of topiramate in primary generalized tonic–clonic seizures. Topiramate YTC Study Group. *Neurology* 1999; **52**: 1330–1337.

Biton V, Vasquez KB, Sachdeo RC, et al. Adjunctive tiagabine compared with phenytoin and carbamazepine in the multicenter, double-blind trial of complex partial seizures. *Epilepsia* 1998; **39**(suppl 6): 125–126.

Bourgeois B, Leppik IE, Sackellares JC, et al. Felbamate: a double-blind controlled trial in patients undergoing presurgical evaluation of partial seizures. *Neurology* 1993; **43**: 693–696.

Brodie MJ. Tiagabine pharmacology in profile. *Epilepsia* 1995; **36**: 7–9.

Brodie MJ. Pregabalin as adjunctive therapy for partial seizures. *Epilepsia* 2004; **45**: 19–27.

Brodie MJ. Zonisamide as adjunctive therapy for refractory partial seizures. *Epilepsy Res* 2006; **68**(suppl 2): S11–S16.

Brodie MJ, Chadwick DW, Anhut H, et al. Gabapentin versus lamotrigine monotherapy: a double-blind comparison in newly diagnosed epilepsy. *Epilepsia* 2002; **43**: 993–1000.

Brodie MJ, Duncan R, Vespignani H, Solyom A, Bitenskyy V, Lucas C. Dose-dependent safety and efficacy of zonisamide: a randomized, double-blind, placebo-controlled study in patients with refractory partial seizures. *Epilepsia* 2005; **46**: 31–41.

Brodie MJ, Mumford JP, 012 Study Group. Double-blind substitution of vigabatrin and valproate in carbamazepine-resistant partial epilepsy. *Epilepsy Res* 1999; **34**: 199–205.

Brodie MJ, Overstall PW, Giorgi L. Multicentre, double-blind, randomised comparison between lamotrigine and carbamazepine in elderly patients with newly diagnosed epilepsy. The UK Lamotrigine Elderly Study Group. *Epilepsy Res* 1999; **37**: 81–87.

Brodie MJ, Perucca E, Ryvlin P, Ben-Menachem E, Meencke HJ, for the Levetiracetam Monotherapy Study Group. Comparison of levetiracetam and controlled-release carbamazepine in newly diagnosed epilepsy. *Neurology* 2007; **68**: 402–408.

Brodie MJ, Richens A, Yuen AW. Double-blind comparison of lamotrigine and carbamazepine in newly diagnosed epilepsy. UK Lamotrigine/Carbamazepine Monotherapy Trial Group. *Lancet* 1995; **345**: 476–479.

Brown P, Steiger MJ, Thompson PD, et al. Effectiveness of piracetam in cortical myoclonus. *Mov Disord* 1993; **8**: 63–68.

Browne TR. Clonazepam. *N Engl J Med* 1978; **299**: 812–816.

Buchthal F, Svensmark O, Simonsen H. Relation of EEG and seizures to phenobarbital in serum. *Arch Neurol* 1968; **19**: 567–572.

Canadian Clobazam Cooperative Group. Clobazam in treatment of refractory epilepsy: the Canadian experience. A retrospective study. *Epilepsia* 1991; **32**: 407–416.

Canadian Study Group for Childhood Epilepsy. Clobazam has equivalent efficacy to carbamazepine and phenytoin as monotherapy for childhood epilepsy. *Epilepsia* 1998; **39**: 952–959.

Chadwick D, for the Vigabatrin European Monotherapy Study Group. Safety and efficacy of vigabatrin and carbamazepine in newly diagnosed epilepsy: a multicentre randomised double-blind study. *Lancet* 1999; **354**: 13–19.

Chadwick DW, Anhut H, Greiner MJ, et al. A double-blind trial of gabapentin monotherapy for newly diagnosed partial seizures. International Gabapentin Monotherapy Study Group 945–77. *Neurology* 1998; **51**: 1282–1288.

Chiron C, Dumas C, Jambaqué I, et al. (1997) Randomized trial comparing vigabatrin and hydrocortisone in infantile spasms due to tuberous sclerosis. *Epilepsy Res* 1997; **26**: 389–395.

Chiron C, Tonnelier S, Rey E, et al. Stiripentol in childhood partial epilepsy: randomized placebo-controlled trial with enrichment and withdrawal design. *J Child Neurol* 2006; **21**: 496–502.

Christe W, Kramer G, Vigonius U, et al. A double-blind controlled clinical trial: oxcarbazepine versus sodium valproate in adults with newly diagnosed epilepsy. *Epilepsy Res* 1997; **26**: 451–460.

Chung SM, Sperling M, Biton V, Krauss G, Beaman M, Hebert D. Lacosamide: efficacy and safety as oral adjunctive therapy in adults with partial-onset seizures. *Epilepsia* 2007; **48**(suppl 7): 57.

Cloyd JC, Fischer JH, Kriel RL, Kraus DM. Valproic acid pharmacokinetics in children. IV. Effects of age and antiepileptic drugs on protein binding and intrinsic clearance. *Clin Pharmacol Ther* 1993; **53**: 22–29.

Cohen LS, Rosenbaum JF. Clonazepam: new uses and potential problems. *J Clin Psychiatry* 1987; **48**(suppl 1): 50–56.

Coppola G, Franzoni E, Verotti A, et al. Levetiracetam or oxcarbazepine as monotherapy in newly diagnosed benign epilepsy of childhood with centrotemporal spikes (BECTS): an open-label, parallel group trial. *Brain Dev* 2006; **29**: 281–284.

Cozza KL, Armstrong SC, Oesterheld JR. *Concise Guide to Drug Interaction Principles for Medical Practice: Cytochrome P450s, UGTs, P-glycoproteins*, 2nd edn. Washington DC: American Psychiatric Press Inc., 2003.

Cramer JA, Fisher R, Ben-Menachem E, et al. New antiepileptic drugs: comparison of key clinical trials. *Epilepsia* 1999; **40**: 590–600.

Crawford PM, Engelsman M, Brown SW. Tiagabine: phase II study of efficacy and safety in adjunctive treatment of partial seizures. *Epilepsia* 1993; **34**(suppl 2): S182.

Cross JH. Topiramate monotherapy for childhood absence seizures: an open label pilot study. *Seizure* 2002; **11**: 406–410.

Dam M, Ekberg R, Loyning Y, Waltimo O, Jacobsen K. A double-blind study comparing oxcarbazepine and carbamazepine in patients with newly diagnosed, previously untreated epilepsy. *Epilepsy Res* 1989; **3**: 70–76.

De Silva M, MacArdle B, McGowan M, et al. Randomised comparative monotherapy trial of phenobarbitone, phenytoin, carbamazepine, or sodium valproate for newly diagnosed childhood epilepsy. *Lancet* 1996; **347**, 709–713.

Dean C, Mosier M, Penry K. Dose–response study of vigabatrin as add-on therapy in patients with uncontrolled complex partial seizures. *Epilepsia* 1999; **40**: 74–82.

Deckers CLP, Czuczwar SJ, Hekster YA, et al. Selection of antiepileptic drug polytherapy based on mechanisms of action: the evidence reviewed. *Epilepsia* 2000; **41**: 1364–1374.

Ding D, Hong Z, Chen GS, et al. Primary care treatment of epilepsy with phenobarbital in rural China: cost–outcome analysis from the WHO/ILAE/IBE global campaign against epilepsy demonstration project. *Epilepsia* 2008; **49**: 535–539.

Dogan EA, Usta BE, Bilgen R, et al. Efficacy, tolerability, and side effects of oxcarbazepine monotherapy: a prospective study in adult and elderly patients with newly diagnosed partial epilepsy. *Epilepsy Behav* 2008; **13**: 156–161.

Dong X, Leppik IE, White J, Rarick J. Hyponatremia from oxcarbazepine and carbamazepine. *Neurology* 2005; **65**: 1976–1978.

Duley L, Henderson-Smart D. Magnesium sulphate versus phenytoin for eclampsia. *Cochrane Database Syst Rev* 2003; **(4)**: CD000128.

Eke T, Talbot JF, Lawdon MC. Severe persistent visual field constriction associated with vigabatrin. *BMJ* 1997; **314**: 180–181.

Elger C, Bialer M, Cramer JA, et al. Eslicarbazepine acetate: a double-blind, add-on, placebo-controlled exploratory trial in adult patients with partial-onset seizures. *Epilepsia* 2007; **48**: 497–504.

Elger CE, Brodie MJ, Anhut H, et al. Pregabalin add-on treatment in patients with partial seizures: a novel evaluation of flexible-dose and fixed-dose treatment in a double-blind, placebo-controlled study. *Epilepsia* 2005; **46**: 1926–1936.

Elterman RD, Shields WD, Mansfield KA, et al. Randomized trial of vigabatrin in patients with infantile spasms. *Neurology* 2001; **57**: 1416–1421.

Eriksson A-S, Hoppu K, Nergardh A, et al. Pharmacokinetic interactions between lamotrigine and other antiepileptic drugs in children with intractable epilepsy. *Epilepsia* 1996; **37**: 769–773.

Faught E, Ayala R, Montouris GG, Leppik IE. Randomized controlled trial of zonisamide for the treatment of refractory partial-onset seizures. *Neurology* 2001; **57**: 1774–1779.

Faught E, Wilder BJ, Ramsay RE, et al. Topiramate placebo-controlled dose-ranging trial in refractory partial epilepsy using 200-, 400-, and 600-mg daily dosages. Topiramate YD Study Group. *Neurology* 1996; **46**: 1684–1690.

Feely M, Calvert R, Gibson J. Clobazam in catamenial epilepsy. A model for evaluating anticonvulsants. *Lancet* 1982; **ii**: 71–73.

Feksi AT, Kaamugisha J, Sander JWAS, Gatiti S, Shorvon SD. Comprehensive primary health care antiepileptic drug treatment programme in rural and semi-urban Kenya. *Lancet* 1991; **337**: 406–409.

Felbamate Study Group in Lennox–Gastaut Syndrome. Efficacy of felbamate in childhood epileptic encephalopathy (Lennox–Gastaut syndrome). *N Engl J Med* **328**: 29–33.

Ferrie CD, Panayiotopoulos CP. The clinical efficacy of vigabatrin in adults. *Rev Contemp Pharmacother* 1995; **6**: 457–468.

French JA, Kanner AM, Bautista JA, et al. Efficacy and tolerability of the new antiepileptic drugs, I: treatment of new-onset epilepsy – report of the TTA and QSS Subcommittees of the American Academy of Neurology and the American Epilepsy Society. *Epilepsia* 2004; **45**: 401–409.

French JA, Kanner AM, Bautista J, et al. Efficacy and tolerability of the new antiepileptic drugs, II: treatment of refractory epilepsy – report of the TTA and QSS Subcommittees of the American Academy of Neurology and the American Epilepsy Society. *Epilepsia* 2004; **45**: 410–423.

French JA, Kugler AR, Robbins JL, et al. Dose–response trial of pregabalin adjunctive therapy in patients with partial seizures. *Neurology* 2003; **60**: 1631–1637.

French JA, Mosier M, Walker S, et al. (the Vigabatrin Protocol 024 Investigative Cohort). A double-blind, placebo-controlled study of vigabatrin 3 g/day in patients with uncontrolled complex partial seizures. *Neurology* 1996; **46**: 54–61.

Friedlander WJ. Putnam, Merritt, and the discovery of Dilantin. *Epilepsia* 1986; **27**(suppl 3): S1–S21.

Gabapentin in partial epilepsy. UK Gabapentin Study Group. *Lancet* 1990; **335**: 1114–1117.

Gaily E, Granstrom M-J, Liukkonen E. Oxcarbazepine in the treatment of epilepsy in children and adolescents with intellectual disability. *J Int Dis Res* 1998; **42**(suppl 1): 41–45.

Gal P, Oles KS, Gilman JT, Weaver R. Valproic acid efficacy, toxicity and pharmacokinetics in neonates with intractable seizures. *Neurology* 1988; **38**: 467–471.

Gamble CL, Williamson PR, Marson AG. Lamotrigine versus carbamazepine monotherapy for epilepsy. *Cochrane Database Sys Rev* 2006: CD001031.

Gastaut H, Low MD. Antiepileptic properties of clobazam, a 1–5 benzodiazepine, in man. *Epilepsia* 1979; **20**: 437–446.

Gelisse P, Genton P, Kuate C, Pesenti A, Baldy-Moulinier M, Crepel A. Worsening of seizures by oxcarbazepine in juvenile idiopathic generalized epilepsies. *Epilepsia* 2004; **45**: 1282–1286.

Genton P, Bureau M. Epilepsy with myoclonic absences. *CNS Drugs* 2006; **20**: 911–916.

Genton P, Bauer J, Duncan S, et al. On the association of valproate and polycystic ovaries. *Epilepsia* 2001; **42**: 295–304.

Genton P, Guerrini R, Remy C. Piracetam in the treatment of cortical myoclonus. *Pharmacopsychiatry* 1999; **32**(suppl 1): 49–53.

Gillham R, Kane K, Bryant-Comstock L, Brodie MJ. A double-blind comparison of lamotrigine and carbamazepine in newly diagnosed epilepsy with health-related quality of life as an outcome measure. *Seizure* 2000; **9**: 375–379.

Glauser T, Ben-Menachem E, Bourgeois B, et al. ILAE treatment guidelines: evidence-based analysis of antiepileptic drug efficacy and effectiveness as initial monotherapy for epileptic seizures and syndromes. *Epilepsia* 2006; **47**: 1094–1120.

Glauser T, Kluger G, Krauss G, Perdomo C, Arroyo S. Short-term and long-term efficacy and safety of rufinamide as adjunctive therapy in patients with inadequately controlled Lennox–Gastaut syndrome. *Neurology* 2006; **66**: 1–96.

Glauser TA, Nigro M, Sachdeo R, et al. Adjunctive therapy with oxcarbazepine in children with partial seizures. *Neurology* 2000; **54**: 2237–2244.

Glazko AJ. The discovery of phenytoin. *Ther Drug Monit* 1986; **8**: 490–497.

Goa KL, Sorkin EM. Gabapentin. A review of its pharmacological properties and clinical potential in epilepsy. *Drugs* 1993; **46**: 409–427.

Goren MZ, Onat F. Ethosuximide: from bench to bedside. *CNS Drugs Rev* 2007; **13**: 224–239.

Grant SM, Heel RC. Vigabatrin. A review of its pharmacodynamic and pharmacokinetic properties, and therapeutic potential in epilepsy. *Drugs* 1991; **41**: 889–926.

Guerreiro MM, Vigonius U, Pohlmann H, et al. A double-blind controlled clinical trial of oxcarbazepine versus phenytoin in children and adolescents with epilepsy. *Epilepsy Res* 1997; **27**: 205–213.

Gupta R, Appleton R. Corticosteroids in the management of the paediatric epilepsies. *Arch Dis Child* 2005; **90**: 379–384.

Halász P, Kälviäinen R, Mazurkiewicz-Beldzińska M, et al. Adjunctive lacosamide for partial-onset seizures: efficacy and safety from a randomized controlled trial. *Epilepsia* 2009; **50**: 443–453.

Hanson JW, Smith DW. The fetal hydantoin syndrome. *J Pediatr* 1975; **87**: 285–290.

Harden C. Safety profile of levetiracetam. *Epilepsia* 2001; **42**: 36–39.

Hart YM, Cortez M, Andermann F, et al. Medical treatment of Rasmussen's syndrome (chronic encephalitis and epilepsy): effect on high dose steroids or immunoglobulins in 19 patients. *Neurology* 1994; **44**: 1030–1036.

Heller AJ, Chesterman P, Elwes RD, Crawford P, et al. Phenobarbitone, phenytoin, carbamazepine, or sodium valproate for newly diagnosed adult epilepsy: a randomised comparative monotherapy trial. *J Neurol Neurosurg Psychiatry* 1995; **58**: 44–50.

Hung SI, Chung WH, Jee SH, et al. Genetic susceptibility to carbamazepine-induced cutaneous adverse drug reactions. *Pharmacogenet Genomics* 2006; **16**: 297–306.

Iametti P, Raucci U, Zuccaro P, et al. Lamotrigine hypersensitivity in childhood epilepsy. *Epilepsia* 1998; **39**: 502–507.

Isojärvi JI, Tauboll E, Tapanainen JS, et al. On the association between valproate and polycystic ovary syndrome: A response and an alternative view. *Epilepsia* 2001; **42**: 305–310.

Jawad S, Richens A, Goodwin G, et al. Controlled trial of lamotrigine (Lamictal) for refractory partial seizures. *Epilepsia* 1989; **30**: 356–363.

Jawad S, Yuen WC, Peck AW, et al. Lamotrigine: single-dose pharmacokinetics and initial 1 week experience in refractory epilepsy. *Epilepsy Res* 1987; **1**: 194–201.

Kale R, Perucca E. Editorial: revisiting phenobarbital for epilepsy. *BMJ* 2004; **329**: 1199–1200.

Kalviainen R, Nousiainen I. Visual field defects with vigabatrin: epidemiology and therapeutic implications. *CNS Drugs* 2001; **15**: 217–230.

Kälviäinen R, Äikiä M, Saukkonen AM, et al. Vigabatrin vs carbamazepine monotherapy in patients with newly diagnosed epilepsy. A randomized, controlled study. *Arch Neurol* 1995; **52**: 989–996.

Kälviäinen R, Brodie MJ, Chadwick D, et al. A double-blind, placebo-controlled trial of tiagabine given three-times daily as add-on therapy for refractory partial seizures. *Epilepsy Res* 1998; **30**: 31–40.

Kalviäinen R, Nousiainen I, Mäntyjärvi M, et al. Vigabatrin, a GABAergic antiepileptic drug, causes concentric visual field defects. *Neurology* 1999; **53**: 922–926.

Kaneko S, Battino D, Andermann F, et al. Congenital malformations due to antiepileptic drugs. *Epilepsy Res* 1999; **33**: 145–158.

Kanner AM, Frey M. Adding valproate to lamotrigine: a study of their pharmacokinetic interaction. *Neurology* 2000; **55**: 588–591.

Katayama F, Miura H, Takanashi S. Long-term effectiveness and side effects of acetazolamide as an adjunct to other anticonvulsants in the treatment of refractory epilepsies. *Brain Dev* 2002; **24**: 150–154.

Knowles SR, Shapiro LE, Shear NH. Anticonvulsant hypersensitivity syndrome: incidence, prevention and management. *Drug Saf* 1999; **21**: 489–501.

Knudsen JF, Thambi LR, Kapcala LP, Racoosin JA. Oligohydrosis and fever in pediatric patients treated with zonisamide. *Pediatr Neurol* 2003; **28**: 184–189.

Kothare SV, Valencia I, Khurana DS, Hardison H, Melvin JJ, Legido A. Efficacy and tolerability of zonisamide in juvenile myoclonic epilepsy. *Epileptic Disord* 2004; **6**: 267–270.

Kutluay E, McCague K, D'Souza J, Beydoun A. Safety and tolerability of oxcarbazepine in elderly patients with epilepsy. *Epilepsy Behav* 2003; **4**: 175–180.

Kwan P, Brodie MJ. Phenobarbital for the treatment of epilepsy in the 21st century: a critical review. *Epilepsia* 2004; **45**: 1141–1149.

Lackner TE, Cloyd JC, Thomas LW, Leppik IE. Antiepileptic drug use in nursing home residents: effect of age, gender, and co-medication on pattern of use. *Epilepsia* 1998; **39**: 1083–1087.

Lee GC, Tam CP, Danesh-Meyer HV, Myers JS, Katz LJ. Bilateral angle closure glaucoma induced by sulphonamide-derived medications. *Clin Exp Ophthalmol* 2007; **35**: 55–58.

Leppik IE. Practical prescribing and long-term efficacy and safety of zonisamide. *Epilepsy Res* 2006; **68**(suppl 2): S17–S24.

Levinson DF, Devinsky O. Psychiatric adverse events during vigabatrin therapy. *Neurology* 1999; **53**: 1503–1511.

Lim L, Foldvary N, Maschs E, Lee J. Acetazolamide in women with catamenial epilepsy. *Epilepsia* 2001; **42**: 746–749.

Lin JH, Yamazaki M. Role of P-glycoprotein in pharmacokinetics: clinical implications. *Clin Pharmacokinet* 2003; **42**: 59–98.

Loiseau P. Review of controlled trials of tiagabine: a clinician's viewpoint. *Epilepsia* 1999; **40**(suppl 9), 145.

Loiseau P, Brachet Liermain A, Legroux M, Jogeix M. Intérêt du dosage des anticonvulsivants dans le traitement des épilepsies. *Nouv Presse Med* 1977; **16**: 813–817.

Loiseau P, Yuen AWC, Duche B, et al. A randomized double-blind cross-over add-on trial of lamotrigine in patients with treatment-resistant partial seizures. *Epilepsy Res* 1990; **7**: 136–145.

Löscher W. Basic pharmacology of valproate: a review after 35 years of clinical use for the treatment of epilepsy. *CNS Drugs* 2002; **16**: 669–694.

Low PA, James S, Peschel T, Leong R, Rothstein A. Zonisamide and associated oligohidrosis and hyperthermia. *Epilepsy Res* 2004; **62**: 27–34.

Lux AL, Edwards SW, Hancock E, et al. The United Kingdom Infantile Spasms Study comparing vigabatrin with prednisolone or tetracosactide at 14 days: a multicentre, randomised controlled trial. *Lancet* 2004; **364**: 1773–1778.

Lux AL, Edwards SW, Hancock E, et al. The United Kingdom infantile spasm study (UKISS) comparing hormone treatment with vigabatrin on developmental and epilepsy outcomes to age 14 months: a multicentre randomized trial. *Lancet* 2005; **4**: 712–717.

McElhatton RR. The effects of benzodiazepine use during pregnancy and lactation. *Reprod Toxicol* 1994; **8**: 461–475.

Mackay MT, Weiss SK, Adams-Webber T, et al. Practice parameter: medical treatment of infantile spasms: report of the American Academy of Neurology and the Child Neurology Society. *Neurology* 2004; **62**: 1668–1681.

Marso MA. Clobazam as an add-on in the management of refractory epilepsy (Review). *The Cochrane Library* 2008, Issue 2.

Marson AG, Al-Kharusi AM, Alwaidh M, et al, on behalf of the SANAD Study Group. The SANAD study of effectiveness of carbamazepine, gabapentin, lamotrigine, oxcarbazepine, or topiramate for treatment of partial epilepsy: an unblinded randomized comparison. *Lancet* 2007; **369**: 1000–1015.

Marson AG, Al-Kharusi AM, Alwaidh M, et al. The SANAD study of effectiveness of valproate, lamotrigine, or topiramate for generalised and unclassifiable epilepsy: an unblinded randomised controlled trial. *Lancet* 2007; **369**: 1016–1026.

Marson AG, Kadir ZA, Chadwick DW. New antiepileptic drugs: a systematic review of their efficacy and tolerability. *BMJ* 1996; **313**: 1169–1174.

Marson AG, Kadir ZA, Hutton JL, et al. The new antiepileptic drugs: a systematic review of their efficacy and tolerability. *Epilepsia* 1997; **38**: 859–880.

Marson AG, Williamson PR, Clough H, Hutton JL, Chadwick DW, Epilepsy Monotherapy Trial Group. Carbamazepine versus valproate monotherapy for epilepsy: a meta-analysis. *Epilepsia* 2002; **43**: 505–513.

Matsuo F, Bergen D, Faught E, et al. Placebo-controlled study of the efficacy and safety of lamotrigine in patients with partial seizures. *Neurology* 1993; **43**: 2284–2291.

Meador KJ, Gevins A, Loring DW, et al. Neuropsychological and neurophysiologic effects of carbamazepine and levetiracetam. *Neurology* 2007; **69**: 2076–2084.

Meadow SR. Congenital abnormalities and anticonvulsant drugs. *Proc R Soc Med* 1970; **63**: 48–49.

Meo R, Bilo L. Polycystic ovary syndrome and epilepsy: a review of the evidence. *Drugs* 2003; **63**: 1185–1227.

Messenheimer J, Ramsey RE, Willmore LJ, et al. Lamotrigine therapy for partial seizures: a multicenter, placebo-controlled, double-blind, cross-over trial. *Epilepsia* 1994; **35**: 113–121.

Mikati MA, Schachter SC, Schomer DL, et al. Long-term tolerability, pharmacokinetic and preliminary efficacy study of lamotrigine in patients with resistant partial seizures. *Clin Neuropharmacol* 1989; **12**: 312–321.

Montouris G. Safety at the newer antiepileptic drug oxcarbazepine during pregnancy. *Curr Med Res Opin* 2005; **21**: 693–701.

Montouris G, Morris GL 3rd. Reproductive and sexual dysfunction in men with epilepsy. *Epilepsy Behav* 2005; **7**(suppl 2): S7–S14.

Mula M, Trimble MR, Lhatoo SD, Sander JW. Topiramate and psychiatric adverse events in patients with epilepsy. *Epilepsia* 2003; **44**: 659–663.

Muller M, Marson AG, Williamson PR. Oxcarbazepine versus phenytoin monotherapy for epilepsy. *Cochrane Database Syst Rev* 2006; (**2**): CD003615.

Mumford JP, Dam M. Meta-analysis of European placebo controlled studies of vigabatrin in drug resistant epilepsy. *Br J Clin Pharmacol* 1989; **27**(suppl 1): S101–S107.

Murphy JV, Sawasky F, Marquardt KM, Harris DJ. Deaths in young children receiving nitrazepam. *J Pediatr* 1987; **111**: 145–147.

Nabbout R, Melki I, Gerbaka B, et al. Infantile spasms in Down syndrome: good response to a short course of vigabatrin. *Epilepsia* 2001; **42**: 1580–1583.

Naritoku DK, Warnock CR, Messenheimer JA, et al. Lamotrigine extended-release as adjunctive therapy for partial seizures. *Neurology* 2007; **69**: 1610–1618.

Nation RL, Evans AM, Milne RW. Pharmacokinetic drug interactions with phenytoin. *Clin Pharmacokinet* 1990; **18**: 131–150.

Noachtar S, Andermann E, Meyvisch P, Andermann F, Gough WB, Schiemann-Delgado J. Levetiracetam for the treatment of idiopathic generalized epilepsy with myoclonic seizures. *Neurology* 2008; **70**: 607–616.

Noyer M, Gillard M, Matagne A, Hénichart J-P, Wülfert E. The novel antiepileptic drug levetiracetam (ucb L059) appears to act via a specific binding site in CNS membranes. *Eur J Pharmacol* 1995; **286**: 137–146.

Ohtahara S. Zonisamide in the management of epilepsy – Japanese experience. *Epilepsy Res* 2006; **68**(suppl 2): S25–S33.

Painter MJ, Scher MS, Stein AD, et al. Phenobarbital compared with phenytoin for the treatment of neonatal seizures. *N Engl J Med* 1999; **341**: 485–489.

Pal DK. Phenobarbital for childhood epilepsy: systematic review. *Paediatr Perinat Drug Ther* 2006; **7**: 31–42.

Patsalos PN. Clinical pharmacokinetics of levetiracetam. *Clin Pharmacokinet* 2004; **43**: 707–724.

Patsalos PN, Perucca E. Clinically important drug interactions in epilepsy: general features and interactions between antiepileptic drugs. *Lancet Neurol* 2003; **2**: 347–356.

Patsalos PN, Perucca E. Clinically important drug interactions in epilepsy: interactions between antiepileptic drugs and other drugs. *Lancet Neurol* 2003; **2**: 473–481.

Patsalos PN, Berry DJ, Bourgeois BF, et al. Antiepileptic drugs – best practice guidelines for therapeutic drug monitoring: a position paper by the subcommission on therapeutic drug monitoring, ILAE Commission on Therapeutic Strategies. *Epilepsia* 2008; **49**: 1239–1276.

Patsalos PN, Froscher W, Pisani F, van Rijn C. The importance of drug interactions in epilepsy therapy. *Epilepsia* 2002; **43**: 365–385.

Pellock JM, Faught E, Leppik IE, et al. Felbamate: Consensus of current clinical experience. *Epilepsy Res* 2006; **71**: 89–101.

Perry S, Holt P, Benatar M. Levetiracetam versus carbamazepine monotherapy for partial epilepsy in children less than 16 years of age. *J Child Neurol* 2008; **23**: 515–519.

Perucca E. A pharmacological and clinical review on topiramate, a new antiepileptic drug. *Pharmacol Res* 1997; **35**: 241–256.

Perucca E. Clinically relevant drug interactions with antiepileptic drugs. *Br J Clin Pharmacol* 2006; **61**: 246–255.

Perucca E. Designing clinical trials to assess antiepileptic drugs as monotherapy: difficulties and solutions. *CNS Drugs* 2008; **22**: 917–

Perucca E, Bialer M. The clinical pharmacokinetics of the newer antiepileptic drugs. Focus on topiramate, zonisamide and tiagabine. *Clin Pharmacokinet* 1996; **31**: 29–46.

Perucca E, Kwan P. Overtreatment in epilepsy: how it occurs and how it can be avoided. *CNS Drugs* 2005; **19**: 897–908.

Perucca E, Beghi E, Dulac O, et al. Assessing risk to benefit ratio in antiepileptic drug therapy. *Epilepsy Res* 2000; **41**: 107–139.

Perucca E, Cloyd J, Critchley D, Fuseau E. Rufinamide: clinical pharmacokinetics and concentration-response relationships in patients with epilepsy. *Epilepsia* 2008; **49**: 1123–1141.

Perucca E, Berlowitz D, Birnbaum A, et al. Pharmacological and clinical aspects of antiepileptic drugs use in the elderly. *Epilepsy Res* 2006; **68**(suppl 1): 49–63.

Peters DH, Sorkin EM. Zonisamide. A review of its pharmacodynamic and pharmacokinetic properties, and therapeutic potential in epilepsy. *Drugs* 1993; **45**: 760–787.

Pina-Garza JE, Espinoza R, Nordli D, et al. Oxcarbazepine adjunctive therapy in infants and young children with partial seizures. *Neurology* 2005; **65**: 1370–1375.

Posner EB, Mohamed K, Marson AG. A systematic review of treatment of typical absence seizures in children and adolescents with ethosuximide, sodium valproate or lamotrigine. *Seizure* 2005; **14**: 117–122.

Posner EB, Mohamed K, Marson AG. Ethosuximide, sodium valproate or lamotrigine for absence seizures in children and adolescents. *Cochrane Database Syst Rev* 2005; (**4**): CD003032.

Privitera MD, Brodie MJ, Mattson RH, Chadwick DW, Neto W, Wang S, EPMN 105 Study Group. Topiramate, carbamazepine and valproate monotherapy: double-blind comparison in newly diagnosed epilepsy. *Acta Neurol Scand* 2003; **107**: 165–175.

Pylvänen V, Pakarinen AJ, Knip M, Isojärvi J. Characterization of insulin secretion in valproate-treated patients with epilepsy. *Epilepsia* 2006; **47**: 1460–1464.

Rambeck B, Wolf P. Lamotrigine clinical pharmacokinetics. *Clin Pharmacokinet* 1993; **25**: 433–443.

Ramsay RE, Pellock JM, Garnett WR, et al. Pharmacokinetics and safety of lamotrigine (Lamictal) in patients with epilepsy. *Epilepsy Res* 1991; **10**: 191–200.

Reife R, Pledger G, Wu SC. Topiramate as add-on therapy: pooled analysis of randomized controlled trials in adults. *Epilepsia* 2000; **41**(suppl 1): S66–S71.

Reinikainen KJ, Keranen T, Halonen T, et al. Comparison of oxcarbazepine and carbamazepine: a double-blind study. *Epilepsy Res* 1987; **1**: 284–289.

Richens A, Chadwick DW, Duncan JS, et al. Adjunctive treatment of partial seizures with tiagabine: a placebo-controlled trial. *Epilepsy Res* 1995; **21**: 37–42.

Richens A, Davidson DL, Cartlidge NE, Easter DJ. A multicentre comparative trial of sodium valproate and carbamazepine in adult onset epilepsy. Adult EPITEG Collaborative Group. *J Neurol Neurosurg Psychiatry* 1994; **57**: 682–687.

Rosenfeld W, Fountain NB, Kaubrys G, Heinzen L, McShea C. Lacosamide: an interim evaluation of long-term safety and efficacy as oral adjunctive therapy in subjects with partial-onset seizures. *Epilepsia* 2007; **48**(suppl 6): 318–319.

Rowan AJ, Ramsay RE, Collins JF, et al. VA Cooperative Study 428 Group. New onset geriatric epilepsy: a randomized study of gabapentin, lamotrigine, and carbamazepine. *Neurology* 2005; **64**: 1868–1873.

Ryvlin P, Rheims S, Semah F, et al. Meta-analysis of add-on treatment in drug resistant partial epilepsy: a comprehensive study of 41 randomized controlled trials among 10 AEDs. *Neurology* 2006; **66**: A36.

Sachdeo R, Edwards K, Hasegawa H, et al. Safety and efficacy of oxcarbazepine 1200 mg/day in patients with recent onset partial epilepsy. *Neurology* 1999; **52**(suppl 2): A391.

Sachdeo R, Kramer LD, Rosenberg A, Sachdeo S. Felbamate monotherapy: controlled trial in patients with partial onset seizures. *Ann Neurol* 1992; **32**: 386–392.

Sachdeo RC, Beydoun A, Schachter SC, et al. Oxcarbazepine (Trileptal) as monotherapy in patients with partial seizures. *Neurology* 2001; **57**: 864–870.

Sachdeo RC, Glauser TA, Ritter F, Reife R, Lim P, Pledger G. A double-blind, randomized trial of topiramate in Lennox-Gastaut syndrome. Topiramate YL Study Group. *Neurology* 1999; **52**: 1882–1887.

Sachdeo RC, Wasserstein A, Mesenbrink PJ, D'Souza J. Effects of oxcarbazepine on sodium concentration and water handling. *Ann Neurol* 2002; **51**: 613–620.

Saetre E, Perucca E, Isojärvi J, et al. On behalf of the LAM 40089 Study Group. An international multicenter randomized double-blind controlled trial of lamotrigine and sustained-release carbamazepine in the treatment of newly diagnosed epilepsy in the elderly. *Epilepsia* 2007; **48**: 1292–1302.

Sander JWAS, Hart YM, Trimble MR, Shorvon SD. Vigabatrin and psychosis. *J Neurol Neurosurg Psychiatry* 1991; **54**: 435–439.

Schachter SC, Vazquez B, Fisher RS, et al. Oxcarbazepine: double-blind randomized, placebo-controlled, monotherapy trial for partial seizures. *Neurology* 1999; **52**: 732–737.

Schapel GJ, Beran RG, Vajda FJE, et al. Double-blind, placebo-controlled, cross-over study of lamotrigine in treatment resistant partial seizures. *J Neurol Neurosurg Psychiatry* 1993; **56**: 448–453.

Schmidt D, Sachdeo R. Oxcarbazepine for treatment of partial epilepsy: a review and recommendations for clinical use. *Epilepsy Behav* 2000; **1**: 396–405.

Schmidt D, Einicke I, Haenel F. The influence of seizure type on the efficacy of plasma concentrations of phenytoin, phenobarbital, and carbamazepine. *Arch Neurol* 1986; **43**: 263–265.

Schmidt D, Gram L, Brodie M, et al. Tiagabine in the treatment of epilepsy – a clinical review with a guide for the prescribing physician. *Epilepsy Res* 2000; **41**: 245–251.

Schmitt B, Kovacevic-Preradovic T, Critelli H, Molinari L. Is ethosuximide a risk factor for generalised tonic–clonic seizures in absence epilepsy? *Neuropediatrics* 2007; **38**: 83–87.

Sewell AC, Bohles HJ, Herwig J, Demirkol M. Neurological deterioration in patients with urea cycle disorders under valproate therapy – a cause for concern. *Eur J Pediatr* 1995; **154**: 593–594.

Shakir RA, Johnson RH, Lambie DG, Melville ID, Nanda RN. Comparison of sodium valproate and phenytoin as single drug treatment in epilepsy. *Epilepsia* 1981; **22**: 27–33.

Shorvon S. Safety of topiramate. *Epilepsia* 1996; **37**: S18–22.

Shorvon S. Pyrrolidone derivatives. *Lancet* 2001; **358**: 1885–1892.

Shorvon SD, Lowenthal A, Janz D, et al. Multicenter double-blind, randomized, placebo-controlled trial of levetiracetam as add-on therapy in patients with refractory partial seizures. European Levetiracetam Study Group. *Epilepsia* 2000; **41**: 1179–1186.

Smith PEM, for the UK Oxcarbazepine Advisory Board. Clinical recommendations for oxcarbazepine. *Seizure* 2001; **10**: 87–91.

Tanaka E. Clinically significant pharmacokinetic drug interactions with benzodiazepines. *J Clin Pharm Ther* 1999; **24**: 347–355.

Tanganelli P, Regesta G. Vigabatrin vs. carbamazepine monotherapy in newly diagnosed focal epilepsy: a randomized response conditional cross-over study. *Epilepsy Res* 1996; **25**: 257–262.

Taylor CP, Angelotti T, Fauman E. Pharmacology and mechanism of action of pregabalin: the calcium channel alpha2-delta subunit as a target for antiepileptic drug discovery. *Epilepsy Res* 2007; **73**: 137–150.

Taylor S, Tudur Smith C, Williamson PR, Marson AG. Phenobarbitone versus phenytoin monotherapy for partial onset seizures and generalized onset tonic–clonic seizures. *Cochrane Database Syst Rev* 2002; (**2**): CD002217.

Terada Y, Fukagawa S, Shigematsu K. Reproduction studies of zonisamide (3). Teratogenicity study in mice, dogs, and monkeys. *Jpn Pharmacol Ther* 1987; **15**: 4435–4453.

Trojnar MK, Wojtal K, Trojnar MP, et al. Stiripentol. A novel antiepileptic drug. *Pharmacol Rep* 2005; **57**: 154–160.

Tudur Smith C, Marson AG, Clough HE, Williamson PR. Carbamazepine versus phenytoin monotherapy for epilepsy. *Cochrane Database Syst Rev* 2002; (**2**): CD001911.

Tudur Smith C, Marson AG, Williamson PR. Phenytoin versus valproate monotherapy for partial onset seizures and generalized onset tonic-clonic seizures. *Cochrane Database Syst Rev* 2001; (**4**): CD001769.

US Gabapentin Study Group No. 5. Gabapentin as add-on therapy in refractory partial epilepsy: a double-blind, placebo-controlled, parallel-group study. *Neurology* 1993; **43**: 2292–2298.

Uthman B, Rowan J, Ahman PA, et al. Tiagabine for complex partial seizures: a randomised, add-on, dose-response trial. *Arch Neurol* 1998; **55**: 56–62.

Vauzelle-Kervroëdan F, Rey E, Cieuta C, et al. Influence of concurrent antiepileptic medication on the pharmacokinetics of lamotrigine as add-on therapy in epileptic children. *Br J Clin Pharmacol* 1996; **41**: 325–330.

Verity CM, Hosking G, Easter DJ. A multicentre comparative trial of sodium valproate and carbamazepine in paediatric epilepsy. The Paediatric EPITEG Collaborative Group. *Dev Med Child Neurol* 1995; **37**: 97–108.

Verrotti A, Trotta D, Morgese G, Chiarelli F. Valproate-induced hyperammonemic encephalopathy. *Metab Brain Dis* 2002; **17**: 367–373.

Vigabatrin Paediatric Advisory Group. Guidelines for prescribing vigabatrin in children has been revised. *BMJ* 2000; **320**: 1404–1405.

Vigevano F, Cilio MR. Vigabatrin versus ACTH as first-line treatment for infantile spasms: a randomized, prospective study. *Epilepsia* 1997; **38**: 1270–1274.

Wallace SJ. Use of ethosuximide and valproate in the treatment of epilepsy. *Neurol Clinics* 1986; **4**: 601–616.

Wilder BJ, Ramsay RE, Murphy JV, Karas BJ, Marquardt K, Hammond EJ. Comparison of valproic acid and phenytoin in newly diagnosed tonic–clonic seizures. *Neurology* 1983; **33**: 1474–1476.

Wilensky AJ, Friel PN, Levy RH, Comfort CP, Kaluzny SP. Kinetics of phenobarbital in normal subjects and epileptic patients. *Eur J Clin Pharmacol* 1982; **23**: 87–92.

Wroe SJ, Yeates AB, Marshall A. Long-term safety and efficacy of zonisamide in patients with refractory partial-onset epilepsy. *Acta Neurol Scand* 2008; **118**: 87–93.

Zaccara G, Franciotta D, Perucca E. Idiosyncratic adverse reactions to antiepileptic drugs. *Epilepsia* 2007; **48**: 1223–1244.

Zhou S, Yung Chan S, Cher Goh B, et al. Mechanism-based inhibition of cytochrome P450 3A4 by therapeutic drugs. *Clin Pharmacokinet* 2005; **44**: 279–304.

Chapter 9

Chapter from: Shorvon SD, Perucca E, Engel J Jr, eds. *The Treatment of Epilepsy*. Oxford: Blackwell Publishing Ltd, 2009

Walker MC, Shorvon SD. Emergency treatment of seizures and status epilepticus, pp. 231–248.

Books

Delgado-Escueta AV, Wasterlain C, Treiman D, Porter R. *Advances in Neurology*, Vol **34**: *Status Epilepticus: mechanisms of brain damage and treatment*. New York: Raven Press, 1983.

Gastaut H, Roger J, Lob H. *Les États de Mal Épileptiques*. Paris: Masson, 1967.

Shorvon S. *Status Epilepticus: Its clinical features and treatment in children and adults*. Cambridge: Cambridge University Press, 1994.

Shorvon SD, Trinka E, Walker MC. *The proceedings of the First London Colloquium on Status Epilepticus* – University College London, April 12–15, 2007. *Epilepsia* 2007; **48** (suppl 8)

Trinka E, Shorvon SD. *Proceedings of the Innsbruck Colloquium on Status Epilepticus*, Innsbruck, Austria, April 2–5, 2009. *Epilepsia* 2009; **50** (suppl 12)

Wasterlain C, Treiman D. *Status Epilepticus: Mechanisms and management*. Cambridge, MA: MIT Press, 2006.

Journal articles/chapters in books

Alldredge BK, Lowenstein DH. Status epilepticus related to alcohol abuse. *Epilepsia* 1993; **34**: 1033–1037.

Alldredge BK, Gelb AM, Isaacs SM, et al. A comparison of lorazepam, diazepam, placebo for the treatment of out-of-hospital status epilepticus. *N Engl J Med* 2001; **345**: 631–637.

Aminoff MJ, Simon RP. Status epilepticus. Causes, clinical features and consequences in 98 patients. *Am J Med* 1980; **69**: 657–666.

Appleton R, Sweeney A, Choonara I, Robson J, Molyneux E. Lorazepam versus diazepam in the acute treatment of epileptic seizures and status epilepticus. *Dev Med Child Neurol* 1995; **37**: 682–688.

Benowitz NL, Simon RP, Copeland JR. Status epilepticus: divergence of sympathetic activity and cardiovascular response. *Ann Neurol* 1986; **19**: 197–199.

Boggs G, Painter JA, DeLorenzo RJ. Analysis of electrocardiographic changes in status epilepticus. *Epilepsy Res* 1993; **14**: 87–94.

Brooks-Kayal AR, Shumate MD, Jin H, Rikhter TY, Coulter DA. Selective changes in single cell GABA(A) receptor subunit expression and function in temporal lobe epilepsy. *Nat Med* 1998; **4**: 1166–1172.

Brown JK, Hussain IH. Status epilepticus. I: Pathogenesis [see comments]. *Dev Med Child Neurol* 1991; **33**: 3–17.

Browne TR. Paraldehyde, chlormethiazole, lidocaine for treatment of status epilepticus. *Adv Neurol* 1983; **34**: 509–517.

Browne TR. Fosphenytoin Cerebyx. *Clin Neuropharmacol* 1997; **20**: 1–12.

Cascino GD, Hesdorffer D, Logroscino G, Hauser WA. Treatment of nonfebrile status epilepticus in Rochester, Minn, from 1965 through 1984. *Mayo Clin Proc* 2001; **76**: 39–41.

Claassen J, Hirsch LJ, Emerson RG, Mayer SA. Treatment of refractory status epilepticus with pentobarbital, propofol, or midazolam: a systematic review. *Epilepsia* 2002; **43**: 146–153.

Cockerell OC, Rothwell J, Thompson PD, Marsden CD, Shorvon SD. Clinical and physiological features of epilepsia partialis continua. Cases ascertained in the UK. *Brain* 1996; **119**: 393–407.

Corsellis JA, Bruton CJ. Neuropathology of status epilepticus in humans. *Adv Neurol* 1983; **34**: 129–139.

Cossart R, Dinocourt C, Hirsch JC, et al. Dendritic but not somatic GABAergic inhibition is decreased in experimental epilepsy. *Nat Neurosci* 2001; **4**: 52–62.

DeLorenzo RJ, Waterhouse EJ, Towne AR, et al. Persistent non-convulsive status epilepticus after the control of convulsive status epilepticus. *Epilepsia* 1998; **39**: 833–840.

Garzon E, Fernandes RMF, Sakamoto AC. Serial EEG during human status epilepticus. Evidence for PLED as an ictal pattern. *Neurology* 2001; **57**: 1175–1183.

Goodkin HR, Joshi S, Kozhemyakin M, Kapur J. Impact of receptor changes on treatment of status epilepticus. *Epilepsia* 2007; **48**(suppl 8): 14–15.

Howell SJ, Owen L, Chadwick DW. Pseudostatus epilepticus [see comments]. *Q J Med* 1989; **71**: 507–519.

Ingvar M, Siesjo BK. Cerebral oxygen consumption and glucose consumption during status epilepticus. *Eur Neurol* 1981; **20**: 219–220.

Kaplan PW. Prognosis in nonconvulsive status epilepticus. *Epileptic Dis* 2000; **2**: 185–193.

Kapur J, Macdonald RL. Rapid seizure-induced reduction of benzodiazepine and Zn^{2+} sensitivity of hippocampal dentate granule cell $GABA_A$ receptors. *J Neurosci* 1997; **17**: 7532–7540.

Lansberg MG, O'Brien MW, Norbash AM, et al. MRI abnormalities associated with partial status epilepticus. *Neurology* 1999; **52**: 1021–1027.

Leppik IE, Derivan AT, Homan RW, Walker J, Ramsay RE, Patrick B. Double-blind study of lorazepam and diazepam in status epilepticus. *J Am Med Assoc* 1983; **249**: 1452–1454.

Lothman EW, Bertram EH, Bekenstein JW, Perlin JB. Self-sustaining limbic status epilepticus induced by 'continuous' hippocampal stimulation: electrographic and behavioral characteristics. *Epilepsy Res* 1989; **3**: 107–19.

McIntyre J, Robertson S, Norris E, Appleton R, Whitehouse WP, Phillips B, et al. Safety and efficacy of buccal midazolam versus rectal diazepam for emergency treatment of seizures in children: a randomised controlled trial. *Lancet* 2005; **366**: 205–210.

Mayer SA, Claassen J, Lokin J, Mendelsohn F, Dennis LJ, Fitzsimmons BF. Refractory status epilepticus: frequency, risk factors, impact on outcome. *Arch Neurol* 2002; **59**: 205–210.

Mazarati AM, Baldwin RA, Sankar R, Wasterlain CG. Time-dependent decrease in the effectiveness of antiepileptic drugs during the course of self-sustaining status epilepticus. *Brain Res* 1998; **814**: 179–185.

Mehta V, Singhi P, Singhi S. Intravenous sodium valproate versus diazepam infusion for the control of refractory status epilepticus in children: a randomized controlled trial. *J Child Neurol* 2007; **22**: 1191–1197.

Meldrum BS. Endocrine consequences of status epilepticus. *Adv Neurol* 1983; **34**: 399–403.

Meldrum BS, Brierley JB. Prolonged epileptic seizures in primates. Ischemic cell change and its relation to ictal physiological events. *Arch Neurol* 1973; **28**: 10–17.

Meldrum BS, Horton RW. Physiology of status epilepticus in primates. *Arch Neurol* 1973; **28**: 1–9.

Meldrum BS, Vigouroux RA, Brierley JB. Systemic factors and epileptic brain damage. Prolonged seizures in paralyzed, artificially ventilated baboons. *Arch Neurol* 1973; **29**: 82–87.

Misra UK, Kalita J, Patel R. Sodium valproate vs phenytoin in status epilepticus: a pilot study. *Neurology* 2006; **67**: 340–342.

Nelligan A, Shorvon SD. History of status epilepticus. *Epilepsia* 2009; **50**(suppl 3): in press.

Okazaki MM, Evenson DA, Nadler JV. Hippocampal mossy fiber sprouting and synapse formation after status epilepticus in rats: visualization after retrograde transport of biocytin. *J Comp Neurol* 1995; **352**: 515–534.

Parent JM, Yu TW, Leibowitz RT, Geschwind DH, Sloviter RS, Lowenstein DH. Dentate granule cell neurogenesis is increased by seizures and contributes to aberrant network reorganization in the adult rat hippocampus. *J Neurosci* 1997; **17**: 3727–3738.

Shaner DM, McCurdy SA, Herring MO, Gabor AJ. Treatment of status epilepticus: a prospective comparison of diazepam and phenytoin versus phenobarbital and optional phenytoin. *Neurology* 1988; **38**: 202–207.

Shorvon S, Walker M. Status epilepticus in idiopathic generalized epilepsy. *Epilepsia* 2005; **46**(suppl 9): 73–79.

Simon RP. Physiologic consequences of status epilepticus. *Epilepsia* 1985; **26**(suppl 1): S58–S66.

Simon RP, Copeland JR, Benowitz NL, Jacob P, Bronstein J. Brain phenobarbital uptake during prolonged status epilepticus. *J Cereb Blood Flow Metab* 1987; **7**: 783–788.

Tomson T, Lindbom U, Nilsson BY. Nonconvulsive status epilepticus in adults: thirty-two consecutive patients from a general hospital population. *Epilepsia* 1992; **33**: 829–835.

Treiman DM, Meyers PD, Walton NY, et al. A comparison of four treatments for generalized convulsive status epilepticus. Veterans Affairs Status Epilepticus Cooperative Study Group. *N Engl J Med* 1998; **339**: 792–798.

Treiman DM, Walton NY, Kendrick C. A progressive sequence of electroencephalographic changes during generalized convulsive status epilepticus. *Epilepsy Res* 1990; **5**: 49–60.

Trinka E. The use of valproate and new antiepileptic drugs in status epilepticus. *Epilepsia* 2007; **48**(suppl 8): 49–51.

Van-Ness PC. Pentobarbital and EEG burst suppression in treatment of status epilepticus refractory to benzodiazepines and phenytoin. *Epilepsia* 1990; **31**: 61–67.

Walker MC. Diagnosis and treatment of nonconvulsive status epilepticus. *CNS Drugs* 2001; **15**: 931–939.

Walker MC, Howard RS, Smith SJ, Miller DH, Shorvon SD, Hirsch NP. Diagnosis and treatment of status epilepticus on a neurological intensive care unit. *QJM* 1996; **89**: 913–920.

Walker MC, Smith SJ, Shorvon SD. The intensive care treatment of convulsive status epilepticus in the UK. Results of a national survey and recommendations [see comments]. *Anaesthesia* 1995; **50**: 130–135.

Walker MC, Tong X, Brown S, Shorvon SD, Patsalos PN. Comparison of single- and repeated-dose pharmacokinetics of diazepam. *Epilepsia* 1998; **39**: 283–289.

Williamson PD, Spencer DD, Spencer SS, Novelly RA, Mattson RH. Complex partial status epilepticus: a depth-electrode study. *Ann Neurol* 1985; **18**: 647–654.

Young GB, Gilbert JJ, Zochodne DW. The significance of myoclonic status epilepticus in postanoxic coma. *Neurology* 1990; **40**: 1843–1848.

Zhang X, Cui SS, Wallace AE, et al. Relations between brain pathology and temporal lobe epilepsy. *J Neurosci* 2002; **22**: 6052–6061.

Chapter 10

Chapters from: Shorvon SD, Perucca E, Engel J Jr, eds. *The Treatment of Epilepsy*. Oxford: Blackwell Publishing Ltd, 2009

Engel J Jr. Overview of surgical treatment for epilepsy, pp. 743–756.

Baca C, Stern J. Scalp EEG in the epilepsy surgery evaluation, pp. 757–766.

Spencer S, Nguyen D, Duckrow R. Invasive EEG in presurgical evaluation of epilepsy, pp. 767–798.

Stefan H, Rampp S, Hopfengärtner R. MEG in presurgical evaluation of epilepsy, pp. 799–804.

Wellmer J, Elger C. MRI in the presurgical evaluation, pp. 805–820.

Van Paesschen W, Goffin K, Laere K. PET and SPECT in presurgical evaluation of epilepsy, pp. 821–828.

Mauguière M, Merlet I, Jung J. Experimental neurophysiological techniques, pp. 829–850,

Jones-Gotman M, Djordjevic J. Neuropsychological testing in presurgical evaluation, pp. 851–864,

Kanner A. Presurgical psychiatric evaluation, p. 865.

Leiphart J, Fried I. Mesial temporal lobe surgery and other lobar resections, pp. 875–886.

Wetjen N, Junna M, Radhakrishnan K, Cohen-Gadol A, Cascino G. Resective surgery of neoplasms, pp. 887–902.

Uff C, Kitchen N. Resective surgery of vascular and infective lesions for epilepsy, pp. 903–924.

Chern J, Comair Y. Surgery of developmental anomalies causing epilepsy, pp. 925–934.

Dorfmüller G, Bulteau C, Delalande O. Hemispherectomy for epilepsy, pp. 935–942.

Roberts D. Corpus callostomy, pp. 943–950.

Smith M, Byrne R, Kanner A. Hypothalamic hamartoma and multiple subpial transection, pp. 951–958.

Kaufman C, Pilcher W. Awake surgery for epilepsy, pp. 959–966.

Hauptman J, Mathern G. Epilepsy surgery in children, pp. 967–974.

McEvoy A, Arnold F. Stereotactic surgery for epilepsy, 975–992.

Polkey C. Complications of epilepsy surgery, pp. 993–1006.

Van de Wiele B. Anaesthesia for epilepsy surgery, pp. 1007–1016.

Schachter S. Vagal nerve stimulation, pp. 1017–1024.

Bergey G. Brain stimulation, pp. 1025–1034.

Yang I, Chang E, Barbaro N. Stereotactic radiosurgery for medically intractable epilepsy, p. 1035.

Cock H, Nilsen K. Future focal treatment approaches to epilepsy, pp. 1043–1050.

Palmini A. Epilepsy surgery in countries with limited resources, pp. 1051–1056.

Books

Engel J Jr, ed. Surgical Treatment of the Epilepsies, 2nd edn. New York: Raven Press, 1993.

Lüders HO, Comair YG, eds. Epilepsy Surgery, 3rd edn. Philadelphia: Lippincott, Williams & Wilkins, 2009.

Miller JW, Silbergeld DL, eds. Epilepsy Surgery: Principles and Controversies. New York: Taylor & Francis, 2006.

Pickard JD, Trojanowski T, Maira G, Polkey CE, eds. Neurosurgical Aspects of Epilepsy. New York: Springer-Verlag, 1990.

Silbergeld DL, Ojemann GA, eds. Neurosurgery clinics of North America. Epilepsy Surgery 1993; 4: 337–344.

Spencer DD, Spencer SS, eds. Surgery for Epilepsy. Cambridge, MA: Blackwell, 1991.

Theodore WH, ed. Surgical Treatment of Epilepsy. Amsterdam: Elsevier, 1992.

Tuxhorn I, Holthausen H, Boenigk H, eds. Paediatric Epilepsy Syndromes and Their Surgical Treatment. London: John Libbey, 1997.

Wieser HG, Elger CE, eds. Presurgical Evaluation of Epileptics: Basics, Techniques, Implications. Berlin: Springer-Verlag, 1987.

Wyler AR, Hermann BP, eds. The Surgical Management of Epilepsy. Boston: Butterworth-Heinemann, 1994.

Zentner J, Seeger W, eds. Surgical Treatment of Epilepsy. New York: Springer-Verlag, 2003.

Journal articles/chapters in books

Agirre-Arrizubieta Z, Huiskamp GJ, Ferrier CH, van Huffelen AC, Leijten FS. Interictal magnetoencephalography and the irritative zone in the electrocorticogram. Brain 2009; 132(Pt 11): 3060–3071.

Anhilde JA, Rosen I, Linden-Mickelsson Tech P, Kallen K. Does SISCOM contribute to favorable seizure outcome after epilepsy surgery? Epilepsia 2007; 48: 579–588.

Anschel DJ, Romanelli P. Epilepsy and radiosurgery. Arch Neurol 2008; 65: 1136–1137.

Assaf BA, Karkar KM, Laxer KD, et al. Ictal magnetoencephalography in temporal and extratemporal lobe epilepsy. Epilepsia 2003; 44: 1320–1327.

Aubert S, Wendling F, Regis J, et al. Local and remote epileptogenicity in focal cortical dysplasias and neurodevelopmental tumours. Brain 2009; 132(Pt 11): 3072–3086.

Barba C, Barbati G, Minotti L, Hoffmann D, Kahane P. Ictal clinical and scalp-EEG findings differentiating temporal lobe epilepsies from temporal 'plus' epilepsies. Brain 2007; 130(Pt 7): 1957–1967.

Barkovich AJ, Kuzniecky RI, Jackson GD, Guerrini R, Dobyns WB. A developmental and genetic classification for malformations of cortical development. Neurology 2005; 65: 1873–1887.

Battaglia G, Chiapparini L, Franceschetti S, et al. Periventricular nodular heterotopia: classification, epileptic history and genesis of epileptic activity. Epilepsia 2006; 47: 86–97.

Bautista RED, Cobbs MA, Spencer DD, et al. Prediction of surgical outcome by interictal epileptiform abnormalities during intracranial EEG monitoring in patients with extra-hippocampal seizures. Epilepsia 1999; 40: 880–890.

Baxendale S, Thompson P, Harkness W, Duncan J. Predicting memory decline following epilepsy surgery: a multivariate approach. Epilepsia 2006; 47: 1887–1894.

Baxendale S, Thompson P, Harkness W, Duncan J. The role of the intracarotid amobarbital procedure in predicting verbal memory decline after temporal lobe resection. *Epilepsia* 2007; **48**: 546–552.

Behrens E, Schramm J, Zenter J, et al. Surgical and neurological complications in a series of 708 epilepsy procedures. *Neurosurgery* 1997; **41**: 1–10.

Bell ML, Rao S, So EL, et al. Epilepsy surgery outcomes in temporal lobe epilepsy with a normal MRI. *Epilepsia* 2009; **50**: 2053–2060.

Benar CG, Grova C, Kobayashi E, et al. EEG-fMRI of epileptic spikes: concordance with EEG source localization and intracranial EEG. *Neuroimage* 2006; **30**: 1161–1170.

Berg AT, Mathern GW, Bronen RA, et al. Frequency, prognosis and surgical treatment of structural abnormalities seen with magnetic resonance imaging in childhood epilepsy. *Brain* 2009; **132**(Pt 10): 2785–2797.

Berkovic SF, Kuzniecky RI, Andermann F. Human epileptogenesis and hypothalamic hamartomas: new lessons from an experiment of nature. *Epilepsia* 1997; **38**: 1–3.

Bernier GP, Richer F, Giard N, et al. Electrical stimulation of the human brain in epilepsy. *Epilepsia* 1990; **31**: 513–520.

Bertram EH, Zhang DX, Williamson JM. Multiple roles of midline dorsal thalamic nuclei in induction and spread of limbic seizures. *Epilepsia* 2008; **49**: 256–268.

Binder DK, Podlogar M, Clusmann H, et al. Surgical treatment of parietal lobe epilepsy. *J Neurosurg* 2009; **110**: 1170–8.

Bingaman WE, guest ed. *Neurosurgery Clinics of North America, Cortical Dysplasias.* Philadelphia: WB Saunders, 2002.

Binnie CD, Marston D, Polkey CE, Amin D. Distribution of temporal spikes in relation to the sphenoidal electrode. *Electroencephalography Clin Neurophysiol* 1989; **73**: 403–409.

Boatman D, Freeman J, Vining E, et al. Language recovery after left hemispherectomy in children with late-onset seizures. *Ann Neurol* 1999; **46**: 579–586.

Bonelli SB, Powell RH, Yogarajah M, et al. Imaging memory in temporal lobe epilepsy: predicting the effects of temporal lobe resection. *Brain* 2010 [Epub ahead of print]

Bourgeois M, Crimmins DW, de Oliveira RS, et al. Surgical treatment of epilepsy in Sturge-Weber syndrome in children. *J Neurosurg* 2007; **106**(1 suppl): 20–28.

Buergermann GJ, Sperling MR, French JA, et al. Comparison of mesial versus neocortical onset temporal lobe seizures: neurodiagnostic findings and surgical outcome. *Epilepsia* 1995; **36**: 662–670.

Burneo JG, Steven DA, McLachlan RS, Parrent AG. Morbidity associated with the use of intracranial electrodes for epilepsy surgery. *Can J Neurol Sci* 2006; **33**: 223–227.

Cambier DM, Cascino GD, So EL, Marsh WR. Video-EEG monitoring in patients with hippocampal atrophy. *Acta Neurol Scand* 2001; **103**: 231–237.

Carne RP, O'Brien TJ, Kilpatrick CJ, et al. MRI-negative PET-positive temporal lobe epilepsy: a distinct surgically remediable syndrome. *Brain* 2004; **127**: 2276–2285.

Cascino GD. Epilepsy and brain tumors: implications for treatment. *Epilepsia* 1990; **31**(suppl 3): S37–S44.

Cendes F, Cook MJ, Watson C, et al. Frequency and characteristics of dual pathology in patients with lesional epilepsy. *Neurology* 1995; **45**: 2058–2064.

Cendes F, Li LM, Watson C, Andermann F, Dubeau F, Arnold DL. Is ictal recording mandatory in temporal lobe epilepsy? Not when the interictal electroencephalogram and hippocampal atrophy coincide. *Arch Neurol* 2000; **57**: 497–500.

Chaichana KL, Parker SL, Olivi A, Quinones-Hinojosa A. Long-term seizure outcomes in adult patients undergoing primary resection of malignant brain astrocytomas. Clinical article. *J Neurosurg* 2009; **111**: 282–92.

Chang EF, Quigg M, Oh MC, et al., Epilepsy Radiosurgery Study Group. Predictors of efficacy after stereotactic radiosurgery for medial temporal lobe epilepsy. *Neurology* 2010; **74**: 165–172.

Chassoux F. Stereo-EEG: the Sainte-anne experience in focal cortical dysplasias. *Epileptic Disord* 2003; **5**: 95–103.

Chassoux F, Semah F, Bouilleret V, et al. Metabolic changes and electro-clinical patterns in mesio-temporal lobe epilepsy: a correlative study. *Brain* 2004; **127**: 164–174.

Choi H, Sell RL, Lenert L, et al. Epilepsy surgery for pharmaco-resistant temporal lobe epilepsy: a decision analysis. *JAMA* 2008; **300**: 2497–2505.

Christodoulou C, Koutroumanidid M, Hennessy MJ, et al. Postictal psychosis after temporal lobectomy. *Neurology* 2002; **59**: 1432–1435.

Chugani DC, Chugani HT, Muzik O, et al. Imaging epileptogenic tubers in children with tuberous sclerosis complex using alpha-^{11}Cmethyl-L-tryptophan positron emission tomography. *Ann Neurol* 1998; **44**: 858–866.

Chugani HT, Shewmon DA, Peacock WJ, Shields WD, Mazziotta JC, Phelps ME. Surgical treatment of intractable neonatal-onset seizures: the role of positron emission tomography. *Neurology* 1988; **38**: 1178–1188.

Chung CK, Lee SK, Kim KJ. Surgical outcome of epilepsy caused by cortical dysplasia. *Epilepsia* 2005; **46**(suppl 1): 25–9.

Chung MY, Walczak TS, Lewis DV, Dawson DV, Radtke R. Temporal lobectomy and independent bitemporal interictal activity: what degree of lateralization is sufficient? *Epilepsia* 1991; **32**: 195–201.

Cohen-Gadol AA, Wilhelmi BG, Collignon F, et al. Long-term outcome of epilepsy surgery among 399 patients with nonlesional seizure foci including mesial temporal lobe sclerosis. *J Neurosurg* 2006; **104**: 513–524.

Cook MJ, Fish DR, Shorvon SD, Straughan K, Stevens JM. Hippocampal volumetric and morphometric studies in frontal and temporal lobe epilepsy. *Brain* 1992; **115**: 1001–1015.

Cooke PM, Snider RS. Some cerebellar influences on electrically-induced cerebral seizures. *Epilepsia* 1955; **4**: 19–28.

Cooper IS, Amin I, Riklan M, Waltz JM, Poon TP. Chronic cerebellar stimulation in epilepsy. Clinical and anatomical studies. *Arch Neurol* 1976; **33**: 559–570.

Cooper IS, Riklan M, Amin I, Wlatz JM, Cullinan T. Chronic cerebellar stimulation in cerebral palsy. *Neurology* 1976; **26**: 744–753.

Cossu M, Cardinale F, Castana L, et al. Stereoelectroencephalography in the presurgical evaluation of focal epilepsy: a retrospective analysis of 215 procedures. *Neurosurgery* 2005; **57**: 706–718.

Cossu M, Cardinale F, Colombo N, et al. Stereoelectroencephalography in the presurgical evaluation of children with drug-resistant focal epilepsy. *J Neurosurg* 2005; **103**(4 suppl): 333–343.

D'Ambrosio R, Hakimian S, Stewart T, et al. Functional definition of seizure provides new insight into post-traumatic epileptogenesis. *Brain* 2009; **132**(Pt 10): 2805–2821.

D'Orci G, Tinuper P, Bisculli F, et al. Clinical features and long term outcome of epilepsy in periventricular nodular heterotopia. Simple compared with plus forms. *J Neurol Neurosurg Psychiatr* 2004; **75**: 873–878.

Devlin AM, Cross JH, Harkness W, et al. Clinical outcomes of hemispherectomy for epilepsy in childhood and adolescence. *Brain* 2003; **126**: 556–566.

Diehl B, Luders HO. Temporal lobe epilepsy: when are invasive recordings needed? *Epilepsia* 2000; **41**(suppl 3): 61–74.

Diehl B, Salek-haddadi A, Fish DR, Lemieux L. Mapping of spikes, slow waves, and motor tasks in a patient with malformation of cortical development using simultaneous EEG and fMRI. *Magn Reson Imaging* 2003; **21**: 1167–1173.

Dubeau F, Palmini A, Fish D, et al. The significance of electrocorticographic findings in focal cortical dysplasia: a review of their clinical, electrophysiological and neurochemical characteristics. *Electroencephalogr Clin Neurophysiol* 1998; **48**(suppl): 77–96.

Duchowny M. Clinical, functional, and neurophysiologic assessment of dysplastic cortical networks: Implications for cortical functioning and surgical management. *Epilepsia* 2009; **50**(suppl 9): 19–27.

Eisenschenk S, Gilmore RL, Cibula JE, et al. Lateralization of temporal foci: depth versus subdural electrodes. *Clin Neurophysiol* 2001; **112**: 836–844.

Eliassen JC, Baynes K, Gazzaniga MS. Anterior and posterior callosal contributions to simultaneous bimanual movements of the hands and fingers. *Brain* 2000; **123**(Pt 12): 2501–2511.

Elsharkawy AE, Behne F, Oppel F, et al. Long-term outcome of extratemporal epilepsy surgery among 154 adult patients. *J Neurosurg* 2008; **108**: 676–86.

Engel J. Surgery for seizures. *N Engl J Med* 1996; **334**: 647.

Engel J Jr. Surgical treatment for epilepsy: too little, too late? *JAMA* 2008; **300**: 2548–50.

Engel J Jr, Shewmon DA. Overview: who should be considered a surgical candidate? In: Engel J Jr, ed. *Surgical Treatment of the Epilepsies*, 2nd edn. New York: Raven Press, 1993: 23–34.

Engel J Jr, Driver MV, Falconer MA. Electrophysiological correlates of pathology and surgical results in temporal lobe epilepsy. *Brain* 1975; **98**: 129–156.

Engel J Jr, Wiebe S, French J, et al. Practice parameter: temporal lobe and localized neocortical resections for epilepsy. *Neurology* 2003; **60**: 538–547.

Eriksson SH, Thom M, Bartlett PA, et al. PROPELLER MRI visualizes detailed pathology of hippocampal sclerosis. *Epilepsia* 2008; **49**: 33–39.

Fauser S, Sisodiya SM, Martinian L, et al. Multi-focal occurrence of cortical dysplasia in epilepsy patients. *Brain* 2009; **132**(Pt 8): 2079–2090.

Feichtinger M, Schrottner O, Eder H, et al. Efficacy and safety of radiosurgical callostomy: a retrospective analysis. *Epilepsia* 2006; **47**: 1184–1191.

Feindel W, Leblanc R, de Almeida AN. Epilepsy surgery: historical highlights 1909–2009. *Epilepsia* 2009; **50**(suppl 3): 131–151.

Fish D, Andermann F, Oliver A. Complex partial seizures and small posterior temporal or extratemporal structural lesions: surgical management. *Neurology* 1991; **41**: 1781–1784.

Foldvary N, Klem G, Hammel J, Bingaman W, Najm I, Luders H. The localizing value of ictal EEG in focal epilepsy. *Neurology* 2001; **57**: 2022–2028.

Foldvary N, Lee N, Thwaites G, et al. Clinical and electrographic manifestations of lesional neocortical temporal lobe epilepsy. *Neurology* 1997; **49**: 757–763.

Fountas KN, Smith JR. Subdural electrode-associated complications: a 20-year experience. *Stereotact Funct Neurosurg* 2007; **85**: 264–272.

Freeman JL, Coleman LT, Wellard RM, et al. MR imaging and spectroscopic study of epileptogenic hypothalamic hamartomas: analysis of 72 cases. *AJNR Am J Neuroradiol* 2004; **25**: 450–462.

Fried I. Anatomic temporal lobe resections for temporal lobe epilepsy. *Neurosurgery Clin North Am* 1993; **4**: 233–242.

Friedlander RM. Clinical practice. Arteriovenous malformations of the brain. *N Engl J Med* 2007; **356**: 2704–12.

Frings L, Wagner K, Halsband U, Schwarzwald R, Zentner J, Schulze-Bonhage A. Lateralization of hippocampal activation differs between left and right temporal lobe epilepsy patients and correlates with postsurgical verbal learning decrement. *Epilepsy Res* 2008; **78**: 161–170.

Frost EA, Booij LH. Anesthesia in the patient for awake craniotomy. *Curr Opin Anesthesiol* 2007; **20**: 331–335.

Ganz JC. Gamma knife radiosurgery and its possible relationship to malignancy: a review. *J Neurosurg* 2002; **97**(suppl. 5): 644–652.

Garcia PA, Laxer KD, van der Grand J, et al. Proton magnetic resonance spectroscopic imaging in patients with frontal lobe epilepsy. *Ann Neurol* 1995; **37**: 279–281.

Gardner AB, Worrell GA, Marsh E, et al. Human and automated detection of high-frequency oscillations in clinical intracranial EEG recordings. *Clin Neurophysiol* 2007; **118**: 1134–1143.

Gilliam F, Bowling S, Bilir E, et al. Association of combined MRI, interictal EEG, and ictal EEG results with outcome and pathology after temporal lobectomy. *Epilepsia* 1997; **38**: 1315–1320.

Gleissner U, Helmstaedter C, Elger CE. Right hippocampal contribution to visual memory: a presurgical and postsurgical study in patients with temporal lobe epilepsy. *J Neurol Neurosurg Psychiatry* 1998; **65**: 665–669.

Glosser G, Zwill AS, Glosser DS, et al. Psychiatric aspects of temporal lobe epilepsy before and after anterior temporal lobectomy. *J Neurol Neurosurg Psychiatry* 2000; **68**: 53–58.

Gonçalves Pereira PM, Oliveira E, Rosado P. Relative localizing value of amygdalo-hippocampal MR biometry in temporal lobe epilepsy. *Epilepsy Res* 2006; **69**: 147–164.

Gonzalez-Martinez JA, Srikijvilaikul T, Nair D, Bingaman WE. Long-term seizure outcome in reoperation after failure of epilepsy surgery. *Neurosurgery* 2007; **60**: 873–880.

Hamandi K, Powell HW, Laufs H, et al. Combined EEG-fMRI and tractography to visualise propagation of epileptic activity. *J Neurol Neurosurg Psychiatry* 2008; **79**: 594–597.

Hamberger MJ. Cortical language mapping in epilepsy: A critical review. *Neuropsychol Rev* 2007; **17**: 477–489.

Hamberger MJ, Seidel WT, Goodman RR, et al. Evidence for cortical reorganization of language in patients with hippocampal sclerosis. *Brain* 2007; **130**: 2942–2950.

Hamer HM, Morris HH, Mascha EJ, et al. Complications of invasive video-EEG monitoring with subdural grid electrodes. *Neurology* 2002; **58**: 97–103.

Harvey AS, Cross JH, Shinnar S, Mathern BW. Defining the spectrum of international practice in pediatric epilepsy surgery patients. *Epilepsia* 2008; **49**: 146–55.

Hasegawa T, McInerney J, Kondziolka D, et al. Long-term results after stereotactic radiosurgery for patients with cavernous malformations. *Neurosurgery* 2002; **50**: 1190–1197; discussion 1197–1198.

Heikkinen ER, Konnov B, Melnikov L, et al. Relief of epilepsy by radiosurgery of cerebral arteriovenous malformations. *Stereotact Funct Neurosurg* 1998; **53**: 157–166.

Helmstaedter C, Elger CE. Cognitive consequences of two-thirds anterior temporal lobectomy on verbal memory in 144 patients: a three-month follow-up study. *Epilepsia* 1996; **37**: 171–180.

Hirsch LJ, Spencer SS, Spencer DD, et al. Temporal lobectomy in patients with bitemporal epilepsy defined by depth electro-encephalography. *Ann Neurol* 1991; **30**: 347–356.

Ho SS, Berkovic SF, Berlangieri SU, et al. Comparison of ictal SPECT and interictal PET in the presurgical evaluation of temporal lobe epilepsy. *Ann Neurol* 1995; **37**: 738–745.

Hodaie M, Wennberg RA, Dostrovsky JO, Lozano AM. Chronic anterior thalamic stimulation for intractable epilepsy. *Epilepsia* 2002; **43**: 603–608.

Holloway V, Gadian DG, Vargha-Khadem F, Porter DA, Boyd SG, Connely A. The reorganization of sensorimotor function in children after hemispherectomy. A functional MRI and somatosensory evoked potential study. *Brain* 2000; **123**: 2432–2444.

Holmes MD, Miles AN, Dodrill CB, et al. Identifying potential surgical candidates in patients with evidence of bitemporal epilepsy. *Epilepsia* 2003; **44**: 1075–1079.

Hoppe C, Poepel A, Sassen R, Elger CE. Discontinuation of anticonvulsant medication after epilepsy surgery in children. *Epilepsia* 2006; **47**: 580–3.

Hsu PW, Chang CN, Tseng CK, et al. Treatment of epileptogenic cavernomas: surgery versus radiosurgery. *Cerebrovasc Dis* 2007; **24**: 116–120.

Huppertz HJ, Wellmer J, Staack AM, Altenmüller DM, Urbach H, Kröll J. Voxel-based 3D MRI analysis helps to detect subtle forms of subcortical band heterotopia. *Epilepsia* 2008; **49**: 772–785.

Jeha LE, Najm I, Bingaman W, Dinner D, Widdess-Walsh P, Lüders H. Surgical outcome and prognostic factors of frontal lobe epilepsy surgery. *Brain* 2007; **130**(Pt 2): 574–584.

Jin K, Nakasato N, Shamoto H, et al. Neuromagnetic localization of spike sources in perilesional, contralateral mirror, and ipsilateral remote areas in patients with cavernoma. *Epilepsia* 2007; **48**: 2160–2166.

Jirsch JD, Urrestarazu E, Le Van P, et al. High-frequency oscillations during human focal seizures. *Brain* 2006; **129**(Pt 6): 1593–1608.

Johnston JM Jr, Mangano FT, Ojemann JG, Park TS, Trevathan E, Smyth MD. Complications of invasive subdural electrode monitoring at St. Louis Children's Hospital, 1994–2005. *J Neurosurg* 2006; **105**(suppl 5): 343–347.

Jonas R, Asarnow RF, LoPresti C, et al. Surgery for symptomatic infant-onset epileptic encephalopathy with and without infantile spasms. *Neurology* 2005; **64**: 746–750.

Jonas R, Nguyen S, Hu B, et al. Cerebral hemispherectomy: hospital course, seizure, developmental, language, and motor outcomes. *Neurology* 2004; **62**: 1712–1721.

Jooma R, Yeh HS, Privitera MD, Gartner M. Lesionectomy versus electrophysiologically guided resection for temporal lobe tumors manifesting with complex partial seizures. *J Neurosurg* 1995; **83**: 231–236.

Kagawa K, Chugani DC, Asano E, et al. Epilepsy surgery outcome in children with tuberous sclerosis complex evaluated with alpha- ^{11}Cmethyl-L-tryptophan positron emission tomography (PET). *J Child Neurol* 2005; **20**: 429–438.

Kaminska A, Chiron C, Ville D, et al. Ictal SPECT in children with epilepsy: comparison with intracranial EEG and relation to postsurgical outcome. *Brain* 2003; **126**: 248–260.

Kan P, Van Orman C, Kestle JR. Outcomes after surgery for focal epilepsy in children. *Childs Nerv Syst* 2008; **24**: 587–591.

Kanemoto K, Kim Y, Miyamoto T, Kawasaki J. Presurgical post-ictal and acute interictal psychoses are differentially associated with postoperative mood and psychotic disorders. *J Neuropsychiatry Clin Neurosci* 2001; **13**: 243–247.

Kanner AM. Depression in epilepsy: prevalence, clinical semiology, pathogenic mechanisms and treatment. *Biol Psychiatry* 2003; **54**: 388–398.

Kanner AM, Byrne R, Chicharro A, Wuu J, Frey M. A lifetime psychiatric history predicts a worse seizure outcome following temporal lobectomy. *Neurology* 2009; **72**: 793–799.

Kanner AM, Kaydanaova Y, deToledo-Morrell L, et al. Tailored anterior temporal lobectomy: relation between effect of resection of mesial structures and postsurgical seizure outcome. *Arch Neurol* 1995; **52**: 173–178.

Katariwala NM, Bakay RAE, Pennell PB, et al. Remission of intractable partial epilepsy following implantation of intracranial electrodes. *Neurology* 2001; **57**: 1505–1507.

Kazemi NJ, Worrell GA, Stead SM, et al. Ictal SPECT statistical parametric mapping in temporal lobe epilepsy surgery. *Neurology* 2010; **74**: 70–76.

Kerrigan JF, Litt B, Fisher RS, et al. Electrical stimulation of the anterior nucleus of the thalamus for the treatment of intractable epilepsy. *Epilepsia* 2004; **45**: 346–354.

Kida Y, Kobayashi T, Tanaka T, et al. Seizure control after radiosurgery on cerebral arteriovenous malformations. *J Clin Neurosci* 2000; **7**(suppl 1): 6–9.

Kim MS, Pyo SY, Jeong YG, Lee SI, Jung YT, Sim JH. Gamma knife surgery for intracranial cavernous hemangioma. *J Neurosurg* 2005; **102**(suppl): 102–106.

Kloss S, Pieper T, Pannek H, et al. Epilepsy surgery in children with focal cortical dysplasia (FCD): results of long-term seizure outcome. *Neuropediatrics* 2002; **33**: 21–26.

Kurita H, Kawamoto S, Suzuki I, et al. Control of epilepsy associated with cerebral arteriovenous malformations after radiosurgery. *J Neurol Neurosurg Psychiatr* 1998; **65**: 648–655.

Lamusuo S, Jutila L, Ylinen A, et al. ^{18}F FDG-PET reveals temporal hypometabolism in patients with temporal lobe epilepsy even when quantitative MRI and histopathological analysis show only mild hippocampal damage. *Arch Neurol* 2001; **58**: 933–939.

Lee SK, Lee SY, Kim KK, Hong KS, Lee DS, Chung CK. Surgical outcome and prognostic factors of cryptogenic neocortical epilepsy. *Ann Neurol* 2005; **58**: 525–532.

Lee SK, Yun CH, Oh JB, et al. Intracranial ictal onset zone in nonlesional lateral temporal lobe epilepsy on scalp ictal EEG. *Neurology* 2003; **61**: 757–764.

Lee TMC, Yip JTH, Jones-Gotman M. Memory deficits after resection from left or right anterior temporal lobe in humans: A meta-analytic review. *Epilepsia* 2002; **43**: 283–291.

Lee YJ, Kang HC, Lee JS, et al. Resective pediatric epilepsy surgery in Lennox-Gastaut syndrome. *Pediatrics* 2010; **125**: e58–66.

Lesser RP, Arroyo S, Crone N, et al. Motor and sensory mapping of the frontal and occipital lobes. *Epilepsia* 1998; **39**(suppl 4): 69–80.

Leung H, Schindler K, Clusmann H, et al. Mesial frontal epilepsy and ictal body turning along the horizontal body axis. *Arch Neurol* 2008; **65**: 71–7.

Levy RM. Brain abscess and subdural empyema. *Curr Opin Neurol* 1994; **7**: 223–228.

Li LM, Dubeau F, Andermann F, et al. Periventricular nodular heterotopia and intractable temporal lobe epilepsy: poor outcome after temporal lobe resection. *Ann Neurol* 1997; **41**: 662–668.

Li LM, Fish DR, Sisodiya SM, Shorvon SD, Alsanjari N, Stevens JM. High resolution magnetic resonance imaging in adults with partial or secondary generalised epilepsy attending a tertiary referral unit. *J Neurol Neurosurg Psychiatry* 1995; **59**: 384–387.

Liegeois F, Cross JH, Gadian DG, Connelly A. Role of fMRI in the decision-making process: epilepsy surgery for children. *J Magn Reson Imaging* 2006; **23**: 933–940.

Lim S-N, Lee S-T, Tsai Y-T, et al. Electrical stimulation of the anterior nucleus of the thalamus for intractable epilepsy: a long-term follow-up study. *Epilepsia* 2007; **48**: 342–347.

Liu KD, Chung WY, Wu HM, et al. Gamma knife surgery for cavernous hemangiomas: an analysis of 125 patients. *J Neurosurg* 2005; **102**(suppl): 81–86.

Loddenkemper T, Holland KD, Stanford LD, Kotagal P, Bingaman W, Wyllie E. Developmental outcome after epilepsy surgery in infancy. *Pediatrics* 2007; **119**: 930–935.

McBride MC, Binnie CD, Janota I, et al. Predictive value of intraoperative electrocorticograms in resective epilepsy surgery. *Ann Neurol* 1991; **30**: 526–532.

McClelland S, III, Hall WA. Postoperative central nervous system infection: incidence and associated factors in 2111 neurosurgical procedures. *Clin Infect Dis* 2007; **45**: 55–59.

Madhavan D, Kuzniecky R. Temporal lobe surgery in patients with normal MRI. *Curr Opin Neurol* 2007; **20**: 203–207.

McGonigal A, Bartolomei F, Régis J, et al. Stereoelectroencephalography in presurgical assessment of MRI-negative epilepsy. *Brain* 2007; **130**: 3169–3183.

McIntosh AM, Kalnins RM, Mitchell LA, Fabinyi GC, Briellmann RS, Berkovic SF. Temporal lobectomy: long-term seizure outcome, late recurrence and risks for seizure recurrence. *Brain* 2004; **127**: 2018–2030.

McLachlan RS, Pigott S, Tellez-Zenteno JF, Wiebe S, Parrent A. Bilateral hippocampal stimulation for intractable temporal lobe epilepsy: impact on seizures and memory. *Epilepsia* 2010; **51**: 304–307.

Maraire JN, Awad IA. Intracranial cavernous malformations: lesion behavior and management strategies. *Neurosurgery* 1995; **37**: 591–605.

Mascott CR. In vivo accuracy of image guidance performed using optical tracking and optimized registration. *J Neurosurg* 2006; **105**: 561–567.

Mathern GW, ed. Pediatric epilepsy and epilepsy surgery. *Develop Neurosci* 1999; **21**: 159–408.

Mathern GW. Challenges in the surgical treatment of epilepsy patients with cortical dysplasia. *Epilepsia* 2009; **50**(suppl 9): 45–50.

Mathern GW. Epilepsy surgery patients with cortical dysplasia: present and future therapeutic challenges. *Neurology* 2009; **72**: 206–7.

Mathieu D, Kondziolka D, Niranjan A, Flickinger J, Lunsford LD. Gamma knife radiosurgery for refractory epilepsy caused by hypothalamic hamartomas. *Stereotact Funct Neurosurg* 2006; **84**: 82–87.

Mehta AD, Labar D, Dean A, et al. Frameless stereotactic placement of depth electrodes in epilepsy surgery. *J Neurosurg* 2005; **102**: 1040–1045.

Merriam MA, Bronen RA, Spencer DD, McCarthy G. MR findings after depth electrode implantation for medically refractory epilepsy. *AJNR Am J Neuroradiol* 1993; **14**: 1343–1346.

Mikati MA, Comair YG, Rahi A. Normalization of quality of life three years after temporal lobectomy: a controlled study. *Epilepsia* 2006; **47**: 928–33.

Mikuni N, Okada T, Enatsu R, et al. Clinical significance of preoperative fibre-tracking to preserve the affected pyramidal tracts during resection of brain tumours in patients with preoperative motor weakness. *J Neurol Neurosurg Psychiatry* 2007; **78**: 716–721.

Miller D, Knake S, Bauer S, et al. Intraoperative ultrasound to define focal cortical dysplasia in epilepsy surgery. *Epilepsia* 2008; **49**: 156–8.

Mintzer S, Sperling MR. When should a resection sparing mesial structures be considered for temporal lobe epilepsy? *Epilepsy Behav* 2008; **13**: 7–11.

Mintzer S, Cendes F, Soss J, et al. Unilateral hippocampal sclerosis with contralateral temporal scalp ictal onset. *Epilepsia* 2004; **45**: 792–802.

Moeller F, Tyvaert L, Nguyen DK, et al. EEG-fMRI: adding to standard evaluations of patients with nonlesional frontal lobe epilepsy. *Neurology* 2009; **73**: 2023–2030.

Mohamed IS, Otsubo H, Pang E, et al. Magnetoencephalography and diffusion tensor imaging in gelastic seizures secondary to a cingulate gyrus lesion. *Clin Neurol Neurosurg* 2007; **109**: 182–187.

Molnar GF, Sailer A, Wennberg R, Lozano AM, Chen R. Effects of anterior thalamus stimulation on motor cortex excitability in epilepsy. *Epilepsia* 2002; **43**(suppl 7): 52.

Moran NF, Fish DR, Kitchen N, et al. Supratentorial cavernous heaemangiomas and epilepsy: a review of the literature and case series. *J Neurol Neurosurg Psychiatry* 1999; **66**: 561–8.

Morino M, Ichinose T, Uda T, Kondo K, Ohfuji S, Ohata K. Memory outcome following transsylvian selective amygdalohippocampectomy in 62 patients with hippocampal sclerosis. *J Neurosurg* 2009; **110**: 1164–1169.

Morrell F, Whisler WW, Bleck T. Multiple subpial transection: a new approach to the surgical treatment of focal epilepsy. *J Neurosurg* 1989; **70**: 231–239.

Najm IM, Tilelli CQ, Oghlakian R, et al. Pathophysiological mechanisms of focal cortical dysplasia: a critical review of human tissue studies. *Epilepsia* 2007; **48**: S21–S32.

Nei M, O'Connor M, Liporace J, Sperling MR. Refractory generalized seizures: response to corpus callostomy and vagal nerve stimulation. *Epilepsia* 2006; **47**: 115–122.

Nguyen DK, Nguyen DB, Malak R, et al. Revisiting the role of the insula in refractory partial epilepsy. *Epilepsia* 2009; **50**: 510–20.

Nobili L, Francione S, Mai R, et al. Surgical treatment of drug-resistant nocturnal frontal lobe epilepsy. *Brain* 2007; **130**(Pt 2): 561–573.

O'Brien DF, Basu S, Williams DH, May PL. Anatomical hemispherectomy for intractable seizures: excellent seizure control, low morbidity and no superficial cerebral hemosiderosis. *Childs Nerv Syst* 2006; **22**: 489–498.

O'Brien TJ, So EL, Mullan BP, et al. Subtraction ictal SPECT co-registered to MRI improves clinical usefulness of SPECT in localizing the surgical seizure focus. *Neurology* 1998; **50**: 445–454.

Ochi A, Otsubo H, Donner EJ, et al. Dynamic changes of ictal high-frequency oscillations in neocortical epilepsy using multiple band frequency analysis. *Epilepsia* 2007; **48**: 286–296.

Oguni H, Andermann F, Rasmussen TB. The syndrome of chronic encephalitis and epilepsy. A study based on the MNI series of 48 cases. *Adv Neurol* 1992; **57**: 419–433.

Oishi M, Kameyama S, Masuda H, et al. H. Single and multiple clusters of magnetoencephalographic dipoles in neocortical epilepsy: significance in characterizing the epileptogenic zone. *Epilepsia* 2006; **47**: 355–364.

Ojemann GA, Corina DP, Corrigan N, et al. Neuronal correlates of functional magnetic resonance imaging in human temporal cortex. *Brain* 2010; **133**(Pt 1): 46–59.

Önal C, Otsubo H, Araki T, et al. Complications of invasive subdural grid monitoring in children with epilepsy. *J Neurosurg* 2003; **98**: 1017–1026.

Pacia SV, Jung WJ, Devinsky O. Localization of mesial temporal lobe seizures with sphenoidal electrodes. *J Clin Neurophysiol* 1998; **15**: 256–261.

Palmini A, Najm I, Avanzini G, Babb T, et al. Terminology and classification of the cortical dysplasias. *Neurology* 2004; **62**: S2–8.

Papanicolaou AC, Pataraia E, Billingsley-Marshall R, et al. Toward the substitution of invasive electroencephalography in epilepsy surgery. *J Clin Neurophysiol* 2005; **22**: 231–237.

Pataraia E, Lindinger G, Deecke L, et al. Combined MEG/EEG analysis of the interictal spike complex in mesial temporal lobe epilepsy. *Neuroimage* 2005; **24**: 607–614.

Paulini A, Fischer M, Rampp S, et al. Lobar localization information in epilepsy patients: MEG-a useful tool in routine presurgical diagnosis. *Epilepsy Res* 2007; **76**: 123–130.

Pondal-Sordo M, Diosy D, Tellez-Zenteno JF, Girvin JP, Wiebe S. Epilepsy surgery involving the sensory-motor cortex. *Brain* 2006; **129**(Pt 12): 3307–3314.

Rahimi SY, Park YD, Witcher MR, Lee KH, Marrufo M, Lee MR. Corpus callostomy for treatment of pediatric epilepsy in the modern era. *Pediatr Neurosurg* 2007; **43**: 202–208.

Raymond AA, Fish DR, Sisodiya SM, et al. Abnormalities of gyration, heterotopias, tuberous sclerosis, focal cortical dysplasia, microdysgenesis, dysembryoplastic neuroepithelial tumour and dysgenesis of the archicortex in epilepsy: clinical, EEG and neuroimaging features in 100 adult patients. *Brain* 1995; **118**: 629–660.

Raymond AA, Fish DR, Stevens JM, et al. Association of hippocampal sclerosis with cortical dysgenesis in patients with epilepsy. *Neurology* 1994; **44**: 1841–1845.

Regis J, Bartolomei F. Comment on: Failure of gamma knife radiosurgery for mesial temporal lobe epilepsy: report of five cases. *Neurosurgery* 2004; **54**: 1404.

Regis J, Bartolomei F, de Toffol B, et al. Gamma knife surgery for epilepsy related to hypothalamic hamartomas. *Neurosurgery* 2000; **47**: 1343–1351; discussion 1351–1342.

Regis J, Hayashi M, Eupierre LP, et al. Gamma knife surgery for epilepsy related to hypothalamic hamartomas. *Acta Neurochir* 2004; **91**(suppl): 33–50.

Regis J, Rey M, Bartolomei F, et al. Gamma knife surgery in mesial temporal lobe epilepsy: a prospective multicenter study [see comment]. *Epilepsia* 2004; **45**: 504–515.

Regis J, Scavarda D, Tamura M, et al. Epilepsy related to hypothalamic hamartomas: surgical management with special reference to gamma knife surgery. *Childs Nerv Syst* 2006; **22**: 881–895.

Regis J, Scavarda D, Tamura M, et al. Gamma knife surgery for epilepsy related to hypothalamic hamartomas. *Semin Pediatr Neurol* 2007; **14**: 73–79.

Rheims S, Fischer C, Ryvlin P, et al. Long-term outcome of gamma-knife surgery in temporal lobe epilepsy. *Epilepsy Res* 2008; **80**: 23–29.

Risinger MW, Engel J Jr, Van Ness PC, Henry TR, Crandall PH. Ictal localization of temporal lobe seizures with scalp/sphenoidal recordings. *Neurology* 1989; **39**: 1288–1293.

Rosenow F, Lüders H. Presurgical evaluation of epilepsy. *Brain* 2001; **124**: 1683–700.

Rugg-Gunn FJ, Boulby PA, Symms MR, Barker GJ, Duncan JS. Imaging the neocortex in epilepsy with double inversion recovery imaging. *Neuroimage* 2006; **31**: 39–50.

Rydenhag B, Silander HC. Complications of epilepsy surgery after 654 procedures in Sweden, September 1990–1995: a multicenter study based on the Swedish National Epilepsy Surgery Register. *Neurosurgery* 2001; **49**: 51–56.

Sabaz M, Lawson JA, Cairns DR, et al. The impact of epilepsy surgery on quality of life in children. *Neurology* 2006; **66**: 557–561.

Sackellares JC. Seizure prediction. *Epilepsy Curr* 2008; **8**: 55–59.

Salanova V, Andermann F, Olivier A, Rasmussen T, Quesney LF. Occipital lobe epilepsy: electroclinical manifestations, electrocorticography, cortical stimulation and outcome in 42 patients treated between 1930 and 1991. Surgery of occipital lobe epilepsy. *Brain* 1992; **115**: 1655–1680.

Salek-Haddadi A, Diehl B, Hamandi K, et al. Hemodynamic correlates of epileptiform discharges: an EEG-fMRI study of 63 patients with focal epilepsy. *Brain Res* 2006; **1088**: 148–166.

Sammaritano M, de Lotbiniere A, Andermann F, Olivier A, Gloor P, Quesney LF. False lateralization by surface EEG of seizure onset in patients with temporal lobe epilepsy and gross focal cerebral lesions. *Ann Neurol* 1987; **21**: 361–369.

Sansur CA, Frysinger RC, Pouratian N, et al. Incidence of symptomatic hemorrhage after stereotactic electrode placement. *J Neurosurg* 2007; **107**: 998–1003.

Sass KJ, Spencer SS, Spencer DD, Novelly RA, Williamson PD, Mattson RH. Corpus callostomy for epilepsy. II Neurologic and neuropsychological outcome. *Neurology* 1988; **38**: 24–28.

Schäuble B, Cascino GD, Pollock BE, et al. Seizure outcomes after stereotactic radiosurgery for cerebral arteriovenous malformations. *Neurology* 2004; **63**: 683–687.

Schevon CA, Trevelyan AJ, Schroeder CE, Goodman RR, McKhann G Jr, Emerson RG. Spatial characterization of interictal high frequency oscillations in epileptic neocortex. *Brain* 2009; **132**(Pt 11): 3047–3059.

Schlienger M, Atlan D, Lefkopoulos D, et al. Linac radiosurgery for cerebral arteriovenous malformations: results in 169 patients. *Int J Radiat Oncol Biol Phys* 2000; **46**: 1135–1142.

Schramm J. Temporal lobe epilepsy surgery and the quest for optimal extent of resection: a review. *Epilepsia* 2008; **49**: 1296–1307.

Schulze-Bonhage A, Trippel M, Wagner K, et al. Outcome and predictors of interstitial radiosurgery in the treatment of gelastic epilepsy. *Neurology* 2008; **71**: 277–282.

Schwartz TH, Jeha L, Tanner A, Bingaman W, Sperling MR. Late seizures in patients initially seizure free after epilepsy surgery. *Epilepsia* 2006; **47**: 567–573.

Scott CA, Fish DR, Smith SJ, et al. Presurgical evaluation of patients with epilepsy and normal MRI: role of scalp video-EEG telemetry. *J Neurol Neurosurg Psychiatry* 1999; **66**: 69–71.

Scoville WB, Milner B. Loss of recent memory after bilateral hippocampal lesions. *J Neurol Neurosurg Psychiatry* 1957; **20**: 11–21.

Shahar E, Goldsher D, Genizi J, Ravid S, Keidar Z. Intractable gelastic seizures during infancy: ictal positron emission tomography (PET) demonstrating epileptiform activity within the hypothalamic hamartoma. *J Child Neurol* 2008; **23**: 235–239.

Shimizu H. Our experience with pediatric epilepsy surgery focusing on corpus callostomy and hemispherotomy. *Epilepsia* 2005; **46**(suppl 1): 30–31.

Siegel AM, Cascino GD, Meyer FB, et al. Resective reoperation for failed epilepsy surgery: seizure outcome in 64 patients. *Neurology* 2004; **63**: 2298–2302.

Siegel AM, Jobst BC, Thadani VM, et al. Medically intractable, localization-related epilepsy with normal MRI: presurgical evaluation and surgical outcome in 43 patients. *Epilepsia* 2001; **42**: 883–838.

Siegel AM, Roberts DW, Thadani VM, et al. The role of intracranial electrode reevaluation in epilepsy patients after failed initial invasive monitoring. *Epilepsia* 2000; **41**: 571–580.

Sillanpaa M, Jalava M, Kaleva O, Shinnar S. Long-term prognosis of seizures with onset in childhood. *N Engl J Med* 1998; **338**: 1715–1722.

Simon SL, Telfeian A, Duhaime A-C. Complications of invasive monitoring in intractable pediatric epilepsy. *Pediatr Neurosurg* 2003; **38**: 47–52.

Skucas AP, Artru AA. Anesthetic complications of awake craniotomies for epilepsy surgery. *Anesth Analg* 2006; **102**: 882–887.

Smyth MD, Limbrick DD Jr, et al. Outcome following surgery for temporal lobe epilepsy with hippocampal involvement in preadolescent children: emphasis on mesial temporal sclerosis. *J Neurosurg* 2007; **106**(3 suppl): 205–210.

So NK, Olivier A, Andermann F, et al. Results of surgical treatment in patients with bitemporal epileptiform abnormalities. *Ann Neurol* 1989; **25**: 432–439.

Spencer SS, Schramm J, Wyler A, et al. Multiple subpial transection for intractable partial epilepsy: an international meta-analysis. *Epilepsia* 2002; **43**: 141–145.

Spencer SS, Williamson PD, Bridgers SL, Mattson RH, Cicchetti DV, Spencer DD. Reliability and accuracy of localization by scalp ictal EEG. *Neurology* 1985; **35**: 1567–1575.

Sperling MR, Harris A, Nei M, Liporace JD, O'Connor MJ. Mortality after epilepsy surgery. *Epilepsia* 2005; **46**(suppl 11): 49–53.

Stefan H, Hummel C, Scheler G, et al. Magnetic brain source imaging of focal epileptic activity: a synopsis of 455 cases. *Brain* 2003; **126**: 2396–2405.

Striano S, Nocerino C, Striano P, et al. Venous angiomas and epilepsy. *Neurol Sci* 2000; **21**: 151–155.

Takaya S, Mikuni N, Mitsueda T, et al. Improved cerebral function in mesial temporal lobe epilepsy after subtemporal amygdalohippocampectomy. *Brain* 2009; **132**(Pt 1): 185–194.

Tandon N, Alexopoulos AV, Warbel A, Najm IM, Bingaman WE. Occipital epilepsy: spatial categorization and surgical management. *J Neurosurg* 2009; **110**: 306–318.

Tassi L, Colombo N, Cossu M, et al. Electroclinical, MRI and neuropathological study of 10 patients with nodular heterotopia, with surgical outcomes. *Brain* 2005; **128**: 321–337.

Taylor DC, Falconer MA, Bruton CJ, Corsellis JA. Focal dysplasia of the cerebral cortex in epilepsy. *J Neurol Neurosurg Psychiatry* 1971; **34**: 369–387.

Tellez-Zenteno JF, Dhar R, Wiebe S. Long-term seizure outcomes following epilepsy surgery: a systematic review and meta-analysis. *Brain* 2005; **128**(Pt 5): 1188–1198.

Tharin S, Golby A. Functional brain mapping and its applications to neurosurgery. *Neurosurgery* 2007; **60**(suppl 2): 185–201.

Trenerry MR, Jack CR, Ivnik RJ, et al. MRI hippocampal volumes and memory function before and after temporal lobectomy. *Neurology* 1993; **43**: 1800–1805.

Uijl SG, Leijten FS, Arends JB, Parra J, van Huffelen AC, Moons KG. The added value of ^{18}F-fluoro-D-deoxyglucose positron emission tomography in screening for temporal lobe epilepsy surgery. *Epilepsia* 2007; **48**: 2121–2129.

Urrestarazu E, Chander R, Dubeau F, et al. Interictal high-frequency oscillations (100–500Hz) in the intracerebral EEG of epileptic patients. *Brain* 2007; **130**(Pt 9): 2354–2366.

Usui N, Mihara T, Baba K, et al. Intracranial EEG findings in patients with lesional lateral temporal lobe epilepsy. *Epilepsy Res* 2008; **78**(1): 82–91.

Valentin A, Alarcon G, Garcia-Seoane JJ, et al. Single-pulse electrical stimulation identifies epileptogenic frontal cortex in the human brain. *Neurology* 2005; **65**: 426–435.

Van Paesschen W, Dupont P, Sunaert S, Goffin K, Van Laere K. The use of SPECT and PET in routine clinical practice in epilepsy. *Curr Opin Neurol* 2007; **20**: 194–202.

Van Paesschen W, Dupont P, Van Driel G, Van Billoen H, Maes A. SPECT perfusion changes during complex partial seizures in patients with hippocampal sclerosis. *Brain* 2003; **126**: 1103–1011.

Van Paesschen W, Dupont P, Van Heerden B, et al. Self-injection ictal SPECT during partial seizures. *Neurology* 2000; **54**: 1994–1997.

Van Roost DV, Solymosi L, Schramm J, et al. Depth electrode implantation in the length axis of the hippocampus for the presurgical evaluation of mesial temporal lobe epilepsy: a computed tomography-based stereotactic insertion technique and its accuracy. *Neurosurgery* 1998; **43**: 819–827.

Varghese GI, Purcaro MJ, Motelow JE, et al. Clinical use of ictal SPECT in secondarily generalized tonic-clonic seizures. *Brain* 2009; **132**(Pt 8): 2102–13.

Velis D, Plouin P, Gotman J, da Silva FL, ILAE DMC Subcommittee on Neurophysiology. Recommendations regarding the requirements and applications for long-term recordings in epilepsy. *Epilepsia* 2007; **48**: 379–84.

Vinton AB, Carne R, Hicks RJ, et al. The extent of resection of FDG-PET hypometabolism relates to outcome of temporal lobectomy. *Brain* 2007; **130**: 548–560.

von Lehe M, Wellmer J, Urbach H, Schramm J, Elger CE, Clusmann H. Insular lesionectomy for refractory epilepsy: management and outcome. *Brain* 2009; **132**(Pt 4): 1048–1056.

Von Oertzen J, Urbach H, Jungbluth S, et al. Standard magnetic resonance imaging is inadequate for patients with refractory focal epilepsy. *J Neurol Neurosurg Psychiatry* 2002; **73**: 643–647.

Warach S, Ives JR, Schlaug G, et al. EEG-triggered echo-planar functional MRI in epilepsy. *Neurology* 1996; **47**: 89–93.

Weber B, Wellmer J, Schur S, et al. Presurgical language fMRI in patients with drug-resistant epilepsy: effects of task performance. *Epilepsia* 2006; **47**: 880–886.

Weiner HL, Carlson C, Ridgway EB, et al. Epilepsy surgery in young children with tuberous sclerosis: results of a novel approach. *Pediatrics* 2006; **117**: 1494–1502.

Wennberg R, Arruda F, Quesney LF, Olivier A. Preeminence of extrahippocampal structures in the generation of mesial temporal seizures: evidence from human depth electrode recordings. *Epilepsia* 2002; **43**: 716–726.

Whittle IR, Midgley S, Georges H, Pringle AM, Taylor R. Patient perceptions of 'awake' brain tumour surgery. *Acta Neurochir (Wien)* 2005; **147**: 275–277.

Widdess-Walsh P, Jeha L, Nair D, Kotagal P, Bingaman W, Najm I. Subdural electrode analysis in focal cortical dysplasia: predictors of surgical outcome. *Neurology* 2007; **69**: 660–667.

Wiebe S, Blume WT, Girvin JP, Eliasziw M, Effectiveness and Efficiency of Surgery for Temporal Lobe Epilepsy Study Group. A randomized, controlled trial of surgery for temporal-lobe epilepsy. *N Engl J Med* 2001; **345**: 311–318.

Wieser HG, ILAE Commission on Neurosurgery of Epilepsy. ILAE Commission Report. Mesial temporal lobe epilepsy with hippocampal sclerosis. *Epilepsia* 2004; **45**: 695–714.

Wieser HG, Bancaud J, Talairach J, et al. Comparative value of spontaneous and electrically induced seizures in establishing the lateralization of temporal seizures. *Epilepsia* 1979; **20**: 47–59.

Wieser HG, Ortega M, Friedman A, Yonekawa Y. Long-term seizure outcomes following amygdalohippocampectomy. *J Neurosurg* 2003; **98**: 751–763.

Williamson PD, Boon PA, Thadani VM, et al. Parietal lobe epilepsy: diagnostic considerations and results of surgery. *Ann Neurol* 1992; **31**: 193–201.

Williamson PD, Thadani VM, Darcey TM, Spencer DD, Spencer SS, Mattson RH. Occipital lobe epilepsy: clinical characteristics, seizures spread patterns and results of surgery. *Ann Neurol* 1992; **31**: 3–13.

Wilson SJ, Bladin PF, Saling MM. The burden of normality: a framework for rehabilitation after epilepsy surgery. *Epilepsia* 2007; **48**(suppl 9): 13–16.

Wong SW, Jong L, Bandur D, et al. Cortical reorganization following anterior temporal lobectomy in patients with temporal lobe epilepsy. *Neurology* 2009; **73**: 518–525.

Wrench J, Wilson SJ, Bladin PF. Mood disturbance before and after seizure surgery: a comparison of temporal and extratemporal resections. *Epilepsia* 2004; **45**: 534–543.

Wurm G, Fellner FA. Implementation of T2*-weighted MR for multimodal image guidance in cerebral cavernomas. *Neuroimage* 2004; **22**: 841–846.

Wyllie E, Lachhwani DK, Gupta A, et al. Successful surgery for epilepsy due to early brain lesions despite generalized EEG findings. *Neurology* 2007; **69**: 389–397.

Yogarajah M, Duncan JS. Diffusion-based magnetic resonance imaging and tractography in epilepsy. *Epilepsia* 2008; **49**: 189–200.

Yogarajah M, Focke NK, Bonelli S, et al. Defining Meyer's loop-temporal lobe resections, visual field deficits and diffusion tensor tractography. *Brain* 2009; **132**(Pt 6): 1656–1668.

Yogarajah M, Powell HW, Parker GJ, et al. Tractography of the parahippocampal gyrus and material specific memory impairment in unilateral temporal lobe epilepsy. *Neuroimage* 2008; **40**: 1755–1764.

Yu JS, Yong WH, Wilson D, et al. Glioblastoma induction after radiosurgery for meningioma. *Lancet* 2000; **356**: 1576–1577.

Yun CH, Lee SK, Lee SY, Kim KK, Jeong SW, Chung CK. Prognostic factors in neocortical epilepsy surgery: multivariate analysis. *Epilepsia* 2006; **47**: 574–579.

Zijlmans M, Huiskamp G, Hersevoort M, et al. EEG-fMRI in the preoperative work-up for epilepsy surgery. *Brain* 2007; **130**: 2343–2353.

Index